The Nutrition and Health Dictionary

The Nutrition and Health Dictionary

PERCY J. RUSSELL
ANITA WILLIAMS

School of Medicine,
University of California at San Diego

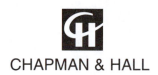

CHAPMAN & HALL

New York • Albany • Bonn • Boston • Cincinnati • Detroit • London • Madrid • Melbourne
Mexico City • Pacific Grove • Paris • San Francisco • Singapore • Tokyo • Toronto • Washington

Art direction: Andrea Meyer, emDASH inc.
Cover design: Saeed Sayrafiezadeh, emDASH inc.

Copyright © 1995
Chapman & Hall

Printed in the United States of America

For more information, contact:

Chapman & Hall
115 Fifth Avenue
New York, NY 10003

Thomas Nelson Australia
102 Dodds Street
South Melbourne, 3205
Victoria, Australia

Nelson Canada
1120 Birchmount Road
Scarborough, Ontario
Canada, M1K 5G4

International Thomson Editores
Campos Eliseos 385, Piso 7
Col. Polanco
11560 Mexico D.F. Mexico

Chapman & Hall
2-6 Boundary Row
London SE1 8HN
England

Chapman & Hall GmbH
Postfach 100 263
D-69442 Weinheim
Germany

International Thomson Publishing Asia
221 Henderson Road #05-10
Henderson Building
Singapore 0315

International Thomson Publishing-Japan
Hirakawacho-cho Kyowa Building, 3F
1-2-1 Hirakawacho-cho
Chiyoda-ku, 102 Tokyo
Japan

1 2 3 4 5 6 7 8 9 10 XXX 01 00 99 97 96 95

Library of Congress Cataloging-in-Publication Data

Russell, Percy J.
    The nutrition and health dictionary / Percy J. Russell and Anita Williams.
        p.   cm.
    ISBN 0-412-98981-6. — ISBN 0-412-98991-3 (pbk.)
        1. Nutrition —Encyclopedias.   2. Health—Encyclopedias.   I. Williams, Anita.   II. Title.
QP141.T88   1994
613.2—dc20   94-17804
                                                                CIP

British Library Cataloguing in Publication Data available

Please send your order for this or any Chapman & Hall book to **Chapman & Hall, 29 West 35th Street, New York, NY 10001, Attn: Customer Service Department.** You may also call our Order Department at 1-212-244-3336 or fax your purchase order to 1-800-248-4724.

For a complete listing of Chapman & Hall's titles, send your requests to **Chapman & Hall, Dept. BC, 115 Fifth Avenue, New York, NY 10003.**

Preface

The growth in the scientific literature of nutrition and the penetration of nutrition research into the disciplines of medicine, biochemistry, economics, sociology, and various applied fields, such as public health, food technology, and government services, have created a need for this book. Nutrition is no longer a descriptive subject. The nutritional sciences have advanced in many directions and have sometimes become so highly technical that it is often difficult for an expert in one field to relate his or her work to other closely allied developments. There is a need for a reference that connects the technical languages among disciplines related to nutrition with one another and with less technical language. We have written this dictionary in the language and style familiar to scientists, but our aim is to make all items understandable to any reader interested in nutrition.

Nearly all entries in this dictionary have extensive cross-references, and our format encourages their use. The cross-references facilitate the integration of basic science information to health and disease, define synonyms, and provide for the progressive expansion of the reader's perspectives. We hope that we are able to show that nutrition rests on a scientific basis limited by the boundaries of our knowledge of related basic sciences.

The selection of items for inclusion was guided to some extent by the first author's background as a teacher of biochemistry and nutrition, and our feeling that no ingested material is adequately described by tables of chemical or nutrient contents alone. However, tables and metabolic map are prominent features of our presentations. Tables allow immediate comparisons with related items; metabolic maps allow tracing of nutrients from ingestion to incorporation and elimination; and additives, natural toxins, and food processings are represented in the text in relationship to health and disease through cross-references.

A word on how to use this book—entries in *italics* that are not scientific names are cross-references. Almost all of the entries have cross-references related directly to the entry or to some other aspects of the subject. We urge the reader to explore.

The
Nutrition
and Health
Dictionary

A

A. The alphabetic symbol for the amino acid *alanine* (Ala).

abalone (*Haliotis*). A red or pink mollusk or shellfish found in the Pacific Ocean off the coast of California. The muscle of the shell is the edible part of the abalone and has a clamlike flavor.

Nutrients in 100 g of abalone

CALORIES KCAL	PROTEIN G	FAT G	CARBOHYDRATE G	THIAMINE MG	IRON MG	CALCIUM MG
98	19	0.5	3	0.2	2	37

absorption. The passage of products of digestion through the lining of the intestines (the intestinal mucosa) into the blood and lymph system. Water, some simple sugars (*monosaccharides*), and many inorganic ions are absorbed in their original form. Carbohydrates must be converted to simple sugars, fats to *fatty acids* and *glycerol*, and *protein* to *amino acids* during digestion to make them absorbable. The products of digestion are used by the body for building tissue and as a source of energy. Though limited amounts of water, alcohol, salts, and *glucose* are absorbed through the stomach (gastric mucosa), the small intestine is by far the most important organ for absorption. The most active absorptive areas of the small intestine are the duodenum and the jejunum. Absorptions of the three food energy sources are very efficient. The percentages absorbed by the gastrointestinal tract are estimated as follow:

Fat, 95%; **Carbohydrate**, 98%; and **Protein**, 92%.

See and *active transport*, *digestive system*, and *food energy*.

acerla. Cherries or berries from the Caribbean islands, a rich source of *ascorbic acid* (vitamin C), sometimes used in "natural vitamin" formulations.

acetaminophen. An *antipyretic* and *analgesic* often used in place of *aspirin*.

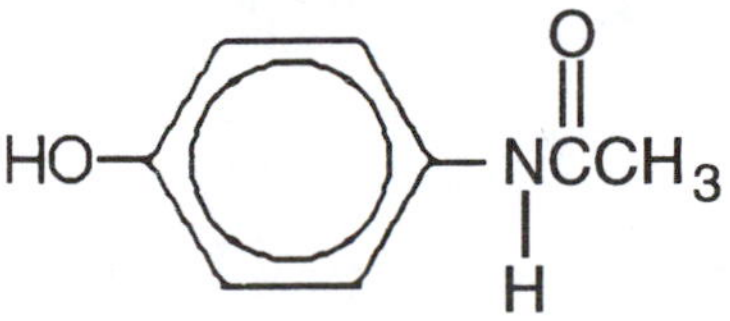

Acetaminophen

1

acetic acid. Mol.Wt. 60. CH₃COOH. A widely used organic acid. Vinegar, for example, is an aqueous solution of 4%–5% acetic acid, plus flavor and colors imparted by the constituents of the alcoholic solutions from which they are made. Ethyl alcohol (ethanol) with certain bacteria and air is oxidized to acetic acid. Various forms of acetic acid are important intermediates in the biochemistry of all living systems. See *acetyl choline* and *coenzyme* A.

$$\underset{\text{Ethanol}}{CH_3\,CH_2\,OH} + \underset{\text{OXYGEN}}{O_2} = \underset{\text{Acetic Acid}}{CH_3COOH} + \underset{\text{WATER}}{H_2O}$$

acetoacetate. The salt of *acetoacetic acid*.

acetoacetic acid. Mol. Wt. 102. A ketone body formed when fats are incompletely oxidized, as in diabetes. Appears in the urine in abnormal amounts in *starvation* or *diabetes*, resulting in *metabolic acidosis*.

$$\underset{\text{Acetoacetic acid (acetoacetate)}}{H_3C-\overset{\overset{\displaystyle O}{\|}}{C}-CH_2-\overset{\overset{\displaystyle O}{\|}}{C}-OH}$$

acetohexamine (Dymelor®). A hypoglycemic agent reported to lower the blood sugar level and to reduce glycosuria in certain diabetics. The drug acts by stimulating the release of *insulin* from the *pancreas*. The insulin appears to exercise its main effect by promoting the uptake of glucose from the bloodstream and storing it as liver and muscle *glycogen*.

acetone. Mol. Wt. 58. Dimethyl ketone, a colorless, volatile, inflammable liquid, miscible with water, useful as a solvent, and having a characteristic sweet, fruity, ethereal odor. Found in the blood and urine in diabetes and other metabolic disorders, or after lengthy fasting; acetone is produced when the fats are not completely oxidized. It is clinically significant because "acetone" or "sweet breath" indicates metabolic acidosis.

$$\underset{\text{Acetone}}{CH_3-\overset{\overset{\displaystyle O}{\|}}{C}-CH_3}$$

acetone bodies. *Acetone, acetoacetic acid,* and β-*hydroxybutyric acid* are collectively called "acetone bodies." They occur in the urine of individuals with *metabolic acidosis* or *ketosis*.

acetylcholine. Mol. Wt. 182. A metabolite fundamental to the mechanism of nerve impulse. An impulse reaching a nerve ending in the normal cycle liberates acetylcholine, which then stimulates a receptor. To enable the receptor to receive further impulses, the enzyme cholines-terase breaks down acetylcholine into *acetic acid* and *choline*. Other enzymes resynthesize these elements into more acetylcholine. The toxins from *Clostridium botulinum* inhibit the synthesis or the release of acetylcholine. See *botulinus poisoning*.

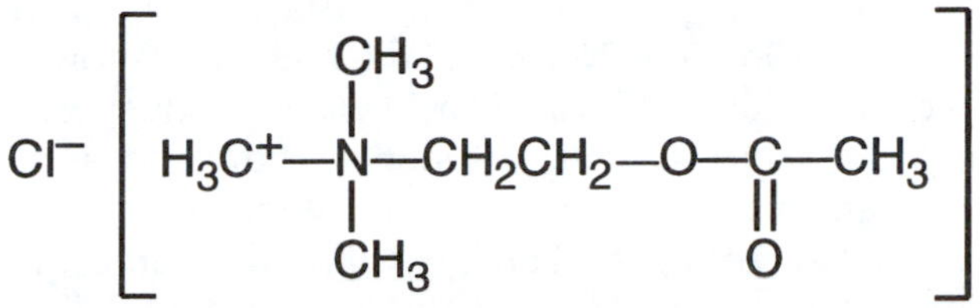

$$Cl^- \left[H_3C^+ - \underset{\underset{CH_3}{|}}{\overset{\overset{CH_3}{|}}{N}} - CH_2CH_2 - O - \underset{\underset{O}{\|}}{C} - CH_3 \right]$$

Acetylcholine chloride

acetyl-CoA. See *acetyl coenzyme A*.

acetyl coenzyme A. A combination of an acetyl group with *coenzyme A*. Previously known as "active acetate," it is a key material in metabolism. See *acetic acid* and *coenzyme A*.

acetylsalicylic acid. See *aspirin*.

achalasia (cardiospasm). A disturbance of normal *peristalsis* of the esophagus which causes foods to stick at the junction of the esophagus and stomach. This area lacks normal ability to "open up" when a *bolus* of food arrives. Chief symptom is difficulty in swallowing food.

achlorhydria. Absence of *hydrochloric acid* in the gastric secretions. It may be due to gastric carcinoma, gastric ulcer, pernicious anemia, adrenal insufficiency, or chronic gastritis.

achylia gastrica. A condition in which the secretion of *gastric juice* is diminished or absent.

acid. A compound that has hydrogen ions that are released in water solutions. Acids are essentially ionized hydrogen donors. In solution, acids provide H ions (H^+) or protons. The pH of a solution is a measure of acidity, neutrality, or alkalinity. A pH 7.0 is neutral, a value below pH 7 is in the acid region of hydrogen ion concentration, and above pH 7 is the alkaline or basic region. See *acid* and *base*.

acid ash residue. The acid ash residue is the total of inorganic acidic anions, chiefly chloride, phosphate, and sulfate in food or tissues reduced to ash by combustion. The acid residue is estimated by the volume of 0.1 N alkali (potassium or sodium hydroxide) required to neutralize the residue.

acid-base balance. The maintenance of the hydrogen ion (H^+) concentration in blood, intersti-tial fluids, and tissues. The H^+ concentration or pH is kept balanced at 7.4 by several *buffers*. Buffers are substances that resist changes in the pH when *acids* or *bases* (alkalis) are added to the system. The metabolisms of most living systems tend to produce acids. The principal buffer systems in humans are bicarbonate-carbonic acid, the phosphate salts, proteins, and hemoglobin-oxyhemoglobin.

acid-forming foods. Foods that have an acid-ash residue after burning. Examples are meat, fish, poultry, eggs, cereals, and some nuts. Certain fruits, such as cranberries and some varieties of prunes and plums, are considered acid forming because they produce organic acids that are not metabolized by the body.

acidemia. A blood pH value below 7.4. Normally, the body tends towards acidemia because of the accumulation of carbon dioxide (CO_2) and acid waste products of metabolism. The acid products are neutralized by *buffer* systems present in the blood and tissue fluids. When acidemia exists, there is an increase in the rate and depth of breathing to remove more dissolved CO_2 from the blood. Later, the kidneys will excrete an acid urine to compensate for the acidemia. Acidemia occurs in starvation and in untreated diabetes. See *acidosis*.

acidity or alkalinity food controls. Substances added to food to control acidity or alkalinity include acids, alkalies, buffers, and neutralizing agents. (See *acid*, *base*, and *buffer*.) Fruit flavors used in various products differ in their levels of acidity. Thus, "fruit" acids may be added to increase flavor intensity. The same "fruit" acids are sometimes added to processed cheese to improve texture and impart tartness. Additives in this group are also used to give an acid or tart taste to soft drinks, to facilitate heat processes of canned vegetables without discoloration, and to compensate for insufficient acid in fruit when making jellies and jams. These additives also facilitate peeling of tubers and fruits, neutralize part of the natural acids (as in tomato soup), and help control the texture of candy.

acidophilus milk. Milk fermented by any of several bacteria, such as *Lactobacillus acidophilus*. Such fermentations hydrolyze the disaccharide *lactose*, making the milk tolerable for persons who lack lactase (lactose-intolerant) and are unable to digest milk. *Yogurt* is similar in this respect. See *fermented milk sources* under *milk*.

acidosis. A condition in which the body's alkaline reserve is lowered due to abnormal loss of alkaline salts or abnormal accumulation of acids. Acidosis may be caused by an accumulation of organic acids (see *metabolic acidosis*) as in diabetic acidosis, or by excess loss of bicarbonates (as in renal disease), or in respiratory disorders that interfere with adequate release of carbon dioxide from the lungs and thereby cause an accumulation of carbonic acid in the blood (*respiratory acidosis*). See *acidemia*.

acidulants or acidifiers. Acids that have many food uses as flavor-enhancing agents, as preservatives to inhibit growth of microorganisms, and as antioxidants to prevent discoloration or rancidity and to adjust the acidity in foods. *Malic acid* is an example of an acidulant.

acinus. Groups of secretory cells in glands such as the salivary glands, the pancreas, and the liver. These organized clusters of cells are called "acini" because their shape resembles that of a bunch of grapes. Their secretions of enzymes and bile feed through ducts which empty into the *gastrointestinal* lumen.

acne. Seen most commonly in the skin of the face, neck, and chest. The characteristic sign is the blackhead or comedo, with the skin surrounding the central blackened area often slightly raised or reddened. Sometimes the central area is white and is called a "whitehead." The blackhead is a plugging of the opening of a hair follicle. This plug consists of a mixture of *sebum*, the normal oily secretion of the sebaceous glands (microscopic glands connected to the shaft containing the root of the hair), and of keratin, the normally present outermost layer of the skin. The sebum produced by these glands serves to lubricate the hair and give it its oily sheen. There is no known cure for acne, nor is there any known way of preventing this common problem. *Retinoic acid* derivatives have been shown to be effective in reducing certain forms of acne.

acne rosacea. An excessive flushing of the blood vessels of the nose and cheeks. A nervous reflex may be a factor in such excessive flushing. Drinking alcohol may encourage the reflex, but it is not essential. With *chronic* abnormal flushing, the blood vessels become more apparent and nose size may increase.

acorn squash. A fall and winter vegetable that belongs to the gourd family. It has a dark green rind, yellow-orange flesh, and many seeds. Acorn squash can grow as large as 8 inches long and 5 inches across. Its flavor is somewhat sweet. An excellent source of *carotene* (vitamin A activity); fair source of *ascorbic acid* (vitamin C), *riboflavin*, and *iron*. See *squash* in the table under *vegetables*.

acquired immune deficiency syndrome. See *AIDS*.

acrolein. Mol. Wt. 56. A substance formed from the glycerol of fat when heated to a high temperature. The acrid odor of overheated fat is caused by acrolein.

$$H-\overset{\overset{\displaystyle H}{|}}{C}=\overset{\overset{\displaystyle H}{|}}{C}-\overset{\overset{\displaystyle H}{|}}{C}=O$$

Acrolein

ACTH. See *adrenocorticotropic hormone*.

actin. One of two proteins in muscle fiber responsible for the contractile process. The other protein is *myosin*. See *muscle*.

active site. That portion of an enzyme surface where combination with the substrate takes place and the chemical or molecular changes in the substrate occur.

active transport. The means by which nutrients and other substances are concentrated within the cell from a lower concentration outside the cell. Active transport is in contradistinction to simple diffusion where the materials, such as water and some salts, pass freely through the membrane in either direction, and to facilitated diffusion where the rate of transfer is increased by enzymes or carriers in the membrane. Both simple diffusion and facilitated diffusion are passive diffusions since the processes are toward equilibrium, that is, concentrations on both sides of the membrane are equal. Active transport requires energy, and the major source of the energy is *adenosine triphosphate* (ATP). How the chemical energy is coupled to the active transport of nutrients across membranes is not clearly understood. Amino acids are actively transported into the intestinal mucosa. Sodium is actively transported in the opposite direction, that is, sodium ions are pumped out of the cell, which in turn is coupled to the active transport of *glucose* and *galactose*. Calcium is an example of facilitated diffusion in the intestines in which *vitamin D* plays a major role. *Cobalamin* (vitamin B_{12}) transport is also facilitated and needs a specific factor, a mucoprotein called "intrinsic factor," to be absorbed. See *absorption*.

acute. Of short duration, a condition or disease; the opposite of *chronic*.

addictive. A substance leading to the habituation of use, usually of a drug, the deprivation of which leads to withdrawal symptoms and an impulse to take the drug again.

Addison's disease. A rare human metabolic disorder in which there is adrenal insufficiency of the hormones of the *adrenal cortex*, either because of infection such as tuberculosis, or a tumor, or general wasting or atrophy following removal of the *pituitary gland* in the treatment of *cancer*. A person with Addison's disease is unable to store sodium chloride and excretes it in the urine in excessive quantities. There is decreased ability to excrete potassium, and the percentage of potassium in the blood rises sharply. With sodium loss, water excretion increases and severe dehydration follows, which can result in a crisis.

additives. See *food additives*.

adenine. A purine base, $C_5H_5N_5$, 6-aminopurine. It is chemically related to *uric acid*. It is one of the two purine bases of *ribonucleic acid* and *deoxyribonucleic* acid. See *adenosine triphosphate*.

adenohypophysis. See *pituitary gland*.

adenosine. A compound containing *adenine* and *ribose*. See *adenosine triphosphate*.

adenosine diphosphate (ADP). Mol. Wt. 427. A compound containing *adenosine* and two phosphoric acid groups. ADP is produced during muscle contraction. It is formed during muscle contraction processes. See *adenosine triphosphate*.

adenosine monophosphate (adenylic acid, AMP). Mol. Wt. 347. See *adenosine triphosphate*.

adenosine triphosphate (ATP). Mol. Wt. 507. The adenosine nucleotides, AMP, ADP, and ATP, are important compounds in terms of *energy balance* and *metabolism*. The *oxidation* of foodstuffs leads through a system called the *terminal respiratory chain* where electrons are donated to oxygen and water is formed. The process is called *oxidative phosphorylation*, because coupled to the oxidation of foodstuffs is the phosphorylation of ADP to form ATP. These reactions take place in the *mitochondria*. ATP is the principal form of chemical energy in the body. It is used in many biosynthetic processes which require energy. The activation of *glucose*, *amino acids*, and *fatty acids* all require the formation of phosphate intermediates, and ATP is the source of the phosphate and chemical energy. The result of these reactions is the formation of AMP or ADP, depending upon the reaction, which can be used to form more ATP by oxidative phosphorylation.

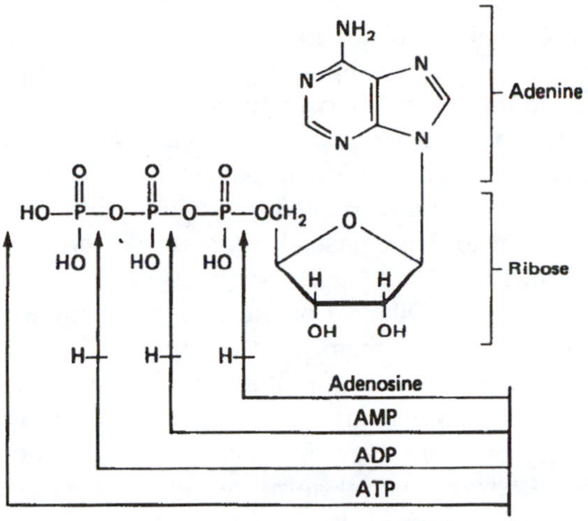

Adenosine triphosphate (ATP)

S-adenosylmethionine. Mol. Wt. 434. A derivative of *adenosine triphosphate* (ATP) involved in the transfer of methyl groups ($-CH3$) in the formation of lecithin (phosphatidylcholine). Other compounds involved in one-carbon transfers are the vitamins *cobalamin* (vitamin B_{12}) and *folacin*.

adenylate cyclase. See *cyclic AMP*.

adequate. Sufficient in amount to meet a specific requirement. The term "adequate diet" is often incorrectly used in reference to an individual diet that provides the dietary allowances of nutrients as recommended by the Food and Nutrition Board of the National Research Council.

ADH. See *antidiuretic hormone (vasopressin)*.

adipic acid (hexanedioic acid). Mol. Wt. 146. Used in bottled drinks and throat lozenges because it has little tendency to pick up moisture, and frequently used to supply tartness to powdered products, such as gelatin desserts and fruit-flavored drinks. Adipic acid is occasionally added to edible oils to prevent them from going rancid.

$$HOOC-CH_2-CH_2-CH_2-CH_2-COOH$$

Adipic acid

adipose tissue. A fatty connective tissue found under the skin and in many other regions of the body. It serves as a padding and insulation around and between organs. It insulates the body by reducing heat loss and serves as a food reserve. See *body fat*.

ADP. Adenosine diphosphate. See *adenosine triphosphate*.

adrenal cortex. The outer layer of the adrenal glands. See *adrenal glands*.

adrenal glands. The two adrenal glands are located one above each kidney (suprarenal). Each adrenal gland actually functions as two separate glands, producing different hormones from its two parts, the medulla (the inner portion), and the cortex (the outer portion). The adrenal medulla is a separate organ from the cortex physiologically. The medulla produces *epinephrine* and *norepinephrine*, which are important in preparing the body for action against external danger or fright. Epinephrine (sometimes called adrenaline) dilates blood vessels so that more blood can flow through them and increase the amount of work done by the heart. Both epinephrine and norepinephrine elevate the blood glucose level by stimulatiing the breakdown of the *glycogen* stored in the liver. Dilation of the tiny coronary arteries in the heart is also engendered by both hormones. Epinephrine and norepinephrine are both derivatives of the *essential amino acid tyrosine*. The medulla is stimulated to release epinephrine by the *sympathetic* branch of the *autonomic nervous* system to give the body the extra energy it needs in emergencies by causing the release of *glucose* from liver *glycogen*. The cortex, the outer part of the adrenal glands, produces a series of adrenocortical hormones including hydrocortisone (*cortisol*). The adrenocortical hormones influence the salt and *water balance* of the body, the metabolism of foods, and the ability of the body to handle stress. The cortex of the adrenal glands requires stimulation by a hormone produced by the pituitary gland, *adrenocorticotropin*.

adrenaline. See *epinephrine*.

adrenocorticotropic hormone (adrenocorticotropin, ACTH). A hormone liberated by the anterior *pituitary gland*, which stimulates the cortex of the *adrenal glands*. The basophilic cells of the hypophyseal pituitary anterior lobe secrete adrenocorticotropin, often referred to as ACTH, a polypeptide with 39 amino acids. ACTH acts upon the adrenal gland cortices. When there is too little ACTH, the cortical layers atrophy. Hyperplasia occurs when excessive quantities of ACTH are given. Under the influence of ACTH, all the adrenal cortical hormones are secreted. In addition, ACTH has a direct lipolytic action. Fat is mobilized and the fatty acid level in the blood increases due to *lipolysis*.

aerobic. Pertaining to air or oxygen. Air or oxygen is required for life or normal function, as in aerobic bacteria.

aflatoxins. Mol. Wt. 312. Several closely related toxic compounds produced by certain molds which cause liver injury in poultry. Some may be extremely carcinogenic.

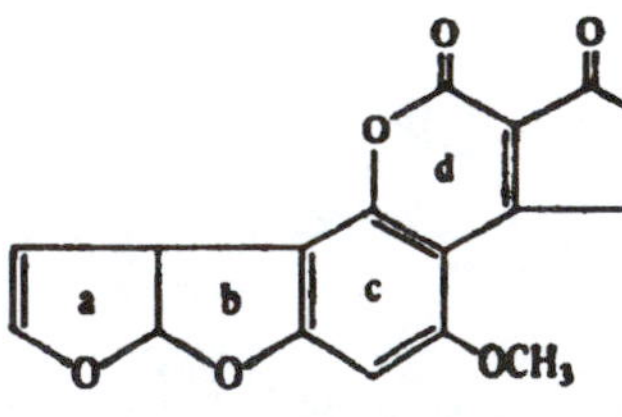

Aflatoxin B$_1$
All aflatoxins contain the same tetracylic ring systems shown above, a, b, c, and d.

agar. A vegetable gelatin made from various kinds of algae or seaweed, used as a jellying agent in home cooking. It is used in the Orient in the preparation of soups and jellies as a thickening agent. It is also used in the commercial manufacture of jams, jellies, ice creams, and mayonnaise. It is used in medicine and is essential in microbiology, where it is used as a solid support on which bacteria are grown in culture. See *carrageenan*.

AIDS. Acquired immune deficiency syndrome (AIDS) is a disease caused by infection with *human immunodeficiency virus (HIV)*. AIDS is the condition of a lack of the capacity to form antibodies against infections. AIDS itself does not kill a person. Persons with AIDS die of secondary infections because of the lack of an immune system. Many of the infections that cause death in persons with AIDS are extremely rare in persons with uncompromised and intact immune systems.

alanine (Ala, A). Mol. Wt. 89. One of the nonessential *amino acids* found in proteins. It is the amino acid derivative of *pyruvic* acid.

$$CH_3—CH—COOH$$
$$|$$
$$NH_2$$

Alanine (Ala, A)

albacore (*Thunnus alalunga*). A type of tuna fish. Albacore has the true white meat of all tuna and is used for the finest canned tuna. Canned tuna labeled "all white meat, solid pack," is albacore. It is an excellent source of protein containing small amounts of *calcium*, *phosphorus*, and *iron*. See *fish*.

albinism. An inborn error of the metabolism of the essential amino acid tyrosine that results in the failure to produce the pigment melanin, causing a congenital, nonpathologic partial or total absence of pigment in skin, hair, and eyes. Albinism is frequently accompanied by astigmatism, photophobia, and nystagmus because the choroid membrane in the eye is unprotected from light as a result of lack of pigment.

albumin. One of a group of simple proteins widely distributed in plant and animal tissues; found in the blood as serum albumin, in milk as lactalbumin, and in the white of egg as ovalbumin. It is soluble in cold water; coagulated on heating, it no longer dissolves in cold or hot water. In general, albumins from animal sources are of higher nutrient quality than those from vegetable sources because animal proteins contain greater quantities and a better balance of the essential amino acids. See *protein*.

albuminoids. The simple proteins characteristic of the skeletal structure of animals (also called scleroproteins) and of the external protective tissues such as skin, hair, etc. *Collagen* is an example of an albuminoid, which when boiled with water yields *gelatin*. See *protein*.

albuminuria. The presence of albumin in the urine. It is an indication of renal dysfunction.

Alcaligenes. A species of bacteria which usually produces an alkaline reaction in the medium of growth. *A. viscolactis* (vicosus) causes ropiness of milk, and *A. meta-caligenes* gives a slimy growth on cottage cheese. These organisms come from manure, feeds, soils, water, and dust.

alcohol. A class of organic compound that contains the hydroxyl (-OH) group. A general term often applied to ethyl alcohol (*ethanol*). Alcohol in its pure form is a transparent, colorless liquid, volatile and very flammable. It is distilled from a great variety of fruits and grains which contain either natural sugar or substances that can be transformed into sugar. By the addition of natural or artificial yeast strains and mineral compounds, the sugar is changed by fermentation into alcohol and other by-products which are used commercially. This is the alcohol commonly known as grain or wine alcohol. Its technical name is ethyl alcohol or ethanol. It is found in beer, whiskeys, wines, brandies, liqueurs, and rum. Alcohol should not be regarded as a single substance. Methanol, or wood alcohol, which is very different from the grain or ethyl alcohol we drink, is the poisonous alcohol most frequently encountered.

Nutritive value of alcoholic and carbonated beverages

BEVERAGE	CALORIES KCAL	CARBOHYDRATES G	ALCOHOL G
100% ethanol	7.1	0	1
beer (8 oz)	75	0	11
brandy, gin, rum, vodka, whiskey (1 jigger)			
80 proof	70	0	10
90 proof	80	0	11
100 proof	90	0	13
liqueurs			
cordial glass	65	6	7
Champagne	75	3	10
Muscatel	160	14	15
Sauterne	85	4	10
table wine	85	—	10
Vermouth			
French	105	1	15
Italian	165	12	18
colas (cup)	95	24	0
ginger ale	75	19	0
flavored soda	105	26	0
root beer	100	25	0
quinine soda	75	19	0

alcohol-nutrient interaction. Alcohol (*ethanol*) and nutrients interact at many levels. Ethanol may directly alter the level of nutrient intake through its effect on appetite, its displacement of food in the diet, or its effect on the gastrointestinal tract, resulting in disturbances of digestion and absorption. Through its effect on various organs, especially the liver, ethanol may alter the transport, activation, catabolism, utilization, and storage of nutrients. As a result, alcoholism remains one of the major causes of nutritional deficiencies. Ethanol is directly toxic to many body tissues, and this effect may be worsened by existing nutritional deficiencies. Because of its widespread use and multiple effects, ethanol has a major impact on overall nutritional status. The question of the roles of alcohol and malnutrition in the pathogenesis of liver disease seen in the alcoholic (fatty liver, alcoholic hepatitis, and cirrhosis) is of utmost importance for the treatment and prevention of the disease. Malnutrition has been proposed as the predominant factor in liver injury because each gram of ethanol provides 7.1 calories, which means that 20 ounces of 86 proof beverage represents about 1500 calories or one-half to two-thirds of the normal caloric requirement. Therefore, the alcoholic has a much-reduced demand for food to fulfill caloric needs. Since alcoholic beverages do not contain significant amounts of protein, vitamins, and minerals, the intake of these nutrients may readily become borderline or insufficient. Alcohol does not mix well with a wide variety of medications, such as antibiotics, anticoagulants, antidiabetic drugs including insulin, antihistamines, high blood pressure drugs, *monoamine oxidase* (MAO) inhibitors, and sedatives. Alcohol combined with antihistamines, tranquilizers, or antidepressants causes excessive drowsiness, and synergistic combinations have resulted in some deaths.

aldosterone. Mol. Wt. 360. One of the three major hormones of the *adrenal glands* (cortex) concerned mainly with the level of sodium ions (Na^+) in the body and the *water balance*. The hormone, a cholesterol derivative, cannot actually increase the amount of Na^+ in the body, it can only prevent excessive loss. It does this by acting directly on the filtering system of the kidneys. The aldosterone modifies the membranes involved in filtration so that Na^+ does not pass into the urine. At the same time, potassium ions (K^+) tend to be excreted in increased quantities. The amount of Na^+ in the body is important both for the activity of certain enzymes and for the normal functioning of the nervous system. See *water balance*.

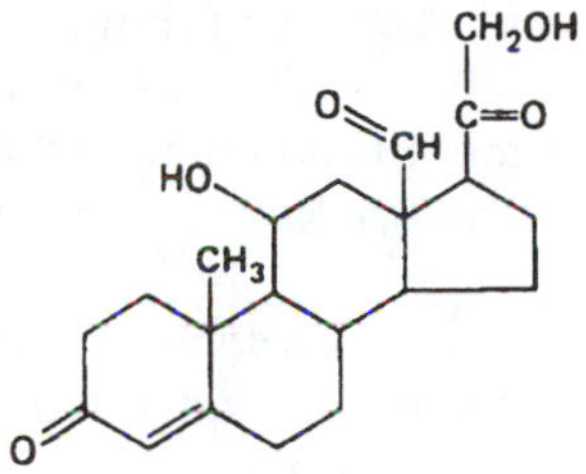

Aldosterone

ale. Ale is fermented malt beverage; beer is its brother. Ale, like beer, is brewed from malt, cereals, and hops, but the method of brewing ale is different from that of brewing beer. Ale is "top fermented," that is, during fermentation at a higher temperature, its yeast rises to the top. The result is a brew with a more pronounced hop flavor than that found in beer. Porter and stout are two well-known varieties of ale, both sweeter and darker than the others. Porter has less hop flavor than stout, which has a full hop flavor with a slightly burnt taste. See *beer* and *yeast*.

alewife (*Alosa pseudoharengus*). An inexpensive edible *fish* belonging to the herring family. Alewives grow to about 10 inches in length and to about a half pound in weight. The fish is rather bony, but the flavor is pleasant and less oily than that of shad. It can be cooked like fresh herring.

alfalfa (*Medicago sativa*). A leguminous plant chiefly used for animal forage, prized by health-food devotees as a rich source of vitamins, usually consumed in the form of alfalfa tablets. Alfalfa sprouts are rich in *ascorbic acid*.

alginate or propylene glycol alginate. As a food additive, it acts as a thickening and stabilizing agent. The most important commercial source of algin is giant kelp. Alginate solutions can be converted to gels by adding calcium. These chemically set gels are extremely stable, and help prevent jellies in pastries from oozing over into the oven. Industry uses algin to help maintain the desired texture in ice cream, candy, cheese, pressure-dispensed whipped cream, yogurt, canned frostings, and many other factory-made goods.

alimentary canal. See *digestive system*.

alimentation. The entire process of nourishing the body, which includes *mastication*, swallowing, digestion, absorption, and assimilation.

alkalemia. As human blood increases above pH 7.4, it becomes more alkaline and the condition is called alkalemia. Alkalemia is less common than acidemia. Alkalemia can occur from loss of acid from the stomach in vomiting or the intake of too much alkaline medicine, for example, in the treatment of gastric or duodenal ulcer. To compensate for alkalemia, *buffer* mechanisms come into action in the opposite direction, and respiration is depressed so that carbon dioxide (*carbonic acid*) is retained and the H ion concentration rises again. The kidneys secrete an alkaline urine and body conditions return toward normal, pH 7.4.

alkali. The chemical opposite of an *acid*. A group of compounds that form salts when combined with acids and soaps when combined with *fatty acids*. An alkali (or base) neutralizes acids by accepting hydrogen ions (H^+). At a more fundamental chemical level, bases are compounds that will donate electron pairs. See *acid-base balance* and *acid* and *base*.

alkaline ash residue. The ash of foods with high concentrations of sodium, potassium, calcium, and magnesium yields an alkaline reaction in water. The alkaline value is determined and expressed as the quantity of 1 N acid required to neutralize the ash. Dairy products are examples of foods that yield an alkaline ash residue. See *acid ash residue*.

alkaline-phosphatase test. An enzyme test performed on blood to screen for bone disease and prostate cancer, and for the diagnosis of obstructive jaundice.

alkaline reserve. The amount of *alkali* or base in the body that is available for neutalizing the acid produced, such as *hydrochloric* or *lactic acid*. A fall in the alkaline reserve results in *acidosis* (*acidemia*). The alkaline reserve is generally measured as the bicarbonate (HCO_3^-) concentration in the plasma, but it also includes phosphate salts and proteins as a part of the alkaline reserve buffer complex.

alkaline tide. The slight change in blood pH toward the alkaline side following a meal. The change is a consequence of the production of hydrochloric acid in the stomach.

alkaloid. An organic nitrogenous base. Many alkaloids are of great medical importance, such as morphine, strychnine, atropine, cocaine, and quinine. They occur in the animal and vegetable kingdoms, and some have been synthesized.

alkalosis. A condition of excessive alkaline substances in the body fluids. Alkalosis (*alkalemia*) can be caused by excessive vomiting, which removes stomach acids, or by hyperventilation, which removes carbonic acid from the blood. Symptoms of alkalosis are shallow respiration, a tingling sensation in the extremities, muscular cramps, and tetanic convulsions. Alkalosis is the physiologic opposite of *acidosis* (*acidemia*).

allergen. Any substance capable of producing an allergy or an allergy reaction. Among common allergens are inhalants (dust, pollens, fungi, smoke, perfumes, vapors from plastics); foods (wheat, eggs, milk, chocolate, strawberries); drugs (antibiotics, serums); infectious agents (bacteria, viruses, fungi, animal parasites); contactants (chemicals, animals, plants, metals); physical agents (heat, cold, light, pressure, radiation). See *allergy*.

allergy. A special type of inflammatory response in various parts of the body to a foreign substance in the environment. Allergic reactions may take several forms, depending upon which part of the body is affected, but all involve the immunologic system. The parts of the body most likely to show allergic responses are the lungs, nose, eyes, skin, middle ear, stomach, and intestines. Depending on the site, allergic reactions can result in asthma, hay fever, conjunctivitis, eczema, hives, sinusitis, and any combination of abdominal pain, nausea, vomiting, or diarrhea. Substances that provoke an allergic reaction are known as *allergens*. An individual who is allergic to grass, for example, produces antibodies which are distributed throughout the body but cause symptoms only where and when they come in contact with their allergen. Allergic symptoms arise from the interaction of an allergen with an antibody made by the allergic individual. The meeting of allergen and antibody sets in progress a reaction that releases various substances, which cause the dilation (opening up) of small vessels and the leaking of fluids through these vessels into the surrounding tissue, resulting in swelling, spasm of the mouth muscles, spasm in air passages, and an outpouring of mucous secretions. The particular resulting symptoms depend upon where the antibody and allergen meet.

almond (*Prunus amygdalus*). The word covers the tree and nut, the seed or kernel of a subgenus which includes the peach tree. The almond closely resembles the peach in its blossom and young unripe fruit, although the almond tree grows larger. The almond tree bears a leathery fruit which, upon maturing, slits open and exposes the nut in its shell. The pitted shell is light tan in color. The nut is covered with a medium-brown skin and is white inside. Basically there are two kinds of almonds, sweet and bitter. Almonds provide some protein, iron, calcium, phosphorus, and B vitamins. They are also high in fat. A 100 g nut, roasted and salted, contains 627 calories.

alpha cells. See *glucagon* and *pancreas*.

alpha (α)-helix. A coiled helical arrangement of the peptide chain of proteins. The helical structure is stabilized by intrachain hydrogen bonding. The α-helix is a common structural feature of proteins. Another important structure of protein stabilized by hydrogen bonding is the β-*pleated sheet*.

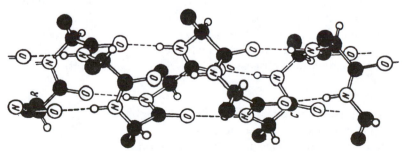

Structure of a right-handed alpha (α)-helix

alpha (α) ketoglutaric acid. Mol. Wt. 86. $C_5H_5O_6$. One of the intermediates in the *Krebs'* (tricarboxylic acid) *cycle*. It is also a product of deamination of *glutamic acid*.

$$HOOC—CH_2—CH_2—\overset{\overset{\textstyle O}{\|}}{C}—COOH$$

Alpha (α) ketoglutaric acid

alpha (α) tocopherol. See *tocopherol*.

alpha or α-tocopherol equivalent (α-T.E.). The α-T.E. is now the standard unit of measurement for designating vitamin E requirements. For greater precision and clarity, a change from the former measure of International Units (I.U.) was made. One α-T.E. of vitamin E activity is defined as one milligram of d,l-α-tocopherol. When only the milligrams of d,l-α-tocopherol is reported in food, that weight is multiplied by 1.2 to account for other tocopherols present—the value approximates the total α-T.E. content. To convert from the old system, 1 α-T.E. is equivalent to 0.7 I.U. of vitamin E activity. See *tocopherol*.

aluminum (Al). Element No. 13. At. Wt. 27. A light silver-colored metal. The amount of aluminum ingested in the average human diet ranges widely from 10 mg to more than 100 mg daily. This element is found in many plant and animal foods. Despite this wide intake and distribution, no clear function in human nutrition has been established. The total aluminum content of the human body is from 50–150 mg.

aluminum hydroxide. Mol. Wt. 78. $Al(OH)_3$. A white, viscous suspension containing aluminum hydroxide and hydrated aluminum oxide; an *antacid* especially useful in treatment of peptic ulcer.

ameba. A minute, one-celled protozoan animal form of life found in soil and water. It constantly changes shape by sending out fingerlike processes of protoplasm (pseudopodia), by which it moves about and obtains nourishment. It possesses an outer translucent substance called the ectoplasm, but the inner substance, endoplasm, is denser and contains a nucleus. It feeds by surrounding its food and enclosing it in the so-called food vacuole. Oxygen is absorbed from the surrounding water, and carbon dioxide is eliminated through the plasma membrane. Some species of *Entamoeba* are parasitic in humans.

amebic dysentery (amebiasis). Disease primarily caused by ameba affecting the colon, but may affect other organs, especially the liver. Severe amebiasis is characterized by diarrhea with blood and/or pus and mucus in the watery discharges. Infection generally takes place following the drinking of water contaminated with sewage containing amebae. Complications of amebic infections are hepatitis, abscesses of the liver, abscesses of the lungs, and perforation of the bowel.

ameboid movement. The method of locomotion of amebae which involves the formulation and contraction of cellular extensions sometimes referred to as pseudopodia (false feet). Many of the cells in the human body, especially the white blood cells, can move about by ameboid movement.

ameloblasts. Special epithelial cells surrounding tooth buds in gum tissue, which form cup-shaped organs for producing the enamel structure of the developing teeth. Insufficient vitamin A (*retinol*) causes faulty production of ameloblasts and therefore impairs the soundness of tooth structure.

amenorrhea. The absence of menstruation. The term is used to cover the absence of regular monthly periods at any time between the onset of puberty and menopause. The classifications are primary amenorrhea, in which the menses have never occurred, and secondary amenorrhea, in which there is an absence of menstrual periods in women who have formerly had normal menstrual cycles.

amination. The addition of an amino group ($-NH_2$) to an organic compound to produce an amine. See *transamination*.

amine. One of a group of nitrogen-containing organic compounds formed when one or more of the hydrogens of ammonia have been replaced by one or more hydrocarbon radicals.

amino acid metabolism. The metabolism of the amino acids follows several directions. The amino acid can be degraded and oxidized as a source of energy, incorporated into proteins, or used for the synthesis of nitrogen-containing compounds. The diagram summarizes and simplifies the various metabolic paths amino acids take. The diagram of intermediates shows the metabolic pathways central to the *Krebs'* (tricarboxylic acid) *cycle*.

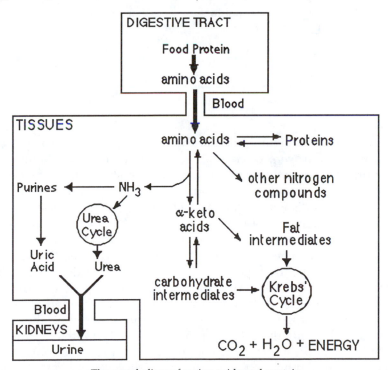

The metabolism of amino acids and protein

In terms of their metabolism, individual amino acids are classified as *glucogenic* (resulting in a net increase in glucose production), *ketogenic* (resulting in a production of *ketone bodies*), or both. The metabolic classification is only important in that it indicates the pathway a given amino acid may take. Most of the amino acids are glucogenic. Only leucine is wholly ketogenic. The diagram shows the metabolic fates of the carbon skeletons of the amino acids.

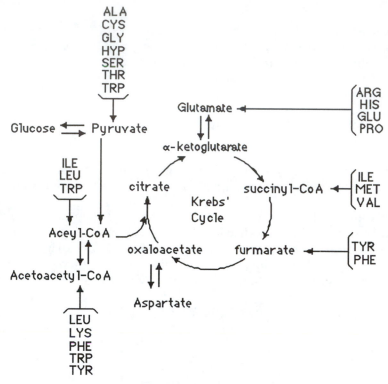

Intermediates formed from the carbon skeletons of amino acids

amino acids. The simplest structural units of the proteins. All amino acids contain carbon, hydrogen, oxygen, and nitrogen; three amino acids contain sulfur. Amino acids have the same relation to proteins that letters have to words. At least 22 different letters make up the amino acid alphabet, and combinations of these amino acids produce a great variety of proteins. The essential or indispensable amino acids for adults are *tryptophan, threonine, methionine, isoleucine, lysine, valine,* and *phenylalaline.* Because *histidine, tyrosine,* and *cysteine* are produced in inadequate amounts in human infants, the body is unable to produce the essential amino acids and they must come from food. The other amino acids, the nonessential amino acids, may be synthesized in the body. The essential amino acids content determines the nutritive or *biological value* (BV) of a protein. A unique feature of the amino acids is the arrangement of their asymmetric carbon, which can exist in two configurations. One configuration is the mirror image of the other (L-form and D-form), based on the configurations of D- and L-glyceraldehyde. Only the L-form of the amino acids occurs in proteins. In general, the body uses only the L-form. Some bacterial nonprotein products contain the D-forms of amino acids. For example, some antibiotics and the cell walls of some bacteria contain D-amino acid forms. Two naturally occurring amino acids, *L-ornithine* and *L-citrulline*, do not occur in proteins. Amino acids are also classified on the basis of their chemical structures. The table shows the classification of the amino acids based on their chemical composition and on their essential or nonessential dietary requirement.

Protein amino acid chemical classification

CHEMICAL CLASSIFICATION	ESSENTIAL	NONESSENTIAL
Neutral		
One -NH$_2$ and one -COOH group	Threonine	Glycine
		Serine
One -NH$_2$, one -COOH and one amide group		Glutamine
		Asparagine
Aliphatic	Alanine	
Contains aliphatic groups	Isoleucine	
	Leucine	
Aromatic		
Contains benzene group	Phenylalanine	Tyrosine
Heterocyclic	Tryptophan	Proline
Contains a heterocyclic ring	HistIdine	Hydroxyproline
Sulfur		
Contains sulfur	Methionine	Cysteine
Basic		
Contains two -NH$_2$ and one -COOH group	Lysine	Hydoxylysine
Contains a guanido group		Arginine
Acidic		
Contains one -NH$_2$ and two-COOH groups		Aspartic acid
		Glutamic acic

The structures of the amino acids are given under the names of the individual amino acids.

amino acid oxidase. The enyzme catalyst for oxidative deamination of D- or L-amino acids. The reactions occur primarily in the liver and kidneys. The enzyme uses *flavin mononucleotide (FMN)* as a cofactor, which is a derivative of the B vitamin *riboflavin*.

amino acid symbols. There is a standard short-hand for the amino acids that is particularly useful when writing the sequences of proteins and peptides. These abbreviations are given in the table.

Amino acid symbols

AMINO ACID	ABBREVIATION*	SYMBOL	AMINO ACID	ABBREVIATION*	SYMBOL
Alanine	Ala	A	Methionine	Met	M
Asparagine			Asparagine	Asn	N
aspartate	Asx	B	Proline	Pro	P
Cysteine	Cys	C	Glutamine	Gln	Q
Aspartate	Asp	D	Arginine	Arg	R
Glutamate	Glu	E	Serine	Ser	S
Phenylalanine	Phe	F	Threonine	Thr	T
Glycine	Gly	G	Valine	Val	V
Histidine	His	H	Tryptophan	Trp	W
Isoleucine	Ile	I	Tyrosine	Tyr	Y
Lysine	Lys	K	Glutamine		
Leucine	Leu	L	glutamate	Glx	Z

* The three-letter symbols may all be capitalized.

aminopterin. A drug used in the treatment of acute leukemias and choriocarcinomas. Aminopterin and the structurally related methotrexate are quite toxic. See chemotherapy and *methotrexate*.

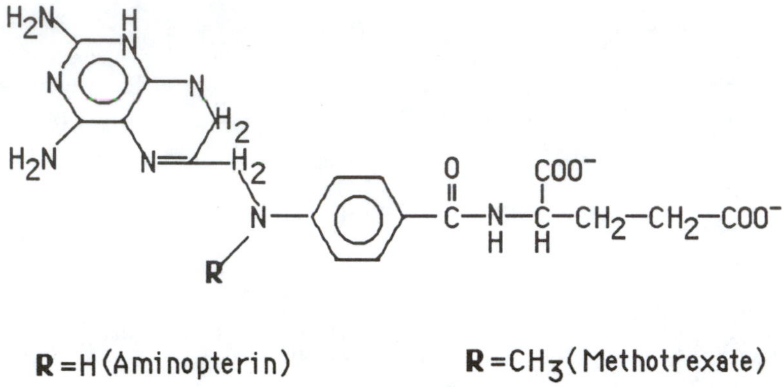

R =H (Aminopterin)   **R =CH₃ (Methotrexate)**

Stuctures of aminopterin and methotrexate

amino sugars. Sugars that contain an amino group ($-NH_2$). An important example of their occurrence is in antibiotics such as the mycin drugs and mucopolysaccharides.

ammoniated glycyrrhizin. A toxic agent having a variety of physiologic effects; it raises blood pressure, alleviates stomach ulcers, and reduces the toxicity of strychnine, carbolic acid, and diptheria toxin. Food companies use it in licorice flavoring and as a component of root beer and wintergreen flavoring in beverages (50 ppm), candy (5–60 ppm), and baked goods (5 ppm). Glycyrrhizin is one of the sweetest natural substances known.

amoeba. See *ameba*.

AMP (adenosine monophosphate). See *adenosine triphosphate* (ATP).

amphetamine sulfate (benzidrine sulfate). Mol. Wt. 369. A synthetic drug that stimulates the central nervous system, reduces appetite, and reduces nasal congestion. Amphetamines are addictive.

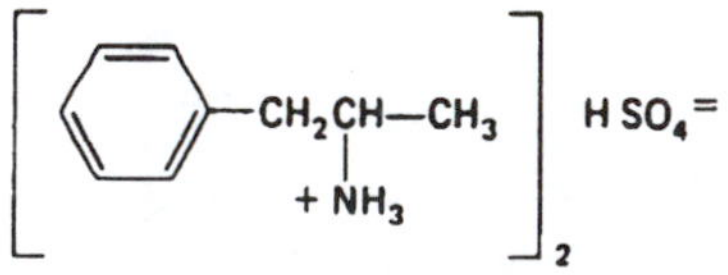

Amphetamine sulfate

amphoteric. A single compound having properties of both an acid and a base, and therefore able to function as either. *Amino acids* have this dual chemical nature because of their structure; they contain both an acid (carboxyl, COOH) group and a base (amino, $-NH_2$) group, as do *proteins*. See *zwitterion*.

amygdalin (vitamin B$_{17}$, laetrile). Mol. Wt. 457. What is believed to be the active principle of laetrile or vitamin B$_{17}$, is shown. It occurs in almond seed extracts and has been controversial in the treatment of cancer.

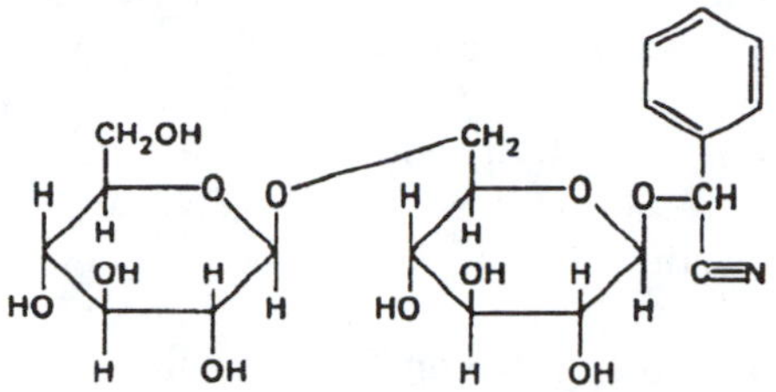

Amygdalin (vitamin B$_{17}$, laetrile)

amylase. A classification of enzymes that digest *starch*, for example, ptyalin in the saliva. To distinguish between the different enzymes, the starch-splitting enzyme found in *saliva* is called salivary amylase, and the one secreted by the *pancreas* is known as pancreatic amylase. The amylases that hydrolyze the starches are classified in various ways, depending on how and where they act on the starch molecules.

amylopectin. The branched chain of linked glucose units, an insoluble form of starch from plants which stains violet-red with iodine and forms a paste with hot water. The animal equivalent of amylopectin is *glycogen*. See *starch*.

amylose. The straight chain of linked *glucose*, a soluble form of *starch* which stains blue with iodine. Potato starch is an example of an amylose.

anabolism. The opposite of *catabolism*. Anabolism includes all chemical changes that build new substances in growth or maintenance. *Metabolism* = anabolism + catabolism. Constructive processes that build up the body substances—the synthesis in living organisms of more complex substances from simpler ones are anabolic processes. Anabolism uses *energy* made available from certain catabolic processes, for example, the oxidation of fat to carbon dioxide + water + energy.

anaerobe. A microorganism living or functioning without air or free oxygen. The opposite is an aerobe. A strict anaerobe is an organism that cannot survive in oxygen. Organisms that can live under either aerobic or anaerobic conditions are called facultative organisms. Most yeasts are facultative.

analgesia. Absence of sensitivity to pain.

analgesics. Analgesics are among the most widely used drugs; painkillers. Narcotics are not classified as analgesics. Narcotics, derivatives of opium such as morphine and codeine sulfate, may cause addiction. *Aspirin* acts as an analgesic and an *antipyretic*. As an analgesic it relieves headache and muscular pain. Aspirin normally is used in 0.324 g per tablets. Often, it is combined with other analgesics such as *phenacetin* and *caffeine*. In large and continued doses, aspirin produces gastric irritation. *Ibuprofen* is a nonsteroidal, anti-inflammatory agent with antipyretic and analgesic properties. Although the exact mechanism of ibuprofen action is unknown, it does not stimulate the *pituitary* or *adrenal* systems. Analgesics are used to treat chronic symptomatic *rheumatoid arthritis* and *osteoarthritis*.

anaphase. The stage in cell division at which the newly formed, duplicated chromosomes separate and go to opposite sides of the dividing cell.

anaphylaxis. An extreme hypersensitivity induced as a result of the presence of an *antigen* to which the animal or individual has been sensitized by injection or some other means of exposure. It is an extreme reaction of the immunologic system.

anastomosis. A natural connection between two vessels. It may be direct or by means of connecting channels. The surgical or pathologic connection of two tubular structures.

androgens (androgenic hormones). A class of steroid hormones that produce secondary male characteristics. They are derivatives of *cholesterol*. The opposites are the female hormones, the *estrogens*. See *testosterone*.

anemia. A condition in which the total quantity of hemoglobin in the circulating blood is less than normal. This deficiency in circulating hemoglobin may be due to a decreased number of red blood cells per unit volume of blood or to a deficient hemoglobin content in the erythrocytes. The various anemias may be classified in the following simplified fashion on an etiologic basis. See *cobalamin, folacin,* and *iron.*

Types of anemias

TYPE	CAUSE	TREATMENT
Hemorrhagic	Acute hemolysis Immune reactions (erythroblastosis, hypersplenism). Toxic reactions (bacteria toxins, drugs).	Transfusion
Aplastic	Bone marrow destruction Infections; chronic diseases; drugs; irradiation; hormonal disorders.	Transfusion Removal of drug or irradiations.
Nutritional	Deficiencies Iron; folacin; cobalamin; ascorbate; other vitamins; protein; minerals.	Administration of deficient nutrient.
Hemolytic	Chronic hemolysis Genetic disorders (Mediterranean; sickle cell anemias). Acquired disorders (paroxysmal nocturnal hemoglobinuria).	Various

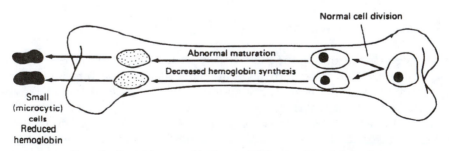

Anemias due to iron, pyridoxine, and other nutrient deficiencies

anemia, aplastic. *Anemia* caused by aplasia, a retardation or incomplete development of bone marrow or its destruction by chemical agents such as benzene, arsenic, or nitrogen mustard, or by physical factors such as x-rays and other sources of ionizing radiation. In this type of anemia, not only are red blood cells reduced in numbers, so too are the white cells. Resistance to infection is reduced, blood platelet count drops as well, and there may be bleeding.

anemia, folacin. *Folacin* is a vitamin necessary for normal red blood cell production. It is active as several derivatives called folates. The folate stores in the body are much smaller than those of *cobalamin* (vitamin B_{12}), so it is much more common to see dietary folate deficiency. This condition occurs in individuals who rarely eat uncooked vegetables or fruits, and in pregnant women or alcoholics. Folic acid requirements are increased in chronic hemolytic anemias and in pregnancy, so individuals with these conditions may develop the characteristic megaloblastic anemia while ingesting an adequate diet. The anemia symptoms of folic acid and cobalamin deficiencies are similar. See *anemias, megaloblastic*.

anemia, hemolytic. If the red blood cells are broken down (hemolyzed) at a faster rate than normal, and before they can be replaced, hemolytic anemia results. Sometimes this is due to a hereditary condition called spherocytosis, in which the red blood cells are small and round (spherocytic), but it may also be caused by antibodies in the blood which attack the red cells, or by various drugs, or by a variety of inherited disorders such as sickle cell anemia and thalassemia. Hemolytic anemia has the same symptoms as other anemias and may also produce jaundice. The breakdown of the red blood cells releases hemoglobin which is converted into the pigment bilirubin, which turns the tissues of the skin and whites of the eyes yellow, a condition known as *jaundice*. The spleen, where most red blood cells are normally destroyed, may become enlarged from an overaccumulation of dead cells, and can be detected on physical examination of the upper-left part of the abdomen. Signs of heart failure and an enlarged liver may indicate that the anemia is severe.

anemia, pernicious. An anemia caused by the deficiency or failure to absorb *cobalamin* (vitamin B_{12}). The gastric mucosa (stomach lining) fails to excrete *mucoproteins*, called *intrinsic factor*, required for absorption. Pernicious anemia is characterized by giant red cells (*macrocytes*), and each red cell appears to be overloaded with hemoglobin (hyperchromic) while the total number of red blood cells is decreased (anemia). Numbness in the fingers and toes is common. The disease occurs generally in males between the ages of 40 and 65 years. Treatment and maintenance usually involves intramuscular injection of a vitamin B_{12} derivative, and the prognosis is excellent. The administration of microgram quantities of cobalamin daily by mouth is sufficient to overcome vitamin B_{12} deficiencies when there is normal production of intrinsic factor. Vitamin B_{12} is required to remove methyl groups ($-CH3$) from folic acid (folacin). Unmethylated folacin is required for the production of red blood cells. See *folic acid deficiency* and *folacin*.

anemias, iron deficiency. A group consisting of a number of chronic *anemias* which are characterized by small pale *erythrocytes*. The basic cause is depletion of iron stores due to a discrepancy between iron intake and iron requirements. In adults, chronic blood loss is the most common cause of iron deficiency anemia. It may be physiologic, as in excessive or prolonged menstruation, or pathologic, as in occult intestinal blood loss due to ulcerations, parasites, or malignancy. Disorders of the gastrointestinal tract such as *achlorhydria* or chronic diarrhea may also lead to iron deficiency anemia because of impaired iron absorption. The symptoms of iron deficiency are similar to those of other types of anemia and include easy fatigability, pallor, dyspnea on exertion, and a constant feeling of tiredness. The skin, mucous membranes, and nails are pale in proportion to the reduction in the circulating hemoglobin. Nails may be brittle; individual blood cells are pale (hypochromic) and smaller than normal (microcytic). See *anemias*.

anemias, megaloblastic. The anemias caused by deficiencies of the *vitamins B₁₂* and *folic acid* show identical bone marrow and peripheral blood changes. This is because both vitamins are essential for normal deoxyribonucleic acid (DNA) synthesis. In each case, the marrow is *hyperplastic* and the precursor erythroid and myeloid cells are large and bizzare; some are multinucleated. But many of these cells die within the marrow, so that the mature cells which leave the marrow are decreased in number. Thus, a pancytopenia (a reduction in all cellular elements of the blood) develops. After the body stores of vitamin B₁₂ or *folate* are used up, signs of anemia begin to appear. The hematologic effects of deficiency are accompanied by effects on other organ systems, particularly the gastrointestinal tract when folate is deficient, and the nervous system when B₁₂ is deficient.

anemias, nutritional. The *anemias* that result from a deficiency of *iron*, proteins, certain vitamins, digestion of *cobalamin* (vitamin B₁₂), *folacin*, *ascorbic acid* (vitamin C), or *copper* are frequently termed nutritional anemias. A deficiency may be caused by defective absorption or imperfect utilization. The vast majority of cases of nutritional anemia seen in the United States are related to iron deficiency. For many years, diet has been recognized as a remedial agent in overcoming nutritional anemia.

angina. A spasmodic choking or suffocating pain. It is also the name of the condition that causes the pain.

angina pectoris. Similar to *myocardial infarction* in that it results from an inadequate oxygen supply to the myocardium. The difference is that myocardial infarction is a result of a rather sudden blockage of a coronary artery, whereas angina pectoris is a more gradual process in which the coronary vessels cannot bring sufficient blood supply (or oxygen) to the myocardium because they are occluded by atherosclerotic plaques and their walls have lost their elasticity. See *atherosclerosis*.

angiocardiogram. A special type of x-ray examination using radiopaque dye to aid in visualizing the heart and large blood vessels leading to and from the heart. The dye is injected through a catheter into an artery. Immediately after the dye is injected, x-rays are taken in rapid sequence. The dye is radiopaque, that is, it does not allow x-rays to pass through, and its passage through the heart can be visualized. This type of examination is done for detection of congenital heart diseases or other structural defects of the heart, its valves, or the large blood vessels.

angiography. Roentgenography (x-ray) of a blood vessel taken in rapid sequence following the injection of a radiopaque substance.

angioneurotic edema. A condition characterized by development of *edema* in areas of the skin, mucous membranes, or viscera. It's benign and thought to be a reaction to a food *allergen*.

angiotensin (vasopressin). A polypeptide hormone that acts as a pressor substance (elevates the blood pressure). Angiotensin is produced in the body by interaction of the enzyme *renin*, produced in the kidneys by the renal cortex, and a serum globulin fraction, angiotensinogen, produced by the liver. Angiotensin also has an effect on water balance since it stimulates the secretion of *antidiuretic hormone* (ADH) by the *adrenal glands*.

angitis. Inflammation of a vessel such as a blood vessel, Iymph vessel, or bile duct.

Angstrom (Å). A linear unit of measure equivalent to 1/100,000,000 of a centimeter. The measure is named after a Swedish physicist.

anion. A chemical group or ion carrying a negative charge. Anions migrate to the anode or positive electrode. The anions include all nonmetals, acid radicals, and the *hydroxyl* ion (OH^-). The *cation* is positive, the opposite of the anion.

anise (*Pimpinella anisum*). A culinary herb belonging to the parsley family, growing to a height of 2 feet, with feathery leaves and tiny grayish brown fruits which are dried for use. The plants and fruits have a distinctive licorice flavor. The dried fruits are called aniseed.

annatto. A yellowish red vegetable dye made from the pulp around the seeds of a small tropical tree, *Bixa orellana*. The tree is a native of the Caribbean. Annatto is widely used in coloring cheese, especially cheddar, and to a lesser extent, butter.

anodyne. A medicine that eases pain.

anomeric carbon. The aldehyde or ketone carbon of a sugar molecule that forms an acetal or ketal by interaction with one of the alcohol groups of the molecule and becomes a chiral or asymmetric carbon capable of rotating polarized light. See *glucose*.

anorexia. Lack or loss of appetite for food. Seen in depression, malaise, commencement of fever and illnesses, also in disorders of the alimentary tract, especially of the stomach.

anorexigenic. Producing anorexia or diminishing the appetite.

anosmia. Lack or loss of sense of smell.

antacid. A substance that counteracts or neutralizes acidity. Aluminum hydroxide and magnesium trisilicate tablets act on the gastrointestinal system, relieving excess acidity in the stomach and the consequent pain of gastritis and peptic ulcer. The tablets should be chewed and swallowed with a small amount of water; unless some fluid is taken, the drug preparation may only coat the esophagus and not reach the stomach. Aluminum hydroxide is often the preferred antacid because it is not adsorbed by the body. Calcium carbonate is also used as an antacid. However, calcium carbonate stimulates acid (HCl) secretion and stimulates *gastrin* secretions. *Magnesium* salts are often added to antacid preparations to prevent constipation.

antagonist. A substance that counteracts the action of another substance. The antagonist often prevents the normal action because its molecular structure is so like that of the first substance that it almost fits into the first substance's position in a metabolic process and prevents the reaction from taking place.

anterior. Situated toward the front.

antibiotics. Substances that are "against life." They are chemical substances produced by certain living cells, such as bacteria, yeasts, and molds that are antagonistic or damaging to other living cells, such as disease-producing bacteria. Antibiotics may kill living cells or prevent them from growing and multiplying. *Penicillin* is an example of an antibiotic that damages certain bacteria that cause disease in humans.

antibodies. Specific serum proteins or *immunoglobulins* formed in more complex organisms, including humans, in response to the intrusion of antigens, substances alien to the body. Each antibody binds itself specifically to an appropriate site (antigenic determinant) on the *antigen*. Antibodies are involved principally in resisting infection.

anticaking agent. A substance that keeps salts and powders free-flowing; used in such products as table salts, garlic and onion salts and powders, powdered sugar, and malted-milk powders. Examples of anticaking agents are calcium silicate, tricalcium phosphate, and magnesium carbonate.

anticoagulant. An agent that prevents coagulation. In blood chemistry, anticoagulants prevent the clotting of blood. Examples of anticoagulants are *dicumarol* and *heparin*. The mechanisms of anticoagulants vary, since different anticoagulants interfere with the blood-clotting mechanism at different stages of the process.

antidiuretic hormone (ADH, vasopressin). A polypeptide hormone secreted by the pituitary gland, which acts upon the distal renal tubule, causing the reabsorption of water. The result is diminished urinary output, hence the term "antidiuretic hormone." The posterior *pituitary gland* secretes ADH in response to body stress. The ADH mechanism is the body's primary water-conserving mechanism and is therefore essential to life. Serum osmolarity is regulated by the effects of ADH. Changes in osmolarity are sensed by receptors located in the *hypothalamus*. When osmolarity is increased, ADH is released and acts on the distal tubules and collecting ducts of the kidneys, so that they become more permeable to water. Thus, more electrolyte-free water is reabsorbed and urine is excreted in a concentrated form. The sensation of thirst is stimulated in a similar fashion, resulting in increased water intake. As a consequence of both processes, osmolarity returns to normal. ADH is also released when the circulating blood volume is severely decreased. This effect is a late attempt to maintain enough blood volume to perfuse tissues. When the serum osmolarity decreases, the secretion of ADH is reduced. The permeability of the distal tubules and collecting ducts of the kidney is decreased so that the excess water can be excreted as urine. See *osmotic pressure*.

antigens. Substances foreign to the body that lead to the formation of specific *antibodies* are called antigens. Most antigens contain several antigenic determinants. Chemically, antigens may belong to the proteins, the polysaccharides, or to other classes of substances.

antihemorrhagic. Preventing *hemorrhage* (bleeding).

antihistamine. A drug that counteracts the effects of *histamine*. It is of value in the treatment of certain allergic conditions such as hay fever, nettle rash, and certain forms of eczema.

antimetabolite. A chemical compound that resembles a substance occurring naturally and prevents its metabolism. Generally, the antimetabolite replaces metabolites in enzyme reactions. Certain antimetabolites are used for medicinal purposes, for example *dicumarol* in the treatment of blood clots. Dicumarol is an antimetabolite of *vitamin K* and is also an antivitamin.

antimicrobial. Destructive to or preventing the development of microorganisms.

antimicrobial preservatives. *Food spoilage* has two effects. One is to become a hazard to health and the other is for a food to lose its attractiveness. In the former, molds, bacteria, fungi, and yeasts growing in foods can cause food poisoning either by producing infections or by producing deadly toxins. Preservatives known as antimicrobial agents protect foods from these microbes. Sodium and *calcium propionate* are used to prevent growth of certain bacteria or molds in bread. The calcium salts also provide a significant source of calcium in the diet. Propionic acid or propionate is probably one of the most innocuous food additives. It is found naturally in some rye breads and Swiss cheese. *Sodium benzoate* is effective under acidic conditions. It is added to foods such as fruit juices, pickles, salad dressing, and preserves, and occurs naturally in many fruits and vegetables. *Sodium nitrite* is added as a curing agent to meat and fish products to enhance color and improve flavor. As a preservative, it prevents the growth of *Clostridium botulinum*, which produces a powerful neurotoxin causing *botulism*. Nitrites are capable of reacting with secondary amines or urea, forming *nitrosamines* that can be carcinogenic. *Antioxidants* are preservatives that are added to foods to prevent oxygen from reacting with components of food. They prevent polyunsaturated oils from oxidizing and also may protect the fat-soluble vitamins. The most common antioxidants are *butylated hydroxyanisole* (BHA), *butylated hydroxytoluene* (BHT), and *propyl gallate*. *Ascorbic acid* is used in foods as both an antioxidant and oxidant. As an antioxidant, it reacts with oxygen, thereby losing its nutritive value, but it maintains the quality of the food. It is often used in combination with BHA, BHT, or propylgallate because it regenerates these primary antioxidants. Ascorbic acid is also added in the baking industry as an oxidant to improve the property of the *gluten* in bread dough.

antimyotic agents. Preservatives used to prevent or control the *food spoilage* organisms such as mold, bacteria, and yeast. Otherwise, foods such as bread become moldy quickly, especially in warm weather. One mold that sometimes appears in bread lacking antimyotics is called "rope," making the bread inedible. Rope is caused by certain bacteria not destroyed during baking. Other antimyotics are used in cheese, including *ascorbic acid*, and sodium and potassium sorbates (*sorbic acid*).

antineuritic. Preventing or relieving inflammation of a nerve. Counteracting neuritis. Often referred to as a characteristic of *thiamine* because it counteracts the neuritis resulting from *B-complex* deficiency (*avitaminosis*).

antioxidant. A substance that prevents or delays *oxidation*. A substance capable of chemically protecting other substances against oxidation. Antioxidants are one of the most common groups of food additives used to prevent change in color or flavor caused by oxygen in the air. For example, some fruits and vegetables containing certain enzymes (such as apples, apricots, bananas, cherries, peaches, pears, and potatoes) darken when exposed to air after being cut, bruised, or allowed to overmature. Antioxidants also are used to prevent rancid taste and odor from developing in fats and oils during storage, and in commercial cake mixes. The vitamins *ascorbic acid* (vitamin C) and the *tocopherols* (vitamin E) act in the body as water-soluble and fat-soluble antioxidants, respectively. The synthetic antioxidants *butylated hydroxy-anisole (BHA)* and *butylated hydroxytoluene (BTH)* are frequently used in foods because they are highly lipophilic, are active at low concentrations, and are not toxic.

antipyresis. The application of remedies against fever. See antipyretic.

antipyretic. Reducing temperature in fever but not affecting normal body temperature.

antirachitic. Preventing, curative, or corrective of *rickets*. *Vitamin D* has antirachitic activity.

antiscorbutic. Preventive or curative of scurvy. *Ascorbic acid* (vitamin C) has antiscorbutic activity.

antivitamin. An *antimetabolite* against a vitamin which it replaces or competes with metabolically. For example, deoxypyridoxine is an antimetabolite to *pyridoxine* (vitamin B_6); oxythiamine and pyrithiamine are antivitamins to *thiamine* (vitamin B_1). The following table shows some of the more common antivitamins.

Antvitamins

VITAMIN	ANTIVITAMIN
Biotin	*avidin* (raw egg white protein)
Folacin	methotrexate and aminopterin (used in cancer chemotherapy)
Niacin	pyridine-3-sulfonic acid; 3-acetylpyridine
Pantothenate	ω-methylpantothenate
Pyridoxine	dioxypyridoxine (Isoniazid) and *INH*: used in the treatment of tuberculosis
Riboflavin	galactoflavin; isoriboflavin
Vitamin K	*Dicumarol* (an anticoagulant)

anus. Opening at the posterior end of the *digestive tract*, through which indigestible solid wastes are expelled.

anxiety. Apprehension, tension, or uneasiness that stems from the anticipation of danger, the source of which is largely unknown or unrecognized. It is primarily of intrapsychic origin, in distinction to fear, which is the emotional response to a consciously recognized and usually external threat or danger.

aortosclerosis. Hardening of the walls of the *aorta*. See *arteriosclerosis*.

A.P. See *As Purchased*.

aphasia. The absence or impairment of the ability to communicate through speech, writing, or signs due to dysfunction of brain centers.

aphrodisiac. Something which excites sexual activity, usually a drug.

apoenzyme. The protein portion of an enzyme to which the *prosthetic group* or *coenzyme* is attached.

apoferritin. The protein base in intestinal mucosa cells that will bind with iron (from food) to form ferritin, the storage form of iron. Apoferritin is the iron-free protein.

appendicitis. The vermiform appendix is a narrow, shallow, blind tube, about 3 inches long, that looks much like an earthworm. It is located at the juncture of the large and small intestines. It serves no known purpose. Appendicitis is an inflammation of the appendix. Appendicitis cannot be caused by swallowing seeds.

appetite. Similar to *hunger* but a less physiologically related activity. The desire for a specific food is related to appetite, whereas when one is hungry, any one of a variety of foods may satisfy. Food intake is regulated by the *hypothalamus*, and many other centers in the brain stem and spinal cord are involved in the actual process of eating. Salivation, chewing, and swallowing are examples. Appetite is very complex and not well understood.

apple (*Malus*). Apples come in many varieties, with an estimated 6500 or more horticultural forms, and in many shapes. They can be round like the McIntosh or egg-shaped like the Delicious. In size, they can vary from a 2-inch crab apple to a 6-inch Rome Beauty. The flesh may be white as a Cortland, yellow as a Golden Delicious. The tastes may be crisp as a Northern Spy, mellow as a Baldwin, sweet as a Grimes, or tart as a young Winesap. The skin is thin and glossy and ranges in color from bright or russet red, to yellow, to green. Fresh apples are a good supplement to the diet, since they contain *carbohydrates* and *carotene* (vitamin A activity) and *ascorbic acid* (vitamin C). Apples contain *cellulose* to maintain body regularity and, when eaten raw, help clean the teeth. See this item in the table under *fruits*.

apple juice. See this item in the table under *fruits*.

apricot (*Prunus arnenuaca*). An oval stone fruit of a golden yellow color that grows on a small tree belonging to the peach family. Excellent source of *vitamin A* and high in natural sugars. See this item in the table under *fruits*.

arachidonic acid. Mol. Wt. 304. Arachidonic acid has four double bonds and 20 carbon atoms. It is an important *unsaturated fatty acid*. It was at one time included as an *essential fatty acid*. It is not actually essential in the diet. It is found in nature only in animal foods but can be readily made in the body from the essential fatty acid *linoleic acid*. Arachidonic acid is a precursor to the *prostaglandins*. See *lipids, classification*.

$$CH_3-(CH_2)_4-(CH=CH-CH_2)_4-(CH_2)_2-COOH$$

Arachidonic acid

areolar tissue. A fibrous connective tissue which forms the subcutaneous layer of tissue. It fills many of the small spaces in the body and helps hold organs in place.

arginine (Arg, R). Mol. Wt. 174. One of the *nonessential amino acids* found in proteins. It is the member of the *urea cycle* from which urea is formed by action of the enzyme arginase. See *amino acids*.

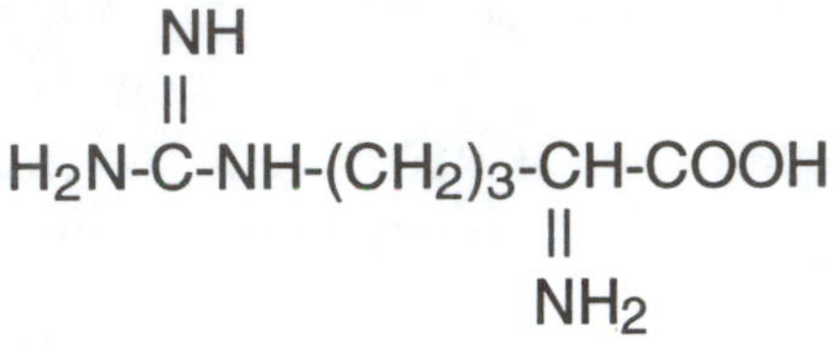

$$NH$$
$$\|$$
$$H_2N\text{-}C\text{-}NH\text{-}(CH_2)_3\text{-}CH\text{-}COOH$$
$$\|$$
$$NH_2$$

Arginine (Arg, R)

ariboflavinosis. A disease resulting from the deficiency of *riboflavin*. It is characterized by lesions of the tongue and at angles of the mouth, dermatitis, and ocular changes. See *vitamin deficiency*.

aroma. The aromas of substances come from highly diversified classes of volatile compounds, usually present in foods in very low concentrations. The term "aroma of substances" is used loosely. The compound responsible for the typical aroma or *taste* of a given food might also be responsible for the *off-flavor* or off-taste in another food. Many of the aromas and tastes of foods are augmented by the direct addition of isolated or synthesized compounds to food. Most aromas and tastes of foods are due to a complex of many compounds that contribute to the sensations of smell or taste. In meat, for example, about 250 volatile compounds have been identified, and there are an equal number that have not been identified. Coffee has about twice the number of volatile compounds in the known and unknown categories. See *tongue* and *flavor*.

aromatic compounds. Chemical compounds containing characteristic ring structures of atoms related to benzene. They are known for their stability and characteristic behavior. Some are known or believed to be carcinogenic.

arrowroot. The starch obtained from the tubers of several kinds of tropical plants. The roots are peeled, washed, and pulped to produce a white fluid. This is made into a powder which is then milled. Arrowroot is an excellent thickening agent and can be used in lieu of flour or cornstarch. It is neutral in flavor and produces soups, sauces, pie fillings, and puddings that are clear and sparkling. Arrowroot is easily digested.

arteriogram. An x-ray test after injecting a radiopaque "dye"; for the diagnosis of brain tumors. See *angiogram*.

arteriosclerosis. One of the most common changes within the brain tissue itself is that known as arteriosclerosis, or "hardening of the arteries." There is primarily a loss of elasticity in the arteries feeding the brain tissue, producing profound physical changes. Almost everyone who reaches old age suffers to some extent from arteriosclerotic involvement. The anatomic changes in the arteries supplying blood to the brain result in major pathologic changes within the brain itself. These are primarily the result of: the decreased amount of oxygen available to the brain cells; waste products of the brain cells not being as readily removed and tending to accumulate; a decreased amount of sugar being furnished to the brain as fuel; and hemorrhages, either minor or major, resulting with the attendant destruction of the brain tissue involved and the possible loss of function.

artery. A blood vessel that carries blood away from the heart.

arthritis. The term is used to cover all inflammatory diseases of the joints. Research has shown there are approximately 100 different types of arthritis, but all are capable of producing disability. The exact cause of arthritis is not well understood, but there are some definitely established predisposing factors. Infection is one, the most common organisms being streptococcus, staphylococcus, and pneumococcus. Also, trauma; overweight and/or poor posture; prolonged physical stress and strain; emotional disturbances; metabolic disorders, such as *gout*; and heredity are among the other contributing factors.

artichoke (*Cynara scolymus*). Globe or common artichokes are the leafy buds from a plant resembling the thistle. The artichokes cultivated in the United States are grown mainly in the midcoastal regions of California. Artichokes may be eaten in many ways. One way is to eat them with the fingers, pulling off the leaves one at a time and dipping them into a sauce. Eventually a core of thin, light-colored leaves is reached; this covers the choke and the heart. Artichokes contain small amounts of vitamins and minerals.

articular cartilage. The covering of the joint surfaces at the ends of a long bone. The cartilage provides a smooth contact surface in joint formation and gives some resilience for shock absorption.

ascariasis (roundworm infection). Usually contracted from eggs reaching the mouth by way of fingers that have been in contact with contaminated soil. The worm inhabits the small bowel. Mild roundworm infection may not bother most people who have it. If the worm migrates to various parts of the body, it may cause serious effects. Ordinarily, symptoms of infection with these worms are nondescript abdominal complaints and *anemias*.

ascites. The accumulation of serous fluid (liquids of the body, similar to blood serum, which are in part secreted serous membranes) in the peritoneal cavity, which contains all the abdominal organs exclusive of the kidneys. It may be caused by interference in venous return as occurs in cardiac disease; obstruction of flow in the vena cava or portal vein; obstruction in lymphatic drainage; disturbance in electrolyte balance as occurs in sodium retention; or the depletion of plasma proteins.

ascorbic acid (vitamin C). Mol. Wt. 176. The reduced form of ascorbic acid and the oxidized form (dehydroascorbic acid) have equal vitamin activity. This level of oxidation should not be confused with oxidations (catalyzed by heavy metals and heat) that inactivate vitamin C by changing the structure irreversibly. Ascorbic acid is related chemically to the sugars. One of its functions in the body is to maintain the connective tissues. Without ascorbic acid, the structure of the connective tissue becomes weakened. The linings of blood vessels, as well as the sheath of connective tissue about them, become weakened so that bleeding occurs. Ascorbic acid serves in several metabolic systems. It is involved in the hydroxylation of *proline* to *hydroxyproline*, an important step in the synthesis of *collagen*, a component of connective tissue; the hydroxylation of tryptophan to 5-hydroxytryptophan, a precursor in the biosynthesis of serotonin; the conversion of 3,4-dihydroxyphenylethylamine to *norepinephrine*; and hydroxylation of p-hydroxyphenylpyruvate to homogentisic acid in the catabolic pathway of *tyrosine*. It has been shown that ascorbic acid lowers the blood *cholesterol* of people with *atherosclerosis*. It also influences the formation of hemoglobin, the absorption of iron from the intestine, and the deposition of iron in liver tissue. Ascorbic acid is found in many parts of the body. Since ascorbic acid is water soluble, it is readily absorbed from the *gastrointestinal tract* into the bloodstream within a few hours after it is ingested and taken up by the tissues. Studies using radioactive ascorbic acid show that it is rapidly taken from the serum and transported to the *adrenal glands*, kidneys, and liver. Tissues that have higher metabolic activity contain the highest concentrations of ascorbic acid.

Ascorbic acid

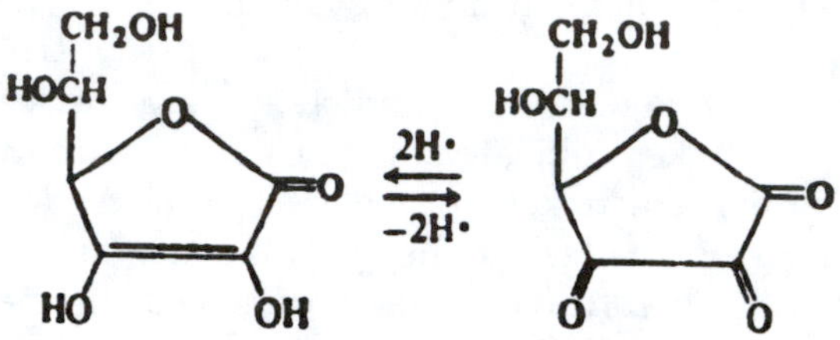

Dehydroascorbic acid

The Food and Nutrition Board of the United States recommends a daily allowance of 60 mg per day for adult males and 55 mg for females. Practically all vitamin C comes from fruits and vegetables. Foods rich in vitamin C are citrus fruits, liver, tomatoes, and most vegetables. Fruits, except citrus fruits, generally have a lower vitamin C content than vegetables. Vitamin C is not destroyed by heat but by the oxidation that heat accelerates. The cooking of vegetables (whether by steaming, boiling, or pressure cooking) looses about half of the ascorbic acid. Freezing, canning, and dehydration also cause some degree of destruction. Citrus fruits and juices, and tomato juice perhaps are the most convenient sources of ascorbic acid. The following table gives the ascorbic acid content of some foods:

Ascorbic acid (ascorbate, vitamin C) in mg/100 g of foods

Banana	10-30	Eggs	Trace	Potato	5-15
Currants	90-300	Meat	Trace	Potato chips	10-30
Broccoli		Vegetables leafy	50-200	Rose hips	70-460
Brussel sprout	70-100	Guava	200	Rose hips syrup	150-200
Cabbage		Mango	10-50	Berries various	25-60
Lettuce	10-60	Melon	1-45	Stone fruits e.g., plums	5-10
Canned fruit various	1-25	Papaya	30-120	Sweet potato	20-30
Citrus fruit fresh, juice	25-60	Pineapple	25		

ascorbyl palmitate. Formed by combining *ascorbic acid* (vitamin C) with *palmitic acid* (a *saturated fatty acid*). This additive functions as an antioxidant in shortening in the same fashion as ascorbic acid. It readily reacts with oxygen, preventing the latter from reacting with unsaturated fats and causing rancidity. It is also used as a source of vitamin C in vitamin pills and fortified foods.

ash. The mineral matter that remains after completely burning the combustible portion of food or any material (the noncombustible residue).

asparagine (Asx, Asn, B, N) Mol. Wt. 132. One of the amino acids found in proteins. Formed from aspartic acid by the addition of ammonia to the free carboxylic acid group to form an amide group. See *aspartic acid*.

$$H_2N-\overset{\overset{\textstyle O}{\|}}{C}-CH_2-\overset{\overset{\textstyle NH_2}{|}}{CH}-COOH$$

Asparagine (Asn, Asx, B, N)

asparagus (*Asparagus officinalis*). A member of the lily-of-the-valley family. The name comes from a Greek word meaning "stalk" or "shoot." Especially prized is the variety of asparagus that yields very thick, white, fleshy stalks that are very tender. These asparagus are grown in little individual mounds and cut when only the green tip shows, so that the stalks are still white. A good source of *carotene* (vitamin A activity), fair for *vitamin B*, and *ascorbic acid* (vitamin C) and *iron*. See table under *vegetables*.

Aspartame®. Aspartame is an artificial sweetener. It was discovered accidentally in 1965 during research for ulcer drugs. G. D. Searle & Co. first sought approval of Aspartame in dry foods and as a tabletop sweetener in 1973, with Food and Drug Administration (FDA) approval in 1974, but challenges over the substance's safety and validity of the company's data kept Aspartame from being marketed. The board of inquiry held its hearings in early 1980. In a report to FDA the following October, the board concluded that the evidence did not support charges that Aspartame consumption posed an increased risk of brain damage that could result in mental retardation or endocrine dysfunction. The FDA board, however, recommended that Aspartame's approval be withheld until more long-term animal tests were conducted on the possibility that Aspartame might cause brain tumors. On July 24, 1981, the FDA approved the use of Aspartame in dry foods. Approval of Aspartame for use in carbonated beverages followed in July 1983. The following December it was also proposed as an "inactive ingredient" in human drug products. Food and beverages containing Aspartame are required by the FDA to include a warning to individuals suffering from a rare genetic disease called *phenylketonuria* (PKU). The warning notes that *phenylalanine*, an amino acid whose intake must be restricted by PKU victims, is present in the product. Aspartame is made by combining a methyl ester of phenylalanine and the amino acid aspartic acid. Aspartame provides 4 calories per g but is approximately 200 times sweeter than sucrose. While it is stable in dry form and would be suitable as a sugar substitute in dry products, it is not suitable for sweetening alkaline or neutral products requiring high-temperature cooking because it is unstable under these conditions. Aspartame loses its sweetness as it undergoes decomposition with heat. Storage for long periods in nonacid products would also cause major losses of its sweetening properties; even in a neutral solution at room temperature, half of the sweetness is lost in a matter of hours. See *cyclamates* and *saccharine*.

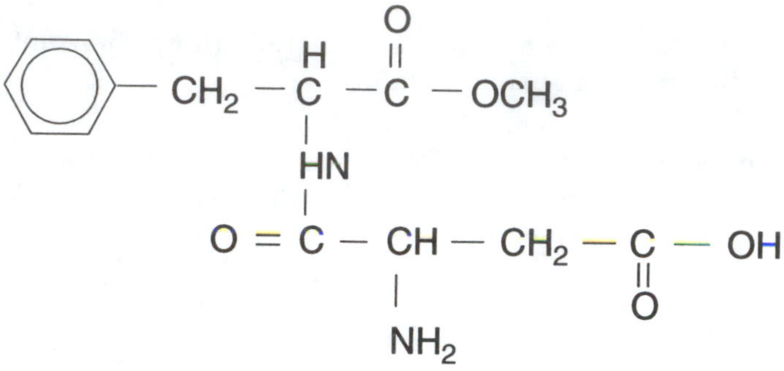

$$\text{C}_6\text{H}_5-\text{CH}_2-\underset{\underset{\text{HN}}{|}}{\overset{\text{H}}{\text{C}}}-\overset{\overset{\text{O}}{||}}{\text{C}}-\text{OCH}_3$$

$$\text{O}=\text{C}-\underset{\underset{\text{NH}_2}{|}}{\text{CH}}-\text{CH}_2-\overset{\overset{\text{O}}{||}}{\text{C}}-\text{OH}$$

Aspartame®
(aspartyl-L-phenylalanine methyl ester)

aspartic acid (Asp, B). Mol. Wt. 133. One of the nonessential amino acids found in proteins. Aspartic acid contains two carboxylic acid groups and is classified as an acidic amino acid. It can be synthesized in the body from *oxaloacetic acid*. See *amino acids*.

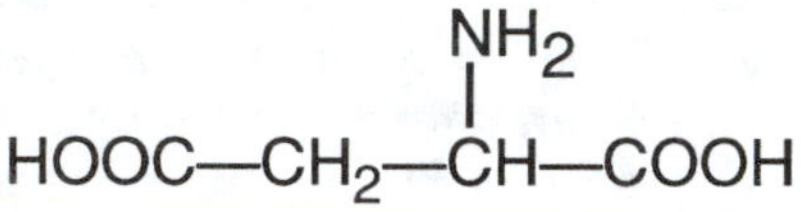

$$\underset{\underset{\text{HOOC—CH}_2\text{—CH—COOH}}{}}{\overset{\text{NH}_2}{|}}$$

Aspartic acid (Asp, B)

Aspergillus flavus. A mold found on corn, peanuts, and certain grains when improperly dried and stored. It is a natural source of *aflatoxin*, a powerful carcinogenic toxin.

aspirin (acetylsalicylic acid). Mol. Wt. 180. A white crystalline solid formed by the action of acetic anhydride on salicylic acid. Aspirin is one of the three most widely used medications for treating mild pain—*acetaminophen* and *ibuprofen* are the others. Evidence from animal studies has shown that these analgesic effects of aspirin and acetaminophen on pain are principally by peripheral blockade of pain. Their primary clinical effects are related to inhibition of *prostaglandin* synthesis. The responses to the prostaglandins have been reported to include hyperalgesia (pain), fever, edema, and *erythema*. In general, nonopiate analgesics alleviate the pain of headache and other pain arising from integumental strictures. Mild to moderate postoperative and postpartum pain, pain from *neoplasms*, and other types of visceral pain may also respond to these drugs. They are generally not useful in severe pain. Aspirin normally is used in 0.324 g tablets, often being combined with other drugs such as phenacetin. Many patients suffer reactions to aspirin that mimic allergic responses, but involve no truly immunologic mechanism. Some people with chronic hives, for example, see their condition worsen after taking aspirin, and a small percentage of asthmatics will suffer acute broncho-spasm. Recently, the mechanism of the multiple effects of aspirin has become better under-stood. Aspirin inhibits the enzyme cyclooxygenase, which is required for the synthesis of prostaglandins and *thromboxanes*, hormone-like substances which are derived from the essen-tial fatty acids (*eicosanoid hormones*), as shown. These hormonelike substances affect blood pressure (vasodilation and vasoconstriction), swelling, and blood clotting. The effect of aspirin on blood clotting is to reduce it by inhibiting the formation of thromboxane A2, a hormonelike substance that promotes the aggregation of platelets. It is the inhibition of platelet aggregation by the action of aspirin that has led to its promotion for the prevention of heart attacks. Aspirin can cause gastric bleeding and anemia. It interferes with the cellular uptake of *niacin* and the utilization of *pyridoxine* and *folacin*. Fever in adults can be controlled by either aspirin or acetaminophen. Aspirin given to children with influenza has shown an increased risk of *Reye's syndrome*, which causes deterioration of the brain and liver. Before giving aspirin to children, a physician should be consulted.

Aspirin

As Purchased (A.P.). Refers to food as offered for sale on the retail market. In tables that give nutritive value for food "as purchased," the nutrient content is stated in terms of the weight of the food before inedible portions, usually discarded, are removed.

asthenia. Without strength. Weakness.

asthma. A respiratory problem whose chief feature is labored or difficult breathing. Often accompanied by a characteristic wheezing or whistling sound. The whistling or wheezing sounds of asthma are loudest when breathing air out. The symptoms of asthma are caused by changes in the respiratory system, the system of passageways that carries air from the mouth into the lungs. In asthma, the small air passageways are the ones chiefly affected. The muscles in these passages go into spasms, narrowing the width of the tubes and thus making the passage of air in and out of the lungs more difficult. In addition to muscle spasm, there is an outpouring of mucus into the small air passages, further obstructing the flow of air. Finally, the mucosa become inflamed and swollen, thus narrowing the air passageways even further, much as an accumulation of rust on the inner surface of a pipe would partially obstruct the flow of water through the pipe. All these changes, the spasms, the swelling, and the outpouring of mucus, occur together, affecting to a greater or lesser degree almost all of the air passages. The resistance to the flow of air, particularly during expiration, or breathing out, is significantly increased, and the individual must work harder to move air in and out of the lungs, which results in a whistling sound. Asthma is considered to be the result of an *allergy*.

astigmatism. A defect in vision in which the lens of the eye is distorted and curved differently in one direction than in the other (like the sides of a football), so that it is impossible to see all of an object in focus at once.

atherosclerosis. The term derives from two Greek words—*athere*, meaning "porridge" or "mush," and *skleros* meaning "hard." A *chronic*, usually progressive, vascular disease characterized by thickening, toughening, stiffening/hardening, and loss of elasticity of arterial walls followed by secondary degenerative changes. The changes may be generalized or more prominent in certain organs or locations such as the heart, kidneys, lungs, brain, and extremities. When a child is born, the inner lining of the arteries is normally smooth, white, and glistening. However, beginning very early in childhood and continuing relentlessly throughout life, there is a gradual deterioration of the arteries' smooth lining of *endothelium* by deposits of fatty substances (mostly cholesterol oleate and *cholesterol*) just beneath the surface of the endothelial cells. Later a process analogous to scar formation causes a progressive thickening and toughening of the lining so that it protrudes into the channel, tending to reduce the flow of blood. Still later, the inner lining of the arteries deteriorates further with the development of ulcerations, calcium deposits in the muscular wall of the artery, and seepage of blood into the damaged area. The cause of the disease has been variously attributed to abnormal fat transport or metabolism (cholesterol especially), dietary habits, disorders of blood flow and blood clotting, hormonal disturbances, and mechanical factors. Heredity also appears to be a factor in individual susceptibility. Long-standing hypertension and diabetes are predisposing factors. Atherosclerosis is often confused with *arteriosclerosis*, a more specific disease of the arteries.

atonic. Descriptive of an organ or part lacking normal tone or vigor.

ATP. See *adenosine triphosphate*.

atrophy. A wasting away or reduction in size of a cell, organ, or part of the body.

auditory nerve. The eighth cranial nerve. It consists of two branches; one concerned with hearing and the other distributed to the vestibule and semicircular canals of the internal ear and concerned with the sense of balance. Disturbance of the former causes deafness; the latter, giddiness.

Aureomycin®. Mol. Wt. 479. A proprietary brand of chlortetracycline, an antibiotic. It generally is prepared as a hydrochloride.

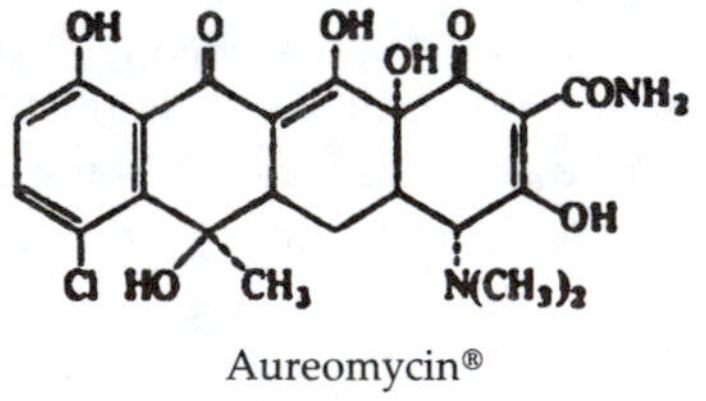

Aureomycin®

auscultation. The act of listening for sounds in the body in order to determine the condition of the organs and also for the detection of pregnancy.

autonomic nervous system. A system of motor nerves, intimately connected with the cerebrospinal nervous system, having centers in the medulla, midbrain, hypothalamus, and cerebral cortex, yet it is to some extent set apart both anatomically and functionally. The autonomic system acts upon the glands and smooth muscles of the viscera and blood vessels. The autonomic nervous system is divided into two subdivisions, the sympathetic and parasympathetic, which have somewhat antagonistic effects. The sympathetic system is mainly concerned with mobilizing the resources of the body for use in work or in emergencies. The parasympathetic division is mainly concerned with conserving and storing the bodily resources. Both divisions of the autonomic nervous system act with less precision and more diffuseness than the cerebrospinal system, sometimes referred to as the voluntary nervous system. The diagram is a schematic representation of the autonomic nervous system. The light lines represent nerve pathways for the sympathetic impulses. The heavy lines are nerve pathways for parasympathetic impulses. The circles are ganglia.

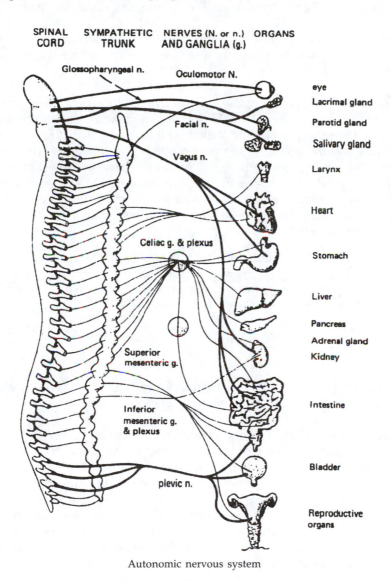

Autonomic nervous system

autosome. Any one of the *chromosomes* other than the sex (X and Y) chromosomes.

autotrophic. Bacteria capable of manufacturing organic nutrients from *carbon dioxide* (CO_2) and water are called autotrophs.

autoxidation. Autoxidation is a complex of interrelated reactions involving a large number of intermediates. Autoxidation of food is affected by the fatty acid composition, the degree of unsaturation, the presence or absense of *antioxidants*, storage and other conditions. There are so many variables associated with autoxidation that rates vary considerably. See *peroxidation*.

avidin. A protein isolated from egg white that can combine with *biotin*, a B vitamin, causing the vitamin to be unavailable to the body. Cooking renders avidin inactive.

avitaminosis. A condition or clinical symptom due to the lack or the deficiency of a vitamin in the diet, or to lack of absorption or utilization of it. The avitaminoses are given under each vitamin's listing. See *vitamin deficiency*.

avocado (*Persea Americana*). A fruit native to Central or South America, also called an alligator pear. In the United States, it grows along the southern sections of the country from California to Florida, especially in the Rio Grande Valley. The fruit may vary from the small, round, bell variety, which is shiny green, to the pear-shaped, slightly russet-coated fruit; the fruit may weigh from 5-6 ounces, to 2-3 pounds. Avocados have a coarse, shell-like skin or a smooth thin skin, depending upon the variety. The flesh is yellowish green and fairly firm, with a single large seed, round or conical. Avocados have fair amounts of *thiamine, riboflavin*, and *ascorbic acid* (vitamin C). Unlike most fruits, they have a high fat content which varies from less than 5% to more than 20%.

Nutrients in 100 g of edible avocado

CALORIES	PROTEIN G	FAT G	CARBOHYDRATE G	VITAMIN A IU	VITAMIN C MG
167	Trace	16.4	6.3	290	14

axon. A fiber of a nerve cell that conducts impulses away from the cell body and can release, but cannot itself be stimulated by, transmitter substances. See *neuron*.

azodicarbonamide. Mol. Wt. 66. A dough-conditioning agent employed by the baking industry. Dough conditioning replaces months of storage as the standard way of aging flour. Natural and chemical aging have identical chemical affects on flour; both produce more manageable dough and lighter, more voluminous loaves of bread. Azodicarbonamide does not bleach flour, so it must be used with a bleach such as benzoyl peroxide. When azodicarbonamide reacts with flour, the additive is rapidly and completely converted to a second compound. In the same chemical reaction the protein (*gluten*) of flour is oxidized, accounting for the changes in the dough's properties. The nutritive value of vitamins and amino acids in bread is not affected by azodicarbonamide.

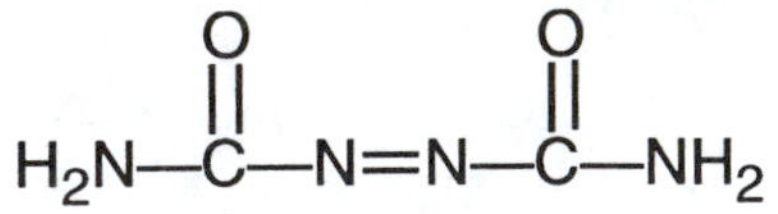

$$H_2N-\overset{\overset{\displaystyle O}{\|}}{C}-N{=}N-\overset{\overset{\displaystyle O}{\|}}{C}-NH_2$$

Azodicarbonamide

B

B. The alphabetic symbol for the amino acids *aspartic acid* and *asparagine* (Asp, Asx).

bacillary dysentery. A common form of dysentery caused by different strains of dysentery bacillus, resulting from poor sanitation. Attacks come on abruptly, with fever, nausea, vomiting, abdominal pain, and cramps and diarrhea. Blood and mucus are present in the watery stools in severe cases. Untreated, it is a self-limited disease, as a rule clearing up in a week or 10 days, but it may become chronic and debilitating and progress to a chronic colitis. Treatment aimed at maintaining salt and *water balance* is very important.

bacon. The cured and smoked fat and lean meat from the side of the pig, after the spareribs have been removed. Canadian-style bacon, which resembles ham rather than ordinary streaky bacon, is the eye muscle that runs along the pig's back. The word "bacon," originally French, meant pork and cured pork products.

Nutrients in 100 g of cooked bacon

TYPE	CALORIES KCAL	FAT G	CARBOHYDRATES G	PROTEIN G	THIAMINE MG	IRON MG
Strips	630	58	2	23	590	280
Canadian	312	30	10	30	860	280

bacteria. Very small one-celled microorganisms, the smallest living things with self-contained metabolic processes. There are many families and strains; some require oxygen in order to multiply and are called *aerobic* bacteria. The anaerobic ones will not grow if oxygen is present. Some strains are *hemolytic* (destructive to red blood cells). Bacteria have different shapes. The cocci are spherical; streptococci grow in chains and are known as "strep germs." There are rod-shaped bacilli, spiral corkscrew-shaped spirilla, and comma-shaped vibrios. Bacteria are widely distributed in the air, water, soil, and animal and plant tissues. Some bacteria have useful functions such as decay of dead matter and fermentation of fruit and vegetable juices; they can also produce disease or cause harmful *food spoilage*.

bacterial toxins. Food poisoning is caused by the ingestion of bacterial toxins that have been produced in food by the growth of specific kinds of bacteria. The powerful toxin is ingested directly, and symptoms of food poisoning therefore develop rapidly, usually within 1 to 6 hours after the food is eaten. See *food poisoning*.

bacteriophage. A *virus* that attacks bacteria.

Baker's yeast (*Saccharomyces cerevisiae*). A microorganism, one of the fungi. Baker's yeast has replaced brewer's yeast in baking. It is composed of strains specially selected for both their flavor and their ability to produce a great deal of *carbon dioxide* and little *alcohol*. See *yeast*.

baking powder. A leavening agent used in batters and doughs to make them rise and become light and porous during baking. In mixtures it produces carbon dioxide, one of the three leavening gases (the other two are air and water vapor or steam). Today, commercial baking powders contain at least three ingredients: (1) baking soda, also known as sodium bicarbonate or bicarbonate of soda, and in less-refined form, saleratus; (2) an acid salt that produces carbon dioxide, the leavening agent, and may be a tartrate compound, a phosphate compound, or sulfate and phosphate combinations; (3) starch, which is used as a stabilizer to keep the powder from caking and reacting in the can. There are three different kinds of baking powders, named according to the type of acid salt used in the formula. The common names sometimes found in recipes are: (1) tartrate, which contains cream of tartar and tartaric acid. This type releases most of its gas quickly in the batter or dough at room temperature; (2) phosphate, which contains calcium acid phosphate and may also be combined with sodium acid pyrophosphate (this type of powder releases two-thirds of its gas (CO_2) at room temperature and the remainder when heat is applied), and (3) double-acting or SAS phosphate in which the acids are sodium aluminum sulfate (SAS) and calcium acid phosphate. This type releases a small portion of gas when the ingredients are combined at room temperature, but the greater amount is released in the oven. Baking can be delayed a few minutes.

baking soda (bicarbonate of soda). Mol. Wt. 84. The chemical formula of this product is $NaHCO_3$. Its home use lies mostly in baking, where it is used to leaven cakes containing acid ingredients such as butter, milk, vinegar, molasses, and fruit juices. It is also used along with cream of tartar or *baking powder* when the amount of acid in the ingredients being combined varies a great deal, as it does when such things as chocolate, brown sugar, honey, sour cream, apples, etc., are used together. The acid in the ingredients combines with the baking soda to produce a gas, *carbon dioxide*, which leavens the dough.

balance. In nutrition, the term balance refers to the relationship between nutrients taken in and subsequently excreted by the body. When the intake and output are the same, the condition is described as balance, or equilibrium. When the intake exceeds the output, the balance is positive and retention of the nutrient has occurred. A negative balance describes the state in which the intake is less than the output and the body stores have been used. The balance study has been a useful tool for measuring protein and mineral metabolism, although the balance is greatly affected by other dietary components and by body stores. See *energy balance, nitrogen balance*, and *water balance*.

balm or lemon balm (*Melissa officinalis*). A hardy perennial reaching a height of 1.5–2 feet. It has broad, dark green leaves, with a faint lemon flavor, and flowers growing in pale yellow clusters. Leaves and tender sprigs lend a subtle flavor to lemonade, teas, meats, sauces, stuffings, soups, and salads. Industrially, balm is used in making perfume and liqueurs.

bamboo shoot (*Bambusa, Arundinaria, and Dendrocalamus*). The inner white part of the young shoot of the tropical bamboo plant. The shoot is prepared by stripping off the tight, tough, overlapping sheaths of the plant. The shoots are then cut into strips and are ready for cooking. Bamboo shoots are a basic ingredient in Chinese, Japanese, and other oriental cooking.

banana (*Musa paradisiaca*). Bananas are seedless fruit grown on a plant that resembles the palm, each plant bearing a single bunch of fruit. The plant is first cousin to the tough, fibrous Manila hemp plant. Bananas are harvested green, and their food value and flavor are the result of carefully controlled conditions and temperatures during ripening, when their starch is converted to sugar. The skin of the partly ripened fruit is usually yellow, but there are also red-skinned varieties. Bananas provide *ascorbic acid* (vitamin C) with good quantities of *carotene* (vitamin A activity) and some *thiamine*. They are low in protein and fat. See this item in the table under *fruits*.

barbital (5,5-diethylbarbituric acid). A crystalline powder and derivative of barbituric acid. It is used as a hypnotic and sedative and is habit-forming.

Barbital

barbiturates. Drugs derived from barbituric acid; one of the most extensive series of sedative, hypnotic, and anesthetic drugs presently in use. Among the better-known barbiturates are barbitone, hexobarbitone, and phenobarbitone. See *barbital*.

barley (*Hordeum*). A hardy cereal grass related to wheat, which it resembles. It comes in a number of varieties and seldom grows higher than 3 feet. Barley is high in nutritive value. It is an essential ingredient in the brewing of beer and in the distillation of Scotch whiskey. Barley is high in carbohydrates with moderate amounts of protein, calcium, and phosphorus, and small amounts of B vitamins.

basal energy expenditure (BEE). In a hospital setting, energy requirements for patients suffering from disease or injury are increased and are often expressed as a percentage above the measured or estimated basal energy expenditure (BEE), or over the resting metabolic expenditure (RME). Basal energy expenditure is an important part of the energy requirement for any person, since it represents the life requirement for the nonactive person. The BEE is defined as the amount of energy—number of calories—needed to perform necessary physiologic work at rest, in the
postabsorptive state (12–14 hours after the last meal), in a thermoneutral environment. The RME does not require the postabsorptive state. The basal energy expenditure can be measured by direct or indirect calorimetry. See *energy balance* and *basal metabolism*.

basal metabolism. The minimum metabolic activity necessary for maintenance of life and vital processes is called the basal metabolism. It is measured as the heat production or energy expenditure of an individual at rest and after a 12-hour fast. This is determined from the oxygen consumption measured over a short period of time. A value of 4.8 calories per liter of oxygen consumed yields the heat production for the period of measurement. The measurement is called the basal metabolic rate or BMR and is normally around 1200–1800 calories (5000–7600 kJ) per day. The BMR may also be expressed as percent above or below normal value for an age and sex. Normal values have a range of plus or minus 20. The basal rate is greatly influenced by secretions of the thyroid gland. A list of the factors that influence the BMR is given. See *energy balance*.

Factors in the Basal Metabolic Rate (BMR) test

EXCLUDED FROM BMR TEST	TAKEN INTO ACCOUNT	OF QUESTIONABLE IMPORTANCE
1. Muscular movements	1. Sex	1. Occupation
2. Recent muscle exertion (within 1 hour)	2. Age	2. Race
3. Food within 12-15 hours	3. Weight and height	3. Diet
4. Emotions, noise, unease	4. Surface area	4. Time of year
5. Temperature extremes	5. Undernutrition or overnutrition	5. Previous day's activity
6. Diseases	6. Athletic training	6. Novety of the situation
	7. Climate	
	8. Altitude	
	9. Sleep	
	10. Body temperature	

base. A base may be defined as a substance that combines with acids to form neutral salts. It may also be defined as a substance that increases the concentration of *hydroxyl ions*, or conversely decreases the concentration of *hydrogen ions* when dissolved in water. The solution has a *pH* greater than 7. See *acid* and *acid and base*.

base pairings. The specific linkage of two nucleotides in the structures of *deoxyribonucleic acid* (DNA) and *ribonucleic acid* (RNA). *Nucleotides* contain nitrogen base derivatives of either purines or pyrimidines. Pairings are either the pyrimidine base thymine in DNA or uracil in RNA with the purine base adenine and the pyrimidine base cytosine, a purine base guanine. In DNA, there are two purine nucleotides, adenine and guanine, and two pyrimidine nucleotides, cytosine and thiamine. In the DNA chain, adenine always forms hydrogen bonds to thiamine, and guanine always forms hydrogen bonds to cytosine. This rule of base pairings is fundamental; along with the amino acid sequence it determines the intracellular double-stranded structure of DNA, the replication of DNA, and the translation of the nucleotide sequence of DNA or of messenger-RNA into the amino acid sequence of protein.

basic food groups. The basic food groups translate the recommended allowances for specific nutrients into a simple guide for meeting multiple nutrient needs by selecting from four basic categories of food. The number of recommended servings differs according to the nutritional needs for various age groups and stages of life. Four kinds of foods are considered basic to meeting nutritional needs: (1) milk and milk products; (2) meat or meat equivalents; (3) fruits and vegetables; and (4) grain (breads and cereals). These four food groups make specific nutrient contributions to the diet. Highlights of the daily food groups include the following: (1) The groups are not applicable for infant feeding. (2) The first four groups contain "essential" foods; another category contains "accessory" foods. (3) Each category includes a variety of foods that contribute important and similar nutrients. (4) No single food group furnishes all the nutrients; at least one essential nutrient is lacking in each food group. (5) Within each group, individual food items have a unique nutritional profile. A modification of the basic four has been developed by the Center for Science in the Public Interest, Washington, D.C.. It takes into account recommendations made in 1977 by the Senate Select Committee on Nutrition and Human Needs, in setting dietary goals for the United States, to modify current diet in the direction of lowered fat, cholesterol, salt, and added sugars, and increased fiber, starches (complex carbohydrates), and natural vitamins and minerals. It permits variety without unbalancing the total nutrient intake by indicating foods that can be used daily, foods that can be used in moderation several times a week, and foods that should be used occasionally. For people requiring dietary modification because of medical conditions, the guide also indicates, by number, foods high in unsaturated fat, saturated fat, cholesterol, and sodium.

The Basic Four Food Groups

FOOD	ONE SERVING IS	SERVINGS PER DAY	
I. MILK GROUP			
Milk, whole or skim	8 ounces	Children 0-9:	2 to 3
Yogurt, plain	8 ounces	Children 9-12:	3
Hard cheese	125 ounces	Teenages:	4
Cheese spreads	2 ounces	Adults:	2
Cottage cheese	16 ounces (2 cups)	Pregnant:	3
Ice cream	12 ounces (1.5 cups)	Nursing:	4

II. MEAT GROUP
THIS SERVING PROVIDES THE AMOUNT OF CALCIUM IN 8 OUNCES OF MILK.

Meat, lean part	2 to 3 ounces	
Poultry	2 to 3 ounces	**Two**
Fish	2 to 3 ounces	If only vegetable protein is used, it must be of adequate
Eggs	2 to 3	nutritional quality as explained in the section on *protein*.
Beans and peas, cooked	1to 1.5 cups	
Nuts and seeds	0.5 to 0.75 cups	
Peanut butter	4 tablespoons	
Hard cheese	2 to 3 ounces	
Cottage cheese	0.5 cup	

III. VEGETABLE & FRUIT GROUP
CHEESE CAN BE COUNTED IN BOTH THE MILK AND MEAT GROUPS;
THUS 0.5 CUP OF COTTAGE CHEESE IS 1 MEAT SERVING AND 0.25 MILK SERVING.

Vegetables, cut up	0.5 cup	**One** vitamin C source, such as orange, grapefruit, or
Fruit, cut up	0.5 cup	equivalent amount of juice.
Grapefruit	0.5 medium	**One** vitamin A source, a deep-yellow or dark-green
Orange	1	vegetable.
Melon	0.5 medium	**Two** other choices to give a total of 4 servings.
Potato	1medium	
Salad	1 bowl	
Lettuce	1 wedge (1/8 head)	

IV. BREAD AND CEREAL GROUP

Bread	1 slice (1 ounce)	**One** whole grain
Cooked cereal	0.5 to 0.75 cup	**Three** whole grain or enriched to give a total of 4 servings.
Pasta, cooked	0.5 to 0.75 cup	
Rice, cooked	0.5 to 0.75 cup	
Dry cereal	1 ounce	

Modified from U.S. Department of Agriculture, U.S. Department of Health, Education and Welfare; *Nutiiton and You: Health Dietary Guidelines for Americans*; Washington, D.C., Government Printing office, Feb. 1980.

basil, sweet (*Ocimum basilicum*). There are five or six varieties of basil, which belong to the mint family, all differing in height, color, and taste. The basils most often used in the United States are sweet basil and dwarf basil. All basil varieties have a unique fragrance and taste that add zest and flavor in cooking. The word basil comes from the Greek *basilikon* meaning "royal" or "king." Sweet basil is a culinary seasoning useful in almost any dish that can be herbed, and is especially pleasant in seafoods, salads, potatoes, vegetable soups, and dishes that contain tomatoes. Basil may be used fresh or dried.

bass. The name covering more than 400 fish that belong mostly to three different fish families, *Serranidae, Moronidae,* and *Centrarchidae,* of the order *Perciformes.* Some bass are freshwater fish; others, saltwater fish. The most common freshwater varieties include white or silver bass and yellow bass. The best-known saltwater bass are common sea bass and striped bass. Bass is a good source of protein and phosphorus.

beach plum (*Prunus maritima*). A member of the prune tree family. Beach plums grow wild. Although highly prized for jams and jellies, the plums are seldom cultivated. The fruit is small and dark purple-blue when ripe, with a thick, tough skin and bullet-hard seed. The flavor is a combination of grape, plum, and cherry, on the bitter and sour side. They are mostly used cooked. See *plum.*

beans. Beans are the seed or seeds of many plants, both trailing vines and erect bushes. They belong to the group of foods called *legumes,* which also includes peas, lentils, and peanuts. When cooked for a short time in a small amount of water, they are a fair source of *carotene* (vitamin A activity) and *ascorbic acid* (vitamin C). See this item in the table under *vegetables.*

beef. Beef is the flesh of an adult animal of the Bovidae family of ruminants. Practically all the beef eaten comes from steers, heifers, and cows. High-quality beef comes from animals that generally weigh from 900 to 1300 pounds each and range in age from 1–3 years. The better-known breeds of cattle are the Shorthorn and Hereford, Aberdeen, Angus, Brahman and Santa Gertrudis. Beef is an excellent source of high-quality protein, and provides good amounts of *iron* and *niacin.* One hundred grams of cooked, boneless, lean beef supplies the following percentages of the recommended daily allowances for a 25-year-old man: 30% *protein,* 27% *iron,* 10% *riboflavin,* 22% *niacin,* and 4% *thiamine.* One hundred grams of raw beef, choice grade, gives the calories shown.

Nutrients in 100 g of beef, chuck, medium fat

CALORIES KCAL	PROTEIN G	FAT G	CARBOHYDRATE G	VITAMIN A RE	NIACIN MG	IRON MG
327	26	24	0	40	4	3

Calories in 100 g of raw beef

Chuck, lean	257	Round	197	Canned, corned	216
Flank, lean	144	Rump	303	Dried, chipped	203
Hamburger	179	Sirloin	313	Canned, corned, hash,	181
Porterhouse	390	Corned	293	with potato	

beer. A foamy, fermented beverage brewed from a malted cereal, with hops added. Beer is brewed from a variety of grains, such as wheat, millet, barley and rice. Today's American beer is brewed from barley, which has been germinated in water and dried, cereal adjuncts such as corn or rye, and hops, the dried cones of the hop vine. In addition, cultured yeast is needed for the fermentation that creates beer's characteristic sparkle. Also needed is pure filtered water which by volume makes up about nine-tenths of the finished beer. There are many varieties of beer, including ale, porter, and stout. The most popular American beer is lager. The word "lager" comes from the German and means "to store," and that is what lager beer is, beer stored for various periods of time to age or mellow. The nutrient content of beer is shown.

Nutrients in 355 mL (12 fluid ounces) of beer

CALORIES KCAL	PROTEIN G	FAT G	CARBOHYDRATE G	THIAMINE MG	NIACIN MG	RIBOFLAVIN MG
150	1	Trace	18	0.01	2	0.1

beet (*Beta*). The enlarged red root of a plant which is first cousin to chard. Beet greens, the tops of the plants, are also edible, and some varieties are purposely grown for this use. Beets are also grown for sugar. Beets have small amounts of vitamins and minerals. Beet greens are an excellent source of carotene (vitamin A activity) and calcium. See this item in the table under *vegetables*.

benign. Not malignant; not having a tendency to recur; having a favorable outcome.

benzoic acid. See *sodium benzoate*.

benzoyl peroxide. Mol. Wt. 232. As a food additive it is an important flour bleach that does not "age" flour, used in conjunction with "aging" agents (*azodicarbonamide, potassium bromide*). Benzoyl peroxide is a powder that bleaches flour within 24 hours after being mixed with it.

As the bleach does its work, most of it decomposes to benzoic acid which remains in the flour after baking. The benzoic acid residue is not hazardous.

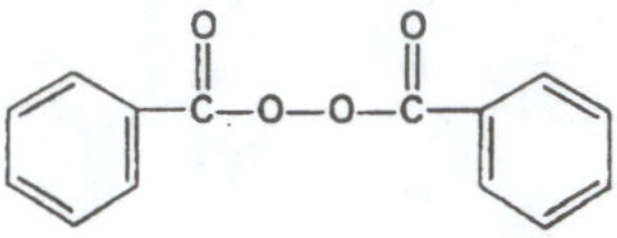

Benzoyl peroxide

bergamot. A name used for three very different plants. (1) A native American herb, (*Monarda*) which belongs to the mint family. The leaves have a pleasant lemon scent. There are several varieties of the herb. The best-known one is the *Monarda didyma*, commonly known in the Eastern states as "Oswego tea," from the tribe of Indians that used it extensively. (2) A pear, one of the oldest to be cultivated in the British Isles. The bergamot pear is a winter pear, with several varieties. (3) A tree of the citrus family cultivated in Italy for the essential oils of the rind of its small, pear-shaped orange. These oils are only used commercially, chiefly in perfumes or as a flavoring.

beri-beri. A nutritional disease of the peripheral nerves caused by a deficiency of *thiamine* (vitamin B_1). It is characterized by pain (neuritis) and paralysis of the extremities, cardiovascular changes, and edema. Beri-beri is common in Asia where diet consists largely of milled rice with little protein.

berry. The word describes not only the fruits that have "berry" as part of their names, but also cherries, tomatoes, and even the hips of roses, for the definition says that berries are any kind of small, pulpy fruit, no matter what the structure may be. In cookery there are certain fruits thought of as strictly berries, such as barberries, bilberries, blackberries, blueberries, cloudberries, cranberries, currants, elderberries, gooseberries, loganberries, mulberries, raspberries, rowanberries, and strawberries.

beta (β)-carotene. See *carotene*.

beta (β)-hydroxybutyric acid. Mol. Wt. 104. A natural metabolic product of fatty acid degradation. It is one of the three compounds known as ketone bodies which occur in *metabolic acidosis* or *ketosis*, the other two being *acetone* and *acetoacetic* acid. Beta-hydroxybutyric acid is the reduced form of acetoacetic acid. See *ketone bodies*.

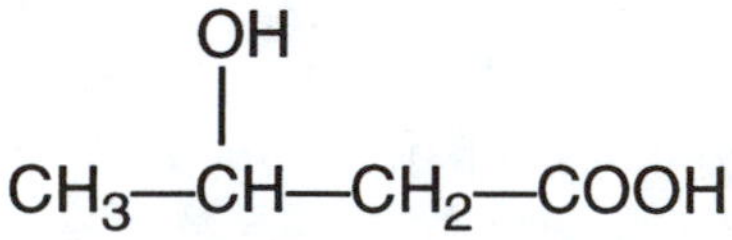

$$CH_3—CH(OH)—CH_2—COOH$$

Beta (β)-hydroxybutyric acid

betaine. Mol. Wt. 118. A methyl donor ($-CH_3$) that derives from *choline* and functions to synthesize the *essential amino acid methionine* from homocysteine.

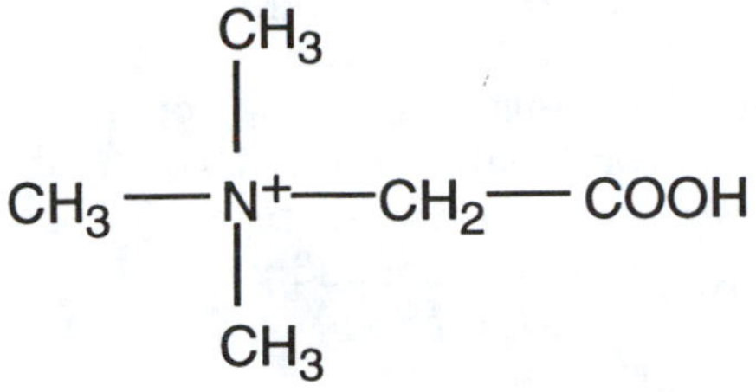

$$CH_3 - N^+ - CH_2 - COOH$$

with CH_3 above the N and CH_3 below the N

Betaine

beta (β)-lipoproteins. Low-density lipoproteins (LDL) carrying about two-thirds or more of the total plasma *cholesterol* in addition to other lipids, and formed in the liver from endogenous fat sources. See *lipoprotein*.

beta (β)-pleated sheets. A common and important structure of protein. It consists of peptide chains running parallel or antiparallel. The β-pleated sheet structures are stabilized by hydrogen bondings among peptide chain sections. The side chain amino acid residues extend above and below the general plane of the pleated sheet. See *alpha (α) helix*.

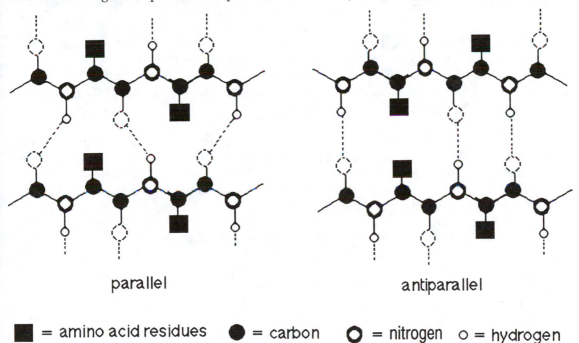

parallel   antiparallel

■ = amino acid residues   ● = carbon   ◯ = nitrogen   ο = hydrogen

β-pleated sheet structures

BHA (tert-butyl-4-hydroxy-anisole) and BHT (2,6-di-tert-butyl-p-hydroxytoluene). BHA and BHT are synthetic antioxidants used in foods to prevent *autoxidation*. They are highly effective at low concentrations and are not toxic at the concentrations used in foods. BHA and BHT are used in many vegetable oils and in almost every processed food that contains fat or oil. These additives may slightly increase the shelf-life of food by preventing *polyunsaturated* oil from oxidizing and becoming rancid. They also protect the fat-soluble vitamins, *retinol* (vitamin

A) and *tocopherol* (vitamin E). BHA and BHT are added to breakfast cereal packaging, chewing gum, convenience foods, vegetable oils, shortening, potato flakes, potato chips, enriched rice, candy, and many other oil-containing products. The total concentration of antioxidants ranges from as low as 0.0001% in gelatin desserts to 0.1% in chewing gums. The usual concentration is about 0.01%. See *autoxidation* and *peroxidation*.

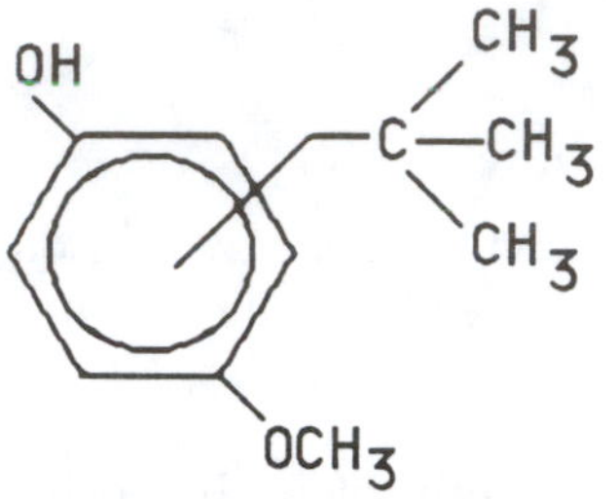

BHA

tert-butyl-4-hydroxy-anisole
butylated hydroxyanisole

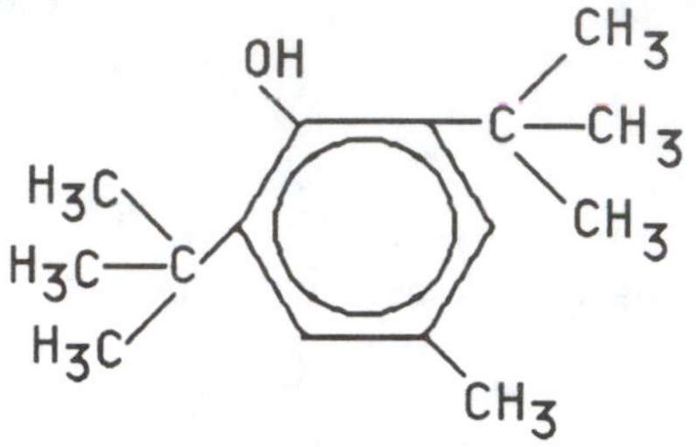

BHT

2,6-di-tert-butyl-p-hydroxytoluene
butylated hydroxytoluene

bicarbonate (HCO$_3^-$). One of the main buffer systems of the human body. Bicarbonate forms by dissolving carbon dioxide (CO_2) in water to form carbonic acid (H_2CO_3). The salts sodium bicarbonate ($NaHCO_3$) and potassium bicarbonate ($KHCO_3$) with carbonic acid form an important *buffer system* in the blood. The pK$_a$ (log of the dissocialtion constant) value of the bicarbonate buffer system is 6.3. See *acid and base*.

bile. An alkaline viscous yellow to green bitter fluid (pH 8 to 8.6) that is secreted continuously by the liver at a rate of 0.5–1 liter per day. It is stored and concentrated in the gallbladder, which contracts when fat enters the *duodenum* and forces bile into the intestine along with the pancreatic juice. The activator for this process is a hormone called *cholecystokinin*, which is secreted by the duodenal wall when fat enters it. Bile is composed of water, *bile pigments*, *bile salts*, *cholesterol*, and electrolytes. The bile salts are largely concerned in the digestion and absorption of fats. They assist in the emulsification of fat globules by the reduction of surface tension. They react with insoluble fatty compounds such as *stearic acid*, cholesterol, and the fat-soluble vitamins to produce *micelles* which are soluble in water and can be absorbed. After absorption, the bile salts are reabsorbed in the bloodstream and carried to the liver where they stimulate further bile secretions. Bile pigments are the waste products of hemoglobin breakdown. Bile is essential for the absorption of *vitamin K* and other fat-soluble vitamins. It also stimulates intestinal motility and neutralizes the acid chyme, creating a favorable hydrogen ion concentration (*pH*) for pancreatic and intestinal enzyme activity. Its secretion into the intestine is the mode of excretion for sterols, numerous drugs, and other waste products.

bile acid. Complex acids, of which cholic, glycocholic and taurocholic acids are examples, that occur as *bile salts*.

bile pigments. Derived from the heme of hemoglobin contained in red blood cells broken down in the liver. The bacterial action on these pigments gives the characteristic brown color to feces. The major bile pigments are *bilirubin* and *biliverdin*. Bilrubin and biliverdin are red and green, respectively, but become brown when oxidized by intestinal bacteria. The position with the asterisk (*) indicates the difference between these two structures.

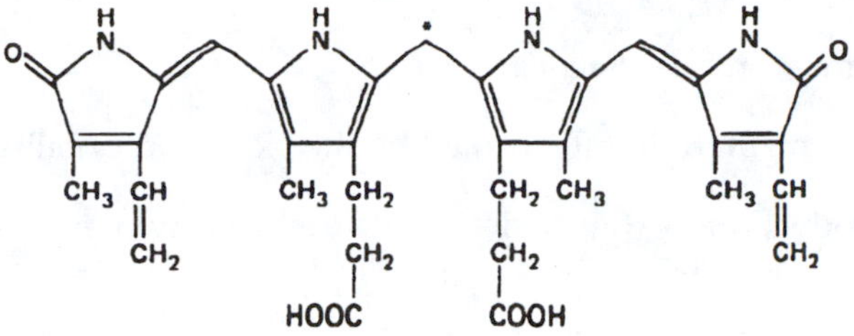

Bilirubin

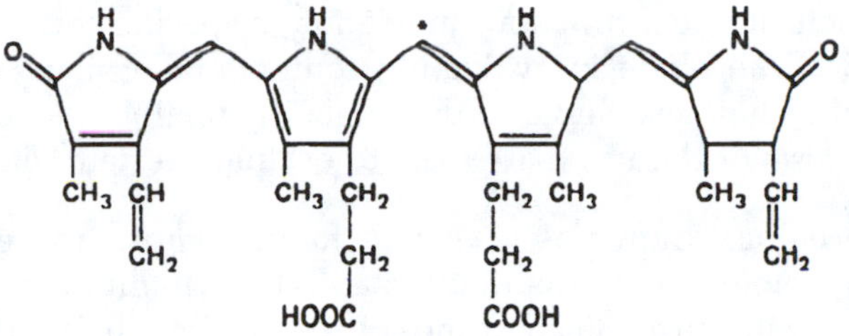

Biliverdin

bile salts. Act as emulsifying agents causing large fat droplets to be broken up into many smaller droplets. Also aid in the absorption of fats by the small intestine. The bile salts are themselves absorbed through the wall of the large intestine and returned to the liver for reuse. The major bile salts are conjugated cholesterol derivatives of the bile acids *cholic acid*, *chenodeoxycholic acid*, *deoxycholic acid* and *lithocholic acid*. The bile acids conjugate with *glycine* and *taurine*. The salts of these conjugated bile acids are the bile salts. As an example, the structure of a bile salt, *cholyltaurine* (taurocholic acid) is given. The bile salts are water-soluble and are powerful *emulsifiers*.

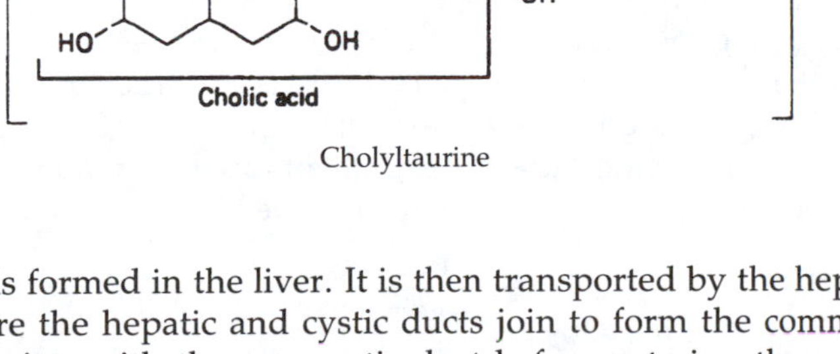

Cholyltaurine

biliary system. Bile is formed in the liver. It is then transported by the hepatic duct from the liver to a point where the hepatic and cystic ducts join to form the common bile duct. The common bile duct unites with the pancreatic duct before entering the small intestine. The opening of the common bile duct is guarded by the sphincter of Oddi. When this sphincter is closed, the bile formed by the liver flows down the hepatic duct and then through the cystic duct to reach the gallbladder.

bilirubin. A red pigment in bile. See *bile pigments*.

biliverdin. A greenish pigment in bile formed by the oxidation of bilirubin. See *bile pigments*.

binary fission. Reproduction by the division of a cell into two essentially equal parts by a nonmitotic process.

biochemical analysis. Biochemical assessments of nutritional status are made primarily in blood and urine. Biochemical tests are designed to measure specific nutrients; some measure only the nutrient, others measure functions in relation to specific body functions. Biochemical methods are applied to the blood in evaluating contents of protein, enzymes, and several vitamins and minerals. They also serve to determine hemoglobin level as an assessment of anemia. Biochemical tests of the urine are used to evaluate certain vitamins.

bioflavin. A substance once known as *vitamin P*, found mainly in the pulp and connective tissue of citrus fruits. Some vitamin distributors add it to vitamin combinations and claim it is useful to help build resistance to infection and colds and is beneficial in cases of hypertension. However, there is no clinical evidence of its need.

biogenesis. Originating from living organisms.

biological catalyst. See *enzymes*.

biological clock. A regular time schedule of biological activitivies. Examples of biological clocks are the menses, the time-regulated release of some hormones, and periods of sleep and wakefulness. Circadian rhythms are physiologic and biochemical activities associated with a 24-hour cycle and are other examples of biological clocks. See *melatonin*.

biological function. The role played by a chemical compound or a system of chemical compounds in living organisms.

biological magnification. Increasing concentration of relatively stable chemicals as they are passed up a food chain from initial consumers to top predators.

biological value (BV). The biological value of a food protein is the efficiency with which that protein furnishes the proper proportions and amounts of the essential or indispensable amino acids needed for the synthesis of body proteins in humans or animals. The more nearly a protein supplies the tissues with the necessary proportion and amounts of these indispensable amino acids, the higher its biological value. Egg protein has the highest biological value and is the standard by which other proteins are measured. The BV is one of several values used to measure the quality of a protein and represents a value obtained under controlled, experimental conditions. The methods for conducting these measurements are not standardized, nor is there full agreement concerning the way to express the result. The BV is defined as:

$$BV = \frac{\text{Nitrogen retained}}{\text{Nitrogen absorbed}} \times 100$$

$$BV = \frac{(\text{dietary N}) - (F - Fm) + (U - Ue)}{(\text{dietary N}) - (F - Fm)} \times 100$$

Where F equals the fecal nitrogen during the testing of a protein; Fm equals the fecal nitrogen on a protein-free diet (endogenous fecal nitrogen); U equals urinary nitrogen excreted during the testing of a protein; and Ue equals urinary nitrogen excreted on a protein-free diet (endogenous urinary nitrogen excretion). The BVs of proteins in food are as follows:

Biological Values of Foods

Food	BV	Food	BV	Food	BV	Food	BV
Eggs	100	Rice	86	Beef	75	Corn	72
Milk	93	Casein	75	Fish	75	Wheat, flour	44

A protein with a BV of 70 or greater is capable of supporting growth (maintaining a positive nitrogen balance) if sufficient calories are also taken. A value below 60 is considered an incomplete protein. The protein to be tested for a BV is fed to the animal as (1) the only source of nitrogen, and (2) at a level just below a predetermined level required for nitrogen balance. The BV makes no allowances for the losses of nitrogen in the digestive process. See *net protein utilization (NPU)*, *net dietary protein value (NDpV)*, *net dietary protein calories percent (NDpCal%)*, and *chemical score*.

biopsy. The removal of a sample of living cells from a living patient for the purpose of diagnosis, or the prognosis of a disease, or of confirmation of normal conditions. The specimen is sent to a specially trained pathologist who examines the cells and determines the type of growth they represent.

biosynthesis. The chemical synthesis of materials in living plants or animals. *Enzymes* usually are the catalysts for biosynthetic reactions.

biotic. Pertaining to life.

biotin. Mol. Wt. 244. A water-soluble vitamin, belonging to the vitamin B-complex group. This vitamin plays an important role as a *coenzyme* for biochemical reactions, in which *carbon dioxide* (CO_2) is incorporated into metabolites. Biotin even in very small amounts appears to function as a coenzyme mainly in carboxylation and deamination reactions. Biotin serves as a coenzyme with active acetate in reactions that transfer carbon dioxide from one compound and fix in onto another. It also serves as a coenzyme in reactions which split off the amino group from certain amino acids (*aspartic acid, serine, threonine*). It has been demonstrated that biotin aids in the synthesis of saturated fatty acids. Biotin has been found necessary also in conversion of *ornithine* into *citrulline*, an important step in *urea* formation, for protein synthesis, *oxidative phosphorylation*, and *carbohydrate metabolism*. The factor is required for purine metabolism, and in the presence of carbon dioxide, for conversion of pyruvate to oxaloacetate and then to aspartate. It interrelates with *folacin, pantothenic acid*, and *cobalamin* (vitamin B_{12}) in metabolic processes. The human requirement for biotin has not been established in quantitative terms, since the amount needed for metabolism is so small. This coenzyme occurs in many natural foods, and is apparently synthesized by intestinal bacteria. Examples of excellent food sources of biotin include egg yolk, liver, kidney, tomatoes, and yeast. In the table are the biotin sources in some foods.

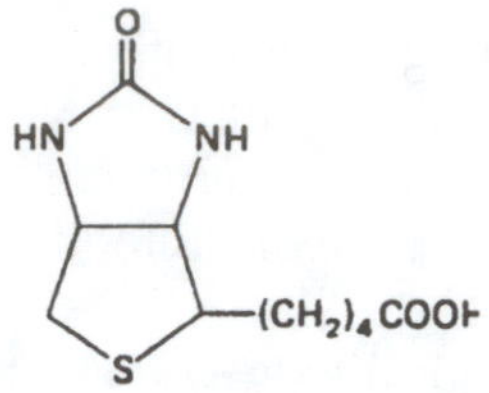

Biotin

Biotin in mg/100 g of foods

Banana	4	Filberts	16	Peas, fresh	12
Beans, lima	10	Grapefruit	3	Peas, dried	19
Beef	4	Halibut	8	Peanuts	39
Carrots	2	Hazel nuts	14	Pork, bacon	7
Cauliflower	17	Liver / Beef	100	Pork, muscle	3
Cheese	2	Milk	5	Salmon	5
Chicken	5-10	Molasses	9	Spinach	2
Chocolate	32	Mushrooms	16	Strawberries	4
Corn	6	Onion, dried	4	Tomatoes	2
Eggs, whole	25	Oysters	9	Wheat, whole	5

birch beer. The sap of the sweet birch, also called black birch or cherry birch, can be fermented into a mild or potent beer. Birches are tapped like maples and their sap is delightful to drink, faintly sweet and tasting of wintergreen.

blackberry (*Rubus*). An oblong, conical fruit composed of many small fruits called drupelets. Blackberries are also called brambles, since they are the fruit of various brambles. Ripe blackberries are purple-black in color, although they are red when they are unripe. Berries contribute to the vitamin and mineral content of the diet. Iron content is fair and the *ascorbic acid* (vitamin C) content is fair to good, depending upon the amount eaten. See this item in the table under *fruits*.

blackhead. See *acne*.

blackstrap molasses. See *molasses* and *sucrose*.

bladder. A vesicle, blister, or hollow structure, normal or pathologic, which contains watery fluid. Gallbladders and urinary bladders are examples of normal bladders. A tube, or ureter, leads from each kidney to the urinary bladder. The bladder empties through the urethra, a tube leading to an external opening called the meatus. The bladder, which functions as a collecting and temporary storage point for urine, expands to accommodate increasing amounts. With the accumulation of about half a pint, reflex contractions lead to a desire to urinate. The contraction stimulates pressure receptors in the muscles of the bladder wall, from which nervous impulses go to the brain. When it is convenient to urinate, the brain sends out signals which cause the bladder's external sphincter to relax. Under *urinary bladder* is a diagram of the urinary bladder and its relationship to that system.

bleaching and maturing agents. Bleaching and maturing agents are used in flour milling and bread baking. Freshly milled wheat flour has a yellowish color and lacks the qualities needed for an elastic, stable dough. When flour is stored and allowed to age for several months, it gradually becomes white due to oxidation and "matures" to make it satisfactory for baking. Natural aging is costly, so the flour millers speed up the bleaching and aging (which modifies the gluten characteristics of the flour) by adding oxidizing and/or bleaching chemicals such as *benzoyl peroxide*, *azodicarbonamide*, the calcium and ammonium phosphates, and chlorine dioxide.

blood. A tissue consisting of cells suspended in a fluid called plasma in the approximate proportion of 45 parts of corpuscles to 55 parts of plasma. Its specific gravity is 1.005, and its reaction is faintly alkaline (pH 7.4). The majority of the corpuscles in blood are red blood cells (erythrocytes), but white blood cells (leukocytes) and platelets are also found. All the oxygen and part of the carbon dioxide are carried by the red blood cells, but everything else travels in the plasma. If blood plasma or whole blood is allowed to stand outside the body, clotting occurs and a protein called fibrin is deposited, leaving a fluid called serum. Plasma is, in fact, serum plus 0.3–0.5 g of fibrinogen per 100 mL, the substance from which fibrin is formed. The blood corpuscles are heavier than the plasma, which has a specific gravity of 1.028. Blood constitutes 5–10% of the total body weight. A reduction in blood volume leads to a fall in the capillary blood pressure, as a result of which fluid is transferred from the tissues and so restores the blood volume but dilutes the blood. The motor functions of blood are all carried out when blood circulates normally through the blood vessels. These functions are: (1) to carry oxygen from the lungs to tissue cells and carbon dioxide from the cells to the lungs; (2) to carry food materials absorbed from the digestive system to the tissue cells and to remove waste products for elimination by excretory organs, the kidneys, intestines, and skin; (3) to carry hormones which help regulate body functions from ductless (endocrine) glands to the tissues of the body; (4) to help regulate and equalize body temperature—body cells generate large amounts of heat, and the circulating blood absorbs this heat; (5) to protect the body against infection; (6) to maintain the fluid balance of the body. The average man has a blood volume of 5–6 liters, the average woman 4–5 liters. The table shows the nutrients associated with normal functioning of the circulatory system. See *Appendix* for the normal constituents of human blood.

Micronutrients associated with the circulatory system

VITAMIN	MINERAL	FUNCTION
—	Fe	Formation of hemoglobin
Pyridoxine	Mn	Red blood cell division and maturation
Folate	Co	
Cobalamin		
Pantothenate	—	Maintain elasticity and strength of capillaries
Ascorbate		
	Mo	Blood clotting. Iron utilization. Mobilization of iron stores
Vitamin K	Cu	
	Ca	

blood-brain barrier. A general term that loosely describes the fact that the number of substances in the blood that transfer into brain cells is limited relative to transfer into other cells. It is a complex phenomenon involving several concepts. The major source of energy for the brain is glucose, which can pass the "barrier;" other sugars cannot. Since the brain depends on glucose, hypoglycemic (low blood sugar) states can bring on convulsions, as in *insulin shock*. The brain can adapt to the utilization of ketone bodies as a source of energy under a prolonged state of *metabolic acidosis* or *ketosis*. Amino acids vary greatly in their ability to be actively taken up (active transport) by the brain cells. *Glutamine* is the amino acid taken up to the greatest extent by the brain. Tyrosine is readily taken up and *glutamic acid*, *lysine*, and *leucine* exchange rapidly between the brain cells and blood but with no net uptake. The blood-brain barrier mechanisms, anatomically and biochemically, are complex and not well understood.

blood cells, red (erythrocytes). Human red blood cells are disks about 7.5 thousandths of a milliliter (mL) or 7.5 microns in diameter. There are about 5.5 million in every milliliter of whole blood from men, and nearly 5 million per mL from women. There are about 25 billion red blood cells in the whole body, and they are constantly being destroyed and replaced at a rate of about 9000 million an hour. The normal red cell lasts approximately 120 days before it is destroyed. Red blood cells are flexible and withstand much bending, squeezing, and deformation as they are pushed through the narrow capillaries. They consist of an intricate, spongy network of protein-filled spaces (sinusoids) in the red marrow. The development of a mature red cell takes about a week, during which the endothelial cell enlarges, divides, forms *hemoglobin*, and finally loses its nucleus. This process is called maturation. The diagram shows the role of *bone* in blood production.

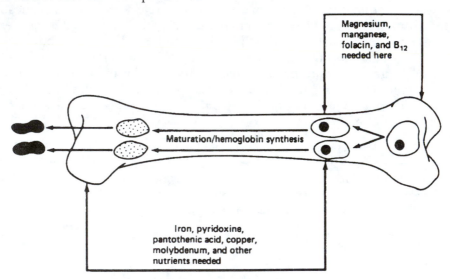

Normal production of red blood cells, red (erythrocytes)

blood cells, white (leukocytes). There are several different kinds of white blood cells, the main ones being the polymorphonuclear leukocytes, the monocytes, and the lymphocytes. There are normally 5000 to 10,000 white cells per milliliter (mL) of blood, but the number varies during the day. There is a rapid turnover with constant destruction and replacement; they live for 7–14 days. There is usually a rise in white blood cells (leukocytosis) after meals, severe exercise, or other forms of stress such as infection. About 70–75% of the leukocytes are polymorphonuclear, less than 5% are monocytes, and the rest are lymphocytes. Their function is primarily one of protection. They can ingest and destroy foreign particles, such as bacteria, in the blood and tissues. This function is called *phagocytosis*, and the white cells performing it are phagocytes. White cells are capable of *ameboid movement* and thus can pass through the walls of capillaries into surrounding tissue. This ability to enter tissue makes them very useful in fighting infection. An area of infection is characterized by a great increase in white cells which gather about the site to destroy bacteria.

blood clotting. The coagulation of blood is a mechanism by which clots of blood plug ruptured blood vessels and repair weakened ones. Clots are formed by threadlike fibers (*fibrin*) that create an interlacing network containing red blood cells. Clots are formed by a complex series of interrelated reactions, an enzymatic *cascade*. The clotting process is divided into an extrinsic pathway, initiated by injury, and an intrinsic pathway linked to a common pathway. The diagram shows the relationships among these pathways and indicates where vitamin K is involved in the clotting mechanism.

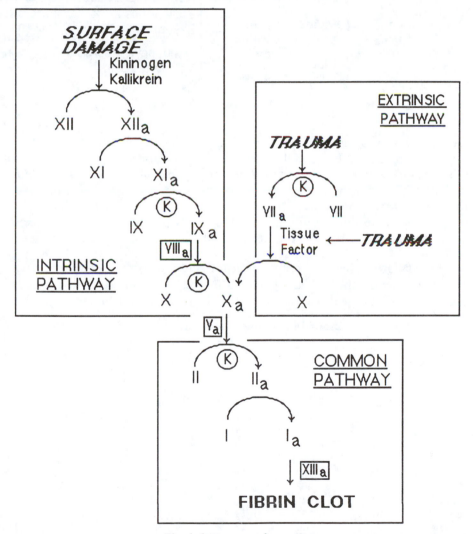

Blood clotting cascade reactions
The Roman numerals represent the various blood clotting factors. I, Ia, II, and IIa represent *fibrinogen*, *fibrin*, *pro-thrombin*, and *thrombin*, respectively. The encircled K represents sites where *Vitamin K* acts.

blood composition.

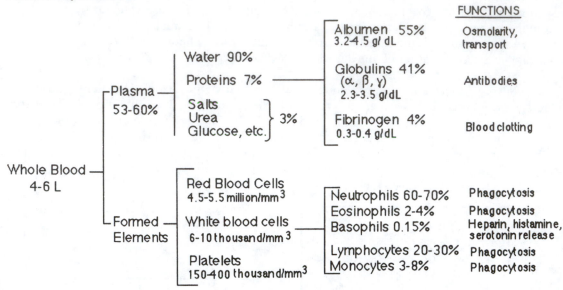

Composition of whole blood

blood count. A laboratory test performed on a drop of blood which measures the number and characteristics of the red blood cells, white blood cells, and platelets. The measurement of these cells is then compared with standards for the normal individual. The red blood count is done in several parts, including the *hematocrit*, the *hemoglobin*, and the blood smear. The hematocrit measures the proportion of red cells in a unit of blood. The blood smear measures a number of things, including the number of white cells per cubic centimeter (cc) of blood and the differential white count (the proportion of the various kinds of white cells present).

blood flow. Blood flows through the tissues of the body, delivering oxygen by way of the arteries. Blood then enters the capillary beds within the tissues and exits the tissues by way of veins that return to the heart oxygenated. The table gives an estimate of the blood flow

Blood flow through human tissues

TISSUES	TISSUE WT. KG	BLOOD FLOW ML/ MIN	ML/ 100 G/MIN	A-V O DIFFERENCE ML/L	OXYGEN USE ML/ MIN.	ML O$_2$/ 100 G/ MIN
Hepatic-Portal	2.6	1,500	58	34	51	2.0
Kidneys	0.3	1,260	420	14	18	6.0
Brain	1.4	750	54	62	46	3.3
Skin	3.6	462	13	25	12	0.3
Skeletal muscle	31	840	3	60	50	0.2
Heart muscle	0.3	252	84	114	29	10
Residual tissue	24	336	1.4	129	44	0.2
Whole body	63	5,400	8.6	46	250	0.4

through various human tissues and of how much oxygen is extracted from the blood as measured by the A-V O difference, the difference in the amount of oxygen on the arterial and venous sides of the blood flow through a tissue. The table also shows how much oxygen is used by the various tissues. See *heart*.

blood plasma. Proteins. Plasma contains 7–8 g% of protein which is made up of *fibrinogen* and *prothrombin* in small amounts, albumin 4–5 g% percent, and globulin 2–3 g%. Fibrinogen and prothrombin are concerned with the clotting of blood. Albumin is a protein of low molecular weight, 68,000, and small particle size, which is responsible for 80% of the osmotic pressure exerted by the blood. Globulin is a mixture of proteins of much larger size, which are of little importance osmotically, but are intimately concerned with the defense mechanism of the body, the antibodies. The plasma proteins are constantly changing because of new formation, especially in the liver, and utilization in the tissues. The plasma proteins are completely renewed about once a week. The following electrolytes are found in solution in blood plasma: sodium (330 mg per deciliter), *potassium* (20 mg per deciliter), *chloride* (360 mg per deciliter), *calcium* (10 mg per deciliter), *bicarbonate* (165 mg per deciliter) and smaller quantities of phosphate, sulfate, and organic radicals. Other constituents found in blood plasma are the following: *glucose* (100 mg per deciliter), *urea* (30–40 mg per deciliter), *cholesterol* (200 mg per deciliter), *uric acid* (3 mg per deciliter), small quantities of lactic acid, amino acids, fatty acids, and traces of many other substances. See the appendix under *Normal Constituents of Human Blood*.

blood platelet (thrombocyte). A minute particle of protoplasm (the basic material of cells) which is much smaller than the red blood cell. The normal platelet count is 180,000 to 350,000 per milliliter of blood. One of the functions of the platelets is to maintain the texture of the smallest blood vessels (capillaries) in proper condition. Without platelets, red cells often leak out from the capillaries, tiny bleeding points may be seen, and blood will not clot.

blood pressure. The force that blood exerts on the walls of vessels through which it flows. All parts of the blood vascular system are under pressure, but the term "blood pressure" usually refers to arterial pressure. Pressure on the arteries is highest when the ventricles contract during systole (systolic pressure). Pressure is lowest when the ventricles relax during diastole (diastolic pressure). The brachial artery in the upper arm is the artery generally used for blood-pressure measurement. Blood pressure is measured in terms of millimeters (mm) of mercury (Hg). A pressure of 120/80 (120 over 80) means a systolic pressure of 120 mm Hg and diastolic pressure of 80 mm Hg. A systolic pressure above 140 mm Hg indicates hypertension. The blood pressure may temporarily rise or fall under various states or conditions. The following represent some normal changes.

Normal changes in blood pressure

MUSCULAR ACTIVITY	SLEEP	EMOTION	WEIGHT	GENDER
Increases systolic pressure 60-80 mm Hg	Systolic pressure falls in quiet sleep, rises during dreams, and rises before awakening.	Increases systolic pressure	Generally a rise in systolic pressure, with increased body weight after age 60	Systolic pressure in men is 8-10 mm Hg higher than in women

blood sugar (glucose). The normal functioning of all the cells in the body depends upon an adequate supply of *glucose* in the blood which reaches them, and the amount present (the blood sugar level) varies from 70 to 100 mg per 100 mL in the fasting state. The blood sugar level is controlled partly by dietary intake and mainly by hormones of the *pancreas* (*insulin* and *glucagon*), the *pituitary*, and the *adrenal glands*. Glucose is a monosaccharide of low molecular weight and diffuses rapidly out of the blood into the tissues because of the differences in concentration and an enzyme-facilitated uptake by the cells. The blood sugar level usually remains relatively constant even in a fasting state, although it is constantly being removed and used by the cells of the various tissues. The glucose needed to maintain the blood sugar level is obtained primarily by absorption from the intestine during *digestion*. If this is inadequate, breakdown of the liver *glycogen* provides a further supply through the influence of the hormone *glucagon*. The level of the blood sugar (glucose) at any moment depends upon the balance between the uptake and utilization by the tissues, its absorption from the intestines, and the mobilization of glycogen in the liver. The following four hormones control these functions: (1) anterior pituitary hormones (*pituitary*), (2) *insulin* and *glucagon* (*pancreas*), (3) *epinephrine* (*adrenal medulla*), and (4) *cortisone* (*adrenal cortex*).

blood types. All human blood may be divided into four main types or groups; O, A, B, AB. This system of typing is used to prevent incompatible blood transfusion, which causes serious reactions and sometimes death. Certain types of blood are incompatible or not suited to each other if combined. Two bloods are said to be incompatible when the *plasma* or *serum* of one blood causes clumping of the cells of the other. Two bloods are said to be compatible and safe for transfusion if the cells of each can be suspended in the *plasma* or *serum* of the other without clumping. Blood typing and cross-matching are done by trained laboratory technicians. Blood types A, B, AB, or O are determined by different mucopolysaccharides on the membrane surface of red blood cells. Red cells in type A blood are clumped (agglutinated) by anti-A serum, those in type B blood are agglutinated by anti-B serum. Type AB blood cells are clumped by both serums and type O blood is not agglutinated by either serum. Blood serum is defined as the watery part of the blood which remains after the clot has been removed. See *RH factor*.

Preferred and permissible blood types for transfusions

RECIPIENT TYPE	PREFERRED DONOR TYPE	PERMISSIBLE DONOR TYPE
A	A	O
B	B	O
AB	AB	A, B, O
O	O	only O

blood vessels. The blood vessels are the closed system of tubes through which the blood flows. The arteries and arterioles are distributors. The capillaries are the vessels through which all exchange of fluid, oxygen, and carbon dioxide takes place between the blood and tissue cells. The venules and veins are collectors, carrying blood back to the heart. The capillaries are the smallest of these vessels but are of greatest importance functionally in the circulatory system. The diagrams show the major arteries and veins in humans.

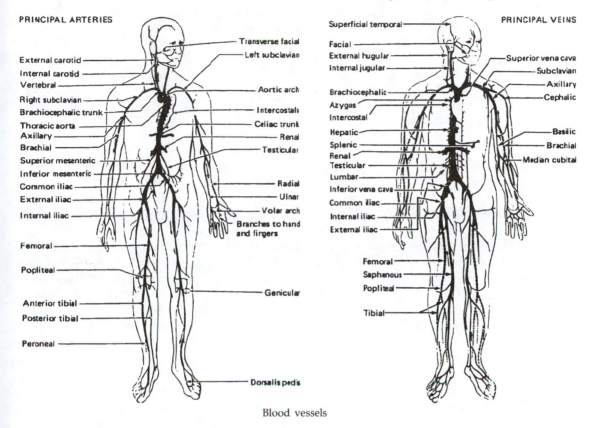

PRINCIPAL ARTERIES

External carotid
Internal carotid
Vertebral
Right subclavian
Brachiocephalic trunk
Thoracic aorta
Axillary
Brachial
Superior mesenteric
Inferior mesenteric
Common iliac
External iliac
Internal iliac
Femoral
Popliteal
Anterior tibial
Posterior tibial
Peroneal

Transverse facial
Left subclavian
Aortic arch
Intercostals
Celiac trunk
Renal
Testicular
Radial
Ulnar
Volar arch
Branches to hand and fingers
Genicular
Dorsalis pedis

PRINCIPAL VEINS

Superficial temporal
Facial
External hugular
Internal jugular
Brachiocephalic
Azygos
Intercostal
Hepatic
Splenic
Renal
Testicular
Lumbar
Inferior vena cava
Common iliac
Internal iliac
External iliac
Femoral
Saphenous
Popliteal
Tibial

Superior vena cava
Subclavian
Axillary
Cephalic
Basilic
Brachial
Median cubital

Blood vessels

blueberry (*Vaccinium*). The edible berry of a plant of the same name. Blueberries belong to the *Vaccinium* genus, and there are many varieties, ranging in color from purplish blue to blue-black. Bilberries and whortleberries are blueberry varieties. Blueberries have fair amounts of *ascorbic acid* (vitamin C) and iron. See this item in the table under *fruits*.

bluefish (*Pomatomus saltatrix*). A vivacious fish, bluish above and silvery below, an important food source along the Atlantic Coast. Bluefish get to be as large as 10 pounds, but those sold in fish markets usually weigh from 3–6 pounds. Bluefish are meaty fish, delicate in flavor. Good sources of protein and phosphorus.

BMR (basal metabolic rate). See *energy balance* and *basal metabolism*.

body cavities. The organs of the body are located in certain cavities, the major ones of which are the dorsal cavity (toward the back part of the body) and the ventral cavity (toward the front part of the body). The dorsal cavity has a cranial area which contains the brain, and a vertebral area which contains the spinal cord. These areas are continuous. The ventral cavity has a thoracic cavity and an abdominopelvic cavity. These areas are separated by the diaphragm.

body, chemical composition. The following is an estimate of the percent chemical composition of the human body on a dry-weight basis. See *trace elements*.

Percent chemical composition of the human body*

C	H	O	N	NA	CL	MG	FE	I
18	10	65	3	0.2	0.2	0.1	0.0004	0.00004

* Minute quantities of the following elements are also present: F, Si, Mn, Zn, Cu, Al, and As.

body fat (adipose tissue). There are two types of adipose tissue — white fat, which is most of the *fat*, and *brown fat*, which is only in the neck and upper part of the back. White fat is stored in adipose cells and serves as an energy store. Brown fat is believed to be for the production of heat (*thermogenic*) instead of chemical energy (*adenosine triphosphate, ATP*). Brown fat decreases with age and increases with increased exposure to cold environments. The amount of body fat is an objective measure of the state of nutrition. There are several methods of making the evaluation. Measurement of the width of the fat layer which lies directly beneath the skin is one method. It takes into account the fact that subcutaneous tissue is a repository for fat. Fat-layer width can therefore be estimated by measuring skinfold thickness with a pincerlike device called a caliper. Skinfold thickness can then be translated into terms of percentage of body fat. The caliper is applied to the designated areas of the body which are considered to be representative of overall fat thickness. The three-headed extensor muscle (triceps) along the back of the upper arm is one such area. *Fats* are compounds which include both fats and oils. Natural oils in the skin provide a radiant complexion, while in the scalp they help nourish the hair. The layer of fat beneath the skin protects the body from extremes of temperature. A pad of hard fat beneath each kidney protects it from being jarred and damaged. The soft fat in the breasts of a woman protects her glands from heat and cold and cushions them against shock. The fat that lards the muscles provides a ready supply of usable energy for their action. The subcutaneous tissue is a layer of connective tissue specializing in the formation of fat. It is unevenly distributed over the body. In addition to providing protection and insulation, it acts as a depository for reserve fuel to be drawn upon whenever the amount of calories taken is less than the amount burned up through activity. Normal activity obtains about 70% of its energy from fat oxidation; with strenuous activity, glucose oxidation provides additional energy. The average 20-year-old American woman needs about 2000 calories a day to meet her energy need. One pound of body fat provides 3500 calories, or enough for almost two days of energy needs. Normally, the brain and nerve cells depend on glucose, not fat, as the major source of energy. During starvation or after a period of glucose deprivation, brain cells develop the ability to metabolize fat for energy and so continue to function. Under these starvation conditions, the body may be in a state of ketosis or metabolic acidosis. The normal fat content is generally considered to be about 15% for a male and about 19% for a female by weight.

body fluids. About 40% of the body's water is found inside the cells, and about 15% bathes the outside of the cells. The remainder is in the blood vessels. Special conditions are needed to regulate the amounts of water inside and outside the cells so that they do not collapse from water leaving them or swell up under the stress of too much water entering them. The cells pump minerals across their membranes and these minerals carry water with them. This dynamic mineral transport activity is how the cells maintain water balance. Minerals, and some positively charged and some negatively charged ions, or electrolytes, maintain water balance and acid-base balance and play many other roles. The total number of positive and negative charges in the body fluids remains equal. The components of water also exist as positive and negative ions: H is a positive or hydrogen ion, and OH is a negative or hydroxyl ion. Excess OH ion in a solution makes it acid; excess OH ion makes it a base. The body protects itself against changes in the *acid-base balance* of its fluids by providing buffers, molecules that can accommodate excess positive or negative ions. The maintenance of the acid-base balance by the body's buffering system permits all other life processes to take place. In the human, the acid-base balance of the circulating blood and lymph is narrowly buffered around a pH value of 7.4; above or below pH 7.4 is considered a condition of *alkalosis* or *acidosis*. See *water balance*.

Fluid percent of body weight

TOTAL BODY WATER	INTRACELLULAR FLUID	INTERSTITIAL FLUID	PLASMA
50-60%	35-40%	11-15%	4-5%

body temperature. Warm-blooded animals maintain an approximately constant body temperature even though their environments may undergo relatively gross temperature changes. Basically, two mechanisms are involved in heat regulation: (1) a metabolic or chemical process which produces heat by breakdown of foods in the body, and (2) physical processes which eliminate heat. The metabolic processes involve to a large extent the oxidation of foods, which results in the production of heat. When more food is consumed than is required for caloric needs, maintenance of the body temperature, and physical activity, the excess food is converted into fat and stored as such. The loss of body heat takes place as follows: (1) About 70% is normally lost to the surrounding environment through radiation, convection, and conduction; (2) about 25% through evaporation of water from the external surface of the skin and internal surface of the lungs; (3) about 3 % of the total heat is used to bring the inspired air and ingested cold foods to body temperature; (4) about 1–2% is lost with the excreta. The normal body temperature for humans is 37°C or 98.6°F, no matter what the temperature of the environment. It should be recognized that the body temperatures given are average values and may vary slightly under normal conditions. See *fever*.

body weight. Many factors determine the body weight. Genetics and environment are usually the most frequently mentioned factors. The determination of a body weight that is healthy and consistent with longer life expectancy is a complex problem. For any given age, sex, and frame density, there is a range of 20–40 pounds that is considered "normal average weight" for a specific individual. However, there appears to be another "safe zone" range of 10–20 pounds above or below the normal average weight that is also healthy and not associated with a shortened life span. See *Weight Ranges for Heights of Men and Women* in the *Appendix*.

boiling point. The temperature at which the vapor pressure of a liquid equals the atmospheric pressure. At the boiling point, bubbles of vapor rise continually and break on the surface. The boiling temperature of pure water at sea level (barometer 30 inches) is 212°F (100°C). At high altitudes, the boiling point of water is lower because the atmospheric pressure is lower. At 5000 feet above sea level, for example, the boiling point of water is 203°F, at 10,000 feet, 194°F.

bologna. A mildly seasoned sausage made of finely ground beef, pork, or veal. The meat is packed into a casing and smoked. Good source of protein and fat with small amounts of *thiamine*, *riboflavin*, and *niacin*. See this item in the table under *meats*.

bolus. The mixture of food particles and saliva that results from mastication (the chewing process). See *deglutition*.

bomb calorimeter. An apparatus for measuring calories stored in foods or any organic material. The apparatus is carefully designed for measuring all the heat produced by the complete oxidation of an accurately measured amount of any food. The apparatus is insulated thoroughly against loss of heat, and the amount of heat produced is measured by the change in temperature of a measured amount of water. In an experiment, a weighed portion of the food whose caloric value is to be determined is placed in the bomb; after the bomb is charged with pure oxygen it is submerged in water. An electric circuit causes combustion to take place. The heat given off into the water is measured by a thermometer calibrated to 100° centigrade or Celsius (°C). The rise in temperature of the water and the total heat capacity of the water bath and bomb are determined; it is then possible to determine the energy released by food.

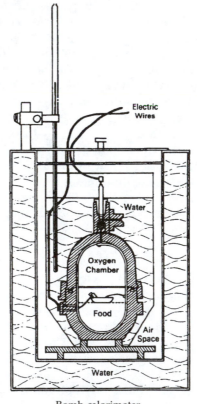

Bomb calorimeter
Davidson, S., et al., *Human Nutrition and Dietetics*, 1975. Reproduced with
permission of Churchill Livingstone, Edinburgh.

bonds. The physical forces that hold atoms together in molecules.

bone. Living tissue containing blood vessels and nerves within the hard bone structure. The living cells that form bones are osteocytes. Bone cells can select calcium and other minerals from blood and tissue fluid and deposit the calcium phosphate and calcium carbonate in the connective tissue fibers between cells. Periosteum, the membrane covering bone surfaces, carries blood vessels and nerves to the bone cells. Two kinds of bone are formed by the bone cells; compact and cancellous. Compact bone is hard and dense, while cancellous bone has a porous structure. The combination of compact and cancellous bone cells produces maximum strength with minimum weight. Bone contains 99% of the body's total metabolic *calcium* pool. Several vitamins are involved in bone development and maintenance. *Vitamin D* has a direct effect on the mobilization of calcium to and from bone. A vitamin D deficiency in a child results in the nutritional disease *rickets*, and the adult counterpart in *osteomalacia*. *Retinol* (vitamin A) is also required for proper bone development which stops if a retinol deficiency continues. *Ascorbic acid* (vitamin C) is also required for a normal skeleton since without it abnormal *collagen* is formed and this leads to an impaired calcium deposition (calcification). Bone is also very important in the maturation of *red blood cells*.

bone marrow. Two kinds of marrow, yellow and red, are found in the marrow cavities of bones. Red bone marrow is active *red blood cell* manufacturing material, producing red blood cells and many of the white blood cells. Deposits of red bone marrow in the adult are in cancellous proteins of some bones—the skull, ribs, and sternum, for example. Yellow bone marrow is mostly fat and is found in marrow cavities of mature long bones.

bonito (*Thunnus*). Any of various medium-sized tuna. A relative of the mackerel and kingfish, it lives in both the Atlantic and the Pacific. A saltwater fish caught commercially on a large scale. More of it is canned in flakes and chunks than is sold fresh. See this item as tuna in the table under *fish*.

boron (B). Element No. 5. At. Wt. 11. Minute traces of boron are found in body tissue, but no clues to its purpose have been discovered. Boron has been found to be essential for plant nutrition and growth, but experiments in animals have not demonstrated any evidence of deficiency after boron deprivation.

botulinus poisoning (botulism). Poisoning due to the ingestion of a toxic substance found preformed in food. Botulism is caused by a potent toxin secreted by different strains of *Clostridium botulinum*, an anaerobic, spore-forming organism which is widely distributed in soils. The bacterium grows readily under anaerobic conditions in improperly sterilized preserved foods which have a near-neutral or slightly alkaline reaction. The toxin of *C. botulinum* is one of the most potent poisons known. The ingestion of even minute quantities will result in a severe syndrome which may be fatal within 2–10 days. The entire human population could be eliminated by 200 g (7 ounces) of the toxin. Symptoms include headache, nausea, prostration, oculomotor abnormalities, blindness, progressive difficulty in swallowing and talking, ascending paralysis, and death. Treatment is primarily supportive in addition to the administration of polyvalent botulinus antitoxin. Inadequately processed home-canned foods are most often the cause of botulism, but preserved meats and fishes also are causes. In general, low- and medium-acid canned foods are most often incriminated. Of canned foods, those most often responsible for botulism have been string beans, sweet corn, beets, asparagus, spinach, and chard. Meats, fish and seafood, and milk products also have been responsible for outbreaks of botulism. Sausage and ham are often involved. The name "botulism" is derived from the Latin word for sausage, *botulus*, because the first recognized European outbreaks were caused by spoiled sausages. See *food poisoning*.

bowels. See *colon*.

bradycardia. Abnormal slowness of the heartbeat and pulse, characterized by a pulse rate that is under 60 beats per minute. The opposite of *tachycardia*.

brain. The brain, a mass of nervous tissue, is the highest level of the nervous system. It coordinates activities of the entire body; carries on the learning, thinking, and reasoning processes; and directs the voluntary movements of the body. The brain may be divided into three parts; the cerebrum, cerebellum, and the brain stem, the last consisting of the forebrain, midbrain, pons, and medulla. See *nervous system*.

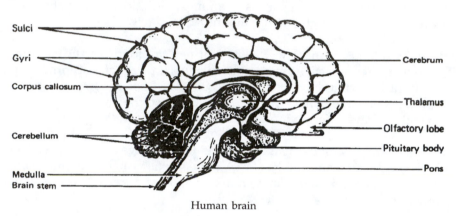

Human brain

brain development. The relationship between nutrition and brain development in humans is very complex and poorly understood. It is generally agreed that proper nutrition during the early years of life is extremely important. The fully developed human brain is so large relative to the body size that most brain development occurs after birth to permit the passage of the head during birth. The table shows that during the first three years of life the human brain almost quadruples in size.

Human brain growth

AGE YR	BRAIN WEIGHT KG (LBS)	% DEVELOPED	AGE YR	BRAIN WEIGHT KG (LBS)	% DEVELOPED
Newborn	340 (0.8)	42	3	1200 (2.7)	86
1	970 (2.2)	69	20	1400 (3.1)	100
2	1150 (2.6)	82			

bran. The outer layers of food grains, obtained during flour making, are called bran. Bran contains carbohydrates, vitamins, and minerals. It adds bulk to the diet and has a laxative effect. Bran is used as a breakfast food and as an ingredient in baking. Pure bran is dark brown in color and sold in the shape of flour, small strips, curls, and buds. Pure bran is often combined with another cereal such as wheat, and then pressed into flakes or little strips. The percentage of bran in these combinations is generally 40%. Bran cereal is a good source of carbohydrates and has fair amounts of *calcium* and *phosphorus*. See *cereals*, *grains*, and *wheat*.

brandy. This colorless, spirituous liquid is obtained by the evaporation, or distillation, of most of the watery portion of wine. The *alcohol* content is usually 50–60%. Wine can be made from grapes and other fruits, although the word "brandy" implies the use of grapes. The word itself comes from the middle English *brandywine* or *brandwine* which mean burnt wine, or wine distilled by high heat.

Brazil nut (*Bertholletia excelsa*). Botanically speaking, the Brazil nut is not a *nut* at all, but the edible seed of a rough-barked giant tree of the Amazon forest of South America. The fruit is globular, 4–6 inches in diameter, hard-walled, and contains 8–24 seeds, arranged like the sections of an orange. These seeds are white. The shell of the individual nut is triangular, dark brown, and very rough. The kernels are white with a rich flavor and are quite oily. Brazil nuts provide some protein, iron, and thiamine. Because of their high fat content, they are high in calories.

bread. A food made from flour or meal, liquid, and shortening. *Leavening* agents are usually added, and the dough or meal is shaped, allowed to rise, and baked. Breads are usually named after the meal or flours from which they are made, for example, corn bread, rye bread, whole wheat bread. The nutritive value of various breads is given in the table that follows.

brewer's yeast. The fungi *Saccharomyces cerevisiae*, which will ferment sugars to alcohol under anaerobic conditions. Brewer's yeast is a concentrated source of high-quality protein and of many B vitamins except *cobalamin* (vitamin B_{12}). Because it is also a good source of iron and phosphorus, it is sometimes prescribed for those needing dietary supplements. See *yeast*.

brine. A strong salt solution used in the preservation of fish, meats, and vegetables, and in pickling. See *curing*.

broccoli (*Brassica oleracea*). A dark-green vegetable that is closely related to cauliflower, cabbage, and brussels sprouts. Broccoli has tight small heads called curds, which sit like buds on a thick stem. Both heads and stems are eaten. One of the richest vegetable sources of *ascorbic acid* (vitamin C) if it is cooked quickly in a small amount of water. Excellent source of β-*carotene* (vitamin A activity), *riboflavin*, *iron*, and *calcium*. See this item in the table under *vegetables*.

bromelain. A proteolytic enzyme (*protease*) from pineapple that digests proteins. See *papain*.

brominated vegetable oil (BVo). Chemically, BVo is vegetable oil (olive, sesame, corn, or cottonseed) whose density has been increased to that of water by being combined with bromine. Flavoring oils are dissolved in BVo, which is then added to carbonated or noncarbonated fruit-flavor drinks. The lighter-than-water oils are dispersed throughout the drink by BVo, without which they would float to the surface and form a ring at the neck of the bottle. BVo also makes a soft drink slightly cloudy, giving the illusion of thickness or "body."

Food, Approximate Measure, and Weight (in grams)			Water	Food Energy	Protein	Fat
Breads:						
Boston brown bread, slice 3 by 3/4 in.	1 slice	48	45	100	3	1
Cracked-wheat bread:						
Loaf, 1 lb.	1 loaf	454	35	1,190	40	10
Slice, 18 slices per loaf.	1 slice	25	35	65	2	1
French or vienna bread:						
Enriched, 1 lb. loaf	1 loaf	454	31	1,315	41	14
Unenriched, 1 lb. loaf.	1 loaf	454	31	1,315	41	14
Italian bread:						
Enriched, 1 lb. loaf	1 loaf	454	32	1,250	41	4
Unenriched, 1 lb. loaf.	1 loaf	454	32	1,250	41	4
Raisin bread:						
Loaf, 1 lb.	1 loaf	454	35	1,190	30	13
Slice, 18 slices per loaf.	1 slice	25	35	65	2	1
Rye bread:						
American, light (⅓ rye, ⅔ wheat):						
Loaf, 1 lb.	1 loaf	454	36	1,100	41	5
Slice, 18 slices per loaf.	1 slice	25	36	60	2	Trace
Pumpernickel, loaf, 1 lb.	1 loaf	454	34	1,115	41	5
White bread, enriched:*						
Soft-crumb type:						
Loaf, 1 lb.	1 loaf	454	36	1,225	39	15
Slice, 18 slices per loaf.	1 slice	25	36	70	2	1
Slice, toasted	1 slice	22	25	70	2	1
Slice, 22 slices per loaf.	1 slice	20	36	55	2	1
Slice, toasted	1 slice	17	25	55	2	1
Loaf, 1½ lbs.	1 loaf	680	36	1,835	59	22
Slice, 24 slices per loaf.	1 slice	28	36	75	2	1
Slice, toasted	1 slice	24	25	75	2	1
Slice, 28 slices per loaf.	1 slice	24	36	65	2	1
Slice, toasted	1 slice	21	25	65	2	1
Firm-crumb type:						
Loaf, 1 lb.	1 loaf	454	35	1,245	41	17
Slice, 20 slices per loaf.	1 slice	23	35	65	2	1
Slice, toasted	1 slice	20	24	65	2	1
Loaf, 2 lbs.	1 loaf	907	35	2,495	82	34
Slice, 34 slices per loaf.	1 slice	27	35	75	2	1
Slice, toasted	1 slice	23	35	75	2	1
Whole-wheat bread, soft-crumb type:						
Loaf, 1 lb.	1 loaf	454	36	1,095	41	12
Slice, 16 slices per loaf.	1 slice	28	36	65	3	1
Slice, toasted	1 slice	24	24	65	3	1
Whole-wheat bread, firm-crumb type:						
Loaf, 1 lb.	1 loaf	454	36	1,100	48	14
Slice, 18 slices per loaf.	1 slice	25	36	60	3	1
Slice, toasted	1 slice	21	24	60	3	1

*Values for iron, thiamin, riboflavin, and niacin per pound of unenriched white bread would be as follows:

	Iron	Thiamine	Riboflavin	Niacin
	Milligrams	Milligrams	Milligrams	Milligrams
Soft crumb	3.2	.31	.39	5.0
Firm crumb	3.2	.32	.59	4.1

	FATTY ACIDS									
		UNSATURATED								
SATURATED (TOTAL)	OLEIC	LINOLEIC	CARBOHYDRATE	CALCIUM	IRON	VITAMIN A VALUE	THIAMINE	RIBOFLAVIN	NIACIN	ASCORBIC ACID
			22	43	.9	0	.05	.03	.6	0
2	5	2	236	399	5.0	Trace	.53	.41	5.9	Trace
			13	22	.3	Trace	.03	.02	.3	Trace
3	8	2	251	195	10.0	Trace	1.27	1.00	11.3	Trace
3	8	2	251	195	3.2	Trace	.36	.36	3.6	Trace
Trace	1	2	256	77	10.0	0	1.32	.91	11.8	0
Trace	1	2	256	77	3.2	0	.41	.27	3.6	0
3	8	2	243	322	5.9	Trace	.23	.41	3.2	Trace
			13	18	.3	Trace	.01	.02	.2	Trace
			236	340	7.3	0	.82	.32	6.4	0
			13	19	.4	0	.05	.02	.4	0
			241	381	10.9	0	1.04	.64	5.4	0
3	8	2	229	381	11.3	Trace	1.13	.95	10.9	Trace
			13	21	.6	Trace	.06	.05	.6	Trace
			13	21	.6	Trace	.06	.05	.6	Trace
			10	17	.5	Trace	.05	.04	.5	Trace
			10	17	.5	Trace	.05	.04	.5	Trace
5	12	3	343	571	17.0	Trace	1.70	1.43	16.3	Trace
			14	24	.7	Trace	.07	.06	.7	Trace
			14	24	.7	Trace	.07	.06	.7	Trace
			12	20	.6	Trace	.06	.05	.6	Trace
			12	20	.6	Trace	.06	.05	.6	Trace
4	10	2	228	435	11.3	Trace	1.22	.91	10.9	Trace
			12	22	.6	Trace				
			12	22	.6	Trace	.06	.05	.6	Trace
8	20	4	455	871	22.7	Trace	2.45	1.81	21.8	Trace
			14	26	.7	Trace	.07	.05	.6	Trace
			14	26	.7	Trace	.07	.05	.6	Trace
2	6	2	224	381	13.6	Trace	13.6	.45	12.7	Trace
			14	24	.8	Trace	.09	.03	.8	Trace
			14	24	.8	Trace	.09	.03	.8	Trace
3	6	3	216	449	13.6	Trace	1.18	0.54	12.7	Trace
			12	25	.8	Trace	.06	.03	.7	Trace
			12	25	.8	Trace	.06	.03	.7	Trace

bronchi. The *trachea* divides to form the two bronchi. One bronchus enters each lung, which divides into many small air passages called bronchioles or bronchial tubes, which lead air into the final air spaces within the lungs. See *respiratory system*.

bronchitis. An inflammation of the bronchi, the passageways of the lungs. It is usually an extension of colds or upper respiratory infections and has many of the same symptoms as pneumonia: cough, fever, and labored breathing. Asthmatic bronchitis is a loose term for the wheezing and cough which occur in allergic individuals who have symptoms, particularly in response to infection. Bronchiolitis is a viral inflammation of the smallest air passageways (bronchioles), usually occurring in infants. Its symptoms and signs are fever, cough, and labored breathing. Bronchitis, upper respiratory infection, laryngitis, and pneumonia may coexist in any given illness. An infection often involves several parts of the respiratory tree to varying degrees.

brown fat. Brown fat is much less abundant in humans than white fat, generally referred to as *body fat* or *adipose tissue*. Its role appears to be the production of heat (thermogenesis) from the oxidation of fat. In adult humans, it occurs in the upper back and neck regions. Infants have more brown fat than adults. Exposure to cold for extended periods appears to increase the brown fat content. White fat is a source of chemical energy, obtained from the energy oxidation of its fatty acids to produce *adenosine triphosphate* (ATP), an important form of chemical energy. In brown fat tissue, heat to warm the body is produced instead of ATP.

brucellosis. Milk from infected cows or goats may transmit the *coccobacilli* that cause brucellosis (undulant fever), transmitted through cuts or scratches in the skin of persons.

Brunner's glands. Mucus-secreting glands in the *duodenum* which provide mucus to protect the mucosa from irritation and erosion by the strongly acid gastric juices entering from the stomach. Emotional tension and stress inhibit these mucus secretions, a major factor in duodenal ulcer formation.

brussels sprouts (*Brassica oleracea gemmifera*). A member of the cabbage family, looking like miniature cabbage. The plant, instead of making one large cabbage head, produces a number of rows of small heads where the leaves are attached. By pulling away the lower leaves, the little heads are given room to develop. Brussels sprouts are high in *carotene* (vitamin A activity) and *ascorbic acid* (vitamin C), and contain fair amounts of iron. See this item in the table under *vegetables*.

BSP test. A chemical measure of liver function in which an injection of Bromsulphalein is given, and some time later a blood specimen is taken for analysis.

buckwheat (*Fagopyrum esculentum*). The triangular seeds of this plant are used as a cereal, although botanically speaking, it is a *herb*. It is not a member of the family of cereal grasses to which wheat belongs. High in carbohydrates, with small amounts of vitamins and minerals.

buffer. A substance that can help a solution resist or counteract changes in free acid or alkali concentration. There are many buffers in the body. The word "buffer" comes from a Middle English root meaning "to protect from blows." In chemistry, a buffer is a combination of a weak acid and its salt, or a weak base and its salt. A solution containing such a mixture is called a "buffer solution." Buffers protect a solution against wide variations in its pH (hydrogen ion or proton concentration), even when strong bases or acids are added. Buffers protect the acid-base balance of a solution by rapidly offsetting changes in ionized hydrogen concentrations. They resist pH change by either acid or base additions. Blood contains many buffer systems which include the *protein, hemoglobin, bicarbonate,* and *phosphate* buffer systems, which maintain a pH of the blood and body fluids at pH value of 7.4. See *acid and base.*

bulgur. A cracked *wheat* that retains the *bran* and germ.

bulk. Fruits, vegetables, and cereals such as bran, in addition to being good sources of carbohydrate and minor sources of protein, also provide bulk. Fruits and vegetables also contain *fiber* which is undigestible and nonabsorbable. As it travels through the intestines, bulk stimulates activity helpful in formation and maintenance of normal bowel habits.

bursa. A sac or saclike structure filled with fluid that acts as a cushion and prevents friction between two moving parts.

bursitis. A bursa is a small fluid-filled sac that permits one part of a joint to move easily over another part or over another structure. Bursae act to facilitate the gliding of muscles or tendons over bony or ligamentous surfaces. They are found throughout the body. In bursitis, a bursa becomes inflamed as the result of injury, gout, or acute or chronic infection.

butter. An edible animal *fat*, obtained from milk and cream which have been made solid by churning. Butter can be made from fresh or slightly acid milk. It can be salted or it can be sweet (nonsalted). Butter is high in fat with moderate amounts of *carotene* (vitamin A activity). Whipped butter contains one-third fewer calories than regular butter. The table on page 68 gives the nutritive content of butter. See *milk products.*

butterfat. Butterfat can be separated into high- and low-melting fractions, achieved by melting butter oil and letting crystallization take place first at a higher and then at a somewhat lower temperature. At the selected temperature, the solidified part of the fat can be easily separated from the liquid portion by pressing. The liquid portion, on further cooling, will again exhibit partial crystallization. Repeated separation of the solidified portion will result in a lower-melting solid fraction. The higher-melting butter components are superior for use in chocolate and ice cream manufacture and spray-dried butter emulsions, whereas the lower-melting fractions blended with unfractionated butter will increase spreadability for table use. Anhydrous milk fat is suitable for bulk distribution and can be used for reconstituted liquid dairy products and in reformations for special-purpose butters or shortenings.

buttermilk. Sour fluid is obtained by separating the *butterfat* from cream or milk which has been churned.

Nutrients in 100 g buttermilk

CALORIES KCAL	PROTEIN G	FAT G	CARBOHYDRATE G	ASCORBATE MG	NIACIN MG	CALCIUM MG
36	4	0.1	5	1	0.1	121

Butter

Food, Approximate Measure, and Weight (in grams)	GM	Water Per Cent	Food Energy Calories	Protein GM	Fat GM	Saturated (Total GM)	Oleic GM	Linoleic GM	Carbohydrate GM	Calcium MG	Iron MG	Vitamin A Value I.U.
Regular, 4 sticks per pound:												
Stick ½ cup	113	16	810	1	92	51	30	3	1	23	0	[21] 3,750
Tablespoon (approx. 1 tbsp. ⅛ stick)	14	16	100	Trace	12	6	4	Trace	Trace	3	0	[21] 470
Pat (1-in sq. ⅓-in high; 90 per lb)	5	16	35	Trace	4	2	1	Trace	Trace	1	0	[21] 170
Whipped, 6 sticks or 2, 8-oz containers per pound:												
Stick ½ cup	76	16	540	1	61	34	20	2	Trace	15	0	[21] 2,500
Tablespoon (approx. 1 tbsp. ⅛ stick)	9	16	65	Trace	8	4	3	Trace	Trace	2	0	[21] 310
Pat (1¼-in sq. ⅓-in high; 120 per lb)	4	16	25	Trace	3	2	1	Trace	Trace	1	0	[21] 130

butternut (*Juglans cinerea*). A native North American nut, also known as a white walnut, used primarily in cakes and cookies. Butternuts are very difficult to shell but do not need blanching. They grow in small clusters inside spongy, hair-covered husks. Butternuts contain some protein and iron and are high in fat.

butternut squash (*Cucurbita*). A winter squash, smooth and hard-shelled, long and slender, with seeds contained in a small hollow in the base. The squash gets its name from its color which, for most of the year, is light brown or dark yellow. The flesh is almost orange. Its flavor is sweet, and it mashes smoothly and is comparatively quick-cooking. Butternut squash is an excellent source of β-*carotene* (vitamin A activity) and also provides fair amounts of *ascorbic acid* (vitamin C), iron, and riboflavin. See squash in the table under *vegetables*.

butylated hydroxyanisole (BHA) and butylated hydroxytoluene (BHT). See *BHA*.

butyric acid. Mol. Wt. 88. A *saturated fatty acid* that occurs as a glyceride to the extent of about 5–6% in butter and in very small amounts in a few other *fats*. Butyric acid is a mobile liquid, mixing in all proportions with water, alcohol, and ether; boiling without decomposition, and readily volatile with steam.

$$CH_3—CH_2—CH_2—COOH$$

Butyric acid

C

C. The alphabetic symbol for the amino acid *cysteine* (Cys).

cabbage (*Brassica*). The word cabbage is an anglicized version of the colloquial French word *caboche*, which means "head." Cabbage comes in many varieties, some with loose heads, some with firm ones, and others with flat, conical, or egg-shaped heads. Some cabbages are white, some green, some red; some have plain leaves and some curly ones. Raw cabbage is a very good source of *ascorbic acid* (vitamin C) and some *carotene* (vitamin A activity). Celery cabbage has a smaller amount. Cabbage also contains the goitrogenic agents *thiourea* and *thiocyanates*. During the cooking process, there may be some vitamin loss. See this item in the table under *vegetables*.

cabbage palm (*Roystonea oleracea*). The name given to several kinds of palm trees, which have edible parts. One of these is *O. oleracea*, which is cut down for food when about 3 years old. The parts eaten are the tender central leaves, used as greens, and especially the terminal bud and the tender inside of the thick stem, the "hearts of palm." The taste of these is bland and delicate.

cacao (*Threobroma cacao*). When taken from the pod, cacao or cocoa beans are covered with a limey or fruity pulp which is removed by means of a fermentation process. The pulp-covered seeds are placed in piles, in pits, or in a "sweating box," where they are covered with banana or plantain leaves. During the 3–13 days of fermentation, the beans are stirred and turned to aerate them and to keep down the temperature. The fermentation removes the adhering pulp from the bean, killing the embryo in the seed, and giving aroma, flavor, and color to the bean.

cactus pear. Prickly pear is another name for this fruit of one of a group of plants known as succulents. There are a number of edible varieties, with a water content that averages 85% and a high sugar content. The two most common varieties are the *Opuntia fiscus-indica* and the *O. tuna*. The *O. fiscus-indica* has an oval fruit and is about 1½–3 inches in diameter, with a yellowish skin and pink or reddish pulp. The fruit of the *Tuna* is pear-shaped or roundish, and measures about 1–1½ inches in diameter. Cactus pears have a mild, sweet flavor and are usually eaten raw.

cadmium (Cd). Element No. 48. At. Wt. 112. Cadmium inactivates certain *enzymes*. In large quantities it is a poison. Cadmium can be absorbed from drinking water that has not run through galvanized pipes in significant quantities. Traces of cadmium are present in body tissues and its existence has been known for some time. However, it was not until 1960 that cadmium was isolated as a definite component of a metal-containing protein. The protein metallothionein, found in the renal cortex of the horse, contains cadmium, zinc, and sulfur. The significance of this cadmium-containing protein is not yet clear, but it points to the possibility that the mineral functions in some basic biologic system as a micronutient. See *minerals*.

caffeine. Mol. Wt. 194. The coffee bean in Arabia, the tea leaf in China, the cola nut in West Africa, the cocoa bean in Mexico, the ilex plant, which provides maté in Brazil, and the cassina or Christmas berry tree in North America all contain caffeine. Caffeine is an alkaloid structurally identified as 1,3,7-trimethylxanthine. It is one of several *xanthine* derivatives which occur naturally in coffee beans, tea leaves, cola nuts, and cocoa beans. Theophylline and theobromine are well-known caffeine derivatives. The most common plants in which caffeine occurs are coffee, tea, chocolate, and cola. Caffeine is readily extracted from plant sources and is very soluble in boiling water, from which it crystallizes as a monohydrate with one molecule of water. Pure caffeine is odorless and has a distinctly bitter taste. Dietary caffeine is consumed almost entirely in beverages. Relatively insignificant amounts enter the diet through other foods, such as coffee-flavored ice cream, chocolate bars, and other chocolate-flavored foods. There are no significant uses of caffeine other than in food and drugs. Definitive tests have shown that caffeine is not adaptive, and regular consumption does not diminish its standard effects. However, caffeine withdrawal is well known. Experiments indicate that caffeine is effective in preventing attention lapses after the first hour and the effect persists for 2 or 3 days. The subjects of testing felt more alert and physically active. Performance of physical tasks, particularly ones involving speed, improved. Most caffeine consumed comes from coffee. Caffeine is absorbed rapidly and reaches peak levels in the body about 1 hour after ingestion. While individual tolerances vary, anywhere from 200–300 mg of caffeine (which is equivalent to three or four cups of coffee per day) appears to be a mild stimulant helpful in temporarily relieving minor fatigue with little risk of any harmful effects. High levels of caffeine, however, are clearly toxic. Ingestion of toxic levels of caffeine has caused convulsions

Caffeine

Caffeine content in foods

PRODUCT	AMOUNT	CAFFEINE MG	PRODUCT	AMOUNT	CAFFEINE MG
Coffee			Tea		
drip	5 oz	115	U.S. brands	5 oz	40
percolator	5 oz	80	import brands	5 oz	60
instant	5 oz	65	instant	12 oz	30
brewed, decaf	5 oz	3	iced	5oz	70
Cocoa	5 oz	4	Chocolate		
Chocolate milk	5 oz	5	semi-sweet	1 oz	20
Milk chocolate	8 oz	20	Baker's choc.	1 oz	26
			Choc. syrup	1oz	4

and vomiting with complete recovery in 6 hours. Protracted abuse of coffee may be responsible for arrhythmia in a small percent of the population. Coffee and tea drinking have been suspected, along with other risk factors, as causes of myocardial infarction and other cardiovascular diseases; however, evidence to support this suspected relationship is lacking.

calciferol (Vitamin D₂). A synthetic form of *vitamin D*, it has the most vitamin D activity of those substances derived from *ergosterol*. It is used for prophylaxis and treatment of vitamin D deficiency, rickets, and hypocalcemic tetany.

calcification. Process by which organic tissue becomes hardened by a deposit of calcium salts.

calcitonin. A *thyroid hormone* concerned with the metabolism of *calcium* in the body. The major effect of calcitonin on calcium metabolism is to increase deposition and to prevent removal of mineral matter from the bones. Calcitonin is antagonistic to the activity of the hormone from the *parathyroid glands, parathormone*. Together the two hormones maintain a steady balance of calcium ion (Ca^{+2}) in the blood. Alone, calcitonin leads to a decrease in the blood Ca^{+2} level. Calcitonin production is regulated by feedback through Ca^{+2}. *Vitamin D* is also involved in this regulatory system since it is needed for the transport of Ca^{+2} through the blood. Calcitonin is a polypeptide consisting of a single chain of 32 amino acids. The sequence of these amino acids has been established and the substance has been synthesized.

calcium (Ca). Element No. 20. At. Wt. 40. Of all the minerals in the human body, calcium is present in the largest amounts. It comprises about 1.4–2.0% of total body weight. About 90% of body calcium is in the skeletal tissues (bones and teeth) as deposits of calcium salts (apatite). The remaining calcium, which occurs in the plasma and other body fluids, performs highly important metabolic tasks. It occurs in three forms: (1) nondiffusible, (2) diffusible, or (3) diffusible, but a constituent of an organic complex. From 10–30% of the calcium in an average diet is absorbed through the intestine. The physiologic function of 99% of the calcium in the body is to build and maintain skeletal tissue, and to form teeth. The remaining 1% of the body's calcium performs several vital physiologic functions. In blood clotting, calcium ions are required for bonding between *fibrin* molecules and for stability of the fibrin threads. Calcium is also required for conversion of *prothrombin* to *thrombin*. Thrombin is an enzyme necessary for blood clotting. *Vitamin K* is also involved in these clotting reactions. Dairy products supply the bulk of dietary calcium. One quart of milk contains about 1 g of calcium, and cheese contains a comparable amount. Secondary sources are egg yolks, green leafy vegetables, legumes, nuts, and whole grains. Calcium in the body is usually associated with phosphorus, which is about 1% of body weight. A man who weighs 154 pounds will have 2.3–3.1 pounds of calcium and 1.2–1.7 pounds of phosphorus in his body. About 99% of the calcium and 80–90% of the phosphorus are in the bones and teeth. The rest is in the soft tissue and body fluids and is important to their normal functioning. Phosphorus is an essential part of all cells and occurs primarily as phosphate, ($-PO_4^{-3}$), taking part in the chemical reaction with proteins, fats, and carbohydrates to give the body energy and vital materials for growth and repair. It is one of the *buffer systems* in the blood and helps the blood neutralize *acids and bases*. Both calcium and phosphorus are essential for the work of the muscles and for the normal response of nerves to stimulation. Calcium and phosphorus and other minerals in food are dissolved as the food is digested. Then they are absorbed from the gastrointestinal tract into the bloodstream. The blood carries them to different parts of the body where they are used for growth and upkeep. *Vitamin D* is essential for the absorption of calcium from the gastrointestinal tract. Egg yolk, butter, fortified margarine, and certain fish oils are the chief sources. Too much vitamin D can be dangerous in that it overloads the blood and tissues with calcium. Two hormones secreted by the *parathyroid gland, calcitonin* and *parathormone*, play an important part in the body's use of calcium. Parathormone and calcitonin in the presence of vitamin D keep the amount of calcium in the blood at a normal level of about 10 mg per 100 mL of blood serum. The amount of calcium absorbed by the body is affected by the body's needs, the amount supplied by the diet, the kind of food that supplies it, and the speed with which the food passes through the gastrointestinal tract. See *blood clotting*.

Calcium content in foods

FOOD	AMOUNT	CALCIUM MG	FOOD	AMOUNT	CALCIUM MG
Meat, fish, poultry			Grain products		
beef	1 oz	3	bread, white	1 slice	21
pork	1 oz	3	whole wheat	1 slice	23
chicken	1 oz	4	biscuits	2 in	42
liver	1 oz	4	doughnut, cake	1 ea	13
fish	1 oz	12	doughnut	1 ea	11
tuna	1/4 cup	2	pancake	4 in	45
sardines, canned	1 oz	86	sweet roll	1 ea	35
salmon, canned	1 oz	74	waffle	5 in	85
luncheon meat	1 oz	3	cereal, cooked	3/4 cup	35
bacon, strip	1-5 g	1	cereal, dry	1/2 cup	14
Meat substitutes			Sweets		
eggs	1 ea	28	candy, sugar	1/2 oz	0
dried beans	1/2 cup	44	chocolate	1/2 oz	26
lentils	1/2 cup	25	honey	1 tbsp	4
peanut butter	1 tbsp	11	jelly	1 tbsp	2
Milk			sugar, white	1 tbsp	0
whole	1 cup	290	sugar, brown	1 tbsp	9
skim	1 cup	302	syrup, maple	1 tbsp	33
buttermilk	1 cup	285	Desserts		
chocolate	1 cup	280	cookies	1/2 in	7
cocoa	1 cup	298	cake, white	2x2x3 in	34
Other dairy products			pie, cream	1/8 pie	62
yogurt, low fat	8 oz	415	pie, fruit	1/8 pie	23
Cheddar cheese	1 oz	204			
Swiss cheese	1 oz	272			
American cheese	1 oz	174			
cottage cheese	1/4 cup	31			
half and half	2 tbsp	32			
ice cream	1/2 cup	88			
sherbet	1/2 cup	51			

calcium propionate. Mol. Wt. 186. The calcium salt of *propionic acid* is a chemical used to prevent growth of mold and certain bacteria in bread and rolls and also provides a calcium supplement to this diet. The sodium salt, sodium propionate, is preferred in pies and cakes because calcium alters the action of chemical leavening agents. Propionic acid occurs naturally in many foods and acts as a natural preservative in Swiss cheese. Propionate is also formed and used as a source of energy when the body metabolizes certain fats and amino acids. Propionates inhibit growth but do not kill bacteria or molds.

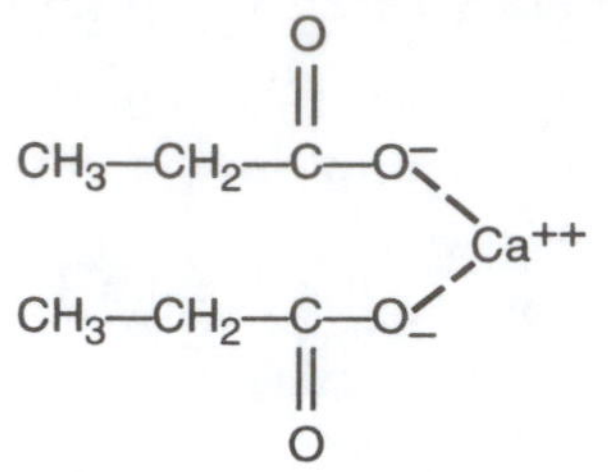

$$CH_3-CH_2-C-O^- \\ \quad\quad\quad\quad\quad Ca^{++} \\ CH_3-CH_2-C-O^-$$

Calcium proprionate

calcium test. A chemical test on blood, used as a screening test and also for the diagnosis of bone disease and certain *parathyroid*, kidney, and pancreatic diseases.

calcium-to-phosphorus ratio (Ca:P ratio). Since calcium and phosphorus are intimately related in metabolism, two ratios between them are significant. (1) The dietary calcium-to-phosphorus ratio affects absorption of these minerals; a 1:1 ratio is ideal for growth, pregnancy, and lactation periods. Otherwise, for adults a 1:1.5 ratio of calcium to phosphorus is required. (2) The serum calcium to phosphorus ratio is the solubility product of two minerals in the serum. An increase in one mineral causes a decrease in the other to maintain a constant product of the two. The normal serum level of calcium is 10 mg per 100 mL; phosphorus is about 4 mg per 100 mL in adults.

calculus. Any abnormal accretion within the body of material which forms a "stone." Calculi are usually composed of mineral salts. The most commonly formed renal calculi are composed of calcium salts. See *tartar*.

caloric equivalent. The number of calories produced per liter of oxygen (O_2) for each oxidizing foodstuff (fat, carbohydrates, and protein) is the caloric equivalent. The values for the three foodstuffs are almost the same—within 10%. Therefore, by determining the amount of oxygen utilized and multiplying it by the caloric equivalent, the number of calories produced can be determined. This is the basis for *indirect calorimetry* measurements. The caloric equivalent value is 4.8 calories per liter of O_2. See *energy balance*.

caloric requirements. The amount of energy required to maintain life is the sum total of calories needed to satisfy requirements for *basal metabolism*, the thermogenic action or *specific dynamic action* of food, as well as for growth, repair, and physical activity. Even minor physical activity adds to caloric requirements above the basal requirement, or BMR. The act of walking on level ground at 2.5 mph requires an expenditure of about 180 calories per hour for an average adult; walking uphill on a 5% grade requires 270 calories per hour, and on a 15% grade, 490 calories. See *energy balance*.

caloric value of food constitutents. Substances such as *carbohydrates* and *fats*, which contain only carbon, hydrogen, and oxygen, yield approximately the same amount of heat when oxidized in the body as when oxidized in a laboratory *bomb calorimeter*. Proteins, which also contain nitrogen, yield smaller caloric values when oxidized in the body. This is due to the fact that 12–17% of the protein molecule is made up of nitrogen, which is not oxidized but eliminated principally as *urea*. At any one time the oxidation of 1 g of glucose in the body yields approximately 3.7 calories—starch yields 4.1 calories and sucrose, 4.0 calories. Since the average diet contains more starch than other carbohydrate constituent, the approximate figure of 4 calories per gram has been taken as the caloric value of the carbohydrates in the diet. The complete oxidation of olive oil in the body yields 9.4 calories per gram of oil, and that of butterfat 9.2 calories. Other fats yield somewhat smaller values, and the approximate figure of 9 calories per gram is generally used as the caloric value of fats in the diet. The average caloric value of protein in the body is 4.1 calories per gram; the round figure of 4 is generally used in dietary calculations. See *caloric equivalent* and *oxidation of food*.

calorie. The commonly used standard for measurement of the energy value of substances is the calorie. The same term is used to express the body's energy requirement. The unit used in nutritional work is the large calorie (Cal) or the kilocalorie (kcal) and is the amount of heat required to raise the temperature of 1 kg of water 1° C. The small calorie (cal), or gram calorie, is one one-thousandth of the value of the large unit and is used when minute amounts of heat are to be considered; 3500 calories equal 1 pound of body fat. The relationship between calorie input and energy output is called "calorie balance." Another unit of energy measurement is the joule, a unit used also in other scientific fields. To convert calories to joules, the factor used is 1 calorie equals 4.184 joules. Calories are derived from the metabolism of carbohydrates, protein, and fat. Proteins and carbohydrates contain 4 calories per gram, fat has 9. All calories are alike, and 4 protein calories are equal to 4 fat calories. So there is really no such thing as a "fattening food."

calorie measurements (values). The original work was done with the *bomb calorimeter* using weighed amounts of pure *fat*, pure *carbohydrate*, and pure *protein*. From the data, average daily calorie value was derived for each food. It became apparent that corrections were necessary when calculating energy values for human diets because some foods are not completely absorbed, and proteins are not completely oxidized to carbon dioxide and water as they are in the calorimeter. Extensive experimentation showed the following rounded figures were suitable for practical use in calculating values of the usually mixed diets eaten: 1 g of pure carbohydrate yields 4 calories; 1 g of pure fat yields 9 calories; 1 g of pure protein yields 4 calories.

calorimeter. An instrument for measuring the heat change in any system, and the *bomb calorimeter* used to measure the *calorie (energy)* value of foods.

calorimetry. The measurement of heat loss. An instrument for measuring heat output of the body or the energy value of foods is called a calorimeter. See *direct calorimetry* and *indirect calorimetry*.

cancer. A malignant *tumor*. Cancer comprises a broad group of malignant neoplasms which are divided into two categories of *carcinomas* and *sarcomas*.

cantaloupe (*Cucumis melo cantalupenis*). A variety of muskmelon, with a sweet and fragrant taste. The cantaloupe was named for a castle in Italy. Cantaloupe is an excellent source of *carotene* (vitamin A activity) and *ascorbic acid* (vitamin C). See this item in the table under *fruits*.

capers (*Capparis*). The unopened flowers of the caper bush. During the flowering season, the buds are picked before the petals can expand and are preserved in vinegar and salt. Capers add liveliness to white and other sauces, to salads and creamed dishes, and act as condiments to appetizers, meats, and seafood.

capillaries. Small microscopic vessels forming networks in all tissues lying between the arterial and venous systems. Somewhat larger than a red cell, thin walled, permitting oxygen, nutrients, and other substances to diffuse through their walls to reach the living tissues. See *blood vessels*.

capillary fluid shift mechanism. The process which controls the movement of water and small molecules in solution (*electrolytes*, nutrients) between the blood in the capillaries and the surrounding *interstitial* area. See *osmosis*.

caproic acid. Mol. Wt. 116. A *saturated fatty acid* occurring in cow and goat butter and coconut fat.

$$CH_3{-}CH_2{-}CH_2{-}CH_2{-}CH_2{-}COOH$$

Caproic acid

caprylic acid. Mol. Wt. 148. A *saturated fatty acid* occurring in coconut oil, goat, and cow butter, and human fat.

$$CH_3{-}CH_2{-}CH_2{-}CH_2{-}CH_2{-}CH_2{-}CH_2{-}COOH$$

Caprylic acid

caramelize. The word "caramel" has two meanings. It describes a candy with a chewy consistency, and it is also a culinary term that refers to the burning of sugar by itself or thinned with water. To caramelize is to heat sugar or foods containing sugar until a brown color and characteristic flavor develop.

caraway (*Carum carvi*). An oval-shaped brown seed named after the ancient district of Caria in Asia Minor. The caraway plant grows to a height of about 2 feet, with feathery green leaves and yellow-white flowers that resemble Queen Anne's lace. Fresh young leaves add flavor to soups, salads, cheeses, vegetables, and meat. The roots may be steamed and eaten as a vegetable. Caraway seeds are used to season soups, meats, vegetables, breads such as rye, cakes, and pastries. Oil extracted from the seed provides the distinctive flavor of the liqueur kümmel.

carbohydrate digestion. *Starches* are complex forms of *sugars*. When starch is eaten, a digestive enzyme in the *saliva* of the mouth, *salivary amylase*, mixes the starch and begins the digestive process. As the food is swallowed, this step continues in the stomach process, where starch is converted to *oligosaccharides* and sugars. In the small intestine, digestive enzymes from the *pancreas*, pancreatic amylases, and from the walls of the intestine itself complete the process. The final products are *monosaccharides*. A similar transformation takes place when sugar replaces starch in the ripening of fruit. *Cellulose*, the carbohydrate that forms the cell walls of vegetables and fruits of all plants, is not digested by humans or mammals. Cellulose is important in the mechanics of the digestive process, however, because it provides fiber bulk and thus aids in discarding residues of *digestion*.

carbohydrate, indigestible. Substances which make up the cell wall structure of plants, consisting of varying amounts of *cellulose, hemicellulose, lignin, pectin* substances, *gums, mucin,* etc., which cannot be hydrolyzed by enzymes of the human *digestive system*. They are not available for *glycogen* formation.

carbohydrate metabolism. The metabolism of *carbohydrates* proceeds in the liver and all body tissues. *Glucose* is carried in the bloodstream from the intestine to the liver. In the presence

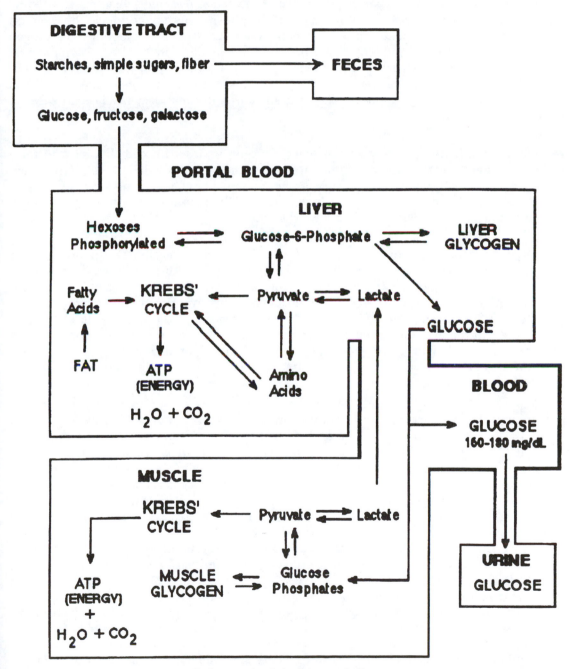

Pathways of carbohydrate metabolism

of the enzyme hexokinase and a high-energy phosphate complex, *adenosine triphosphate* (ATP), glucose is phosphorylated to glucose-6-phosphate, then to glucose-1-phosphate, and is finally stored as *glycogen*. The high-energy compound *uridine triphosphate* (UTP) is involved in the latter reactions. This *polysaccharide* glycogen is found in muscle tissue as well as in the liver, heart, brain, and other tissues. The liver glycogen acts as an *energy reserve* for the other tissues. For carbohydrate metabolism to proceed normally, several B vitamins, as well as the minerals magnesium and phosphorus, are required. *Niacin, riboflavin, thiamine, pyridoxine*, and *pantothenic acid* function as *coenzymes*, and magnesium and phosphorus as cofactors in the chemical reactions involved in the metabolism of carbohydrates. When energy is required, glycogen is broken down to glucose and is oxidized. Hormones are involved in this breakdown process, notably *epinephrine* or *glucagon*. The hormones initiate the formation of the "second messenger," cyclic 3', 5'-*adenosine monophosphate* (*cyclic AMP*) which in turn initiates the breakdown of *glycogen* to glucose-1-phosphate. The diagram traces the major metabolic pathways of carbohydrates in humans.

carbohydrate oxidation. The process in which oxygen unites with carbohydrates to form carbon dioxide, water and heat, and chemical energy, ultimately through the *terminal respiratory chain*. Heat represents the energy available for the maintenance of body temperature. Chemical energy, mainly in the form of *adenosine triphosphate* (ATP), is used for synthetic, mechanical, electrical, and physical work. See *carbohydrate metabolism*.

carbohydrate storage. Carbohydrate is stored in the liver and other cells as the polysaccharide *glycogen*. In the liver, glycogen is not only stored as fuel for other tissues, but also serves two other important functions. First, it exerts a protective action by being present as glycogen and by participating in specific detoxifying metabolic pathways. Second, carbohydrate has a regulatory influence on protein and fat metabolism. Sufficient carbohydrates for energy demands prevent the oxidation of too much protein for this purpose. This protein-sparing effect of carbohydrates allows a major portion of protein to be used for its basic structural purposes of tissue building. The amount of carbohydrate present also determines how efficiently fat will be broken down.

carbohydrates. The name derives from the elemental composition of carbon, hydrogen, and oxygen. The hydrogen and oxygen are in the same ratio as in water, 2:1, hence the name hydrate. Carbohydrates divide into three groups, according to their size and complexity. The complex carbohydrates degrade by digestive enzymes into simple sugars before the body absorbs them. Carbohydrates classify as simple sugars or *monosaccharides*, such as *glucose* or *fructose*; *disaccharides* (composed of two simple sugars); *oligosaccharides* (composed of several simple sugars); and *polysaccharides* (composed of many simple sugars). Carbohydrates supply about 20% of daily energy requirements. The simple sugars and the disaccharides are sweet, a general characteristic of the polyalcohols. The larger polysaccharides may contain more than 1000 monosaccharides in a branched chain array. *Glycogen* and *amylopectin* are examples. Other polysaccharides have a simple linear structure. The starches are examples. Mucilage, plant gums, and cellulose are other common examples of polysaccharides. Polysaccharides serve as energy sources and perform structural functions, depending upon their compositions. Glucose is the most common of the monosaccharides. Carbohydrates function as a primary energy source in human nutrition, yet there are no specific nutritional requirements for carbohydrates. The oxidation of glucose facilitates the oxidation of fat, the major energy source. The starches, which consist of glucose units only, are the only carbohydrates that humans use very efficiently. Important sources of starches for human nutrition are wheat, rice, corn, sorghum, millet, and rye; they contain about 70% starch. Potatoes and other tubers and roots are also rich sources of starch. Under ordinary circumstances, about 97% of the carbohydrates ingested by humans absorb through the digestive tract. A constant source of glucose is necessary for the proper functioning of the brain and the central nervous system. Brain cells, unlike most cells, contain little or no stored supply of glucose and are dependent on a constant supply of glucose from the blood. Sustained, profound hypoglycemic shock, such as in insulin shock, may cause irreversible brain damage.

Classification of carbohydrates

CARBOHYDRATE	% OF TOTAL CARBOHY-DRATE INTAKE	MAJOR FOOD SOURCES	REMARKS
Monosaccharides			
Glucose	5	Fruits, honey, corn syrup, starches.	Biosynthesized by most animal and plant cells. Produced by the liver in humans.
Fructose	5	Fruits, vegetables.	Biosynthesized in humans in a phosphorylated form.
Galactose		Milk (lactose).	Galactose derivatives are important in some genetic diseases.
Carbohydrate derivatives			
Ethanol	Varies	Fermented liquors.	All are naturally occurring products and readily absorbed.
Lactate	Trace	Milk, milk products.	
Malate	Trace	Fruits.	
Citrate	Trace		
Disaccharides			
Sucrose	25	Beet/cane sugars sugars, maples syrup.	
Lactose	10		
Maltose	Trace	Milk, milk products.	In adults, digestive enzyme *lactase* is often absent.
Trehalose	Trace	Malt products, breakfast cereals.	
Levulose	—	Mushrooms, yeast.	
		Synthetic.	Used in some laxatives. Indigestible.
Polysaccharides			
Celluloses		Stalks, leaves, seeds.	
Pectins	3	Fruits.	Indigestible.
Gums	Total		
Mucilages		Seeds, plant saps.	
—		—	—
Inulin		Mushrooms, onions, garlic.	
Galactans		Snails.	This group is partially digestible. Enteric bacteria may degrade further. Raffinose and stachyose produce flatus.
Mannosans	2	Legumes.	
Raffinose	Total	Sugar beets, lentils, navy beans, kidney beans.	
Stachyose		Beans.	
Pentosans		Fruits, gums.	
—		—	
Starches		—	
Dextrins	50		—
Glycogen		Grain, vegetables.	This group is the most important carbohydrate source for humans.
		Meats, seafoods.	

carbon (C). Element No. 6. At. Wt. 12. This chemical element is present in all substances designated as organic. These include proteins, carbohydrates, and fats. When a compound containing carbon combines with oxygen in the body, energy is liberated and carbon dioxide is formed. Compounds that do not contain carbon are classed as inorganic. Carbon has several chemical features that make it unique as a foundation for life. Its four *valences* and tetrahedral structure allow a wide variety of compounds to be formed with a carbon backbone, and the compounds themselves can be stereospecific. Living reactions involving carbon are stereospecifically selected. For example, all proteins contain only L-amino acid forms. Biochemical reactions then differ from chemical reactions by the specificity that the structure of carbon allows.

carbon dioxide. Mol. Wt. 44, CO_2. A colorless gas, heavier than air, generally produced in the combustion or decombustion of carbon or its compounds. It is the metabolic product of carbon compounds present in foods. In plants, CO_2 is important for photosynthesis. The fixation of CO_2 by chlorophyll-containing plants to synthesize starch is a process on which most of life ultimately depends. Fatty acid synthesis in animals also depends on the presence of CO_2 in the formation of the intermediate *methyl malonyl-CoA*.

carbonic acid. Mol. Wt. 62. Carbonic acid is a part of the important bicarbonate *buffer system* in the body. Carbonic acid is formed when carbon dioxide dissolves in water: *Acid* drives the reaction to the left and carbon dioxide (CO_2) is formed. In the equation shown, *base* drives the reaction to the right and *bicarbonate* salts (HCO_3^-) are formed. The exchanges are important in respiration at the cellular level, in hemoglobin chemistry, and in the lungs.

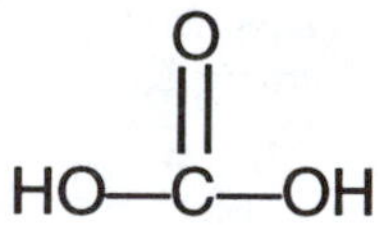

$$HO-\overset{\overset{\textstyle O}{\|}}{C}-OH$$

Carbonic acid

$$CO_2 + H_2O \rightleftharpoons H_2CO_3$$

carbonyl group. A functional chemical group found in *aldehydes*, *ketones*, and *saccharides*. This group is found in all *monosaccharides* (sugars).

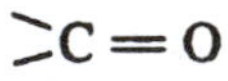

$$>\!C = O$$

Carbonyl group

carboxyl group. The acid group of organic compounds. The structure $-COOH$ dissociates a hydrogen ion (proton, H^+) in aqueous solution and is therefore an *acid*. Carboxyl groups are weak acids because there is a tendency to associate with a proton, that is, the reaction tends toward the left. A weak acid and its salt form a buffer system that resists change in the hydrogen ion concentration in its solution.

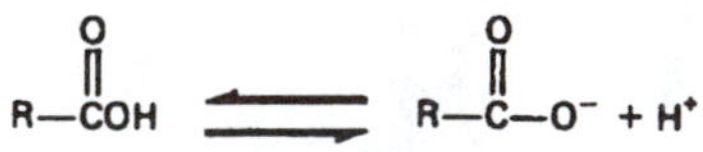

$$R-\overset{\overset{\textstyle O}{\|}}{C}OH \rightleftharpoons R-\overset{\overset{\textstyle O}{\|}}{C}-O^- + H^+$$

Carboxyl group

carboxylation. Reactions which involve the addition of *carbon dioxide* (CO_2) to an organic compound. The reactions are often referred to as carbon dioxide (CO_2) fixation in plants. The vitamin *biotin* is often involved in CO_2 *fixation* reactions. For example, biotin is a coenzyme for the reaction of methyl malonyltranscarboxylase that forms methylmalonyl *coenzyme A*, an intermediate in fatty acid synthesis that requires CO_2 fixation. *Vitamin K* is also involved in the carboxylation of a terminal glutamic acid residue in the formation of normal *prothrombin*.

carboxylic acid. An organic compound containing a *carboxyl group*.

carboxypeptidase. A digestive *enzyme* formed initially from an inactive state called procarboxypeptidase. Carboxypeptidase is specific and differs from other proteolytic digestive enzymes. It hydrolyzes only peptide bonds that are adjacent to the free carboxylic acid end of the peptide chain. Each molecule of the enzyme contains an atom of *zinc*, which is involved in the active site of the enzyme. When the zinc atom is removed, all enzyme action is lost. See *digestion*.

carcinogen. A substance that can cause the development of cancer cells. Over 400 different carcinogens have been identified. See *food toxins*.

carcinoma. A form of *cancer* that consists of a malignant *tumor* originating in the epithelial tissues and tending to spread (*metastasis*) to other tissues. See *epithelium*.

cardamom (*Elettaria cardamomum*). A plant growing to a height of 8–12 feet, the seeds of which are used as a flavoring and grow in groups within a pod which resembles a capsule. The capsules are sun-dried and marketed whole. Cardamom is said to be the world's second most precious spice, the costliest one being *saffron*. Cardamom seeds are brown, and they have an odor and a warm, spicy taste. They are used in curries and in such meats as frankfurters and sausages, in pickling-spice blends, and in baked foods.

cardiac. Pertaining to the heart.

cardiac muscle. A specialized form of *heart* muscle in which the individual cells are joined together by bridges of protoplasm forming a network (syncytium). It has intrinsic rhythmical properties, and if any part of the cardiac muscle contracts, the wave of contraction spreads throughout the muscle as a whole. Conditions that affect the cardiac muscle include: (1) the length of the muscle when it contracts (degree of diastolic filling); (2) the neurohumoral background, a general term for the degree of activity exerted by the autonomic nervous system and the level of hormones such as *epinephrine* and *norepinephrine* circulating in the blood; (3) the concentration of electrolytes such as *potassium* and *calcium* in the blood circulating through the heart. The metabolism of cardiac muscle is essentially the same as that of skeletal muscle, but it has far fewer reserves and is unable to contract in without oxygen (anaerobically) for more than a few seconds. See *skeletal muscle* and *smooth muscle*.

cardiac output. The amount of blood pumped by the *heart* from the left ventricle into the aorta in 1 minute. An average person has a cardiac output of 5–6 liters per minute with an average pulse of 66 per minute. Stroke volume is output of left ventricle during one contraction.

cardiovascular disease (CVD). Arterial disease may result from obstruction impeding the flow of blood; from disorders of the arterial muscles causing them to either constrict or dilate; or from aneurysms, which are weakened vessel segments that fill with blood and balloon outward. The formation of atherosclerotic plaques or fatty deposits along the inner arterial walls is the most common arterial disease. Cardiovascular disease accounts for more than 54% of all causes of death combined. A major contributor to CVD is *atherosclerosis*, which is associated with high blood *cholesterol*. In about one-third of heart attacks, death is the first indication of CVD.

Risk factors for cardiovascular disease

1. Hyperlipodemia (high LDL)	5. Obesity
2. Hypertension	6. Age
3. Cigarette smoking	7. Sex (male)
4. Diabetes mellitus	8. Low HDL level

cardiovascular system. This system, which maintains the *heart* and all *blood vessels*, is a closed system, transporting blood to all parts of the body. Blood flowing through the circuit brings heat, oxygen, food, and other chemical elements to tissue cells and removes *carbon dioxide* and other waste products resulting from cell activity.

cardoon (*Cynara cardunculus*). A thistlelike, silver-green, prickly plant closely related to the artichoke but looking more like an outside stalk of celery. Cardoons are grown from the leafy midribs of the plant, which are fleshy and tender. The flavor is delicate and resembles that of the related *artichoke* and the oyster plant.

carnitine. A chemical, γ-trimethylamine-β-hydroxybutyrate, important in metabolizing *palmitic* and *stearic acids*. A growth factor for the mealworm, but synthesized by other animals from *lysine* and *methionine*. In animals it forms esters with *fatty acids* that allow passage through the membrane of *mitochondria*.

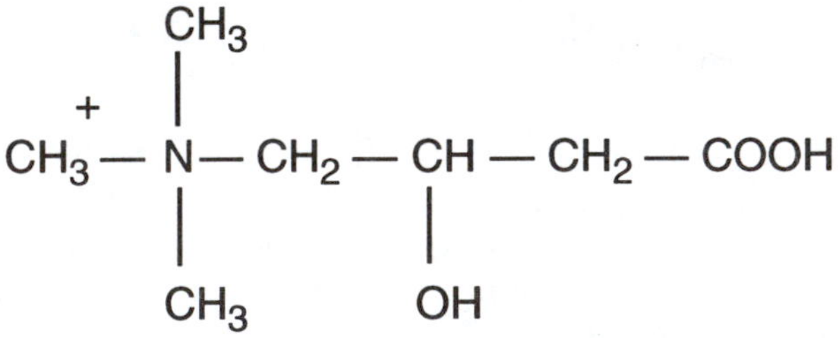

$$CH_3 - \overset{\displaystyle CH_3}{\underset{\displaystyle CH_3}{\overset{+}{N}}} - CH_2 - \underset{\displaystyle OH}{CH} - CH_2 - COOH$$

Carnitine

carob (*Ceratonia siliqua*). The carob tree is native to the Mediterranean region. Known since biblical times as St. John's bread, the powder made from the seed pods tastes something like *chocolate*. Carob is popular as a health food, and as a chocolate substitute in candy because of its low fat content. Carob has 180 calories and 1.4 g of fat per 100 g (3.5 ounces) compared to 528 calories and 35 g of fat for the same amount of sweet chocolate.

carotene (provitamin A). Mol. Wt. 537. A group of yellow, orange, or red plant pigments occurring in many fruits and vegetables, as well as in animal fat, that yield *vitamin A* upon oxidative scission. The digestive tract converts carotene to *retinol* (vitamin A) in animals. Food manufacturers add carotene to margarine, nondairy coffee whiteners, shortenings, butter, milk, cake mix, dessert topping, and other products as artificial coloring, nutritional supplement, or both. *Retinol* is obtained from fish oil and requires no conversion. The average adult should consume 5000 I.U. of vitamin A. Carotene in food has about one-sixth the activity of retinol. Approximately two-thirds of the vitamin A activity of the average American diet is provided by carotene. The most common form of carotene is beta (β)-carotene. Other forms exist, but they are not so active as β-carotene. Chard, kale, spinach and other greens, beans, broccoli, carrots, yellow squash, apricots, and sweet potatoes are rich sources of β-carotene. The carotenoid pigments are comparatively heat-stable compounds but are labile on exposure to radiation and oxidation, especially when in liquid form and when associated with free radicals or peroxides. Other carotenoid pigments also possess vitamin A activity. The table shows the vitamin A activity of other carotenes relative to most the common form, β-carotene.

Natural carotenes

CAROTENE	β-CAROTENE	α-CAROTENE	γ-CAROTENE	3,4-DEHYDROCAROTENE	β-ZEACAROTENE
Percent vitamin activity	100	50	45	75	30

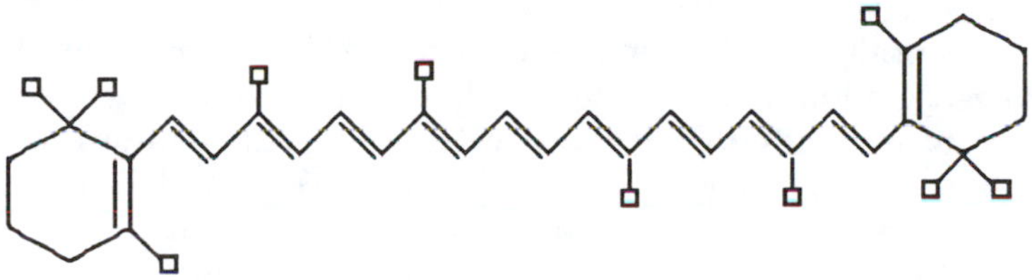

□ = CH₃

β-Carotene

carrageenan. Carrageenan is a complex of various polysaccharides (galactans) obtained from Irish moss and red sea weeds. It is used in foods to stabilize emulsions and to increase the viscosity. In chocolate milk, carrageenan stabilizes the suspension of cocoa particles. It adds "body" to soft drinks; stabilizes the foam in beer; thickens ice cream, jellies, sour cream, syrups; prevents fats and oils from separating out from frozen whipped toppings; and serves as the gelling component for milk puddings and gelatin-like deserts. Carrageenan has no nutritive value. See *agar*.

carrots (*Daucus carota*). Orange root plants which are a good source of β-carotene, a provitamin A. See this item in the table under *vegetables*.

cartilage tissue. A tough, resilient connective tissue found at the ends of the bones, between bones, and in the nose, throat, and ears. It contains large quantities of the protein *collagen*.

casaba. Any of several large winter melons, globular in shape with pointed stem ends and round, furrowed rinds. When ripe, the flesh is creamy white, soft and juicy, but almost without fragrance. It has a distinctive, mild, cucumber-like flavor. The rind is yellow and, although wrinkled, is not netted. See *melon*.

cascade. A sequential series of biochemical reactions related to the production of a specific product. Examples of cascades are the *blood clotting* mechanism and *glycogenolysis*.

casein. The principal protein of milk and the basis of cheese. It is a phosphoprotein. Casein is a nutritious protein because it contains adequate amounts of all the *essential amino acids*. Food manufacturers add casein to ice cream, ice milk, frozen custard, and sherbet to improve their texture. In nondairy coffee creamers, casein adds body and acts as a whitener.

caseinogen. The principal protein in milk from which casein is derived. It is the substance in solution, and casein is the result of its precipitation. Its conversion into casein is the essential process in the curdling of milk.

cashew (*Anacardium occidentale*). A sweet, plump, white kidney-shaped nut, the edible seed of a tropical evergreen tree related to the sumac, native to tropical America and found widely in India and equatorial Africa. Cashews contain some protein, iron, and various B vitamins. They are high in fat content; 100 g contain 561 calories.

cassava. See *manioc*.

catabolism. Processes by which nutrients, reserve tissue material, and cellular substances are broken down into chemically simpler compounds with the liberation of energy. In catabolism, nutrients are oxidized gradually, ultimately yielding carbon dioxide and water and *energy* plus some nitrogen compounds from protein catabolism. Part of the energy released by catabolism is converted to chemical energy (*adenosine triphosphate*), and the remainder is usually converted to heat. The overall process may be summarized as catabolism + anabolism = metabolism. See *metabolism, anabolism, oxidative phosphorylation* and *Krebs' cycle*.

catalase. An enzyme found in most animal cells and the mold *Micrococcus lysodeitikus*, from which the enzyme is often prepared. The enzyme catalyzes the degradation of *hydrogen peroxide*, a potent and destructive by-product of many cellular oxidase reactions.

$$H_2O_2 \longrightarrow H_2O + 1/2O_2$$
$$\text{Catalase}$$

In animal cells, catalase is found in *organelles* called *peroxisomes*.

catalyst. A substance that increases the speed of a chemical reaction without being used up as a result of the reaction. Catalysts only affect the reaction rate and have no effect on the end point (equilibrium) of a reaction. Biochemical catalysts are called *enzymes*.

cataracts. A loss of the lens protein's transparency due to an alteration protein structure. Cataracts only affect vision when they are in the line of sight. Cataracts may result from injury, exposure to radiation, medications (especially steroids), eye diseases, and other metabolic disorders, especially *diabetes*.

catecholamine test. A chemical test on blood or urine; used for diagnosis of tumors of the *adrenal gland*.

catecholamines. Biologically active amines derived from the amino acid *tyrosine*. They have a marked effect on the *nervous* and *cardiovascular systems*, metabolic rate, temperature, and smooth muscle. Two catecholamines with widespread biological effects are *epinephrine* (adrenaline) and *norepinephrine* (noradrenaline).

catfish. A freshwater fish that derives its name from its barbels, or feelers, which resemble a cat's whiskers. Catfish live in streams. The best eating is the channel cat, which weighs from 5–10 pounds. The smaller bullhead is the most common. The channel cat is usually baked; the bullhead is fried.

cathepsins. Enzymes within the cell that have hydrolytic activity. The cathepsins have activities similar to the *digestive enzymes* but are contained within the cell.

cation. A chemical group or ion carrying a positive charge. Cations migrate to the cathode or negative electrode. The cations include all metals and the *hydrogen* ion or proton (H^+). The *cation* is the opposite of the *anion*.

cauliflower (*Brassica oleraccea botrytis*). The word "cauliflower" is a combination of the Latin *caluis*, meaning "stalk," and *floris*, "flower." A member of the cabbage family, cauliflower is a good source of *ascorbic acid* (vitamin C) and a fair source of *iron*. See this item in the table under *vegetables*.

caustic. A burning or corrosive substance, such as strong acids or alkalis.

caviar. Fish roe (eggs) which has been sieved, lightly pressed, and treated with salt. It may come from any of the following fish: beluga (a member of the sturgeon family), sterlet, sturgeon, carp, herring, whitefish, or cod, among others.

cayenne. A hot, pungent red pepper prepared by grinding the dried ripe fruit of several species of the *Capsicum* plant, chiefly *Capsicum frutescens* and *C. annum*. Cayenne is an ingredient of sausage seasonings and curry powders.

cecum. A blind pouch or cul-de-sac that forms the first portion of the large intestine, located below the entrance of the *ileum* at the ileocecal valve. It averages about 6 cm in length and 7.5 cm in width. At its lower end is the vermiform appendix. See *digestive system*.

celeriac (*Apium*). A dark, turnip-rooted European variety of celery that also goes by the names celery root or celery knob. Only the root is eaten. It is eaten hot or used as a cold salad and as a flavoring for soups and stews.

celery (*Apium graveolens*). A stalk vegetable which is a cultivated version of a white-flowered herb that grew wild in both Europe and Asia. The leaves, stalk, and root of cultivated celery are all edible. See this item in the table under *vegetables*.

celiac disease. A disease characterized by fatty diarrhea (steatorrhea) malnutrition, bleeding tendency, and *hypocalcemia*, and caused by intolerance to *glutin*; similar to nontropical *sprue*.

cellobiose. Mol. Wt. 343. The basic *dissacharide* unit of the plant polysaccharide *cellulose*. Cellobiose is composed of two glucose molecules. It is digestible by micoorganisms but not by humans. *Maltose* is digestible. The difference between cellobiose and maltose is in the α- and β-configurations of the linkages between the glucose molecules.

(β 1→4) D-Glucopyranosyl-glucopyranose
Cellobiose

cells. The basic functioning units in the composition of the human body. The human body is composed of millions of cells varying in shape and size and microscopic, the largest being only about 1/1000 of an inch. A group of cells is called a "tissue" when it associates and coordinates to perform particular functions. The interior of cells composed of a substance called *protoplasm*. A typical cell is made up of a cell membrane and two main parts, the *nucleus* and the *cytoplasm*, which are types of protoplasm. The nucleus contains the genetic determinants, *chromosomes*, and controls all activities of the cell, including growth and reproduction. The cytoplasm is the matter surrounding the nucleus and is responsible for most of the work done by the cell. The cytoplasm contains formed elements such as *lysosomes, mitochondria*, and the *endoplasmic reticulum*. The cell membrane encloses the protoplasm and permits the passage of fluid and specific materials into and out of the cell. This specific permeability of the cell membrane is an important structural feature of the cell. It is through the cell membrane that all materials essential to metabolism are received and all products of metabolism are discarded. The bloodstream and tissue fluid which constantly circulate around the cell transport the materials to and from the cells. The diagram shows a schematic representation of a "typical" cell. It is a composite of several animal cell types.

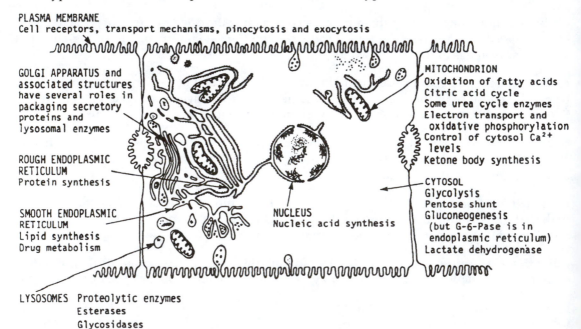

PLASMA MEMBRANE
Cell receptors, transport mechanisms, pinocytosis and exocytosis

GOLGI APPARATUS and associated structures have several roles in packaging secretory proteins and lysosomal enzymes

ROUGH ENDOPLASMIC RETICULUM
Protein synthesis

SMOOTH ENDOPLASMIC RETICULUM
Lipid synthesis
Drug metabolism

MITOCHONDRION
Oxidation of fatty acids
Citric acid cycle
Some urea cycle enzymes
Electron transport and oxidative phosphorylation
Control of cytosol Ca^{2+} levels
Ketone body synthesis

CYTOSOL
Glycolysis
Pentose shunt
Gluconeogenesis
(but G-6-Pase is in endoplasmic reticulum)
Lactate dehydrogenase

NUCLEUS
Nucleic acid synthesis

LYSOSOMES Proteolytic enzymes
            Esterases
            Glycosidases

(Campbell, P.N., and Smith, A.D., *Biochemistry Illustrated*, 1982. Reproduced with permission of Churchill Livingstone, Edinburgh.)

cellulose. Mol. Wt. 20,000 to 400,000. $(C_6H_{10}O_5)_n$. The most common organic compound on earth. A plant *polysaccharide* of *glucose* units connected by β 1→4 linkages in a linear array. Cellulose is not digestible by animal enzymes. Ruminants, such as cattle, depend on intestinal bacteria to digest the cellulose in fodder. *Cellobiose* is considered the building block of cellulose.

central nervous system. The central nervous system (CNS) consists of the *brain* and spinal cord. These are delicate structures which are protected by two coverings, bones and special membranes. The brain is encased by the bones of the skull that form the cranium; the spinal cord by the vertebrae. The membranes enclosing both brain and spinal cord are the meninges. See *nervous system*.

ceramide. A class of *lipids* which do not contain glycerol. They are derived from a sphingosine. See *sphingolipids*.

cereals. Edible seeds, also called *grain*, of the grass family. Rice, wheat, and corn are the mainstays of nutritious diets, followed by rye, barley, millet, and oats. The common grains have a roughly similar composition. They contain from 7–14% protein, and about 75% carbohydrates. The proteins are of low biologic value, but when supplemented with protein sources containing the amino acids in which they are deficient, such as legumes, they are capable of supplying the protein requirements of humans. The vitamin and mineral constituents of grains are held mostly in the outer layers of the kernel or in the embryo (germ). Since much of this is lost in the process of milling, phosphorus remains the major mineral contribution of most grains. Consumption of whole grains or enriched flour ensures intake of *thiamine*, *riboflavin*, *niacin*, and *iron* from the cereals. See table under *grains*.

cerebellum. The second largest part of the *brain*, located above the medulla at the back of the cranial cavity and covered dorsally by the cerebral hemispheres.

cerebral cortex. The outer layer of the cerebrum, consisting of cells known collectively as gray matter, where the principal *brain* centers are located; these are the motor, sensory, visual, auditory, olfactory, and association centers. See *brain*.

cerebral hemisphere. The two halves of the *brain* are known as the cerebral hemispheres, and fill the major part of the skull. Each hemisphere is largely responsible for the sensation and movement of the opposite half of the body. Certain automatic processes, such as swallowing, breathing, and some trunk movements, are doubly controlled from both hemispheres. The cerebral hemispheres consist of an outer layer of nerve cells or gray matter, called the cortex, surrounding a complex network of nerve fibers or white matter. The two cerebral hemispheres are each divided for descriptive purposes into four lobes: (1) frontal, (2) parietal, (3) occipital, and (4) temporal.

   1. *Frontal lobe*: The frontal lobe extends forward and contains nerve cells which transmit impulses of the brain stem and spinal cord on to all the voluntary muscles of the body. Much of the frontal lobe is concerned with emotional expression and experience, but its functions are not well understood. The production of words, phrases, and sentences in correct order and balance depends on the activity of this part of the brain.

   2. *Parietal lobes*: The parietal lobes are the middle part of the cerebral hemispheres behind the fissure of Rolando. They are mainly concerned with the reception of a response to nerve

impulses from sensory nerve endings all over the body. The detailed appreciation, assessment, integration, and judgment of sensation depend on the parietal lobes.

3. *Occipital lobes*: The posterior parts of the cerebral hemispheres form the occipital lobes, which contain the nervous structure necessary for vision. The neuronal equipment necessary for the recognition of light, shade, shape, and color is localized at the back, and the more forwardly placed structures are responsible for the appreciation and interpretation of visual patterns.

4. *Temporal lobes*: The cerebral hemispheres jut out to form the temporal lobes, which are their lower parts. The lobes are especially concerned with hearing, but their other functions are not understood, although they seem to be concerned with memory to some extent.

cerebral thrombosis. Formation of a clot in the brain artery, eventually leading to occlusion of the artery. The result is a stroke or a cerebrovascular accident.

cerebrosides. See *glycolipids* and *lipids*.

cerebrospinal. Pertaining to the brain and spinal cord.

cerebrospinal fluid (CSF). The cerebrospinal fluid fills ventricles of the brain and the subarachnoid space which surrounds the brain and spinal cord. The *central nervous system* is suspended in this collection of fluid whose chief function is to protect the delicate nervous tissue from jarring and injury. It is possible that the cerebrospinal fluid may also be of value for the transfer of biologically important protective substances to various parts of the central nervous system. The cerebrospinal fluid is formed both by filtration and by active secretion by the choroid plexus which lies in the lateral ventricles of the brain. It is a clear, colorless, alkaline fluid which is slightly modified blood plasma free of protein. At any one time, an adult has about 135 mL of this fluid circulating, although over 500 mL is produced daily. If anything interferes with its circulation or its reabsorption, the fluid accumulates. Hydrocephalus (water on the brain) is an abnormal accumulation of cerebrospinal fluid.

cerebrum. The dorsal anterior part of the vertebrate *brain* consisting of two hemispheres. It is the largest region of the human brain and is considered to be the seat of emotions, intelligence, and other nervous activities.

ceroid pigment. Ceroid pigment, also called old-age pigment or liver spots, is believed to result from the long-term oxidations and peroxidations of polyunsaturated fats and proteins. The pigment is the result of formation of insoluble long-chain polymers. The pigments appear as brown spots on skin surfaces. Ceroid pigments are also found in the coronary arteries. Under some circumstances, the pigment may interfere with the normal dissolving of blood clots.

ceruloplasmin. A glycoprotein, blue in color, to which most of the copper in the blood is attached. It is an alpha globulin of blood plasma. It catalyzes the oxidation of *ascorbic acid*, *amines*, and *phenols*.

chard (*Beta vulgaris cicla*). This vegetable is a variety of *beet*, of which the leaves and stalk, not the root, are eaten. Chard, also called Swiss chard, has all the attributes of the green leafy vegetables. It is an excellent source of *carotene* (vitamin A), a very good source of *iron*, and a good source of *ascorbic acid* (vitamin C).

Nutrients in 100 g of cooked chard

CALORIES KCAL	PROTEIN G	FAT G	CARBOHYDRATE G	ASCORBATE MG	VITAMIN A IU	CALCIUM MG	IRON MG
18	2	trace	4	16	5,500	74	2

chayote (*Sechium edule*). The gourdlike fruit of a trailing vine of tropical America, which is eaten as a vegetable, chayote has a deeply ribbed, greenish white rind and one soft seed. It is an extremely bland *squash* and its main virtues are that it is low in starch and that it keeps its shape even when overcooked. Peeled or unpeeled, it can be boiled, fried, baked, stuffed, or combined with other foods such as meats and vegetables.

cheese. See *milk products*.

cheese powders. Cheese powders and cheese-flavored dairy powders make it convenient for food manufacturers to put cheese flavors into baked goods and convenience items. Cheese powders are produced by dispersing the selected cheese type in skim milk or in whey as a 50% slurry. This slurry is heat-treated for *emulsification, homogenized,* and finally spray-dried. Expected storage life is approximately 1 year under suitable conditions. Spray-dried cheese powders can be produced at various flavor levels with salt added, and in addition, other compatible ingredients such as whey or other dairy ingredients may be blended. Many foods such as salad dressings, soups, and various kinds of baked goods are flavored by powdered cheese.

chelate. A chemical compound capable of incorporating a metallic ion onto its molecular structure and thus removing it as an available ion in solution. The characteristic is called "sequestering." Desterrioxamine is a chelating agent developed for the treatment of *hemochromatosis* and *hemosiderosis* diseases in which excess iron is stored in body tissues. The desterrioxamine removes iron from the tissue and transports it to excretion sites.

chelation. Combining of metallic ions to form ring structures so that the ions are held (sequestered) by chemical bonds as a part of the ring.

chelation therapy. The treatment of a variety of symptoms, diseases, and conditions by the administration of chelates. Except in some special instances, chelation therapy is not considered within the bounds of general medical practice. See *chelate*.

chemical additives. Synthetic or natural substances added to foods to improve their flavor, color, and texture or keeping quality. See *food additives*.

chemical score. The chemical score is a value which quantifies the quality of proteins. In this regard, the chemical score is similar to the *biological value* (BV), and the *net protein utilization* (NPU) value. The BV and NPU are based upon animal test systems for value determination.

The chemical score is based upon the amino acid analysis. Specifically, the chemical score is a measure of the percent concentration of the *essential amino acids* in a protein relative to the percent concentration of the essential amino acids in eggs. The amino acid with the lowest percent concentration relative to its concentration in eggs is taken as the chemical score. Because of the lower relative cost and convenience, most biological values of proteins are determined as chemical scores. The relative agreements between the chemical scores, BV, and NPU are generally good. The table shows comparisons of the chemical score, the BV, and the NPU of some foods.

Nutritive measures of food proteins

PROTEIN	CHEMICAL SCORE	NPU	BV
Egg	100	94	100
Beef	67	80	75
Cow's milk	60	59	95
Rice	53	75	86
Corn	49	52	72
Wheat	53	48	44

chemogenic disorders. Disorders resulting from the effects of various chemical agents upon the brain tissue. These include reactions resulting from poison taken into the body (such as alcohol, morphine, carbon monoxide, etc.), poisons resulting from internal physiologic malfunctioning (such as endocrine disturbances), and the toxic effects of various disease processes (such as encephalitis). Severe reactions to the continued use of alcohol are usually classified among the chemogenic disorders, although it is the effect of physical and mental dysfunctions combined with the oral intake of alcohol which produce certain physiologic results, and unconscious needs that explain the total behavior.

chemotherapy. Chemotherapy is the treatment of cancers and other diseases with drugs. Most chemotherapeutic drugs used in cancer depend on the differential toxic effect that tumor cells absorb the toxic drugs at a much faster rate than do normal cells. The toxicity of the drugs to normal tissues is responsible for side effects. The development of resistance to chemotherapy is a problem that arises with long-term treatment. See *aminopterin*.

chenodeoxycholic acid. Mol. Wt. 393. A bile-acid derivative of cholesterol that occurs in bile as a conjugate of *glycine* or *taurine*. See *bile salts*.

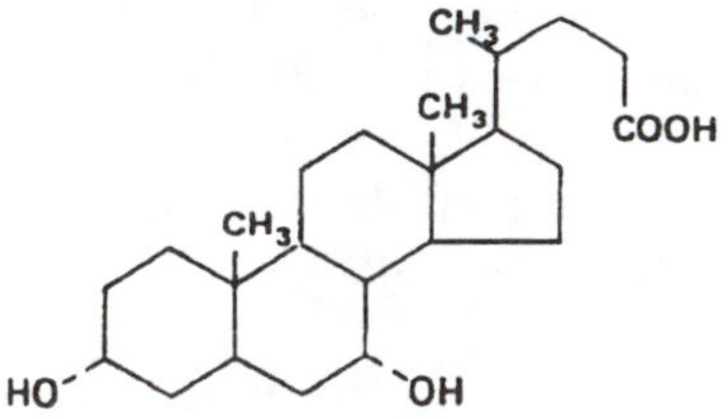

Chenodeoxycholic acid

cherry (*Prunus*). The small, smooth, long-stemmed, round-stoned fruit of a tree that has a birchlike bark and pink or white flowers. Cherries are divided into two groups: sweet and sour. Sweet cherries are the larger of the two, heart-shaped and firm, yet tender. Sour cherries are rounder, softer-textured fruit. Fresh cherries, both sweet and sour, contain small amounts of vitamins and minerals. Canned and frozen cherries are similar in food value, except that those processed with sugar contain more calories. See this item in the table under *fruits*.

cherry liqueur. A number of well-known European liqueurs and brandies are made from special strains of cherries cultivated for the purpose. The best known ones are kirsch, a strong colorless spirit, made in France, Switzerland, and Germany; Cherry Heering, a rich, red cordial made in Denmark; and cherry brandy made in Holland and England.

chervil (*Anthriscus cerefolium*). A delicate herb used to flavor soups, salads, and stews. Chervil is an annual and grows to a height of 2 feet. In appearance, it resembles a delicate parsley with lacy leaves. The flowers are tiny and white. Chervil may be used fresh or dried.

chestnut (*Castanea*). The edible nut of a tree of the same name. Chestnuts are peeled (both the hard brown outer shell and the thin, bitter, brown inner peel), and are eaten in a variety of ways. They may be boiled or roasted. Chestnuts provide some protein, iron, and B vitamins, but their main contribution is calories: 100 g of fresh chestnuts contain 195 calories.

chicken (*Gallus gallus*). An excellent source of high-quality protein, very good to excellent for *niacin*, and a fair source of *iron*. Broiler-fryers are lower in fat and calories than most other meats. The light meat of chicken has a lower fat content and is higher in niacin than the dark meat; however, it is lower in iron.

Nutrients in 100 g of skinless cooked chicken

TYPE	CALORIES	PROTEIN G	FAT G	CARBOHYDRATE G	IRON MG	NIACIN MG
Roast	144	34	2	0	1	6
Broiler	142	24	4	0	2	9
Fryer	223	28	11	3	2	8
Fricasee	153	15	9	3	1	2

chick-pea (*Cicer arietinum*). The chick-pea, also known as garbanzo bean, Spanish bean, or ceci pea, is a branching, bush annual which is well adapted to arid and semiarid regions. The sparse foliage is poisonous, eliminating any use of the plants as forage. Large green pods produce one or two edible seeds, or peas, that wrinkle as they dry and are described as looking like "ram heads." Peas vary in size and color (white, red, and black) in the different varieties. They are a good source of protein, *iron*, and *thiamine*.

Nutrients in 100 g of dry, raw chick-peas

CALORIES KCAL	PROTEIN G	FAT G	CARBOHYDRATE G	CALCIUM MG	IRON MG	NIACIN MG
305	4	5	61	150	7	2

chicory (*Cichorium intybus*). A salad green which is a member of the endive family, with finely cut, feathery leaves that have dark green edges and almost white centers. Some varieties of chicory are cultivated for their roots, which are roasted, then ground and added to certain coffees as stretchers. An excellent source of *carotene* (vitamin A).

chief cells. Specialized cells in the *stomach* which produce the proenzyme pepsinogen. See pepsin and *digestive system*.

chili (*Capsicum frutescens*). A tropical American plant from whose small, elongated pods or peppers we get *cayenne* (red) *pepper* and hot pepper sauce. Chili powder is a blend of dried ground chili pepper pods, which may or may not contain other powdered *herbs* and *spices*.

chitterlings. The intestines of young pigs that have been emptied, turned inside out, and scraped clean while still warm. They are then soaked for 24 hours in cold salted water and washed at least six times before being cut up into 2-inch lengths. Chitterlings are either boiled or deep fried.

chive (*Allium schoenoprasum*). A member of the *onion* family, it grows in clumps of slender, green, tubular leaves. Chives may be used to flavor any food in which a mild onion flavor is desired.

chloride ion (Cl^-). The major *anion* in the extracellular fluid, occurring for the most part in combination with the *cation* sodium (Na^+). Less than 15% of the total body chloride is *intracellular*. Chloride in the blood transfers easily among the various compartments of body fluids. This chloride shift is a primary *homeostatic* mechanism for the control of blood pH and the maintenance of osmolarity of the *extracellular fluid*. Chloride ions form *hydrochloric acid* (HCl), the major stomach acid in the gastric juice, which is required for the proper absorption of *cobalamin* (vitamin B_{12}) and ferrous ion (iron). The stomach acid serves to kill or suppress the growth of bacteria present in ingested food and drink. The chloride ion is also an activator of salivary amylase. See *sodium chloride*.

chlorine (Cl). Element No. 17. At. Wt. 35. Chlorine is a gas, Cl_2. It is a common water purifier and bleach. It is highly toxic and corrosive. Chlorine gas is one of the best aging agents for flour; at a level of about 400 ppm, it instantly ages and bleaches flour white. Chlorine affects the flour by causing changes in the flour proteins and interactions with the unsaturated oils.

chlorine dioxide (ClO_2). A bleaching and maturing agent that works by releasing oxygen which causes changes in the protein fraction of flour and bleaches the yellow pigments.

Fourteen parts per million of chloride dioxide has an immediate bleaching and maturing effect and is the normal amount used to treat flour. Chlorine dioxide and other bleaching agents reduce the *tocopherol* (vitamin E) content of flour.

chlorpropamide. A hypoglycemic agent. Reported to lower the blood sugar level and to reduce *glycosuria* in certain *diabetics*. The drug acts by stimulating the release of *insulin* from the pancreas. The insulin appears to increase its main effect on the liver by promoting a decrease in the output of glucose from the liver into the bloodstream.

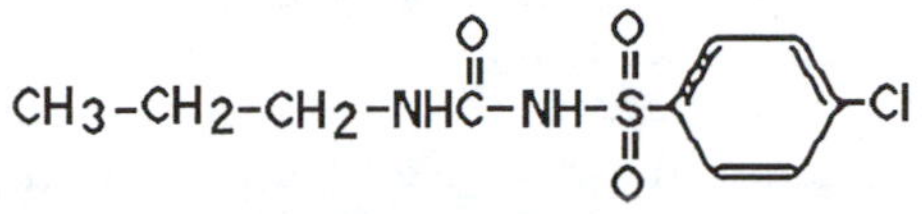

$$CH_3-CH_2-CH_2-NH\overset{O}{\overset{\|}{C}}-NH-\overset{O}{\underset{O}{\overset{\|}{\underset{\|}{S}}}}-\!\!\!\!\bigcirc\!\!\!\!-Cl$$

Chlorpropamide

chocolate. Chocolate and *cocoa* are made from the beans of the *cacao* tree, a perennial evergreen tree of the cola family. Chocolate is a mixture of roasted *cocoa*, cocoa butter (also obtained from the cacao bean), and very fine sugar. The word comes from the Mexican Indian *choco*, "foam," and *atl*, "water." Chocolate, apart from its palatability, has a considerable stimulating effect on the heart and the general musculature of the body. Chocolate contains an appreciable amount of fat and carbohydrates. It is a good source of quick energy.

Nutrients in 100 g of unsweetened chocolate

CALORIES KCAL	PROTEIN G	FAT G	CARBOHYDRATE G	CALCIUM MG	IRON MG	VITAMIN A IU
505	11	53	29	78	7	60

Calories in 100 g of chocolate

Unsweetened	505
Semisweet	508
Sweet	528
Milk chocolate	520

choke cherry (*Prunus virginiana and Prunus demissa*). A small, wild *cherry* that grows on a large shrub and is a native of North America. The flowers are white, and the fruit turns from red to black as it matures. Chokecherries have a puckery taste, and they are best used for jams and jellies.

cholecalciferol (vitamin D$_3$). The first crystalline *vitamin D* was obtained in 1931 and was synthesized shortly thereafter. Soon it became evident that there are at least ten natural substances which exert vitamin D-like activity in varying degrees, but only two of these are of practical importance from the standpoint of their occurrence in foods; *ergocalciferol* (vitamin D_2) which is found in yeast, and *cholecalciferol* (vitamin D_3). See *vitamin D*.

cholecystitis. An inflammation of the *gallbladder*, usually resulting from a low-grade chronic infection. The infectious process produces changes in the gallbladder mucosa which affect its absorptive powers. Normally, the cholesterol, which is insoluble in water, is kept in solution by action of the *bile salts* and especially the *bile acids*. However, when mucosa changes occur in cholecystitis, the absorptive powers of the gallbladder may be altered, affecting the solubility ratios of the *bile* ingredients. Excess water may be absorbed, or excess bile acids may be absorbed, increasing the likelihood of *gallstone* formation.

cholecystokinin. A hormone produced in the wall of the *duodenum* in the presence of fat, which stimulates the contraction of the *gallbladder*, with the emission of *bile*. Bile is necessary to emulsify fat before digestion.

cholesterol. Mol. Wt. 387. A pearly, fatlike substance which crystallizes in the form of circular crystals. When stored in the intima (lining) of the arteries, it begins to irritate and, over a period of time, sets up an inflammatory reaction which may damage the arterial lining and lead to narrowing of the arteries due to atheroma. Cholesterol is found in all animal fats and oils, brain, whole milk, yolk of eggs, liver, kidneys, adrenal glands, and pancreas. It combines with protein to form *lipoproteins* within the cells. From the cells, it circulates through the blood and through the entire body. Cholesterol is also an important component of all cell membranes. Cholesterol has many important functions, such as an insulator of nerve and brain tissue; as a precursor of *bile acids*; as a precursor of *vitamin D*; as a structural unit of tissue membranes; and as a precursor of various sex and *adrenal hormones*. The body needs cholesterol, ensuring its supply by synthesizing it in most tissues other than the brain. The liver is the most active site of cholesterol synthesis. Cholesterol is transported through the blood as a part of several lipoproteins. *Very low density lipoprotein* (VLDL) carries cholesterol from the liver into the bloodstream. VLDL is a very large particle, 500 to 800 A, composed of *triglyceride* mostly, a small amount of cholesterol, more cholesterol oleate, and a very small amount of special proteins called apoproteins Cl, C,ll, E, and B-100. Another cholesterol form, the smaller 200-

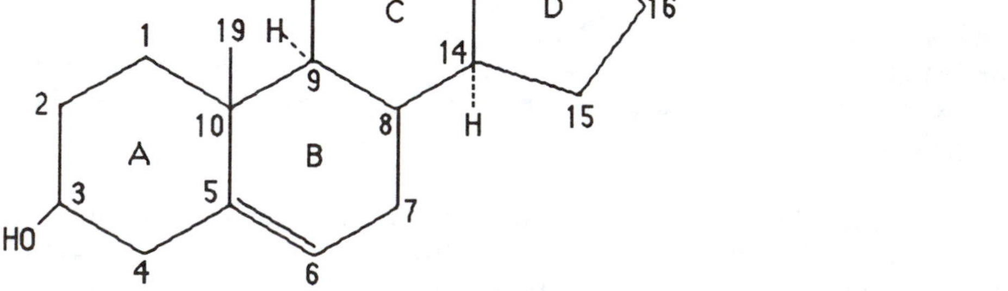

Cholesterol

A *low density lipoprotein* (LDL), derived from VLDL by the action of the lipoprotein lipases, supplies most parts of the body with cholesterol. Moderate levels of LDL in the blood are necessary for health.

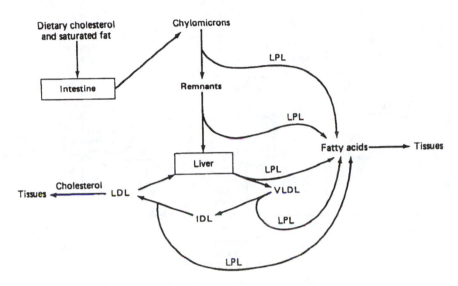

LPL: Lipoprotein lipase
IDL: Intermediate-density lipoprotein
VLDL: Very low density lipoprotein

Transport of cholesterol to tissues

It appears that the greater the level of LDL in the blood, the greater the rate at which cholesterol is deposited by LDL on the walls of the arteries, thus favoring the development of *atherosclerosis* and the risk of *cardiovascular disease*. LDL returns to the liver and is taken up by the special LDL receptors. *High density lipoprotein* (HDL) has a different and apparently beneficial role. It carries cholesterol away from the cells back to the liver and thus promotes its excretion from the body. The process is referred to as reverse cholesterol transport. The diagram shows this relationship.

The more HDL there is in the blood, the less the risk of heart attack, because HDL removes cholesterol from the artery walls. This explains why high LDL levels and low HDL levels both increase the risk of heart attack. As a rule, women are lower cardiovascular risks, generally having higher levels of HDL than men. In both sexes, HDL cholesterol levels can be increased by regular physical exercise. HDL levels tend to be low in obese people. During weight reduction they do not change much; but there is evidence that after weight restabilization at a lower level, the HDL levels rise. The table shows factors that are associated with high and low levels of HDL. The maintenance of low LDL blood levels is a preventive for cardiovascular disease. The tables show the prevailing opinions about cholesterol lipoprotein blood levels relative to a cardiovascular disease (CVD) risk. In addition to the levels of HDL and LDL in the blood, the LDL/HDL ratio is also important in assessing CVD risk.

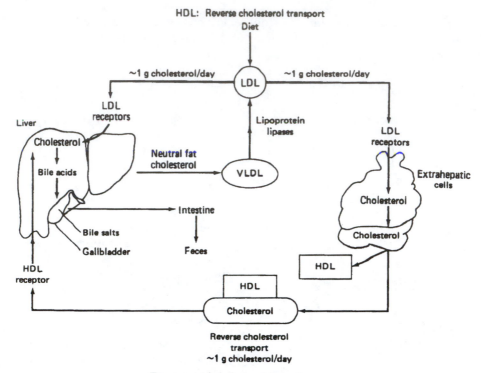

Transport of cholesterol from tissues

Cholesterol-lipoprotein levels blood levels relative to a CVD risk.

TOTAL CHOLESTEROL RANGES MG/DL		NORMAL LIPOPROTEIN RANGES MG/DL	
RANGE	DESIRABILITY	LIPOPROTEIN	NORMAL RANGE
Below 200	Desirable	HDL	30-70
200-240	Borderline	LDL	40-130
Above 240	High risk	LDL/HDL ratio	0-3.0

There are many causes of high levels of cholesterol or *triglycerides* in the blood plasma. Genes play a part and account partially for the differences between individuals; high or low levels tend to run in families. Diet has a major effect on cholesterol and triglyceride, one important factor being the amount and type of fat in the diet. The more *saturated fat* (hard fats, often derived from animal products, such as lard, butter, and hard margarine) in the diet, the higher the blood cholesterol level. Conversely, a low-fat diet in which most of the food energy comes from starches and other carbohydrates (such sources as cereals, vegetables, fruits) leads to a lower blood cholesterol. *Polyunsaturated* (PUFA) and *monounsaturated* (MUFA) *fats*, which tend to be liquid vegetable oils, also reduce blood cholesterol and blood triglyceride levels. The reason for the difference in the effect of saturated and unsaturated fats on blood cholesterol is not known. The amount of cholesterol in the diet has an effect on the increasing blood cholesterol, but the amount and kind of saturated fat appears to be a more important factor. People vary in their sensitivity to food cholesterol and the degree to which a low-cholesterol diet will reduce the cholesterol level in the blood. Some types of insoluble food *fibers* also reduce the blood cholesterol, possibly by binding bile salts and cholesterol derivatives. In particular, in the digestive tract, the pectins present in apples, bananas, and most forms of fruit and vegetables bind cholesterol. The grainy fiber in oat bran is even more effective at lowering blood cholesterol. Blood cholesterol levels about 120 mg/dL are above the threshold risk for cardiovascular disease. The average in the United States is above 150 mg/dL; this means that more than 50% of the United States population is in the risk level of cardiovascular disease. The body's cholesterol control mechanisms remove about 1100 mg of cholesterol per day, about 850 mg coming from endogenous synthesis and about 250 mg absorbed from the average of more than 600 mg ingested per day.

Cholesterol, fat, and unsaturated fat in 100 g food

FOOD	CHOLES-TEROL MG	FAT G	UNSAT'D FAT G	FOOD	CHOLES-TEROL MG	FAT G	UNSAT'D FAT G
White fish, clams, scallops,	66	1	0.2	Organ meats	200-300	5	2
Can tuna (water)				Egg whites	0	0	0
Shrimp, lobster, crab	112	2	0.2	Whole egg	500	12	3
Salmon	75	7	2	Egg substitute	0	4	1
Chicken, turkey (no skin)	87	5	1.3	Cheddar, Roquefort,	100	35	21
Duck, goose (skin)	91	33	8	Swiss, Brie, Jack, cream			
Veal (10% fat)	99	11	5	cheese, Velveeta,			
(15% fat)	99	17	7	spreads			
Beef, pork, lamb				Ice cream, 10% fat	40	11	7
(10% fat)	90	10	4	Whole milk, 3.5% fat	11	4	2
(15% fat)	90	15	6	skim, 0.1% fat	2	0.1	0.1
(20% fat)	90	19	8	1% fat	3	1	1
(30% fat)	90	31	13	2% fat	6	2	2
(40% fat)	90	39	11	Nondairy creamers	0	11	9

cholesterol therapy. In attempts to control blood cholesterol levels, diet and exercise are the best initial approaches. Drug therapy is potentially useful if diet and exercise are without significant effect. The vitamin *niacin (nicotinic acid)* used as a drug in gram quantities (more than 500 times the recommended daily allowance) may raise the HDL and lower the LDL. It is not known how niacin works. As a drug, niacin has side effects, most frequently hot flashes and rashes. Niacin therapy is contraindicated with gout, peptic ulcers, and diabetes. Cholestyramine and colestipol are also used in drug therapies. They are synthetic resins, taken in liquid suspensions, that firmly bind the bile salts and acid derivatives of cholesterol, preventing their reabsorption in the intestinal tract. The resins are sucessful in lowering cholesterol but have constipation, heartburn, and a feeling of fullness as side effects. Additionally, the resins will bind other medications. Lovastatin is an effective drug that lowers the blood cholesterol by inhibiting the production of cholesterol in the liver. Other drugs that have been used to lower blood cholesterol are clofibrate and gemfibrozil, but their primary effect appears to be on elevated *triglycerides*.

cholestyramine. A drug used for the control of blood cholesterol. See *cholesterol therapy*.

cholic acid. A *bile acid*. See *bile salts*.

choline. Mol. Wt. 121. A trimethyl amino ethanol which occurs in biological tissues in the free form and as a component of *acetylcholine* and certain of the *phospholipids* such as *lecithins, plasmogens,* and *sphingomyelins*. Choline is important as a source of labile methyl groups. A choline deficiency has never been demonstrated in humans, and it is not known if a dietary supply is required in addition to that formed by biosynthesis. Choline has many important functions in the body, as a constituent of several phospholipids. As a constituent of *acetylcholine*, choline plays a role in normal functioning of nerves. It is estimated that an average mixed diet for adults in the United States contains 500 to 900 mg per day of choline, or about 0.1–0.18% of the diet. Choline is present in all foods in which phospholipids occur liberally, as in egg yolk, whole grains, *legumes*, meats of all types, and wheat germ. Fresh egg yolk contains about 1.5% choline; beef liver contains 0.6%; legumes such as soybeans, peas, and beans contain from 0.2–0.35%; vegetables and milk have moderate amounts of choline.

$$CH_3$$
$$+ |$$
$$CH_3\text{-}N\text{-}CH_2\text{-}CH_2OH$$
$$|$$
$$CH_3$$

Choline

chondroitin and chondroitin sulfates. Polysaccharides containing *D-glucuronic acid* and acetyl galactosamine. Their general structure is similar, but they differ in content and location of sulfate ester groups in the molecule. Chondroitin contains only a small number of sulfate ester groups. Chondroitin sulfates have a high viscosity and a capability for binding water, and in connective tissue apparently play a role similar to that of *hyaluronic acid*. In addition, these compounds are distinguished by the ion-binding capacity of the sulfate groups. Chondroitin is a component of the cell coat, and chondroitin 4-sulfate is the principal organic component of the ground substance of *cartilage* and *bone*.

chromatin. A complex structure that contains, in addition to *deoxyribonucleic acid* (DNA), large amounts of *histone* and nonhistone proteins and small amounts of *ribonucleic acid* (RNA). It is packaged as distinct bodies called chromosomes in the nucleus. The total chromosomal DNA of any cell is its *genome*.

chromium (Cr). Element No. 24. At. Wt. 52. Chromium has been reported to activate *insulin* action. Chromium has a variety of functions, including the stimulation of the synthesis of fatty acids and cholesterol in the liver; an involvement in insulin metabolism; and a role as part of several other enzymes, including one of the protein-digesting enzymes in the intestine. The human body contains only a small amount of chromium, less than 6 mg, with a decline in age. A typical daily intake ranges between 50–130 mg. Only a small amount of that ingested is absorbed (1–5%). The biologically active form is quite nontoxic and is rapidly secreted. Good food sources of chromium are meats, black pepper, brewer's yeast, mushrooms, beef liver, and bread. See *minerals*.

chromosome. A structure in the nucleus of a cell containing *deoxyribonucleic acid* (DNA), which transmits genetic information. Chromosomes contain the genes or hereditary determiners.

The normal number of chromosomes is constant for each species, being 46 in humans (23 pairs in all somatic cells), constituting the diploid number. In the formation of the gametes (ovum and spermatozoon) the number is reduced to one-half (haploid number), that is, the ovum and sperm each contain 23, or one of each of the 23 pairs. Of these, 22 are considered *autosomes* and one is the sex chromosome (X or Y). At time of fertilization the chromosomes from the sperm unite with the chromosomes from the ovum. This random union determines the sex of the embryo.

chronic. Of long duration; denoting a disease or condition of long duration. The opposite of *acute*.

chyle. The milklike contents of the lacteals and lymphatic vessels of the intestine. It consists principally of absorbed fats. Chyle is carried from the intestine by the lymphatic vessels to the cisterna chyli. The cisterna chyli (the cistern or receptacle of the chyle) is a dilated sac at the origin of the lymphatic vessels. The cisterna chyli lies in the abdomen between the second lumbar vertebra and the aorta. It receives the lymph from the intestinal trunk, the right and left lumbar lymphatic trunk, and two descending lymphatic trunks. The chyle, after passing through the cisterna chyli, is carried upward to the chest through the *thoracic duct* and empties into the venous blood at the point where the subclavian vein joins the left internal jugular vein. See *chylomicrons* and *lymphatic system*.

chylomicrons. A relatively large blood *lipoprotein* containing about 90% *triglycerides*, some *phospholipids*, and a small amount of proteins. The proteins are very important as recognition factors of cell receptors and activators of enzymes that process chylomicron. The important proteins are called Apo-B, Apo-C, and Apo-E. Chylomicrons are synthesized by the intestinal mucosa, vary in size, and are a part of *chyle*. The chylomicrons enter the *lymphatic system* that eventually enters the blood. See *lipoproteins, lipids*.

chyme. The thick, grayish, semiliquid mass into which food is converted by gastric (stomach) digestion. In this form it passes into the small intestine.

chymotrypsin. One of the proteolytic enzymes of the *pancreatic juice*. A *digestive enzyme*, it occurs initially in an inactive zymogen state called chymotrypsinogen. Chymotrypsin continues the hydrolytic action begun by pepsin, and together they break molecules into smaller and smaller peptide fragments. Chymotrypsin has a specificity that hydrolyzes proteins at the amino acids *phenylalanine* and *tyrosine* peptide linkages. See *trypsin*.

cider. See *apple juice*.

cider vinegar. A mild, yellow-brown vinegar, made from hard (fermented) cider. Vinegar results from the oxidation of *ethanol* to *acetic acid*.

cinnamon (Cinnamomum). A reddish brown spice which comes from the dried bark of the shrublike evergreen trees which belong to the laurel group. It is one of the very few spices not obtained from the seeds, flowers, or fruits of a plant. The kinds of cinnamon most commonly used are cassia and Ceylon cinnamon. Cinnamon is sold both ground and whole in sticks.

circadian rhythm. See *biological clock*.

cirrhosis. Scarring of the liver which interferes with its normal function and with blood flow through the liver. The most common cause of the scarring is repeated injury to the liver from drinking large amounts of alcoholic beverages; but other known causes include poor nutrition, hepatitis, rare metabolic disease in which large amounts of iron or copper are deposited in the liver, and the long, continued effects of irritating or toxic drugs. The treatment for cirrhosis involves, first, the complete abstinence from alcohol and other agents known to damage the liver. Additional important measures include eating a well-balanced, nutritious diet and getting plenty of rest.

cis- and *trans-***isomerism**. Any fatty acid which contains a double carbon bond (ethylene linkage) can exist in either of two geometrically isomeric forms. For example, the *trans*-isomer of the natural *unsaturated fatty acid*, *oleic acid*, is elaidic acid. They are structurally related as follows:

$$CH_3(CH_2)_7 \quad H$$
$$\diagdown C \diagup$$
$$\|$$
$$C$$
$$\diagup \diagdown$$
$$HOOC(CH_2)_7 \quad H$$

Oleic acid
(*Cis-form*)

$$CH_3(CH_2)_7 \quad H$$
$$\diagdown C \diagup$$
$$\|$$
$$C$$
$$\diagup \diagdown$$
$$H \quad (CH_2)_7 \; COOH$$

Elaidic acid
(*Trans-form*)

Oleic acid is an oily substance, elaidic is a solid. This is known as *cis-* and *trans*-isomerism. When two carbon atoms are held together by the double bond, there is no freedom of rotation for these groups about the axis of the bond. The natural unsaturated fatty acids exist in the *cis*-form, with their molecules bent back at each double bond. *Trans*-isomers of polyunsaturated acids do not have essential fatty acid activity and lack the ability possessed by *cis*-isomers to lower the level of *lipoproteins* in plasma.

cistron. The genetic unit of biochemical function; the sequence of *nucleotide* pairs in *deoxyribonucleic acid* (DNA) that specifies the amino acid sequence of a single peptide chain.

citric acid. Mol. Wt. 192. An important intermediate in the citric acid or tricarboxylic acid or *Krebs' cycle*, the pathway by which foodstuffs are oxidized. Citric acid is a metabolic product of living systems. Most citric acid is produced by fermentation. *Aspergillus niger* is the principal mold used in commercial citric acid production. Most citric acid is made by the fermentation of *molasses*, with beet molasses preferred over cane. In the food industry, citric acid is added to flavoring extracts, soft drinks, and candies. It has been added to fish to adjust the pH to about 5.9 to aid in its preservation. A large portion of citric acid produced is used for medicinal purposes. Citric acid is an important food additive because it is a strong acid, inexpensive, has a tart flavor, and serves as an antioxidant. The food industry uses it on ice cream, sherbet, fruit juice drinks, carbonated beverages, jellies, preserves, canned fruits, and vegetables, cheeses, candies, and chewing gum. In soft-centered candy, citric acid has the added function of solubilizing the sugar. Manufacturers use citric acid as an antioxidant in instant potatoes, wheat chips, and potato sticks. Citric acid prevents spoilage by *chelation* of metal ions which might otherwise promote reactions that spoil or discolor the food. Humans produce their own citric acid as in the citric acid cycle (*Krebs' cycle*).

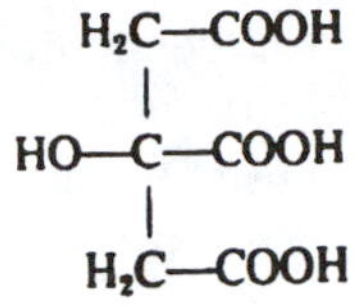

$$H_2C-COOH$$
$$|$$
$$HO-C-COOH$$
$$|$$
$$H_2C-COOH$$

Citric acid

citric acid cycle. See *Krebs' cycle*.

citron (*Citrus medica*). The oldest of the citrus fruits; it grows on a small, thorny tree whose flowers are purple and white. The citron resembles a lemon, and grows to a length of 6–9 inches. It has a greenish yellow, tough and warty, fragrant peel, and a scanty, acid pulp. The fruit is grown for its peel, which is used in baking, and it is a most important ingredient of fruitcakes. The peel is first treated with brine, to remove the bitter oil, to bring out the flavor, and to prevent spoilage. Then it is candied in sugar and glucose.

citrovorum factor (CF). A biologically active form of *folacin* found in bacteria. The bacterium *Leuconostoc citrovorum* required CF for growth.

citrulline. Mol. Wt. 175. One of two naturally occurring L-amino acids that do not occur in proteins, *ornithine* being the other. Both of these amino acids are a part of the *urea cycle* which leads to urea formation.

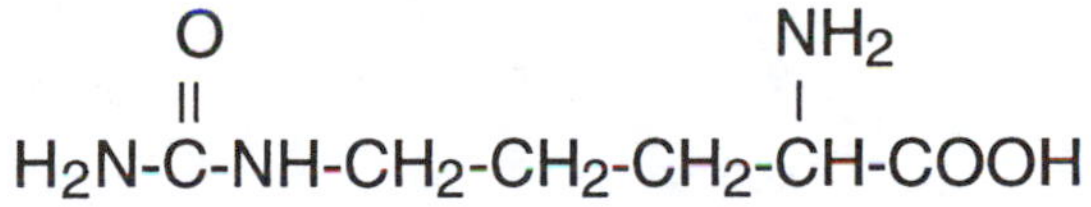

$$\overset{\displaystyle O}{\overset{\displaystyle \|}{}} \qquad \overset{\displaystyle NH_2}{\overset{\displaystyle |}{}}$$
$$H_2N-C-NH-CH_2-CH_2-CH_2-CH-COOH$$

Citrulline

clarifying agents. Clarifying agents remove all particles of mineral elements such as iron and copper from liquids. Vinegar, for example, may turn "cloudy" unless a clarifying agent is added to settle out traces of minerals.

clone. A group of cells or organisms derived asexually from a single ancestor and hence genetically identical.

clove (*Eugenia aromatica*). The dried, unopened flower bud of the evergreen clove tree, which belongs to the myrtle family. The name originated from the fact that the flower buds resembled small nails, and in French, the word for nail is *clou*, in Latin, *clavus*. Cloves are sold whole or ground and are one of the most useful spices. They are used in gingerbreads, spice cakes, fruitcakes, chili sauce, and pickles. They are good for flavoring cooked beets and meat loaves.

coagulated proteins or derived proteins. Insoluble products which result from (1) the action of heat on protein solutions, or (2) the action of alcohol in the proteins. Examples are cooked egg albumin, or egg albumin precipitated by means of alcohol.

coagulation. The change from a fluid state to thickened jelly, curd, or clot by denaturation of a protein with heat, change in pH, or ion concentration. See *blood clotting*.

coagulation time test. A blood-clotting test used for diagnosis of individuals having a tendency to hemorrhage, and also as a guide to treatment in those receiving anticoagulant drugs. See *blood clotting*.

coal tar dyes. Coal, when heated without air, is converted to coke, coal gas, and coal tar. The coal tar, a viscous black liquid, is a mixture of many organic compounds. The synthetic substances made by chemists from coal tar are known as coal tar dyes and are used widely by the food, fabric, and cosmetic industries. Over 95% of these dyes are used in foods, particularly beverages, candy, ice cream, dessert powder, baked goods, and sausages. Levels used range from approximately 10 parts to 500 parts per million, the lower levels being used in liquid foods (beverages, gelatin desserts), the higher level in solid foods (pet food, breakfast cereals).

cobalamin (*extrinsic flavor, vitamin B$_{12}$*). Mol. Wt. 1355. Cobalamin is a generic name for the various forms of vitamin B$_{12}$. Cyanocobalamin is one of the most active forms. Cobalamin has two forms that function as coenzymes in two separate reactions.

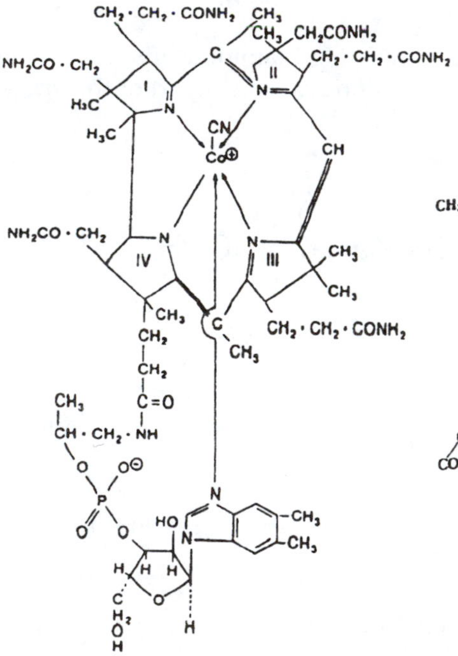

Vitamin B$_{12}$ (cyanocobalamin). 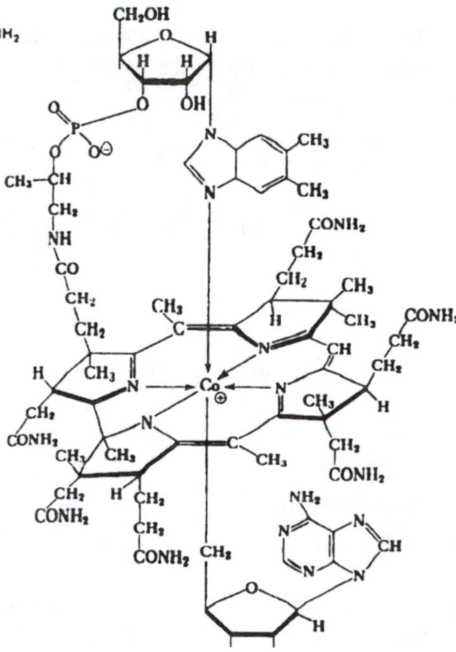   Coenzyme B$_{12}$

Cobalamin (2 forms of vitamin B$_{12}$)

In one reaction, cobalamin reacts with a *folacin* derivative, N^5 methyl $(-CH_3)$ *tetrahydrofolic acid*, to yield a CH_3-vitamin B_{12} derivative and free tetrahydrofolic acid. The CH_3-vitamin B_{12} can then react with homocysteine to form the *essential amino acid methionine*. This last reaction is important in the symptom of vitamin B_{12} deficiency, *pernicious anemia*. In another set of reactions, an adenosine derivative of cobalamin called coenzyme B_{12} serves in a reaction that converts a fatty acid synthesis intermediate into succinyl-coenzyme A, an intermediate of the Krebs' cycle. Coenzyme B_{12} is also required for the synthesis of the *nucleic acids*. A lack of cobalamin results in a nutritional disease called *pernicious anemia*, a rare disease that results from the failure of the intestinal mucosa to produce a mucoprotein required for cobalamin absorption. The mucoprotein is called *intrinsic factor*. The same symptoms of pernicious anemia become evident on a cobalamin-free diet. Hence, cobalamin is called the *extrinsic factor* in the disease. It has been found that one of the symptoms, macrocytic anemia, can be alleviated by high doses of folacin even in the absence of cobalamin, but the neurologic and other symptoms remain. It is clear that red blood cell synthesis requires methyl $(-CH_3)$ free folacin, and cyanocobalamin is required to remove the methyl $(-CH_3)$ group. The reactions involving these two vitamins are closely interwoven. A deficiency of cobalamin then results in a deficiency in another vitamin, the folacin derivative (tetrahydrofolic acid). Cobalamin occurs only in animal food sources. Therefore, strict vegetarianism for a long term (years) may result in an *avitaminosis*, and in the case of a pregnant female, an avitaminosis in the infant. Recovery is rapid and the levels of cobalamin required for good health are in the few micrograms (µg) range. Cobalamin is stable to heat but is inactivated by *acids* or *alkalies*. Good sources of cobalamin are any animal tissues and foods derived from milk. Daily needs are met by the average diet supplying 3 to 5 µg, vitamin B_{12}; major sources are liver, kidney, and muscle meats. See this item in the table under *water-soluble vitamins*.

Cobalamin (Vitamin B_{12}) in µg/100 g of Foods

Beans, green	0	Bread, wheat	0.2-0.4	Egg, whole	0.3	Oats	0.3
Beef		Carrots	0-0.1	Haddock	0.6	Peas	0
kidney	18-55	Cheese		Ham	1.4	Scallops	0.7
liver	31-120	American	0.6	Milk		Sole, filet	1.3
round	4-5	cream	0.2	evaporated	0.2	Soybean	0.2
Beets	0	Swiss	0.9	powder, skim	3	Wheat	0.1
Bread, white	0-0.3	Corn	0	powder, whole	2		
				whole	0.4		

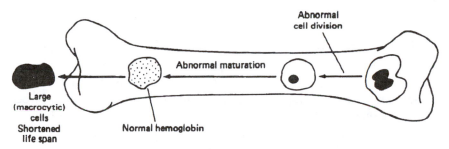

Vitamin B_{12} (cobalamin) or folacin deficiency

cobalt (Co). Element No. 27. At. Wt. 59. Cobalt stimulates the production of *red blood cells* in many animals. A most important function of cobalt is as a metallic component in several enzyme systems which convert enzymes into forms probably necessary in cell metabolism. Cobalt, obtained by humans through animal materials in their diet, is found in liver, kidneys, and bones. A diet containing a moderate amount of meat probably supplies the small amount needed. There is no evidence that humans must ever be concerned about their intake of inorganic cobalt. Cobalt is an important part of *cobalamin* (vitamin B_{12}).

cocarboxylase. Another name for the coenzyme derivative of *thiamine*, thiamine pyrophosphate.

coccus. A type of bacteria which is spherical or ovoid in form. When cocci appear singly they are designated micrococci; in pairs, diplococci; in clusters like bunches of grapes, staphylococci; in chains, streptococci. Many are pathogenic, causing such diseases as septic sore throat, pneumonia, gonorrhea, meningitis, and puerperal fever.

cochlea. Part of the inner ear; a spirally coiled tube of two-and-a-half turns, resembling a snail's shell.

cocoa. The word comes from the Mexican Indian *cacahuatl* and describes a beverage and dessert flavoring made from the beans of the cacao tree which grows only in tropical climates. The cacao or coca bean is the source of chocolate. Cocoa differs from chocolate in fat and sugar content. After the beans are cleaned, dried, roasted, and ground, some of the fat, or cocoa butter, is removed. It is then ground again to form the powder known as cocoa. In Dutch process cocoa, cocoa is treated with an alkali which gives it a darker color and a richer flavor. Instant cocoa is a mixture of cocoa, sugar, flavoring, and an emulsifier, to be added to hot or cold water or milk for use as a beverage. See *cacao*.

Nutrients in 100 g of powdered cocoa

CALORIES KCAL	PROTEIN G	FAT G	CARBOHYDRATE G	NIACIN MG	CALCIUM MG	IRON MG
444	8	24	49	2	125	12

cocoa beans. See *cacao* and *coca*.

cocoa butter. The fat removed from coca beans during their conversion into chocolate and cocoa. It is used primarily in making candy and pharmaceutical products. Cocoa butter is whitish-yellow and smells of *cocoa*.

coconut (*Cocos nucifera*). The fruit of a palm, native to Malaya, which has been transplanted to all parts of the tropical and subtropical world. The fruit is 12–18 inches in length and 6–8 inches in diameter. It takes about a year to mature. The outer covering is smooth, the husk fibrous, and a woody brown shell encases a layer of firm, white meat with a milky fluid at its center.

Nutrients in 100 g of shredded, sweetened coconut

CALORIES KCAL	PROTEIN G	FAT G	CARBOHYDRATE G	CALCIUM MG	IRON MG
579	4	39	53	2	2

Percent composition of coconut oil fatty acids by chain length

CHAIN LENGTH	C_6	C_8	C_{10}	C_{12}	C_{14}	C_{16}	C_{18}
Percent	0.2	8	7	50	18	8	11

cod (*Gadus morrhua*). A soft-finned saltwater fish averaging from 3–4 feet in length and 7–10 pounds in weight. The cod is brownish on the upper body and sides and cream below, with small brown and yellow spots. The roe (eggs) sometimes constitutes a full half of the weight of the female fish. The flesh is firm and white. Cod is a lean fish, a good source of protein, some iron, calcium, and B vitamins. See this item in the table under *fish*.

cod liver oil. Intended for medicinal purposes, derived from the fresh liver of the cod. Cod liver oil is the most important of the fish-liver oils. The better qualities are valued for their content of *retinol* (vitamin A), and *vitamin D*, and are used as medicinal oils and for animal feeding. The lower grades (cod oils) are used in the leather industry.

coenocytic. Having more than one *nucleus* in a single mass of *cytoplasm*.

coenzyme. A nonprotein organic substance that works with or is bound to the protein part of an *enzyme*, which part is called an *apoenzyme*. The complete enzyme is called a holoenzyme. Many enzymes do not work unless the coenzyme is attached. Coenzymes are often necessary for the enzyme to function as a biological catalyst. Most of the vitamins, the water-soluble vitamins in particular, function as coenzymes in some chemically modified form. For example, *thiamine* functions as a coenzyme *thiamine pyrophosphate*; *niacin* functions as the coenzyme *nicotinamide adenine dinucleotide* (NAD); *riboflavin* functions as the coenzyme *flavin adenine dinucleotide*; and *pyridoxine* (vitamin B$_6$) functions as the coenzyme *pyridoxal* or *pyridoxamine phosphate*.

coenzyme A (CoA). A complex *nucleotide* containing *pantothenic acid*. Coenzyme A combines with acetyl groups to yield active acetate, acetyl coenzyme A, which can enter the *Krebs' cycle* for oxidation or serve as an intermediate in fatty-acid synthesis and *cholesterol* synthesis. Coenzyme A is a central biochemical intermediate in many anabolic and catabolic reactions. Acid derivatives with CoA, such as acetyl-CoA, amino acid-CoA, or acyl-CoA are high-energy compounds and are capable of doing synthetic work. To form these CoA derivatives, energy must be put into the reaction. That source of chemical energy is usually *adenosine triphosphate* (ATP) or a nucleoside triphosphate equivalent. The pantetheine portion, shown in the diagram, is also the active portion of the complex enzyme *fatty acid synthetase*.

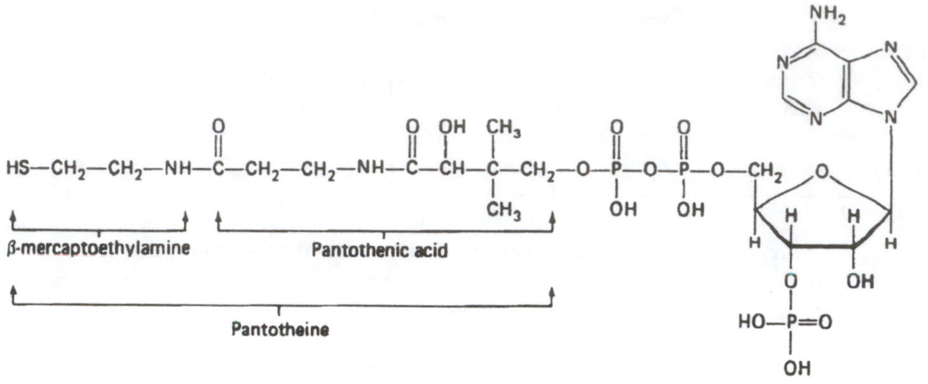

Coenzyme A (CoA)

coenzyme B$_{12}$. See *cobalamin*.

cofactor. A relatively low molecular weight organic compound required for enzyme activity. Metal ions and *coenzymes* are examples of cofactors.

coffee. A substance brewed from roasted and ground coffee beans. The beans themselves, whole or ground, are also known as coffee. The two chief methods of curing coffee are: (1) the dry method, in which the berries or "cherries" are spread out and air-dried in the sun or artificially; and (2) the wet, or "washed coffee" method in which the berries, after removal of the outer skin, are soaked in water. The removal of pulpy material is accomplished primarily by pectolytic bacteria, mostly coliforms, although fungi may be present. This is followed by an acid fermentation by lactic acid bacteria such as *Leuconostoc mesenteroides*, *Lactobacillus brevis* and *L.plantarum*, and *Streptococcus faecalis*. The acids produced may be degraded by oxidizing organisms. After the pulp and its residues have been washed away, the beans are dried and hulled.

cola or kola. The word covers a tree, a nut, and a complex syrup used for making a carbonated beverage. The cola tree (*Cola nitida*) produces fruit containing numerous seeds. These brownish, bitter seeds are the cola nuts from which the cola extract is obtained. Containing a small amount of *caffeine*, the cola nut is a mild stimulant. In the United States the extract of the cola nut is widely used in the drug and beverage industries.

colchicine. An *alkaloid* drug used in the treatment of *gout*. It interferes in the metabolic pathway of *uric acid*.

colectomy. The removal of the diseased portion of the *colon*.

colitis. Inflammation of the *colon*.

collagen. A protein, the main organic constituent of connective tissue and of the organic substance of bones. Collagen in the native state is insoluble in water and changes into gelatin by boiling. *Proline* and *glycine* are the major amino acids of collagen. *Ascorbic acid* (vitamin C) is required for a reaction that adds a hydroxyl group onto proline and *lysine* residues in procollagen to yield the hydroxyproline and g-hydroxylysine residues required for normal collagen. The synthesis of normal collagen is vital for proper wound healing. In ascorbic acid deficiency, wound healing is greatly diminished. See *scurvy*.

collard (*Brassica oleracea*). Collards are a member of the *cabbage* family and most closely related to *kale*. Their leaves are smooth, tall, and broad, but they do not form a head as cabbage does. The usual method of cooking them is to boil them with a piece of bacon or salt pork. The resulting juice is known as "pot likker" and is taken with corn bread. Collards can also be cooked like spinach, chard, cabbage, or kale. Excellent source of *carotene* (vitamin A), iron, calcium, and *ascorbic acid* (vitamin C); fair source of *thiamine*, riboflavin, and *niacin*. See this item in the table under *vegetables*.

colloid. (1) A two-phase system in which particles of one phase ranging in size from 1–100 millimicrons are dispersed in the second phase. The dispersion of particles less than 11 μM is usually considered a solution, and above 100 μM, it is a suspension. (2) A gelatinous material secreted by cuboidal epithelial cells, arranged in hollow spheres one cell thick, as in the *thyroid* tissue. Proteins dissolved in water are examples of colloidal solutions.

colon. The large intestine. The colon extends from the ileocecal sphincter in the right iliac fossa, around the outer portion of the abdominal cavity to end at the anus. When food enters or leaves the stomach, there is a reflex discharge of intestinal contents from the lower ileum into the colon through the ileocecal sphincter. This is called the "gastrocolic reflex." There is also a passive filling of the colon from the ileum about 4–5 hours after the ingestion of food. Normally, about 350 g of fecal matter pass into the colon daily. Water is absorbed by the colon and the feces become formed or semisolid in the next 36 hours. See *digestive system*.

color additives. Food colors can be synthetic or of natural origin, but more than 90% of the colors now in use are synthetic. Sometimes these are called *coal tar dyes* because originally they were made from a chemical obtained from coal tars. Synthetic colors are used in soft drinks, candy, or confectionary products, frozen desserts, gelatin desserts and puddings, maraschino cherries, meat casings, prepared mixes, and some dairy and bakery products. A color, natural or synthetic, added to foods is *carotene* (vitamin A activity), often used to color dairy products as well as margarine. See *food additives*.

colostrum. A clear, watery fluid produced by the *mammary glands* toward the end of a pregnancy. It differs from milk in that it has a very low fat content. Colostrum is believed to give the new born child immunity to most of the common infectious diseases during the first few months of life. Colostrum disappears and milk appears after about the fourth day after delivery. See *lactation* and *mammary gland*.

combustion. The combination of substances with oxygen accompanied by the liberation of energy, usually as heat. The combustion of food involves an indirect combination with oxygen, resulting in the liberation of heat and synthesis of *adenosine triphosphate (ATP)*.

complete protein. A protein that contains the *essential amino acids* in quantities sufficient for maintenance of the body and for a normal rate of growth. Such proteins are said to have a high *biological value* (BV). Egg, milk, cheese, and meat are complete-protein foods.

condensed milk. See *milk*.

congenital. Existing at or before birth with reference to certain physical or mental traits.

conjugated proteins. Conjugated proteins with some nonprotein substances attached to their structure. Protein molecules may be conjugated with fat such as the *lipoproteins* in the blood, or carbohydrates, such as the *glycoproteins*, which are found in the *mucus* secreted into the *digestive system*. Other important conjugated proteins are formed by linkage with phosphoric acid (*phosphoproteins*); with the lipid *lecithin* (*fibrin* in clotted blood and vitellin in egg yolk); with an iron-containing compound (*heme*) to form the oxygen-carrying substance *hemoglobin* in the blood.

conjugation. The process of genetic recombination between two organisms (e.g., yeast, bacteria and algae) through a cytoplasmic bridge between them.

conjunctivitis. An inflammation of the conjunctiva, the membrane lining the inner eyelid and whites of the eyes. Its characteristics are redness, discharge, discomfort (itching and/or burning), and sensitivity to light. The conjunctiva can be inflamed as a result of exposure to chemicals, bacteria, viruses, or allergens, and conjunctivitis is a common feature of *retinol* (vitamin A) deficiency. The well-known pinkeye is an example of conjunctivitis caused by bacteria. Viruses are common causes of conjunctivitis. The watery, slightly reddened eyes seen in many colds result from an attack on the conjunctiva by the cold viruses. Conjunctivitis associated with retinol (vitamin A) deficiency is marked by dryness. One virus, herpes simplex, is notoriously dangerous when it affects the cornea of the eye. See *eye*.

connective tissue. Tissues that support and connect other *tissues* and tissue parts.

contact dermatitis (allergic eczema). An inflammation of the skin resulting from exposure to or contact with some substance in a person's environment. The substance may be animal, mineral, or vegetable in origin and must be a substance to which the person has developed a sensitivity. See *allergy*.

contracture. A combination in which there is fixed resistance to the stretching of a muscle. It results from *fibrosis* of the tissues surrounding a joint or from disorders of the muscle fibers.

contraindicated. Not recommended or advised against use.

copper (Cu). Element No. 29. At. Wt. 64. The human body contains 1.5–2.5 mg per Cu/kg fat-free body weight. The mineral is distributed in all body tissues, but liver, brain, heart, and kidneys contain the highest amounts. In blood, copper appears to be equally divided between plasma and erythrocytes; plasma contains about 110 μg/100 mL. Symptoms of copper deficiency include *anemia*, hypopigmentation, changes in the texture of hair, abnormalities in bone structure, failure of myelination, and central nervous system defects. Copper occurs along with other mineral elements in most natural foods. The richest sources are organ meats, crustaceans, shellfish, nuts, dried legumes, and cocoa. Human milk contains an adequate amount. Only 30% of the copper consumed is absorbed. This occurs in the stomach and upper intestine in an acid medium. From the intestine, copper moves into the bloodstream. About 93% of the serum copper is bound tightly to *ceruloplasmin* and is released from it only when this protein is catabolized. Ceruloplasmin is considered the molecular link in copper and iron metabolism and has been shown to be directly involved in *hemoglobin* biosynthesis. About 7% of the serum copper is loosely bound to albumin and amino acids, and is transported to the various body tissues in these forms. The liver is the main organ for copper storage. The liver also synthesizes ceruloplasmin and prepares the mineral for biliary excretion.

Copper in µg/100 g of Food

Almonds	1210	Cheese,		Halibut	230	Pork chops	310
Apple	120	American	180	Kale	328	Prunes	291
Asparagus	141	Chicken, dark	410	Liver, beef	2450	Rye, whole	656
Avocado	690	Chicken, white	270	Lobster	730	Shrimp	430
Bananas	200	Chocolate, bitter	2670	Mackerel	230	Spinach	197
Beans, dry	960	Cocoa	3340	Mushrooms	1790	Sweet potatoes	184
Beans, lima	915	Corn	449	Oats	739	Turkey	
Beef, round	80	Eggs	253	Oranges	80	dark meat	200
Bread, white	205	Flour,		Oysters	3623	white meat	150
Cabbage	50	whole wheat	435	Peas, dried	802	Walnuts	1000
Carrots	80	white	170	Pecans	1360	Wheat	787

corn or maize (*Zea mays*). One of the cereal *grains*. It originated in the Americas and is now grown worldwide. It is a hardy crop, more resistant to drought and predation by birds than most cereal grains. The nutrient value is similar to that of other cereal grains. Corn has more *retinol* (vitamin A) activity than most of the cereals, and while it appears to contain adequate amounts of *niacin*, it appears to be in a bound form and unavailable for absorption. Consequently, in those poor societies or economic groups that depend on corn as a major source of food, the nutritional disease due to a niacin deficiency, pellagra, is widespread, as it was among the poor in the southern United States several decades ago. Interestingly enough, pellagra was once thought to be a heritable disease associated with other "traits" of the poor, such as laziness and slowness of wit. The Mexican Indians who are poor and who depend on corn as a major source of food never develop pellegra. It is believed that their customary treatment of corn flour with slaked lime (an alkali) in the preparation of tortillas releases the bound niacin in corn and the tryptophan, which has some niacin activity, and so niacin deficiencies never develop. See this item in the table under *vegetables*.

cornmeal. Corn, coarsely ground. In "new-process" cornmeal, the corn is ground after the hull and germ of the kernel are removed. In "old-process" cornmeal, the whole grain is ground into meal. Although old-process cornmeal is richer in *carotene* (vitamin A activity), new-process cornmeal keeps better because it has a lower fat content.

corn oil. The fruits of *corn* (kernels), a large number of which are united with a fleshy stalk to form the "cob", are commercially divided into (1) bran (testa and the pericarp), (2) hominy (endosperm), and (3) germ (scutellum). Oil is obtained only from the germ, which is commercially separated from the endosperm by various processes (steaming, rolling, and sifting) before pressing. It is also obtained as a by-product in starch making. The theory that the *polyunsaturated fatty acids* contained in vegetable oils are "essential" to human metabolism and that they tend to combat the onset of *thrombosis* has made vegetable and seed oils' high content of polyunsaturated acids highly recommended as substitutes for butter and for use in the diet generally. In the same class are *safflower* and *sunflower oils*. They are also used for salads and in margarine.

cornstarch. A starch obtained from the endosperm portion of the kernel. It is used as a thickener in sauces, gravies, and puddings. It is also the basis of laundry starch and talcum powder. Much of it today is converted into high *fructose* corn syrup used in place of *sucrose* in beverages.

corn syrup. Corn syrups are products of partial hydrolyses of starches. Their composition is intermediate between the high-molecular-weight starch itself and *glucose* (dextrose), the product of complete hydrolysis. Corn syrups are manufactured by acid or enzymatic hydrolysis of starch or by a combination of both. The enzymes employed are amylases of bacterial, fungal, and plant origin. After hydrolyzing to the desired degree, the syrups are refined by filtration, carbon treatment, and sometimes by ion exchange to remove traces of salts and to reduce soluble protein. The refined syrups are then concentrated and shipped as a liquid containing 70–85% solids. The wet-milling industry defines corn syrup as starch hydrolysates having a dextrose equivalent (DE) of 28 or higher. DE is a measure of reducing sugar calculated as a percentage of dextrose. Syrups are also available with higher dextrose levels or with high levels of specific *saccharides*, depending on the enzyme used in the processing. Food manufacturers use corn syrup to sweeten and thicken foods and beverages. In some foods, such as candy, icings, and fillings, it retards crystallization of sugar, and it prevents the loss of moisture from cakes, cookies, and whipped foods. There are two kinds of syrup, light and dark. Light corn syrup has been clarified and decolorized. Dark syrup has a stronger flavor.

Functional properties of corn syrups

HIGH DE CORN SYRUPS		LOW DE CORN SYRUPS
1. Browning reaction	5. Flavor enhancement	1. Bodying (mouth feel)
2. Ferment ability	6. Sweetness	2. Foam stabilization
3. Freezing point depression	7. Hydroscopicity	3. Prevents sugar crystallization
4. Osmotic pressures		4. Viscosity

Classification of corn syrups

DEGREE OF CONVERSION	LOW	REGULAR	INTERMEDIATE	HIGH	EXTRA HIGH
(DE)Dextrose Equivalent	28-37	38-47	48-57	58-67	68 or higher

coronary arteries. The heart gets its blood supply from the right and left coronary arteries. These arteries branch off from the aorta just above the heart, then subdivide into many smaller branches within the heart muscle. If any part of the heart muscle is deprived of its blood supply through interruption of blood flow through the coronary arteries and their branches, the muscle tissue deprived of blood cannot function and will die. This is called *myocardial infarction*. Blood from the heart tissue is returned by coronary veins to the right atrium.

coronary heart disease. Although the heart muscle itself may be normal, the circulation to it is reduced or cut off by narrowing or blocking of branches of the coronary arteries. There is a constantly changing pattern of the circulation in the complex branching distribution of the coronary arteries, some of which become thickened and blocked with clots or fatty deposits, which narrow the caliber. In some, a clot in the artery may become partially dissolved, and nature then attempts to open up new channels to replace those which have degenerated. The following factors are known to increase the risk of coronary heart disease, but are not necessarily "abnormalities" *per se* and are not readily amenable to preventive intervention: (1) male hormones, (2) increasing age, (3) a family history of premature vascular disease, (4) endomorphic body fluid, and (5) certain behavior patterns and personality traits. The following abnormalities are known to increase the risk of coronary heart disease: (1) hyperlipemias, (2) *hypertension*, (3) *diabetes mellitus*, (4) *obesity*, (5) *hyperuricemia* and *gout*, (6) certain electrocardiographic abnormalities. The following factors, which are primarily due to culture and environment, are known to increase the risk of coronary heart disease: (1) cigarette smoking, (2) dietary habits (high intake of saturated fats, etc.), (3) lack of physical exercise, and (4) occupational hazards. Elevated serum cholesterol greatly increases the risk of coronary artery disease. Serum *cholesterol* level is raised by diets high in cholesterol and saturated fats. High-cholesterol, high-saturated-fat diets are believed generally to contribute to *atherosclerosis*. The degree of dietary contribution of cholesterol and saturated fats remains controversial, as cholesterologenesis is essentially unaffected by diet. High blood pressure is an important coronary artery disease risk factor. It appears to accelerate the atherosclerotic process and precipitate myocardial ischemia, heart failure, and stroke. Life-style habits contributing to coronary heart disease include cigarette smoking, physical inactivity, obesity, weight gain, and emotional stress. See *cardiovascular disease*.

coronary occlusion. Obstruction or narrowing of one of the coronary arteries which hinders blood flow to some part of the heart muscle.

cortex. Outer layer of an organ, for example, adrenal cortex and cerebral cortex. In plants, it is the tissue beneath the epidermis.

corticosterone. A hormone of the adrenal cortex. Corticosterone influences carbohydrate, potassium, and sodium metabolism. It is essential for normal absorption of glucose, the formation of glycogen in the liver and tissues, and the normal utilization of carbohydrates by the tissues. See *adrenal glands*.

corticotrophin. A hormone of the anterior pituitary gland that specifically stimulates the adrenal cortex. See *adrenal glands*.

cortisol (hydrocortisone) and cortisone. Cortisol and cortisone belonging to a class of steroid hormones, synthesized in the cortex of the *adrenal glands*, known as glucocorticoids. They have a primary effect on carbohydrate, protein, and lipid metabolism. Increased concentrations of cortisol or cortisone may cause a stimulation of appetite and a negative calcium balance (antagonistic to *vitamin D* effects). The production and liberation of cortisol and cortisone are under the control of *adrenocorticotropin* (ACTH). Four of the cortical hormones, including cortisol and cortisone, affect carbohydrate, protein, and fat metabolism in many ways antagonistic to *insulin*. They elevate blood glucose and increase production of glucose from protein, and they slow the growth of connective tissue cells and the formation of complex polysaccharides in these tissues. Injections of cortisone give relief from pain and crippling effects in some cases of rheumatoid arthritis. Cortisone is addictive in some individuals.

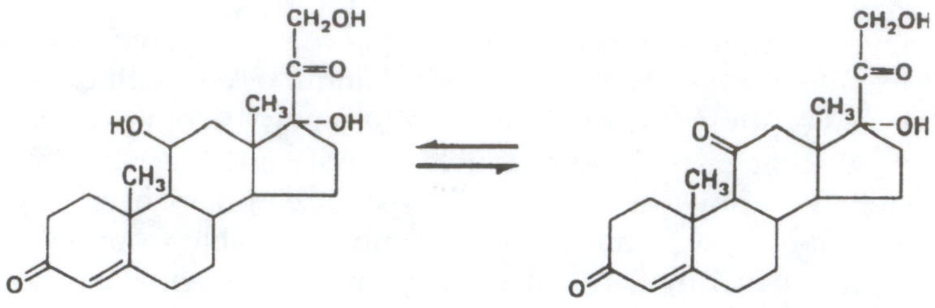

Cortisol (hydrocortisone and cortisone)

coumarin. A compound found in sweet clover. A derivative of coumarin, *dicumarol* is an *antivitamin* of *vitamin K* and is used clinically to prevent blood clotting.

cranberry (*Vaccinium*). A bright red-berry of the heath family, *Ericacae*. Cranberries are high in *ascorbic acid* (vitamin C). See this item in the table under *fruits*.

cream. The rich, fatty part of whole milk which rises to the top and which can be separated from the milk. The longer sweet cream stands, the thicker it becomes. There are different kinds of cream, regulated by their butterfat content. Cream can be sweet or sour. See this item in the table under *milk*.

cream of tartar (sodium acid tartrate). Mol. Wt. 172. The common name for potassium acid *tartaric acid*, an acid salt that is used in angel cake to stabilize the eggwhite foam, to whiten the color, and to increase the tenderness of the cake. It is also used as an acid ingredient in the tartrate baking powder. See *tartaric acid*.

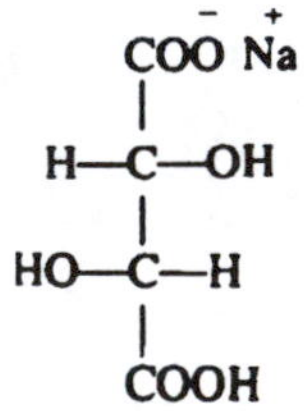

Cream of tartar (sodium acid tartrate)

creatine. Mol. Wt. 131. A crystalline substance that can be isolated from various animal organs and body fluids. It combines readily with phosphate to form phosphocreatine (*creatine phosphate*) which serves as a source of high-energy phosphate released in the anaerobic phase of muscle contraction. See *phosphocreatine, creatinine*.

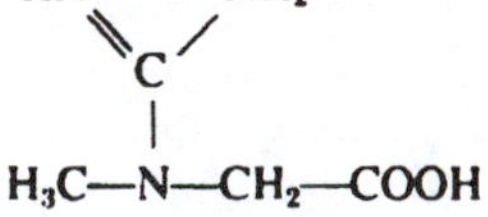

Creatine

creatine phosphate (phosphocreatine). Mol. Wt. 211. $C_4H_{10}N_3O_5P$. A compound of *creatine* and *phosphoric acid* that is found especially in vertebrate muscle, where it is an energy reserve for muscle contraction. It is energetically equivalent to *adenosine triphosphate*. See *creatine phosphokinase* and *muscle*.

creatine phosphokinase (CPK, CK). An enzyme present in skeletal and cardiac muscle and the brain. It catalyzes the reversible transfer of high-energy phosphate between *creatine* and *adenosine triphosphate* (ATP) and between phosphocreatine and *diphosphate* (ADP).

$$\text{Creatine} + \text{ATP} = \text{Creatine} \sim \text{phosphate} + \text{ADP}$$

creatinine. Mol. Wt. 131. A nitrogen-containing substance derived from *creatine* catabolism and present in urine. It is the end product of creatine. Creatinine is excreted at a relatively constant rate that varies roughly in proportion to the muscle mass. Because of the relatively constant excretion rate, it is often used as an index of *kidney* function since a kidney malfunction will sometimes show decreased creatinine excretion rates.

Creatinine

cretinism. A glandular disease, cretinism is easily recognizable within the first 4 months of an infant's life. It is due to insufficient secretion of the *thyroid gland*. Two types of cretinism have been identified, sporadic and endemic. The child may be born with a rudimentary thyroid gland, or the thyroid gland may be absent. In either case, the child is not able to furnish his or her body with sufficient *thyroxin*. Cretinism is recognized by symptoms such as small stature (dwarfism) accompanied by short, thick legs; disproportionally large head; short, broad hands and fingers with square ends; dry and coarse or scaly skin with an edematous appearance; coarse and scant hair; peg-shaped and chalky teeth, with delayed dentition; half-shut eyes and swollen eyelids; low *basal metabolic rate* (BMR), and little perspiration; short and thick neck; delayed sexual development; hoarseness and strident voice. In personality these infants and later these children tend to be restive and stubborn; they lack spontaneity. They are not troublesome in behavior, usually being placid and tactiturn rather than quarrelsome and aggressive. In intelligence, cretins range from the idiot level through the moron level and some reach the borderline-normal classification.

cryptoxanthin. The yellow pigment of corn. Three provitamin A *carotenoids* are known as *carotenes* (α-, β-, and γ-*carotene*), and a fourth is cryptoxanthin.

cucumber (*Cucumis sativus*). The succulent fruit of a rough-stemmed trailing vine belonging to the gourd family. Cucumbers come in a number of varieties, from thick, stubby little fruit 3–4 inches long, to greenhouse giants. The most popular cucumbers have a smooth, dark-green rind. Pickles called gherkins are made from small cucumbers. They are soaked in brine, treated with boiling vinegar, and flavored with dill or spices. See this item in the table under *vegetables*.

cumin (*Cuminum cyminum*). The cumin plant, source of the aromatic cumin seed, is a delicate member of the parsley family, an annual which rarely grows more than 5–6 inches high. The seed is tiny and oval, with a strong, warm, and slightly bitter taste. Since cumin seed resembles caraway seed in flavor as well as looks, its uses are much the same.

curd. Semisolid mass formed when *milk* comes in contact with an acid, such as the acid secretion in the stomach, or with an enzyme.

curing. Curing or pickling is the treatment of meats with high concentrations of salt solutions or by rubbing salt on the meat surface. Curing inhibits the actions of tissue *enzymes* that degrade proteins, and it inhibits the growth of bacteria. The most common salts used in curing are *sodium chloride* (brine) and a combination of *sodium nitrates* and *sodium nitrites*. The concentrations of brine are between 5–20%. The more concentrated brine solution causes some shrinkage of the meats with retention of red color. Additives, spices, sugar, and microflora (bacteria) enhance the flavor of the meat. In addition to enchancing the flavor of the meat, the addition of microflora contributes to the stabilization of the red or pink meat color. See *food storage*.

currant (*Ribes* and *Vitis*). The name is applied to two totally different fruits. One, a fresh currant, is a berry of the genus *Ribes*, a member of the gooseberry family; the other, a dry currant, is a dried grape of the genus *Vitis*. Currants are sweet, tart berries which come in red, white, or black varieties. Red currants are the best known and most frequently used. Red currants are eaten fresh as a fruit, as well as cooked in jams and jellies. White currants are used in salads and fruit cups, and black currants are used primarily in jams, jellies, and beverages. They contain small amounts of *carotene* (vitamin A) and *ascorbic acid* (vitamin C).

Nutrients in 100 g of raw red currant

CALORIES KCAL	PROTEIN G	FAT G	CARBOHYDRATE G	VITAMIN A IU	ASCORBATE MG	CALCIUM MG
55	1	Trace	14	121	41	32

Cushing's syndrome (hyperadrenalism). A result of an increased production of glucocorticoids from the adrenal cortex. It may be caused by a tumor or other disease of the adrenal gland, or it may result from overstimulation of the *adrenal glands* by the *pituitary gland*. See *cortisol*.

custard apple (*Annona reticulata*). Aside from the common custard apple, the name covers several fruits of tropical and subtropical America, such as the cherimoya and the sweetsop, or sugar apple, all of which have a sweet, soft pulp. They do not taste like apples. The outside of the true custard apple looks scaly, rather like an artichoke. The fruit is 4–6 inches in length and heart-shaped, and the pulp is cream-colored. All custard apples have a bland taste, with the pulp eaten directly from the fruit or spooned into a serving dish.

Nutrients in 100 g of raw custard apple

CALORIES KCAL	PROTEIN G	FAT G	CARBOHYDRATE G	VITAMIN A IU	ASCORBATE MG	CALCIUM MG
101	2	1	25	121	19	30

cyanocobalamin (cobalamin, vitamin B$_{12}$). See *cobalamin*.

cyanogens. Hydrogen cyanide (HCN) is a constituent of a large number of edible plants. Cyanogens or the cyanogenic glucosides, which on hydrolysis in the human intestine yield cyanide, are found in such garden variety foodstuffs as lima beans, sweet potatoes, yams, sugar cane, peas, cherries, plums, and apricots. The initial symptoms of acute cyanogen poisoning have been described as numbness in fingertips and toes and giddiness or light-headedness. Small, nonfatal doses often produce headache sensations or tightness in both throat and chest, perceptible heart beating (palpitations), and general weakness. Full recovery is usual as the body processes eliminate the offending chemical.

cyclamates. The sodium or calcium salts of cyclohexylsulfamic acid. They are water soluble, with a *sweet* taste (30 times that of sucrose), and are used as a noncaloric sweetener. In 1968 the National Academy of Sciences (NAS) told the Food and Drug Administration (FDA) that although consumption of reasonable quantities of cyclamate probably posed no hazard to humans, additional studies were needed to resolve various aspects of cyclamate's safety. Further questions arose in 1969 after bladder tumors developed in rats and mice that were fed a mixture of cyclamate and saccharin. That prompted the FDA to remove cyclamate from its *GRAS* (generally regarded as safe) list and to propose phasing it out of general food use. At the FDA's request, the National Academy of Science (NAS) and the National Research Council (NRC) recently undertook an independent review of the carcinogenicity data relating to cyclamate. On June 10, 1985, the NAS panel of scientists issued a report that concluded that the scientific evidence did not indicate that cyclamate or its major derivative, cyclohexy-lamine, was carcinogenic. However, the NAS committee recommended repeating animal studies that suggested that cyclamate may act as a tumor promoter, that is, as a substance that may enhance the development of tumors when fed with other carcinogens. The FDA continues to review cyclamate, including resolution of such safety issues as to whether cyclamate may cause genetic damage and testicular atrophy. See *aspartame* and *saccharin*.

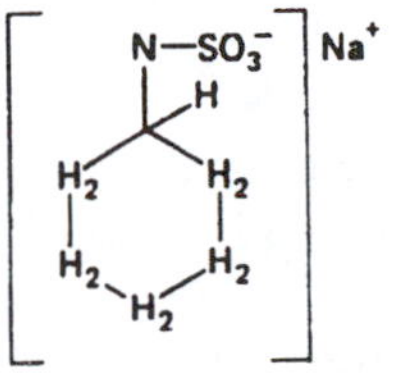

$$\left[\begin{array}{c} N-SO_3^- \\ | \\ H \end{array}\right] Na^+$$

Cyclamate

cyclic AMP (c-AMP). Mol. Wt. 329. A compound produced by *adenosine triphosphate* (ATP) through the action of an enzyme, adenylate cyclase, which is stimulated by a vast number of hormones, including *epinephrine, catecholamines, glucagon,* luteinizing *hormone* (LH), *vasopressin,* *parathormone, prostaglandins,* and *thyrocalcitonin* as well as other biologically active agents such as *histamine* and *serotonin*. It is believed that c-AMP mediates the effects of hormones and other active agents, and plays a regulatory role in cellular metabolism by stimulating the phosphorylation of enzymes and controlling the rate of a number of cellular reactions as varied as the synthesis and activity of proteins, *glycogenolysis, lipolysis,* steroidogenesis, and *active transport.* Because of the role that c-AMP plays, it is often referred to as the "second messenger." Hormones are the primary messengers. In general, the effects of c-AMP oppose the effects of *insulin.*

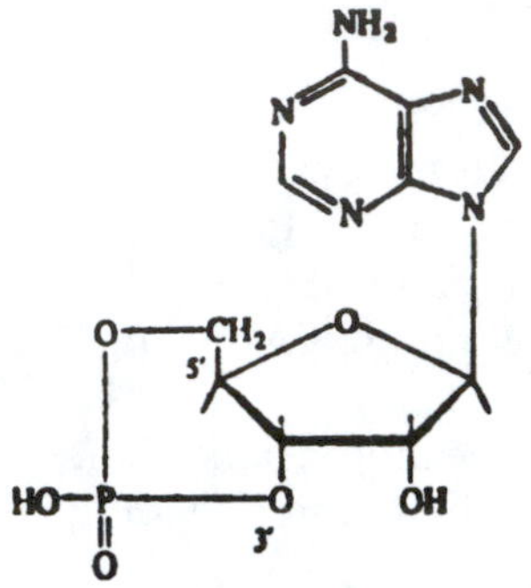

Cyclic AMP

cyst. A sac or saclike structure, usually abnormal, containing liquid or semisolid matter and often caused by blockage of a passage.

cysteine (Cys, C). Mol. Wt. 121. An amino acid and one of two principal sources of sulfur in the human diet. The other source is the *essential amino acid methionine.* The body can make cysteine from methionine but not the reverse. *Cystine* is formed when two molecules of cysteine are reduced and linked by a disulfide or S-S bond. Cystine is present in the *keratin* of hair and in *insulin,* in each of which it forms about 12% of the protein molecule molecular weight.

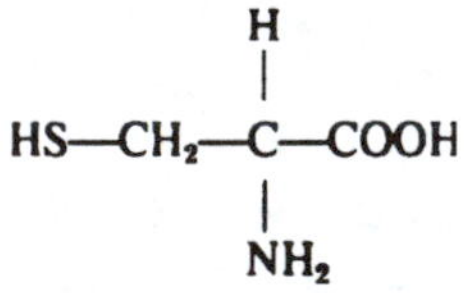

Cysteine (Cys, C)

cysticerosis. Infestation of the body with a form of tapeworm called cysticerus, which is sometimes present in raw beef. Beef should be cooked at least to 140°F to avoid danger.

cystine (Cys-Cys). Mol. Wt. 240. Cystine is the oxidative condensation product of two molecules of the amino acid *cysteine.* Cystine as a separate compound has no major important function. However, the condensation of two cysteine residues within protein chains to form cystine residues is very important to the structure and conformation of a large number of proteins and enzymes. Some examples are *chymotrypsin* and *insulin,* both of which require peptide chains held together by cystine residues for their biologic activity.

$$HOOC - \underset{\underset{NH_2}{|}}{\overset{\overset{H}{|}}{C}} - CH_2 - S - S - CH_2 - \underset{\underset{NH_2}{|}}{\overset{\overset{H}{|}}{C}} - COOH$$

Cystine

cystinuria (cystine stones). Cystinuria is an inborn error of metabolism characterized by faulty absorption of the amino acids cystine, ornithine, arginine, and lysine in the renal tubules; slightly retarded growth; and the appearance of the four amino acids in the urine, due to defective tubular reabsorption. Of these, cystine is the least soluble. It will precipitate when there is increased concentration in the urine, and form stones.

cystitis. An inflammation of the bladder and one of the most common disorders of the urinary tract. It is rarely a primary disease and is often a symptom of some other disturbance in either the urinary tract or the genital tract.

cytochromes. Respiratory enzymes consisting of a number of hemochromogens which are similar to the *heme* in *hemoglobin*. The iron-containing heme proteins of the electron transport system or *terminal respiratory chain* that are alternatively oxidized and reduced in biological oxidation. The electron transport system in cells uses oxygen to form water in an *oxidative phosphorylation* process.

cytokinesis. The division of the cytoplasm during *mitosis* or *meiosis*.

cytoplasm. The material within the *cell*, with the exception of the nucleus. Contains a variety of structures and *organelles*, as well as pigment granules, secretory granules, and nutrients such as protein and carbohydrate particles.

cytosine. One of the *pyrimidine* nitrogenous bases found in the *nucleic acids*.

cytosol. The liquid portion of the *cytoplasm* after the *organelles* and other formed elements have been removed, usually by high-speed centrifugation. It is essentially a colloidal suspension of the soluble proteins of the *cell*.

D

D The alphabetic symbol for the amino acid *aspartic acid* (Asp).

D. A symbol to denote a configuration about an asymmetric carbon relative to D-glyceralde-hyde. The mirror image is the L-configuration. All naturally occurring asymmetric carbons are either all L- or all D-. For example, all amino acids found in proteins have the L-configuration.

d- The designation that an optically active compound is dextrorotatory. It rotates polarized light to the right. It is the opposite of levorotatory (*l-*).

damson (*Prunus*). A variety of plum tree and its fruit, which, like all plums, belongs to the great rose family. The word "damson" is derived from Damascus, capital of Syria, where the plums were cultivated before the time of Christ. Damson plums are small, firm, oval, purple plums. There is a variety with yellow flesh. These are spicier and more acid than ordinary plums. Damson plums are not eaten raw, but are used for cooking and are made into pies, compotes, jams, and preserves. See this listing under plum in the table under the *fruits*.

dandelion (*Taraxacum officinale*). A familiar weed of the chicory family. The name comes from the French *dent de lion* or "lion's tooth," which the sharply indented leaves of the plant are said to resemble. Wild or cultivated, dandelion leaves are eaten as a vegetable, raw or cooked. They have a somewhat bitter flavor. The roots can be eaten as vegetables or roasted and ground and made into a root coffee. Dandelion greens are an excellent source of *carotene* (vitamin A activity), very good for iron, and good for calcium.

Nutrients in 100 g of cooked dandelion greens

CALORIES KCAL	PROTEIN G	FAT G	CARBOHYDRATE G	VITAMIN A IU	ASCORBATE MG	CALCIUM MG
33	2	<1	6	11,700	18	140

dasheen (*Colocasia*). A starch root vegetable with large and small tubers side by side on one plant. It is a variety of *taro* and in southern and tropical climates is used as a substitute for potatoes. The larger tubers (corms) weigh up to 6 pounds; the smaller tubers (cormels) are egg-sized. Both have brown, fibrous skins. When peeled and cooked, the flesh becomes cream-colored, and mealy, with a nutty flavor. Dasheens have more carbohydrates and proteins than potatoes.

date (*Phoenix dactylifera*). The fruit of the date palm. The date is a one-seeded *berry* and grows in thick clusters. Unripe, it is green; ripe, it is yellow or red, with thick and very sweet flesh. Depending upon the variety, dates can be soft, or hard and dry. Dates are ripened off the tree and dried before shipping. Dates are a good source of iron and sugar, as well as protein.

Nutrients in 100 g of natural, dry date

CALORIES KCAL	PROTEIN G	FAT G	CARBOHYDRATE G	VITAMIN A IU	CALCIUM MG	IRON MG
274	2	<1	73	50	73	3

deamination. Removal of an amino group ($-NH_2$) from an *amino acid* or other organic compound. Usually, the first step in the catabolism of amino acids is a deamination, which is accomplished by transfer of the amino group (*transamination*) to another compound. All amino acids are ultimately catabolized in humans to carbon dioxide, water, urea, and energy. After removal of the nitrogen (deamination) to form an alpha keto acid, the nonnitrogenous fraction of the amino acid molecule has one of several uses, depending on the need: (1) Some circulate directly to the tissues to form tissue protein by recombining with amino groups to reform the amino acid; (2) the α-keto acid is metabolized to carbon dioxide, water, *urea*, and energy at that time; or (3) converted to fat or carbohydrate and stored to be metabolized at a later time; or (4) incorporated into other compounds.

decalcification. The withdrawal of *calcium* from the bones where it has been deposited. It may be caused by an inadequate supply of calcium in the diet so that calcium has to be taken from the bones to help meet the body's needs. It may be caused by an imbalance in some of the hormone activity in the body. *Parathormone, calcitonin,* and *vitamin D* are involved in calcium metabolism.

decarboxylation. The removal of a carboxyl group from an amino acid. It is necessary for the formation in the body of at least three vital physiologic regulators (hormones or similar compounds) from the amino acids, *histidine* to form *histamine, tryptophan* to form, *serotonin* and *tyrosine* to form *epinephrine* and *norepinephrine*, as well as for the oxidation of amino acids for energy. The pyridoxine (vitamin B$_6$), as the coenzyme *pyridoxal phosphate*, is involved in the decarboxylation reactions of the amino acids, with the exception of the decarboxylation of histidine. *Thiamine* as the coenzyme *thiamine pyrophosphate* is involved in the oxidative decarboxylation of *pyruvic acid* and α-*ketoglutaric acid*.

deglutition. The act of swallowing is termed deglutition. After food has been grasped and divided by the anterior teeth, it is ground into fine particles by the posterior dentition. At the same time it is tossed about by the tongue and thoroughly mixed with saliva. Saliva makes it possible to swallow the mass of food called a *bolus*. In the first stage, food is ground and rolled into a bolus which has been thoroughly soaked with saliva. The tongue then directs the bolus to the back of the mouth and forces it to enter the pharynx. In the second stage, the bolus passes through the pharynx to enter the esophagus. In the third stage, the food traverses the esophagus to enter the stomach.

dehydrated foods. Products from which most of the water has been removed in order to improve stability during storage. See *lyophilization*

dehydration. (1) Removal of water from food or tissue; or the condition that results from undue loss of water. (2) Excessive loss of water or losses without replacement. Common causes of dehydration in humans are *diarrhea* and *vomiting* (emesis).

dehydrocholesterol (7-dehydrocholecalciferol). The *cholesterol* derivative in the skin that is converted to vitamin D_3. See *vitamin D*.

dehydrogenase. A class of *enzymes* that facilitates the transfer of hydrogen from one compound to another. The vitamins *niacin*, as the *coenzymes nicotinamide adenine dinucleotide* (NAD) and *nicotinamide adenine dinucleotide phosphate* (NADP), and *riboflavin*, as the coenzyme *flavin mononucleotide* (FMN) and *flavin adenine dinucleotide* (FAD), serve in many dehydrogenase reactions.

denature. (1) Denature may refer to the alcohol *ethanol* when a poison is added to make it unsuitable for consumption. It is referred to as denatured alcohol. *Methanol* (wood alcohol) does not have to be denatured since it is a poison. (2) Denature or the process of denaturation most frequently refers to proteins when they lose the natural physical, chemical, or biological characteristics by any means. Proteins are denatured by heat. The coagulation of egg white when boiled is an example of denaturation, that is, one of the physical properties of the protein have changed from soluble to insoluble. Enzymes lose their catalytic activity when denatured and yet may remain soluble proteins. Proteins may be denatured by a wide variety of substances or conditions including heat, acid, alkali, organic solvents, and mechanical agitation. Most cooking or preparation for meals causes denaturation of proteins which only alter their internal structure and has no effect on the quality of protein in general. One clear exception is dry heat, such as occurs in the formation of "puffed wheat" and "puffed rice" type cereals. Dry heat tends to destroy the *essential amino acid lysine*.

denatured alcohol. See *denature*.

deoxycholic acid. Mol. Wt. 393. One of the *bile acids* that forms *bile salts* in bile. The bile salt is conjugated with *taurine* or *glycine* to form deoxycholyltaurine (taurodeoxycholate) and deoxycholylglycine (glycodeoxycholate). The bile salts are powerful emulsifiers.

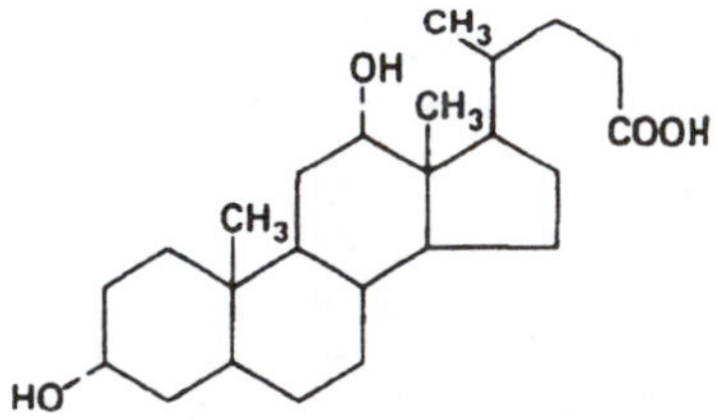

Deoxycholic acid

11-deoxycorticosterone. Mol. Wt. 330. A steroid hormone produced by the cortex of the *adrenal glands*. It is a precursor to the more powerful hormones *aldosterone* and *corticosterone*. The 11-

deoxycorticosterone has about 4% of the activity of aldosterone in its influence on salt and *water balance*.

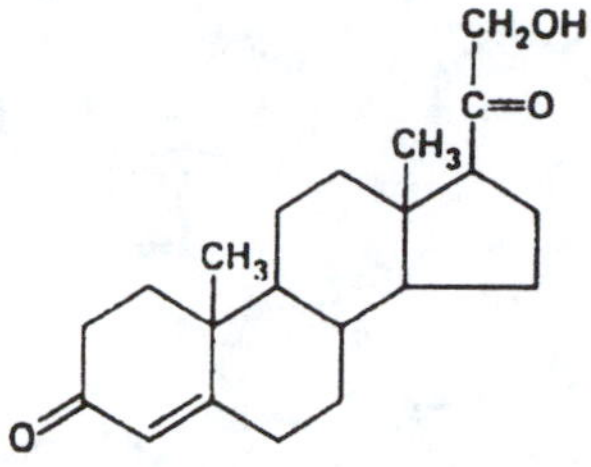

$$CH_2OH$$
$$C=O$$

11-deoxycorticosterone

deoxypyridoxine. Mol. Wt. 154. An *antivitamin* (antimetabolite). A compound similar in structure to *pyridoxine* that is antagonistic to the action of *pyridoxine* (vitamin B_6).

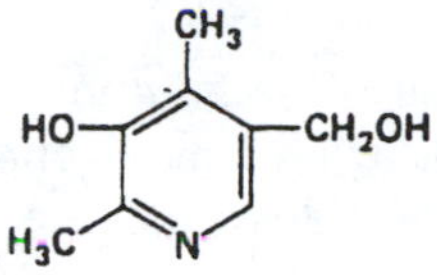

Deoxypridoxine

deoxyribonucleic acid (DNA). A substance found in the *nucleus* of living cells that functions in the transfer of genetic characteristics. The primary genetic material of the cell consists of long chains of nucleic acid called DNA or deoxyribonucleic acid. These chains contain genes. DNA is organized into larger units called *chromosomes* which contain protein and other substances, that are microscopically visible components of cell nuclei. It has been established that DNA molecules consist of a pair of polymeric chains of alternate units of a particular sugar (*deoxyribose*) and a phosphate group. Attached to each sugar is any one of four nitrogenous bases, two *purines* and two *pyrimidines*. The arrangement of these bases along the strand is the key factor that gives each DNA molecule its identity. The strands of DNA are complementary strands in that each base specifically pairs with another. Adenine and thymine are one specific pairing, and guanine and cystosine are the other specific pairing. The two complementary strands entwine naturally to form a double helix. DNA is the hereditary material (*gene*) of the cell, and there exists a biochemical process by which the DNA in a cell can be replicated and passed to successive generations. The position of a particular amino acid in the polypeptide chain is given in each case by the sequence of three nucleotides (a *triplet code*). The sequence of deoxyribonucleotides in DNA fixes the sequence of ribonucleotides in *messenger-ribonucleic acid* (m-RNA), which in turn determines the sequence of amino acids in proteins.

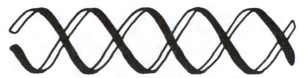

The double helix of DNA
(Campbell, P.N., and Smith, A.D., *Biochemistry Illustrated*, 1982. Reproduced with permission of Churchill Livingstone, Edinburgh.)

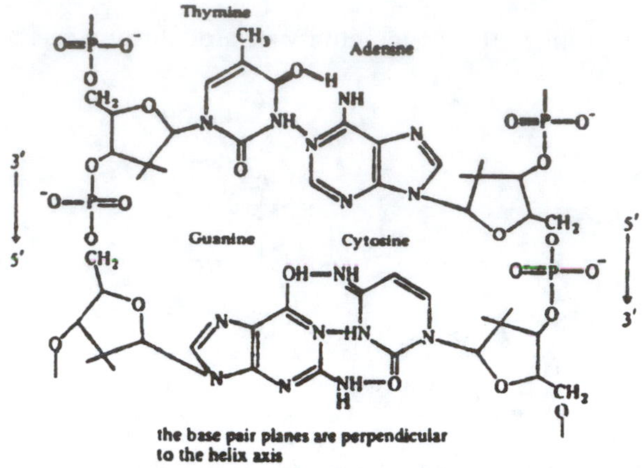

Deoxyribonucleic acid (DNA) base pairing

deoxyribonucleotides. Building blocks of *deoxyribonucleic acid* (DNA), each consisting of a sugar, *2-deoxyribose*, a phosphate group, and nitrogenous bases, the deoxyribonucleotides. There are four different deoxyribonucleotides, all containing deoxyribose and phosphate and differing in the bases, deoxyadenosine monophosphate (dAMP); deoxythymidine monophosphate (dTMP); deoxycytosine monophosphate (dCMP); and deoxyguanosine monophosphate (dGMP).

2-deoxyribose. Mol. Wt. 134. A five-carbon sugar with one less oxygen atom than the parent sugar, ribose. It occurs as a constituent of DNA. See *deoxyribonucleic acid* and *ribose*.

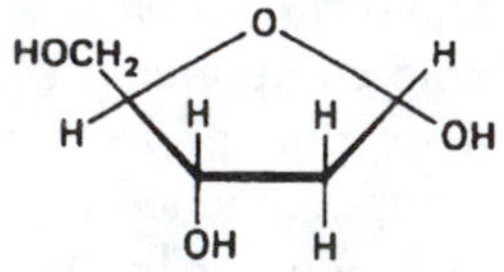

2-deoxyribose

derived proteins. See *coagulated proteins*.

dermatan sulfate. Contains largely L-iduronic acid in place of the acid sugar D-*glucuronic acid*. Dermatan sulfate generally occurs in tissues that are rich in *collagen*. Its biological role appears to be different from the chondroitin sulfates, and it is present mainly in the skin.

dermatitis. An inflammatory, recurring skin reaction, caused by contact with an irritating agent that is ingested or found in the environment. Dermatitis is usually associated with hereditary allergic tendencies and may be aggravated by emotional stress and fatigue. A primary symptom of dermatitis is eczema, a type of skin eruption characterized by tiny blisters that weep and erust. Chronic forms are characterized by scaling, flaking, and eventual thickening and color changes of the skin. Itching is almost always present. Deficiency of any of the B vitamins can cause dermatitis. A protein deficiency can cause chronic eczema.

dessicate. To dry.

dessicated liver. Dehydrated liver, a powder sold in health food stores and supposed to contain, in concentrated form, all the nutrients found in liver. Though probably not dangerous, this supplement has no special nutritional merit. Desiccated means "totally dried."

detoxification. The reduction of the toxic properties of a substance. In living systems, detoxification is accomplished by a wide variety of biochemical reactions. The liver plays an important role in many detoxification processes.

dewberry. Closely related to the *blackberry*, dewberries differ from blackberries by growing on trailing rather than upright vines. There are many different species. Berries contain a fair amount of *iron* and *ascorbic acid* (vitamin C).

dextran. $(C_6H_{10}O_5)_n$. A *polysaccharide*, made by the bacteria *Leuconostoc mesenteroides* from a molasses- or refined-sucrose medium. Dextran serves as a stabilizer for sugar syrups, ice cream, or confections. Dextrans are characterized by (β 1→2) glycosidic linkages as contrasted with the (α 1→4) linkages in *starch*.

dextrin. Formed from *starch* by the action of certain enzymes, acids, or heat. The term dextrin designates a group rather than an individual substance. Malt *diastase*, acting for some time upon starch in fairly concentrated solutions, usually yields about one part of dextrin to four of *maltose*. Dextrins formed by partial hydrolysis of starches are sometimes called "hydrolytic dextrins." Commercial dextrin, the principal constituent of British gum, is obtained by heating starch either alone or with a small amount of a dilute or a weak acid. The dextrins formed essentially by dry heating are sometimes called torrefaction dextrins. The dextrins are much more soluble than the starches. Dextrin molecules, while very large and complex, are smaller than the starch molecules from which they are derived.

dextrose. Another name for *glucose*. Food manufacturers use dextrose primarily as a sweetener, but it serves additional functions in certain foods. Dextrose (and other sugars) turn brown when heated and contribute to the color of bread crust and toast. The same browning reaction accounts for the brown color of caramel. In soft drinks, dextrose contributes "body." It is only three-fourths as sweet as table sugar and may be used in place of table sugar (*sucrose*).

diabetes insipidus. A type of diabetes that is characterized by the excretion of large volumes of water resulting from a lack of *antidiuretic hormone* (ADH) from the *pituitary gland*.

diabetes mellitus. A group of diseases in which the body cannot use *glucose* properly because of a lack of *insulin* or its improper function. It is a disturbance of metabolism, not fully understood, in which the body behaves as if it were partially or entirely deficient in insulin. In diabetes mellitus, the blood sugar (glucose) is abnormally high and there is no apparent secretion of insulin in response to a carbohydrate meal. There is also increased breakdown of liver *glycogen*, defective storage of glucose as glycogen in muscle, and therefore a defective utilization of glucose in the tissues for energy. Although the cause and cure of this disease are not known, heredity is a predisposing factor. With proper medical attention, the disease can often be controlled by diet, insulin, and exercise. Common symptoms include polydipsia (extreme thirst), polyphagia (constant hunger), and polyuria (excessive urine), which may cause bed-wetting and "accidents" during the day. Complications include *ketosis* or diabetic *acidosis*. The extreme of an uncompensated diabetic condition may result in a diabetic coma. Acidosis from diabetes often causes the face to flush, the lips to become red, the breath to have a characteristic sweet odor due to *acetone*, the respiration to increase and become labored, and dehydration to occur. Hypoglycemia, which can be caused by too much insulin, is characterized by irritability, hunger, weakness, double vision, tremors, and pyogenic infections. An extreme of insulin administration may result in insulin shock. The condition of hypoglycemia in an individual is often considered an indication of a predisposition for later diabetes. The condition of diabetes leads to an alteration of both normal glucose and fat metabolism. There are two broad types of diabetes. Juvenile diabetes (Type I) is characterized by a lack of insulin production and Adult Onset Diabetes (Type II) is characterized by a relative insensitivity to insulin. About 90% of the population has Type II diabetes. See *food exchange lists*.

Characteristics of diabetes mellitus types

TYPE I DIABETES (INSULIN-DEPENDENT DIABETES)	TYPE II DIABETES (NONINSULIN DEPENDENT DIABETES)
Cause: Damage or destruction of the beta cells of the *pancreas* for one of the following reasons. (1) Destruction by viral disease. (2) Auto-immune destruction. (3) Other causes. Little or no insulin is secreted.	Cause: Resistance to response to insulin at the cellular level. The exact cause(s) is not known but it is obesity-related. Obese 80%, nonobese 20% of this group.
Treatment: Daily insulin injections.	Treatment: Diet for weight reduction. Drugs to stimulate insulin secretion.
Metabolic ketosis: Not uncommon.	Metabolic ketosis: Rare.

dialysis. A method for separating lower-molecular-weight components from macromolecules. A thin membrane in the form of a tube is filled with the solution containing the molecules to be separated. The pore size of the membrane allows the diffusion of small molecules such as salts or amino acids; larger molecules such as *proteins* or *nucleic acids* cannot pass through the pores and so remain inside the dialysis tube. Dialysis is a convenient method of exchanging solvents in the isolation of enzymes or other macromolecules. It is also used to carry out the cleansing function of the kidney to eliminate urea and other waste products from the blood.

diarrhea. A medical term for liquid stools, the color of the stools varying from light brown to green. Flecks of blood, mucus, or partially digested food may appear in the bowel movement. Most diarrhea results from viral infections of the intestines and stomach (*gastroenteritis*). The inflamed and irritated intestine affected by an infection is less able to absorb food and liquids. It leaks fluid, is overactive, and tends to pass its contents through and out of the body more rapidly than normal. Bacteria can also cause diarrhea. *Salmonellosis* and *shigellosis* are among the more common types of bacterial infections. These can be transmitted from humans and from animals as well. Because there is no cure for viral diseases and therefore for most cases of diarrhea, health professionals usually concern themselves mainly with treating the effects of diarrhea, especially the dehydration, rather than the ailment itself.

diastase. A specific enzyme or ferment in plant cells, such as in sprouting grains, malt, and in the digestive juice. It was the first enzyme to be discovered. It converts *starch* into sugars and *dextrins*. "Diastases" is a general term for enzymes that hydrolyze starches.

diastole. The normal period in the *heart* cycle during which the muscle fibers lengthen, the heart dilates, and the cavities fill with blood; diastole of the atria occurs before that of the ventricles. Roughly the period of relaxation alternating with *systole* or contraction.

diastolic blood pressure. Minimum arterial pressure when left ventricle relaxes after contracting. Average, 75 mm of mercury; normal range, 60 to 90 mm Hg.

diastolic hypertension. Results from an excessive constriction or narrowing of the arterioles throughout the body. The greater the degree of arteriolar narrowing, the greater is the diastolic blood pressure elevation.

diathermy. The therapeutic use of high-frequency electric current to generate heat within some part of the body. The frequency is greater than the maximum frequency for neuromuscular response and ranges from several hundred thousand to millions of cycles per second. It is used to increase blood flow to specific areas.

diazepam (Valium®). A tranquilizer effective in the management of certain individuals with anxiety. Used more than any other benzodiazepine, it also treats fatigue, nausea, and ataxia. Valium has addictive qualities.

dicoumarin. An anticlotting factor first isolated from sweet clover. It is an *antivitamin* structurally related to *vitamin K*.

Dicumarol®. Mol. Wt. 336. An antivitamin and anticoagulant. The registered name of *dicoumarin*, a coumarin derivative isolated originally from spoiled sweet clover and later made synthetically. It is used clinically as an anticoagulant in thrombotic states, and acts to depress the factors concerned with the formation of *thrombin* because of its anti-*vitamin K* activity.

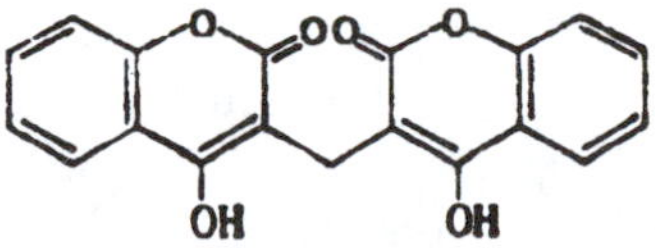

Dicoumarol®

diet. Any combination of foods that constitutes a regular proportion of basic foodstuffs and beverages over a specified period of time. Usually, even though the individual foods may vary from day to day, the ratios of the basic foodstuffs do not vary. For example, the relative proportions of fats, protein, and carbohydrates have not changed radically over the last 80 years. However, within the carbohydrates there has been a radical change in type, in that starch has been largely supplanted by table sugar (*sucrose*). The calories in the average American diet come from approximately 45% fat, 35% carbohydrate, and 15–20% protein. The table shows some variations of diets and the purposes for which such diets are prescribed.

Therapeutic dietary regimens

DIET TYPE	PURPOSE
Bland	Prescribed for chronic diarrhea; peptic ulcers; dyspepsia
High carbohydrate	Nausea; hepatitis; obstructive jaundice (see Low fat)
High caloric	Prescribed for purposes of weight gain; trauma; burns
Low caloric	Prescribed for purposes of weight loss; obesity
Low cholesterol	Prescribed for high blood cholesterol levels
Low fat	Prescribed for pancreatic disease; biliary obstruction; liver disease; gallbladder disease; malabsorption syndromes
Modified fat	Used in the treatment of persons with vascular disease
High fiber	Prescribed for high blood cholesterol levels; constipation
	Prescribed for persons with *diverticulitis*
Galactose-free	Prescribed for *galactosemia*
Lactose-free	Prescribed for *galactosemia*; lactose intolerance
Low protein	Prescribed for chronic renal failure; acute hepatic encephalopathy
High protein	*Nephrotic syndrome* ; hypoalbuminemia
Low sodium	Prescribed for heart failure; renal disease; liver disease
Low sugar	Diabetes mellitus
Semifluid	Diseases of the pharynx and esophagus
Wheat-free	*Celiac disease*

dietary fiber. See *fiber, dietary*.

diffusion. The word diffusion comes from the Latin word *diffundere* meaning "to spread" or "pour forth." It is the process by which particles in solution spread across or throughout the solution and across separating membranes, from the place of highest soluble concentration to all spaces of lesser soluble concentration. It may be simple passive diffusion or it may be carrier-mediated, which increases the rate of the diffusion process. See *active transport* and *osmotic pressures*.

digestibility, coefficient of apparent. The percentage of an ingested nutrient which cannot be recovered in the feces; hence the percentage of an ingested nutrient which is assumed to have been absorbed. The coefficient of digestibility of protein, fat, and carbohydrate in a mixed American diet has been estimated to be 92%, 95%, and 97%, respectively.

digestion. Includes all the changes, physical and chemical, which food undergoes in the body, making it absorbable. In some instances, no change is necessary. For example, water, minerals, and certain carbohydrates are absorbed without modification. In other instances, the cooking process initiates chemical changes in food before it enters the body. The digestive processes are controlled by both neural (nerve) and hormonal mechanisms. Strong, unpleasant sensations may affect the nervous system and thus inhibit the secretion of the digestive fluids, which in turn interferes with digestion. Pleasurable sensations, on the other hand, aid digestion, hence there is value in attractively served food, pleasant surroundings, and cheerful conversation.

SITE OF SECRETION	IMPORTANT CONSTITUENTS	ACTION
Mouth: saliva		
Salivary glands	Mucin	Lubrication
Submaxillary	Amylase (ptyalin)	Cooked starch—dextrins, maltose
Sublingual		Enzyme activity in the mouth is not important
Parotid		
Stomach: gastric juice		
Parietal cells	Hydrochloric acid (HCl)	Bactericidal
Chief cells	Pepsinogen	Pepsinogen→pepsin
	Mucin	Proteins→ peptones, polypeptides
		Reduces Fe^{+3} to Fe^{+2}
Liver: bile	Bile salts	Emulsifies fats for action of lipase
	Bile acids	Facilitates absorption of fats and fat-soluble vitamins
	Bile pigments	Neutralizes acid chyme
Pancreas: pancreatic juice	Thin, watery, alkaline	Neutralizes acid chyme
	Amylases	Starch → dextrins, maltose
	Chymotrypsinogen	→Chymotrypsin
		Proteins → proteoses, peptones, polypeptides.
	Trypsinogen	→Trypsin
		Proteins → proteoses, peptones, polypeptide
Small intestine: intestinal juice (succus entericus)	Mucin	Lubrication: protects duodenum
	Enterokinase	Trypsinogentrypsin
	Proteases	Proteins—proteoses, peptones, polypeptides.
	Peptidases	Polypeptides—small peptides, amino acids
	Lipases	Fats—monoglycerides, fatty acids, glycerol
	Lecithinases	Lecithin→diglycerides + choline phosphate
	Nucleases	Nucleic acid→Nucleotides
	Nucleotidases	Nucleotides→nucleosides + phosphoric acid
	Nucleosidases	Nucleosides→pyrimidines, purines+ribose, deoxyribose
(within mucosal cells)	Digestive hormones	See table under *digestive hormones*
	Sucrase (invertase)	Sucrose → glucose + fructose
	Maltase	Maltose → glucose + glucose
	Lactose	Lactose → glucose + galactose

DIGESTIVE HORMONE	SECRETED FROM	AFFECTED ORGAN	MAJOR EFFECTS
Cholecystokininpancreozymin	Duodenum	Gallbladder	Causes contraction
		Pancreas	Increases secretions
		Small intestine	Increases motility
Enterocrin	Small intestine	Small intestine	Increases secretions
Enterogastrone	Duodenum	Stomach	Inhibits gastric juice secretions
			Reduces motility
Gastrin	Gastric and jejunum mucosa	Stomach	Stimulates HCl and pepsinogen secretions
Gastric inhibitory protein (GIP)	Small intestine	Stomach	Inhibits HCl secretion
		Pancreas	Stimulates insulin secretion
Secretin	Duodenum	Stomach Duodenum	Reduces gastric and duodenal motility
		Pancreas	Inceases water, bicarbonate, and some enzymes

digestive hormones. Among the factors that influence the digestive process are a number of hormones. The relationships among these hormones are not well understood. Listed in the table are some of the digestive hormones and some of their known effects.

digestive system. The digestive system is made up of the alimentary canal or tract (food passage) and the accessory organs of digestion. Its main functions are to ingest and carry food so that digestion and absorption can occur and to eliminate unused waste material. The products of the accessory organs help to prepare food for its absorption and use (*metabolism*) by the tissues of the body. Digestion consists of two processes, one mechanical and the other chemical. The mechanical part of digestion may be broadly divided into chewing and swallowing, *peristalsis*, and defecation. The chemical part of digestion consists of breaking foodstuffs into simple components which can be absorbed and used by the body. In this process, foodstuffs are broken down by enzymes, or digestive juices, formed by digestive glands. *Carbohydrates* are broken into simple sugars. *Fats* are changed into *fatty acids*. *Proteins* are converted to *amino acids*. The accessory organs that aid in the process of digestion are the salivary glands, pancreas, liver, gallbladder, and intestinal glands. A simple diagram of the digestive tract is given.

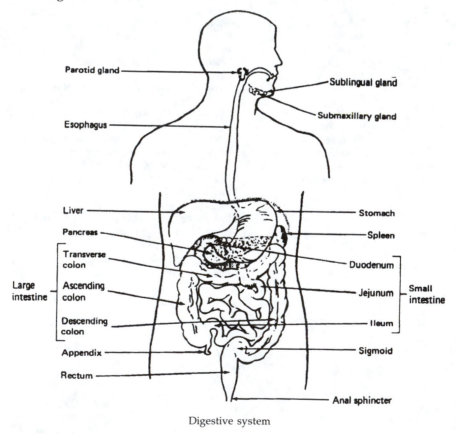

Digestive system

digitalis. A drug derived from leaves of the foxglove (*Digitalis purpurea*) which strengthens contractions of the heart muscles, slows rate of contractions, and promotes the elimination of fluid from body tissue.

diglyceride. A fat containing two *fatty acid* molecules as esters with *glycerol*.

dill (*Anethum graveolens*). A hardy aromatic annual herb plant which reaches a height of about 3 feet. The branches have feathery leaves, and the flowers are yellow and very small. Dill seed is the dried fruit of the herb; dillweed is its dried leaves. Dill is used in preparing and serving soups, cheese, fish, meats, poultry, vegetables, potatoes, breads, and apple pie.

dioctyl sodium sulfosuccinate (DSS). A chemical involved in getting certain powdered foods to dissolve in water by coating the powder with a very small amount of a detergent-like chemical or emulsifier such as DSS. It is used in powdered soft drink mixes in which it helps *fumaric acid* dissolve in water. Manufacturers also use it in some canned milk beverages containing cocoa fat, and in foods that contain a hard-to-dissolve *thickening agents*.

dipeptidase. An enzyme that catalyzes the hydrolysis of dipeptides to amino acids. See *digestive system*.

dipeptide. The condensation of two amino acids through a *peptide linkage* or bond.

diploid. Having two sets of *chromosomes*. In human beings a fertilized egg, normally with 46 chromosomes, or 23 pairs, is in the diploid state. All body cells (somatic tissue) are diploid except for the sperm and the unfertilized egg. The opposite of the *haploid*.

direct calorimetry. The direct measurement of the actual energy expended by the body throughout a given period. It is measured by placing a human subject in a special *calorimeter*. The heat given off by the subject is absorbed by the water in the coils surrounding the well-insulated chamber, where by an accurate mechanism, the total heat may be measured directly. Direct calorimetry is used only for scientific research.

disaccharidase. An enzyme which hydrolyzes *disaccharides*. *Sucrase* is a disaccharidase. See *digestive system*.

disaccharide. A carbohydrate that yields two *monosaccharides* or simple sugars upon hydrolysis. *Sucrose*, *maltose*, and *lactose* are examples of disaccharides. The general formula, $C_{12}H_{22}O_{11}$, shows that disaccharides consist of two monosaccharides or simple sugar groups. During the process of digestion they are split into their component monosaccharides. For example, sucrose splits into *glucose* and *fructose*; *lactose* splits into glucose and *galactose*; and maltose splits into two molecules of glucose.

disodium guanylate (G), and disodium inosinate (IMP). Belong to the same family of *food additives* as *monosodium glutamate*, the flavor enhancer. Flavor enhancers have little or no taste of their own but accentuate the natural flavor of foods. They are used by manufacturers in place of more expensive natural ingredients. Disodium guanylate and disodium inosinate are found in powdered soup mixes, ham and chicken salad spread, sauces, and canned vegetables. Manufacturers often use them together with monosodium glutamate, because of a synergistic action that exists between the three chemicals. They cannot be used in many moist foods, because enzymes in the foods slowly convert the flavor enhancers to inert substances. See *guanosine triphosphate* (GTP) and *inosine triphosphate* (ITP).

disodium inosinate. The disodium salt of IMP. See *inosine triphosphate* (ITP).

distill. The process of vaporizing a liquid by heat or reduced pressure and collection of the vapors by cooling. The resulting liquid is called the distillate.

distilled liquors. Liquors or spirits produced by distillation of an alcoholically fermented product. Rum is the distillate from alcoholically fermented sugar cane juice, syrup, or molasses. Whiskeys are distilled from sugared and fermented grain mashes; for example, rye whiskey is from wheat mash, and rums and whiskeys are made from mashes fermented by special distillers' yeast, strains of *Saccharomyces cerevisiae* var. *ellipsoideus,* which give high yields of alcohol. The grain mashes usually are acidified to favor the yeasts. The aging of the distilled liquors in charred oaken barrels or tuns is a chemical rather than a biological process. See *yeast.*

disulfide bond. A chemical bond formed between two sulfur atoms or sulfhydryl groups ($-SH$). In protein chemistry, disulfide bonds form between *cysteine* residues and hold together separate polypeptide chains or separate parts of the chain. An example of disulfide bond is in *cystine.*

diuresis. The secretion and passage of large amounts of urine. This occurs in *diabetes mellitus* or can also be an early sign of *nephritis.* May also be due to hysteria, result of fear and anxiety, ingestion of large quantities of liquids, *diabetes insipidus,* or the action of drugs. See *antidiuretic hormone.*

diuretics. Diuretics are substances or chemicals that increase urine output. *Hydrochlorothiazide* (HCTZ) is an example of a *thiazide* diuretic that is used to control high blood pressure. See *antidiuretic hormone.*

diverticula. See *diverticulitis.*

diverticulitis. From Latin *divertere,* "to turn aside." Diverticula are outpouchings or sacs that protrude from the intestinal lining into the intestinal wall. There can be scores of such outpouchings or diverticula, especially in the colon. Diverticulosis is always benign at the outset and usually remains so. When inflammation develops and when the inflammation is severe, the result is acute diverticulitis. The condition is sometimes aided by a high-fiber diet.

DNA. See *deoxyribonucleic acid.*

doughnut. A small cake, deep-fried or baked and leavened with yeast or baking powder. Doughnuts are ring-shaped with a hole in the center. Crullers and fried cakes are closely related to them. Both are made of the same kind of dough and deep-fried, but technically crullers are shaped in a twist and fried cakes are made round or square, without a hole. One doughnut contains between 168 and 200 calories.

dried fruits. Fruits of which the solids have been greatly concentrated by evaporating a large portion of the original water content. The purpose of drying is preservation. Dried fruits have a great variety of uses. They may be eaten as is; cooked and used as a sauce; used in pies, puddings, and stuffings; or served as meat accompaniments. In the drying, over 50% of the water is removed, but practically all the food nutrients remain. Dried fruits contain a variety of vitamins and minerals. The caloric value per pound of dried fruit is four to five times that of the fruit when fresh. However, this is true only if the dried fruit is eaten as purchased. When cooked, the fruit regains much of the water lost and approximates the fresh fruit in composition.

Calories in one cup of dried fruit

FRUIT	CALORIES	FRUIT	CALORIES	FRUIT	CALORIES	FRUIT	CALORIES	FRUIT	CALORIES
Apples	315	Currants	536	Figs	453	Peaches	424	Prunes	375
Apricots	423	Dates	505	Nectarines	424	Pears	405	Raisins	429

drug-nutrient interaction. Several therapeutic drugs have direct effects on nutritional status. In many instances the drugs counteract vitamin activities and lead to symptoms of vitamin deficiencies. Drugs in common use that can cause nutrient malabsorption include *antacids*, *laxatives* (including *mineral oil* and phenolphthalein), the antibiotic neomycin, and cholchicine, which is used in the treatment of gout, as well as *cholestyramine*, currently being used to reduce serum cholesterol in individuals with atherosclerotic heart disease. Abuse of antacids can lead to phosphate depletion and, in some people, to the development of osteomalacia. Mineral oil diminishes absorption of all fat-soluble vitamins. Abuse of mineral oil may lead to rickets in a child and osteomalacia in an adult. Abuse of laxatives containing phenolphthalein can cause a malabsorption syndrome with the development of multiple nutrient deficiencies as well as excessive loss of potassium from the body, leading to *hypokalemia* and protein losses. Under certain conditions, the desired therapeutic effect of a drug is by deliberate interference with the utilization of a particular nutrient. Anticoagulants used to treat or prevent blood clots are antivitamin K compounds. Anticonvulsant drugs, which can also cause anorexia, may alter the metabolism of several nutrients including *vitamin D, ascorbic acid, folacin,* and *pyridoxine*. In documented cases of vitamin D deficiency and folic acid deficiency associated with the intake of anticonvulsant drugs, effects have been shown to be due to decreased absorption of these vitamins in individuals already consuming a marginal diet. Drugs may affect nutrition. A number of drugs have been implicated in the production of nutritional deficits through malabsorption of vitamins, increased excretion of vitamins or minerals, and altered nutrient metabolism. The following tables summarize the effects of drugs most commonly encountered:

Effect of food on drug absorption

REDUCED BY FOOD		INCREASED BY FOOD	DELAYED BY FOOD
Penicillin G	Erythromycin[a]	Griseofulvin	Cephalosporins
Penicillin V	stearate[a]	Erythromycin estolate	Digoxin
Phenethicillin	Lincomycin	Nitrofurantoin	Sulfonamides
Ampicillin	Levodopa	Methoxsalen	
Amoxicillin	Tetracyclines[b]	Propranolol	
Aspirin	Theophylline	Metoprolol	
		Phenytoin	

[a] Uncoated, [b] Except Doxycycline

Effect of drugs on nutrients

THERAPEUTIC CLASS	MAJOR DRUGS	NUTRITIONAL EFFECT	POSSIBLE CLINICAL EFFECT
Alcohol	Ethanol	Thiamine deficiency Folacin deficiency Magnesium excretion accelerated Impaired pyridoxine activation	Congenital defects Peripheral neuropathy Anemias Delerium tremens
Antibiotics	Neomycin Kanamycin Griseofulvin	Decreased lactase Decreased synthesis of vitamin K by enteric bacteria Decreased cobalamine and biotin absorption	Lactose intolerance Slowed blood clotting
Anticonvulsants Sedatives	Diphenylhydantoin Phenobarbitol Glutethimide Phenytoin	Accelerated vitamin D metabolism Accelerated vitamin K metabolism Folacin deficiency	Rickets Neonatal hemorrhages Neurologic deterioration Gingivitis Congenital defects
Antiinflammatory	Aspirin Indomethacin Phenylbutazone	Intestinal bleeding Folacin deficiency	Megaloblastic anemia
Antilipoproteinemic	Chlofibrate Cholestyramine	Decreased absorption of cobalamin	
Antitubercular	Isoniazid	Pyridoxine deficiency Niacin deficiency	Polyneuritis Pellagra symptoms
Corticosteroids	Cortisone Prednisone	Accelerated vitamin D metabolism Increased ascorbate, zinc, potassium, and amino acid excretions Lowered serum calcium Increased pyridoxine requirement	A negative nitrogen balance Muscle wasting Slow wound healing Abnormal glucose tolerance
Diuretics	Chlorthiazide Spironolactone	Increased potassium and magnesium excretion Reduced potassium excretion	Muscle weakness Magnesium depletion Hyperkalemia
Hypotensives	Hydralazine	Pyridoxine depletion	Polyneuritis
Laxitive	Mineral oil	Decreased absorption of fat soluble vitamins A, D, E, and K	
Oral contraceptives	Mestranol Ethinyl estradiol Conjugated estrogen	Deficiencies of folacin and the B-vitamins Accelerated ascorbate metabolism Folacin deficiency Reduced calcium excretion	Abnormal glucose tolerance Megaloblastic anemia Reduced bone loss

dulcitol. Mol. Wt. 182. Obtained by hydrogenation or reduction of *galactose* in the same manner as *sorbitol* from *glucose*. A sugar which has a variety of industrial uses, sometimes employed in the manufacture of foods as an improver.

duodenal drainage test. A test in which an intestinal specimen is obtained via a swallowed tube and examined for diagnosis of gallbladder and pancreas diseases.

duodenal ulcer The ulcer is a defect in the duodenum wall, commonly about the size of a dime. The etiology of the disease is controversial. It was commonly believed to be caused by the digestive action of acidic gastric juice. Recent evidence suggests that a large number of ulcers are caused by bacteria. Epigastric pain is the most characteristic symptom. Pain usually occurs an hour or two after meals or when the stomach is empty. Pain is generally chronic and recurs frequently. When the ulcer is chronic, there is often a deformity of the duodenum that can be detected by x-ray.

duodenum. The first portion of the small intestine, extending from the pylorus to the jejunum. See *digestive system*.

durum wheat (*Triticum durum*). A variety of wheat, often called "hard" or "macaroni" wheat, with hard, translucent kernels. It is often used chiefly for making macaroni and other pastas. Pasta products made from it do not disintegrate in cooking, but become tender while remaining firm.

dyspepsia. Indigestion or upset stomach.

dysphagia. Difficulty in swallowing.

dyspnea. Difficult or labored breathing.

dyssebacia. The appearance of enlarged follicles around the sides of the nose, sometimes extending over the cheeks and forehead. The follicles are plugged with dry sebaceous material which often has a yellow color. Commonly found in Africans with pellagra and may be related to *riboflavin* deficiency.

dysuria. Painful or difficult urination.

E

E. The alphabetic symbol for the amino acid *glutamic acid* (Glu).

eczema. See *dermatitis*.

edema. An abnormally large volume of fluid in the intertissue (interstitial) spaces. Swelling of a part of or the entire body due to an excess of water. Edema is most noticeable at the end of the day around the ankles, which increase in size. Edema is a common condition of many nutritional diseases or conditions such as wet *beri-beri* and *marasmus*.

edible portion (E.P.). As used in food tables, the term refers to that part of a food which is most commonly eaten. Some parts, such as parings of potatoes which are edible but not usually eaten, are excluded.

EEG. See *electroencephalogram*.

EFA. See *essential fatty acids*.

eggplant (*Solanum melongena*). An erect, branching plant closely related to the potato. It is cultivated for its fruit, which is eaten as a vegetable. The fruit, which in reality is a berry, varies in length from 2–12 inches. Its shiny surface may be dark purple, white, red, yellowish, or even striped, depending upon the variety. Eggplant is grown in different sizes and shapes: round, oblong, pear-shaped, and long. Little nutritive value can be found in eggplant, but it adds variety to the menu.

eggs. Eggs are rich in essential nutrients. An average chicken egg contains 6 g of protein and 6 g of fat and yields 80 kcal. The proteins, most of which come from albumin in the white

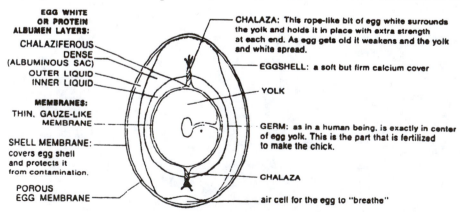

of the egg, have the highest *biological value* (BV) for human adults of all food proteins and serve as a standard for comparison with other proteins. Most of the yellow color of yolks is xanthophyll (lutein), which is *carotenoid* but not a *retinol* (vitamin A) precursor. There is little or no *ascorbic acid* (vitamin C). A medium egg contains about 300 mg of *cholesterol* and when eaten in large numbers may raise the blood cholesterol level. The anatomy of an egg is shown.

The fatty acid, cholesterol, and nutrient value content are given in the tables that follow.

Fat, cholesterol, protein, and carbohydrate in one medium chicken egg

PORTION	CALORIES KCAL	WT. G	TOTAL FAT G	TOTAL SFA G	MFA G	UFA G	CHOLES-TEROL G	PROTEIN G	CARBO-HYDRATE G
Whole	82	50	6	3	3	<1	255	7	Trace
Yolk	54	17	6	3	3	<1	255	3	Trace

Nutrients in one medium chicken egg

PORTION	CALCIUM G	IRON G	VITAMIN A IU	COBALAMIN μG
Whole	27	1	590	2
White	3	Trace	0	—
Yolk	24	1	580	—

eicosanoid hormones. The eicosanoid hormones derive from the essential fatty acid, *arachidonic acid*. The prefix *eicosa-* refers to the number 20, the number of carbons in these compounds. There are three families of local hormones under this classification. They are *prostaglandins, thromboxanes,* and *leukotrienes*. They are called local hormones because they are short-lived and alter the activities of the cells in their immediate vicinity and the cells from which they are derived. Their activities vary from cell to cell and from one derivative to the next. The diagram shows the relationship of the eicosanoid hormones.

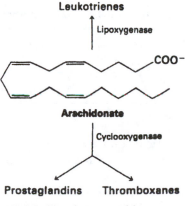

Relationship of eicosanoid hormones

eicosapentaenoic acid (omega(ω)–3 fatty acid). Eicosapentaenoic acid, a fatty acid which is a precursor of *prostaglandins* of the 3 series, decreases platelet aggregation *in vitro*. Unlike *arachidonic acid*, eicosapentaenoic acid does not induce platelet aggregation in human plasma, probably because it forms thromboxane A, which does not have platelet-aggregating properties of the thromboxane A2 from arachidonic acid. These findings suggest that high levels of eicosapentaenoic acid coupled with low levels of arachidonic acid in the diet may prevent *thrombosis* or *atherosclerosis*. Eicosapentaenoic acid is abundant in many foods consumed by Greenland Eskimos, and it is conceivable that its effects may explain the apparently low incidence of ischemic heart disease in Greenland Eskimos. The studies with another omega (ω)-3 fatty acid, dihomo-γ-linolenic acid, and eicosapentaenoic acid indicate that it is possible to manipulate platelet prostaglandin biosynthesis in humans using natural prostaglandin precursors.

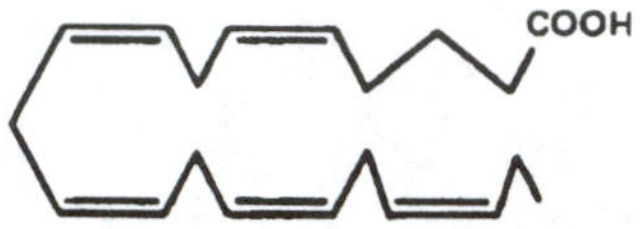

Δ 5, 8, 11, 14, 17-Eicosapentaenoic acid

EKG. See *electrocardiogram*.

elastic tissue. A fibrous connective tissue composed of elastic (*elastin*) fibers and found in the walls of blood vessels, in the lung, and in certain ligaments. The protein content of elastic tissue is mostly elastin and collagen. See *tissues*.

elastin. The insoluble yellow elastic protein of connective tissue.

elderberry. A fruit of the elder (*Sambucus*), a wild shrub of the *Sambucus* family, with white flowers and purple-black or red berries. There are several varieties, with the flowers growing in saucerlike flat clusters, and the berries growing in heavy clusters. Elderberries lack acid and, eaten raw, have a rank flavor and odor. When properly prepared with the addition of lemon juice, crab apples, or sour grapes, they are excellent. They are used for making jellies and jams, and most famous for homemade wines. Elderberries can also be dried or stewed and used for making muffins and pies.

Nutrients in 100 g of raw elderberries

CALORIES KCAL	PROTEIN G	FAT G	CARBOHYDRATE G	VITAMIN A IU	ASCORBATE MG	CALCIUM MG
72	3	trace	16	600	36	40

electrocardiogram (EKG). An electric test used both as a screening test for heart disease and as a diagnostic test in heart disease. The K in EKG derives from the German spelling of heart.

electroencephalogram (EEG). An electric test based on "brain waves;" used in neurologic examinations.

electrolytes. Chemical compounds that dissociate in water, breaking up into separated hydrated particles carrying charges called *ions*, are known as electrolytes, and the process is referred to as ionization. Salts, acids, and bases are electrolytes. Compounds such as *glucose* and *urea* are called nonelectrolytes because they are molecules that do not ionize, that is, they carry no charge. Each ion, the dissociated particle of an electrolyte, carries an electric charge, either negative or positive. Positive ions (cations) in the body fluids include *sodium* (Na^+), *potassium* (K^+), *calcium* (Ca^{+2}), and *magnesium* (Mg^{+2}). The negative ions (anions) include *chloride* (Cl^-), *bicarbonate* HCO^{-3}), *phosphate* (PO_4^{-3}), and sulfate (SO_4^{-2}) ions or organic acids such as *lactate pyruvate*, and *acetoacetate*. Proteins are polyelectrolytes (carry many charges) and may be positively or negatively charged (ampholytes). Sodium ion (Na^+) is the major cation in plasma and *interstitial fluid*, and chloride ion (Cl^-) is the major ion. The major cation in intracellular fluid is potassium ion (K^+), and the major anion is phosphate (PO_4^{-3}). Other ions are present in varying amounts in the different body fluids.

electron transport (terminal respiratory chain). A complex sequence of enzymes that transfers electrons to oxygen to reduce it to and form water immediately. The oxygen comes from the respiration (the air breathed) and the electrons come from the food and from metabolites being oxidized to carbon dioxide (CO_2), water (H_2O), and *energy*. See *terminal respiratory chain*.

electrophoresis. A method of separating molecules, compounds, or metals based upon their electric charge (positive or negative) under a given set of conditions. The rate of migration of a molecule in an electric field is determined by its size and the number and kind (positive or negative) of charged groups per molecule.

elemental analysis. The elemental analysis of the average human adult is given in the table.

Elemental analysis of the average adult human

ELEMENT	PERCENT DRY WEIGHT	ELEMENT	PERCENT DRY WEIGHT	ELEMENT	PERCENT DRY WEIGHT
Oxygen	65	Phosphorus	1	Magnesium	0.05
Carbon	18	Potassium	0.4	Iron	0.004
Hydrogen	10	Sulfur	0.3	Manganese	0.0003
Nitrogen	3	Sodium	0.2	Copper	0.00015
Calcium	2	Chlorine	0.2	Iodine	0.00004

emaciation. A wasted condition of the body.

Embden-Meyerhof pathway. See *glycolysis*.

emboli. Blood clots which form inside a blood vessel, contract, and tend to adhere to the vessel wall. When the free margin comes in contact with fluid blood, fresh blood clots may form. At this stage the clot is very liable to break away. Free-floating blood clots are called emboli, and obstructions of a blood vessel by emboli are called "embolic obstructions." Such embolic obstructions in the heart are called *myocardial infarctions*, and in the brain are called *strokes*.

embolism. The obstruction of a blood vessel by a clot, plug of fat, or other substance brought there by the blood. An obstruction due to a bubble of air or gas is an air embolism.

emesis. See *vomiting*.

emollients and protectives. Drug preparations used on the skin and mucous membranes for a soothing effect. Emollients are fatty preparations that soften the skin. An example is cold cream. Protectives are preparations that form a film on the skin. An example is the compound tincture of benzoin.

emphysema. From Greek words meaning "overinflated." The overinflated structures are microscopic air sacs of the lungs. Tiny bronchioles through which air flows to and from the air sacs have muscle fibers in their walls. These structures may become hypertrophied and lose elasticity. The air flows into the air sacs but cannot flow out easily because of the narrowed diameter of bronchioles. As pressure builds up in the air cells their thin walls are stretched to the point of rupture. The ultimate result is shortness of breath, overwork of the heart, and sometimes death.

empyema. When the fluid within the pleural cavity becomes infected, the exudate becomes thick and purulent and the individual is said to have empyema. The organisms often causing the infection are Staphylococcus, Streptococcus, or Pneumococcus.

emulsification. A process of breaking up large particles of liquid into smaller ones, which remain suspended in another liquid. Emulsification may be done mechanically, as in the homogenization of milk. It may be hastened by chemicals, as by the use of acid and lecithin (from egg yolk) in emulsification of oil for mayonnaise. Emulsification occurs naturally in body processes, as when bile salts emulsify fats during digestion.

emulsifiers. A group of additives used in the processing of food which permit the dispersion of tiny particles or globules of one liquid in another liquid. For example, oil and vinegar used in a salad dressing will begin to separate as soon as mixing stops. With the addition of an emulsifier, they stay combined long after mixing stops. Similarly, an emulsifier enables oil and water to mix and stay mixed. Emulsifiers, sometimes called surfactants (for surface active agents), are used to improve keeping qualities and homogeneity of certain candies and confections. Emulsifiers usually contain water-soluble and fat-soluble portions in the same molecule. *Lecithin*, for example, contains fatty acid as the fat-soluble portion and phosphate and *choline* as the water-soluble portion, and is a commonly used emulsifier.

emulsify. To make into an emulsion. When small drops of one liquid are finely dispersed (distributed) in another liquid, an emulsion is formed. These drops are held in suspension by *emulsifiers*, which surround each drop and make a coating around it. Soap's cleansing action results from emulsifying oily dirt.

emulsion. A system of two immiscible liquids, such as oil and water, in which one is finely divided and held in suspension by another. The fine division may be by mechanical means as in homogenization or by the action of an *emulsifier*.

endergonic. A reaction that proceeds only with an input of energy. The opposite of exergonic. Most anabolic (biosynthetic) reactions are endergonic.

endive (*Cichorium endivia*). A salad green which is a member of the family of plants to which *chicory* also belongs. The endive is a plant with narrow, finely divided, curly leaves and is often called "curly endive." It grows in a loose-leaved head. Two other salad greens closely related to endive are *escarole*, which has broad, waved leaves and a blanched heart, and witloof, or Belgian endive, which is 4–6 inches long and 1–2 inches thick. The leaves of Belgian endive are white with light-green tips pressed closely together to form a cylinder which tapers off to a point. Endive has a slightly bitter flavor and is used almost only in salads. A good source of vitamin A and a fair source of iron.

Nutrients in 100 g of raw, curly endive

CALORIES	PROTEIN G	FAT G	CARBOHYDRATE G	VITAMIN A IU	ASCORBATE MG	CALCIUM MG
20	2	Trace	4	3,300	10	30

endocrine glands. All glands are organs made up of a variety of tissues that aid in secretion of substances needed by the body. The endocrine glands, or ductless glands, have no "pipe-

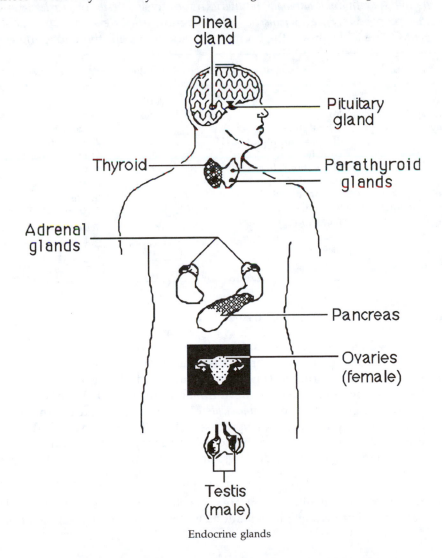

Endocrine glands

lines" for their secretions. Endocrine glands discharge their secretions directly into the blood vessels that pass through them. The endocrine gland secretions, called *hormones*, are carried throughout the body by the circulatory system. Depending on the nature of the hormone produced and the characteristics of the cells it encounters, an endocrine gland may affect the functioning of cells, organs, and tissues in widespread locations throughout the body. Therefore, a gland is endocrine if it produces a hormone that (1) is specific to that gland, (2) is distributed by the blood-stream throughout the body, and (3) has a specific influence on some other part of the body, a target tissue or organ. See *endocrine system*.

endocrine system. The endocrine system is made up of the *endocrine glands* (ductless glands). These glands are located in different parts of the body. Secretions produced by endocrine glands are *hormones*, which are secreted directly into the circulatory blood, reach every part of the body, and influence the activities of specific organs and tissues as well as the activities of the body as a whole. Small in quantity but powerful in action, hormones are part of the body's chemical coordination and regulatory system. There are six recognized endocrine glands; the *thyroid, parathyroid, adrenals, pituitary* (hypophysis), *testes* or *ovaries* (the male and female gonads, respectively), and *pancreas*. The diagram under *endocrine glands* shows the endocrine organs. The table shows the hormones associated with the endocrine glands.

GLAND	HORMONE	GLAND	HORMONE
Pituitary		Adrenal	
Adenohypophysis	Growth	Cortex	Cortisol
(anterior pituitary)	Thyroid stimulating (TSH)		Corticosterone
	Adrenocorticotropic (ACTH)		Aldosterone
	Prolactin		Deoxycorticosterone
	Follicle stimulating (FSH)	Medulla	Epinephrine
	Luteinizing (LH)		Norepinephrine
Neurohypophysis	Antidiuretic (ADH)	Pancreas	Insulin
(posterior pituitary)	Oxytocin		Glucagon
Thyroid	Thyroxine (T_4)	Testes	Testosterone
	Triiodothyronine (T_3)	Ovaries	Estradiol
	Calcitonin		Progesterone
Parathyroids	Parathyroid		

endogenous. Originating in the cells or tissues of the body.

endogenous carbohydrate. Endogenous carbohydrates are synthesized from materials within the tissues. The major storage form of carbohydrate is *glycogen*, a polymer of *glucose*, that is present in nearly every cell. Synthesis of endogenous carbohydrate, principally glucose, occurs even when dietary (exogenous) sources are the major supplers. Fat cannot lead to a net synthesis of glucose or glycogen. The *amino acids* of proteins can lead to a net synthesis of glucose or glycogen by way of a metabolic process called *gluconeogenesis*. Most of the amino acids are gluconeogenic. Under conditions of moderate activity, about 20% of energy expenditure is from the oxidation of glucose. Under stress or acute exercise, the percent of carbohydrate oxidized for energy increases sharply.

endoplasmic reticulum. Found within many areas of cytoplasm as a network of vesicles. These are pairs of parallel membranes sometimes studded with *ribosomes* which contain *ribonucleic acid*

(RNA). In certain *cells*, ribosomes are present without the endoplasmic reticulum. They are the site of protein synthesis and are crucial elements in the cells.

endosperm. The nutritive substance within the embryo sac of plants. The starchy portion within the kernel of *wheat*, corn, or other cereal, from which refined flour is produced after the germ and fibrous outer layers are removed.

endosteum. The narrow cavities and haversian canals in bony tissue are lined with a membrane called endosteum. During bone growth, it is formed by a delicate layer of connective tissue. Beneath it lies a layer of *osteoblasts*. After bone enlargement ceases, the cells become flattened and the two layers are indistinguishable. A stimulus for bone formation, such as an injury, activates these cells.

endothelium. A smooth, thin, glistening tissue made up of flat pavementlike cells which, in continuity, line the chambers of the heart, arteries, arterioles, capillaries, and veins of the entire body.

energy. The capacity of a system for doing work; available power. Energy is manifested in various forms: motion, position, light, electric, heat, chemical, and sound. Energy is interchangeable among the various forms and is constantly being transformed and transferred among them. Energy metabolism may be defined as the chemical reactions in the oxidation of the foodstuffs (protein, fat, and carbohydrate) by which energy is interchanged, produced, and used, and heat given off. The energy or caloric value of foods depends primarily upon the chemical composition, that is, upon the relative amounts of the three primary energy nutrients, *carbohydrates*, *fats*, and *proteins*, that they contain. The energy value of food is determined either by complete combustion in a *calorimeter* experimentally or by calculations from its content of the primary energy nutrients. The average heat of combustion of pure energy nutrients experimentally determined in kilocalories per gram are as follows: carbohydrate, 4.1; fat, 9.45; protein, 5.65; and alcohol, 7.1. In the body, the energy retained by combustion is slightly less, due to incomplete absorption or incomplete combustion or both. Foods with high energy value on the basis of a unit of weight are either rich in fat or low in water content. Thus, all the fatty foods, such as butter, nuts, cream cheese, mayonnaise, and bacon, are relatively high in calorie value, as are foods low in moisture content, such as dried fruits, cookie, candy bars, etc. Foods of low energy value include most fresh fruits and vegetables, especially green leafy vegetables, since these foods have a high content of both water and fiber. Lean meats, cereal foods, and starchy vegetables are intermediate in energy value.

energy balance. In metabolism, the energy balance follows the first law of thermodynamics, which states that under ideal conditions the work energy done is equal to the heat energy produced. It is a statement of the law of the conservation of energy. In an elegant study by Atwater and Benedict, it was shown that a balance exists between the energy taken in as food and the various energy-forms used by humans. In other words, the first law of thermodynamics applies to humans. When the energy balance is perfect, there is a balance of weight, that is, the weight remains constant. When the energy in foodstuffs (fat, carbohydrates, and proteins) exceeds the *energy expenditure*, the excess energy is stored in the body in the form of fat, and there is a gain in weight. When the energy in foodstuffs is less than the energy expenditure, there is a weight loss. During a diet, for example, the energy intake is less than the energy used and the difference is made up by burning the fat in the body, and there is a weight loss equivalent to the fat metabolized. While in practice weight loss follows these simple conditions, the observed weight loss, in particular, or weight gain in an individual is often complicated by water retention. Water retention is influenced by the type of diet, and the tendency to retain water varies among individuals. In computing an energy balance, the energy intake is easily determined by measure of the total calories in the food ingested. The energy used up or expended is more difficult to determine exactly. A *basal metabolic rate* (BMR) must be determined, plus the energy consumed by the activities of the individual which produce heat. Unlike the Recommended Daily Allowance (RDA) for nutrients, there is no margin for error in the energy allowance since increased intake results in increased weight. See *water balance*.

energy expenditure. The table shows estimates of average expenditures in calories for various activities.

Energy expenditures by a 155 lb (70 Kg) person

LIGHT ACTIVITY	KCAL/HR	MODERATE ACTIVITY	KCAL/HR	VIGOROUS ACTIVITY	KCAL/HR
Rest or Sleep	80	Bicycling (5.5 mph)	210	Table tennis	360
Sitting	100	Walking (2.5 mph)	210	Ditch digging (shovel)	400
Driving (car)	120	Gardening	220	Ice skating (10 mph)	400
Standing	140	Canoeing (2.5 mph)	230	Wood chopping	400
Housework	180	Golf	250	Tennis	420
		Lawn mowing (power mower)	250	Water skiing	480
		Lawn mowing (hand mower)	270	Hill climbing	490
		Row boating	300	Skiing (10 mph)	600
		Swimming (0.25 mph)	300	Squash or handball	600
		Walking (3.5 mph)	300	Bicycling (5.5 mph)	660
		Horseback riding (trot)	350	Scull racing	840
		Square dancing	350	Running (10 mph)	900
		Volleyball	350		
		Rollerskating	350		

energy reserve. Energy reserve is the total amount of calories in fat, carbohydrate, and protein available in the body for energy expenditures.

Energy reserves of a normal 155 lb (70 Kg) adult

ENERGY FORM	LOCATION	WEIGHT LBS (KG)	KCAL AVAILABLE
Fat	Adipose tissue	33 (15)	141,000
Glycogen	Muscle	39 (12)	480
	Liver	0.2 (0.07)	280
Glucose	Extracelluar fluid	0.04 (0.02)	80
Protein	Muscle	13 (6)	24,000
Total energy available*			165,840

* Total caloric starvation, without activity, would allow survival for just over 3 months, using 1500 kcal/day as the basal metabolic rate.

energy sources. The major sources of energy from food are *fats*, *carbohydrates*, and *proteins* (amino acids). Alcohol is also a source of energy which is used in place of fat. The following are the numbers of **kilocalories per gram** that the body derives from the food energy sources:

$$\text{Fat} = 9.0; \textbf{Carbohydrate} = 4.0; \text{and } \textbf{Protein} = 4.0.$$

These values are used in calculations to convert the weight of food in grams to kcal of energy available. On a weight basis, fat has more than twice the energy of carbohydrates or proteins. Fats, not carbohydrates, are the major energy source under ordinary conditions of activity. During acute stress or vigorous activity, the total energy expenditure increases. Under such conditions, the percentage of carbohydrates oxidized for energy increases greatly relative to fats oxidized. As shown in the table, the distribution of energy from food is very different from the expenditure of energy from food. This redistribution of the energy in food means a considerable conversion of carbohydrate to fat, for example. The table also shows what is generally considered as a moderately healthy diet for the prevention of heart disease. A healthier diet preserves the distribution for the kinds of fat but lowers the caloric contribution of fat to 20%.

The percent sources of energy as food and as expenditure

FOOD	CURRENT AMERICAN DIET	AMERICAN DIETARY GOALS	INTERNAL ENERGY SOURCE	FOOD	CURRENT AMERICAN DIET	AMERICAN DIETARY GOALS	INTERNAL ENERGY SOURCE
Fat				Carbohydrates			
SFA	16	10		Complex sugar (starches)	22	48	
MUFA	12	10	70	Simple sugars (refined)	18	10	
PUFA	14	10		Natural sugars	6	—	20
Total fat	42	30		Total carbohydrate	46	58	
Protein	12	12	10				

Abbreviations: SFA, saturated fatty acid; MUFA, monounsaturated fatty acid; PUFA, polyunsaturated fatty acid.

enriched. A food may be labeled "enriched" if it contains added nutrients in kinds and amounts meeting standards established by the Food and Drug Administration (FDA). Enriched bread may be made from enriched flour or by the addition of the required substance to the baker's formula or by the use of special high-vitamin yeast and iron. Enriched flour is white flour enhanced in *thiamine*, *riboflavin*, *niacin*, and *iron* value by changing the milling process

Minimum to maximum requirements for 1 pound of bread product

NAME OF FOOD	THIAMINE MG	RIBOFLAVIN MG	NIACIN MG	IRON MG
Bread & rolls	1.l-1.8	0.7-1.6	10.0-15.0	8.0-12.5
Flour	2.0-2.5	1.2-1.5	16.0-20.0	13.0-16.5
Cornmeal grits	2.0-3.0	1.2-1.8	16.0-24.0	13.0-26.0
Macaroni-noodles	4.0-5.0	1.7-2.2	27.0-34.0	13.0- 16.5

Source: U.S. National Archives, Code of Federal Register, Title 21, Food and Drug, 1955, with supplement to 1957

to return these constituents or by the addition of chemicals to white flour. The minimum levels in the standards of identity promulgated under the Food, Drug and Cosmetic Act are given in the table. Certain levels of *vitamin D* and calcium are permitted as optional ingredients. See *fortified* and *wheat*.

enteritis. Inflammation of the intestine.

entero. Combining term denoting intestine.

enterohepatic circulation. The circulation of *bile* from the liver to the *gallbladder*, then into the intestine, from which it is absorbed and carried by the blood back to the liver to be returned to circulation. This continual circulation efficiently conserves the bile which is required. For the 20–30 g of bile used daily by the body, only about 0.8 g is eliminated in the *feces* and must be replenished by the liver.

enterokinase. A proteolytic enzyme which activates the *trypsin* by a partial hydrolysis of *trypsinogen* of the pancreatic fluid. Trypsin is one of several proteolytic enzymes (proteases) involved in the digestion of food protein.

enteropathy. Any disease of the intestine.

enterotoxin. A toxin specific for the cells of the intestinal mucosa and arising in the intestine.

enzymatic. Related to that class of protein substances called *enzymes*, which serve as biological catalysts.

enzymes. Biological catalysts. Enzymes speed up the rate of chemical reactions in the body. They are *proteins* and have all of the properties of proteins in general. The shape and the *amino acid* composition in enzymes determines their physical, chemical, and catalytic properties. Enzymes range in size from molecular weights of a few thousand to a few million. The structural complexity of enzymes also varies from simple *polypeptide* chains composed only of amino acids to complex proteins which may contain metals, carbohydrates, lipids, or other smaller organic molecules as integral parts of the structure. Many enzymes require a *cofactor* or *coenzyme* to be active. Many of the coenzymes derive from *vitamins*. The protein of an enzyme that lacks its coenzyme is called an apoenzyme. When the coenzyme is present, it is called a holoenzyme. When the coenzyme is attached, the enzyme is called apoenzyme. Each cell in the body contains a few thousand different enzymes. Without enzymes, the complex chemical changes which constitute the metabolism of the body would be impossible. They are responsible for a variety of chemical processes such as *oxidation, reduction, hydrolysis*, and the building up or synthesis of simpler molecules into more complex structures. Some of these processes involve numerous enzymes, each one performing one step in turn, until the end product is reached. Most enzymes act within their parent cells, but some leave the cell to act in the surrounding fluids, such as the enzymes of the *digestive system*. Enzymes are highly specific and react upon a limited number of chemical substances called *substrates* to produce specific end products. Enzymes are usually named by adding "ase" to the name of the substrate or sometimes adding "ase" to the particular chemical reaction which they produce. Some important groups of enzymes are: (1) *esterases*, (a) *lipases* digest *fats*; (b) cholinesterase hydrolyzes *acetylcholine*, (c) phosphatases remove phosphate (PO_4); (2) carbohydrates, (a) amylase hydrolyses *starch*, (b) maltase hydrolyses *maltose*, (c) lactase hydrolyses *lactose*; (3) Proteases, (a) proteinase, *pepsin*, and *trypsin* break down proteins, (b) *peptidases* attack partially digested proteins (peptides). The major digestive enzymes are given in the table under *digestive system*. Many of the digestive enzymes occur in inactive forms and are given the general name *zymogen*. For example, *trypsinogen* is an inactive form (a zymogen) of trypsin. With *enterokinase*, a proteolytic enzyme, a polypeptide is removed from trypsinogen, thereby converting it to the active enzyme trypsin. The trypsin, will in turn, degrade the protein in food to *polypeptides* during the digestive process. Several enzymes and *hormones* have active and inactive forms.

epidermis. A stratified squamous *epithelium*, consisting of a variable number of layers of cells. It varies in thickness in different parts, being thickest on the palms of the hands and on the soles of the feet. It forms a protective covering over every part of the true skin and is closely molded on the papillary layer of the corium. The four regions of the epidermis, going from the outside inward, are the stratum corneum, the stratum lucidum, the stratum granulosum, and the stratum germinativum (mucosum).

epiglottis. The cartilage in the throat which guards the entrance to the *trachea*. It prevents fluid or food from entering it and the lungs when a person swallows.

epinephrine (adrenaline). Mol. Wt. 183. The "emergency" or "flight-or-fight hormone" is an enzyme activator *AMP-cyclase* which in turn initiates a series of enzyme activations. In times of stress, small amounts of epinephrine are discharged from the adrenal glands into the bloodstream. Epinephrine ultimately causes the release of a flood of glucose molecules from the liver into the bloodstream for quick energy for the muscles. One epinephrine molecule is thought to cause the release of about 30,000 molecules of glucose. Epinephrine is one of a pair of optical isomers. Only the isomer that rotates polarized light to the left, L-epinephrine, is effective in starting a heart that has stopped beating or in giving a person more energy during times of great emotional stress. Epinephrine is synthesized from the essential amino acid *tyrosine* and also requires *ascorbic acid* (vitamin C) for its synthesis.

Epinepherine (adrenaline)

epithelium. The outermost layers of the skin and the mucous membranes, consisting of cells of various forms and arrangements. The epithelium lines all the portions of the body that have contact with external air (such as the eyes, ears, nose, throat, lungs), and those that are specialized for secretions such as the *liver, kidneys*, and *urinary* and *reproductive systems*. Plain columnar epithelium consists of cells that have a cylindrical shape and are set upright on the surface which they cover. Columnar epithelium is found in its most characteristic form lining the stomach, small and large intestines, digestive glands, and gallbladder. The chief functions of the columnar epithelium are the secretion of digestive fluids and adsorption of digested food and fluids. See *tissues*.

ergocalciferol (vitamin D$_2$, calciferol). Mol. Wt. 397. Vitamin D$_2$ derived from *ergosterol* by the action of light. *Ergosterol* comes from yeast. The first crystalline *vitamin D* was obtained in 1931 and was synthesized shortly thereafter. Soon it became evident that there were at least ten natural substances that exert vitamin D-like activity in varying degrees, but only two of these are of practical importance from the standpoint of their occurrence in foods: ergocalciferol (vitamin D$_2$) and *cholecalciferol* (vitamin D$_3$).

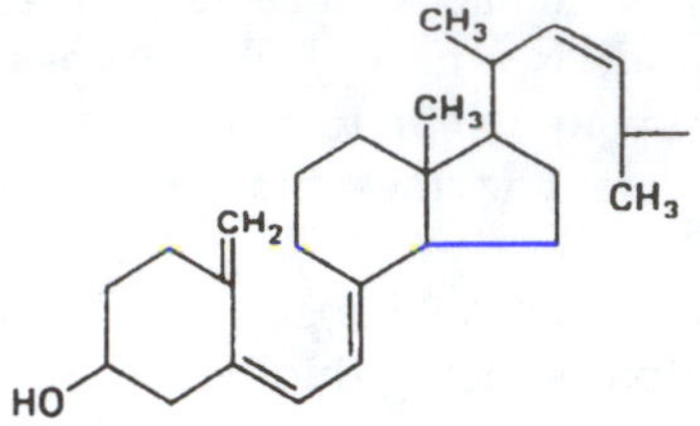

Ergocalicerol (vitamin D$_2$, calciferol)

ergosterol. Mol. Wt. 397. A substance belonging to the class of sterols that is found chiefly in yeasts and molds. It is white and crystalline and similar in appearance to the material of which candles are made. On exposure to ultraviolet light it is converted to vitamin D$_2$ (*ergocalciferol*). See *vitamin D*.

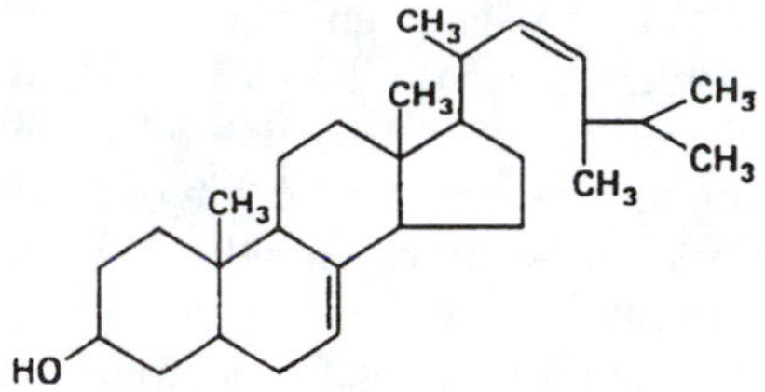

Ergosterol

ergot. A drug obtained from *Claviceps purpurea*, a fungus which grows parasitically on rye. Several valuable *alkaloids*, such as ergotamine, are obtained from ergot. Ergot poisoning may result from eating bread made with grain contaminated with the *Claviceps purpurea* fungus.

erucic acid. An omega (ω)–6 fatty acid, long known as obtainable from the seed oils of cruciferous plants, such as the commercial oils of rapeseed and mustard seed. It also has been found in marine animal oils. Oleic and erucic acids are the best known members of the series $C_nH_{2n}O_2$.

erythema. Redness of the skin produced by congestion or dilation of the capillaries.

erythrocyte. A mature *red blood cell* or corpuscle. Each is a nonnucleated, biconcave disk averaging 7.7 microns (μ) in diameter.

erythropoiesis. The formation of red blood cells.

escarole (*Cichorium*). A salad green which is a type of *endive* with broad, waved leaves. Often the heart is blanched. Its flavor is somewhat bitter. Escarole and endive can be used interchangeably in salads and in cooking. As a green, leafy vegetable it provides a fair amount of iron, is rich in *retinol* (vitamin A), and has small amounts of other vitamins and minerals.

Escherichia coli. E. coli belong to a group of true rod-shaped bacteria which normally lives in the human intestinal tract. This bacillus is found in the intestinal tract and on the skin in the perineal area. When introduced into wounds, it produces infection characterized by light-brown pus with a fecal odor. *E. coli* and other intestinal flora serve humans by providing *vitamin K* and some of the B vitamins. Within the intestines and on the skin, *E. coli* are not a health threat. A systemic *E. coli* infection, however, is very dangerous and generally difficult to treat. It is believed that toxins from *E. coli* in various countries are frequently the cause of gastrointestinal distress experienced by foreign visitors.

esophagus. A muscular tube about 10 inches long, lined with a mucous membrane. It runs parallel with the *trachea* and leads from the pharnyx through the chest to the upper end of the stomach. Its function is to complete the act of swallowing. The involuntary movement of material down the esophagus is carried out by the process known as *peristalsis*, which is the wavelike action produced by contractions and relaxations of the muscular wall. Peristalsis is the method by which food is moved throughout the *gastrointestinal tract*.

essential amino acids. There are some 22 amino acids, in proteins. Eight of these 22 are known as "essential" for adult human beings, because they must be supplied ready-made in foods. The others can be synthesized by the body. The body cannot synthesize essential amino acids at the rate needed. The eight essential amino acids are *lysine, tryptophan, phenylalanine, methionine, threonine, leucine, valine,* and an additional one, *histidine*, which appears to be essential for infants. Practically all of the 22 amino acids are present in most proteins in greater or lesser amounts, but the amounts and proportions of the eight essential amino acids determine whether proteins are of high or low quality. See *biological value*.

essential fatty acids (EFA). Fatty acids which are necessary for normal nutrition and which cannot be synthesized by the body from other substances. *Linoleic* (C18:2), an (ω)–6 fatty acid, and *linolenic* (an (ω)-3 fatty acid) (C20:3) are essential fatty acids; both are polyunsaturated and serve as precursors to *prostaglandins*, *thromboxanes*, and *leukotrienes*, which produce a variety of physiologic effects on blood aggregation, vasodilation, and vasoconstriction. *Arachidonic* acid is sometimes classified as essential but it can be synthesized from linoleic acid.

essential nutrients. Certain compounds that are absolutely indispensable to life processes and that the body cannot make for itself. Many of the compounds the body makes for itself are necessary for good health; however, essential nutrient means a necessary nutrient that can be obtained only from the diet. The nutrients now known to be essential for human beings are certain *essential fatty acids, essential amino acids,* 13 known *vitamins,* 15 known minerals, and water. There are about 40 essential nutrients.

esterase. An enzyme that catalyzes the hydrolysis of *esters* to form an *organic acid* and an *alcohol. Acetylcholine esterase*, for example, hydrolyzes *acetylcholine* to form *acetic acid* and *choline,* an amino alcohol.

esters. *Organic acids* react with *alcohols* to form a class of compounds called esters. Esters are neutral. When ethyl alcohol is mixed with acetic acid in the presence of sulfuric acid, sweet-smelling ethyl acetate is formed. This reaction is a dehydration in which sulfuric acid acts as a catalyst. Ethyl acetate is a common solvent and is used in fingernail-polish remover. Some of the odors of common fruits are due to mixtures of naturally formed volatile esters. In contrast, higher-molecular-weight esters often have a distinctly unpleasant odor. *Fats* and *waxes* are examples of esters with high molecular weights.

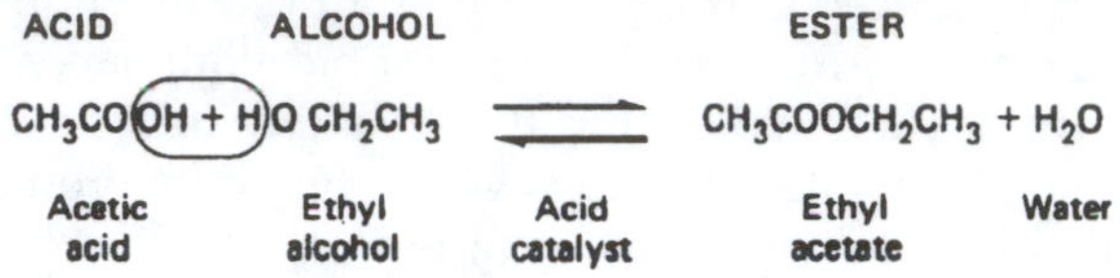

ACID	ALCOHOL		ESTER	
$CH_3CO(OH$ + $H)O\ CH_2CH_3$		⇌	$CH_3COOCH_2CH_3$ + H_2O	
Acetic acid	Ethyl alcohol	Acid catalyst	Ethyl acetate	Water

estradiol–17β. Mol. Wt. 272. One of the class of steroid hormones called estrogens or female sex hormones. The steroid hormones are *cholesterol* derivatives. See *estrogens* and *estrone*.

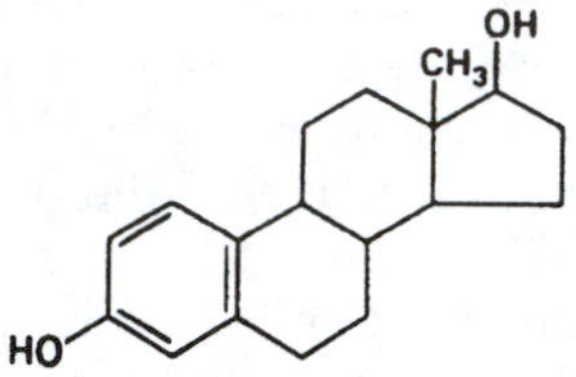

Estradiol-17 B

estrogens. A class of steroid hormones that control the appearance of secondary female characteristics. They are the biological opposites of *androgens*, the male sex hormones. Estrogens are produced by the follicles of the ovaries. The compounds *estradiol* and *estrone* are examples of estrogens. The estrogens promote protein synthesis; cause a marked increase in *phospholipid* metabolism; cause elevation of serum calcium and phosphorus with prolonged administration; and retard bone loss.

estrone. Mol. Wt. 270. One of a class of steroid hormones called *estrogens* or female sex hormones. The steroid hormones are *cholesterol* derivatives. See *estrogens* and *estradiol*.

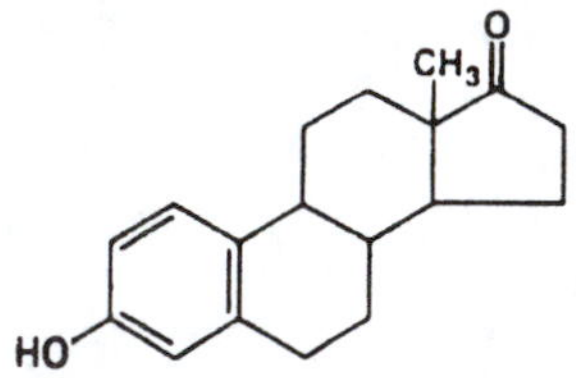

Estrone

ethanol (ethyl alcohol, grain alcohol). Mol. Wt. 46. CH_3CH_2OH. An *alcohol* that is distilled from the products of anaerobic fermentation of carbohydrate by microorganisms, *yeast* in particular, that yields about seven calories per gram, of which more than 75% is available to the body. Sugar or some form of carbohydrate is also frequently added to alcoholic beverages. A pint of beer, 4% alcohol, yields about 200 calories; a glass of wine, 10% alcohol, has about 75 calories; and an ounce of distilled liquor, such as whiskey, brandy, gin, or rum, yields from 75 to 80 calories. Ethanol is considered "fattening" because it is burned in preference to fat. No individual substance is fattening, however; weight gain or loss depends upon total caloric uptake and *energy expenditure*. Ethyl alcohol is rapidly absorbed from the stomach and small intestine, uniformly distributed throughout the body water, and rapidly oxidized with little or none stored. Small amounts are lost into the urine and into the respired air by diffusion. In the liver, ethyl alcohol is converted to acetaldehyde by the enzyme alcohol dehydrogenase and then to *acetyl-CoA*, which may be readily utilized for energy. The rate of metabolism of alcohol is increased by *fructose*. The metabolism of alcohol varies with the individual and with the amount ingested. Small amounts are metabolized by the above-described system, while larger amounts are metabolized by another mechanism which may be inducible and therefore more active in heavy drinkers.

etiology. The cause of a disease.

evaporated milk. See *milk products*.

excretion. The process by which the body rids itself of waste products. The pathways for the removal of waste products are the lungs, skin, kidneys, and intestines. True waste products fall into four general categories: materials that cannot be digested and absorbed; materials that, although absorbed, cannot be utilized; materials that are consumed or produced in the body in larger amounts than the body can use or is able to store; the end products of the metabolism of foodstuffs, chiefly *urea* and excess *carbon dioxide*. Urea and other soluble nitrogenous substances leave the body almost entirely in the *urine* through the *kidneys*. Excess carbon dioxide is excreted by the lungs. Solids are excreted in the *feces*.

exergonic. A reaction that proceeds with a release of energy. The opposite of *endergonic*. Many catabolic reactions (degradations) are exergonic.

exocrine. The external secretion of a *gland*.

exogenous. Originating or produced from an outside source. The opposite of *endogenous*.

extracellular. Situated or occurring outside the cells.

extracellular fluid (ECF). The body water is not a continuous mass, but is divided roughly into two main compartments, the *intracellular fluid* (ICF) and extracellular fluid (ECF). About 60% of the total body water is found within the cells (the intracellular fluid); the other 40% is in various compartments outside the cells (the extracellular fluid). Less than one-fifth of the extracellular fluid is found in the circulatory system, which is composed mainly of the *lymph* and *blood*.

extrinsic factor. *Cobalamin* (vitamin B_{12}). A term used prior to identification of the dietary factor that was required to prevent pernicious anemia, in association with an intrinsic factor. Literally it means a constituent from the outside. See *anemia, pernicious*.

exudate. Material that has escaped from blood vessels and has been deposited in or on tissue, usually as a result of inflammation. Pus is the more common name.

exudation. Most often associated with infection and the presence of large numbers of *leukocytes* and dead bacterial cells. The exudate is then known as pus and is composed of plasma and debris from the site of the *inflammation*. It is helpful in the removal of dead bacteria, tissue cells, and blood cells. It also brings antibodies into the area as well as necessary enzymes, all of which are helpful in removing the debris.

eye. The eye is specialized for the reception of light. Each eye is located in a bony socket or cavity called the orbit, which is formed by several bones in the skull. The orbit provides protection, support, and attachment for the eye and its muscles, nerves, and blood vessels. The interior of the eye is divided into the anterior cavity (anterior to the lens), where a clear watery solution, the aqueous fluid, is formed and circulated. A transparent, semifluid material, the vitreous fluid, is contained in the posterior cavity. The globular form and firmness of the eyeball is maintained by its fluid contents, which also function in the transmission of light. The *retina* contains the rods (night vision) and cones (color vision). It is the rods that contain *rhodopsin* (visual purple) which is early affected by a *retinol* (vitamin A) deficiency known as night blindness (nyctalopia). Retinol (vitamin A) deficiency will also cause a condition known as *conjunctivitis* or inflammation of the conjunctiva.

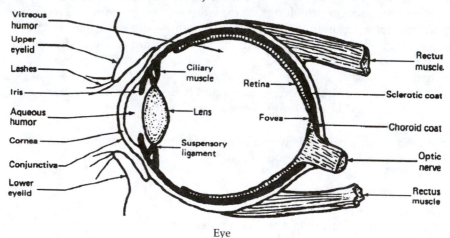

Eye

F

F. The alphabetic symbol for the *essential amino acid phenylalanine* (Phe).

factor. In nutrition, any chemical substance found in foods. A factor might be a vitamin, a mineral, or any other nutrient or nonnutrient. Usually it has some effect on animal growth or reproduction.

facultative. The ability of some microorganisms to live under *aerobic* or *anaerobic* conditions. *Yeast* is an example of a facultative organism.

FAD. See *flavin adenine dinucleotide*.

farina. A *cereal* made from hard (but not durum) *wheat*, from which the *bran* and most of the germ have been removed. It is creamy-colored, rich in protein, and very easily digested. Farina is used as a breakfast cereal, cooked in either water or milk.

Nutrients in 100 g of unriched, cooked farina

CALORIES KCAL	PROTEIN G	FAT G	CARBOHYDRATE G	IRON MG	CALCIUM MG
50	2	Trace	11	26	13

fat (neutral fats, triglycerides, and oils). Fats in foods have the common properties of digestibility, insolubility in water, solubility in organic solvents such as ether and gasoline, and a greasy feel. Each molecule of a fat (a triglyceride) yields one molecule of *glycerol* and three molecules of a *fatty acid* upon *hydrolysis*. Hydrolysis of fat with strong alkali is called *saponifi-*

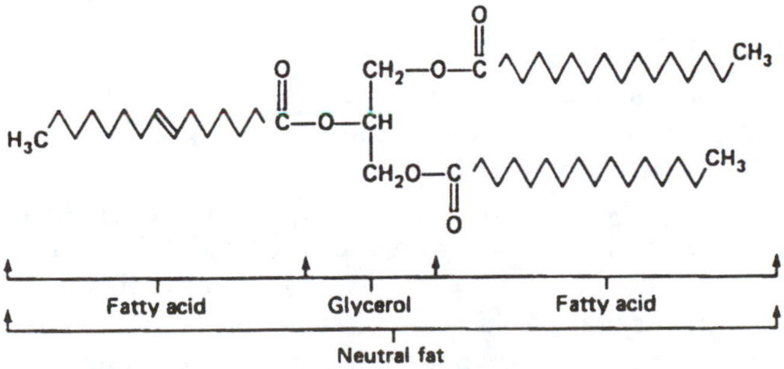

Fat (neutral fat, triglyceride)

151

cation and produces *soap* as a product. In nutrition, the term "fat" refers to both the solid forms of fat and the liquid forms of fat, called oils. Similarly, hard soaps and soft soaps come from the saponifications of solid fat and oils, respectively. Oils are liquids at room temperature because they are composed of *unsaturated fatty acids*. The solid fats contain *saturated fatty acids*. *Palmitic* and *stearic* acids are largely in the solid fats from animal sources. The polyunsaturated fatty acids *linoleic, linolenic,* and *arachidonic* have two, three, and four unsaturated double bonds, respectively, and occur in oils frequently. See *adipose tissue, brown fat,* and *lipids*.

Listed are some of the important fats and oils and some of their fatty acid compositions.

Common neutral fats and oils

FAT OR OIL	SOURCE	MAJOR FATTY ACID CONTENT
Fish		
Cod-liver oil	Livers of Cod	Oleic, myristic, palmitic, and stearic
Menhaden	Body of Menhaden fish	Palmitic, myristic, stearic and a variety of unsaturated fatty acids
Sea Mammals		
Sperm oil	Sperm blubber	Oleic, palmitic, waxes
Whale oil	Whale blubber	Linoleic, isolinoleic, waxes
Land Mammals		
Butterfat	Cow's milk	Butyric, caproic, capric, palmitic, stearic, oleic
Human fat	Human body fat	Stearic, palmitic, oleic, butyric, caproic
Lard	Swine body fat	Stearic, palmitic, oleic, linoleic
Neat's foot oil	Hoofs of cattle	Stearic, palmitic, oleic
Tallow	Ox, sheep fat	Stearic, palmitic, oleic
Plants		
Almond oil	Almonds nuts	Oleic, palmitic, linoleic
Cacao butter	Cacao seed nibs	Palmitic, oleic, stearic, myristic
Castor oil	Castor bean seed	Rincinoleic, stearic, oleic
Coconut oil	Coconut kernels	Caproic, caprylic, capric, oleic
Cotton seed oil	Cotton seeds	Oleic, stearic, palmitic, linoleic
Hemp oil	Hemp seeds	Isolinoleic, oleic
Linseed oil	Flax seeds	Linoleic, lenolinic, oleic, palmitic, myristic
Maize oil	Corn seeds	Arachidic, stearic, palmitic, oleic
Mustard oil	Mustard seeds	Erucic, arachidic, stearic, oleic
Olive oil	Olive fruit	Linoleic, oleic, arachidic
Palm oil	Palm seeds	Palmitic, lauric, oleic
Peanut oil	Peanuts	Arachidic, linoleic, hypogaeic, palmitic
Poppy oil	Poppy seeds	Linoleic, isolenolinic, palmitic, stearic
Rape oil	Rape seeds	Erucic, arachidic, stearic
Soybean oil	Soybean	Oleic, linoleic, lenolinic

fat digestion. Digestion of fats takes place chiefly in the small intestine, where the emulsifying action of bile from the liver assists in bringing the fat into contact with fat-splitting digestive enzymes from the *pancreas* and from the intestinal walls. The final products of these actions are two simpler elements, *fatty acids* and *glycerol*. These are absorbed through the walls of the small intestines and resynthesized within the intestinal cells to reform fat. During the passage, some of the fat enters the circulation as microscopic droplets called *chylomicrons*. Some small portions of dietary fat pass into the circulation without hydrolysis. The droplets of fat are not in true solution in the blood but are in suspension, much like fat in homogenized milk. The end products of fat digestion pass into the *lymph* vessels and are carried by the blood directly to the body tissues. In the tissues, fat oxidation is used to supply energy for work and the internal activities of the body. Fats from all sources are digested easily, and almost entirely, if eaten in moderation. Fat that is not needed immediately is stored as *body fat*. When needed, it is moved into the bloodstream again and is available to the cells for energy. Body weight gains and losses due to diet are almost entirely gains and losses in fat and/or water. The satiety value of fats depends on slow digestion and the emptying time of the stomach; meals that contain considerable fat remain longer in the stomach and prevent the early recurrence of "hunger pangs" which occur when it is empty.

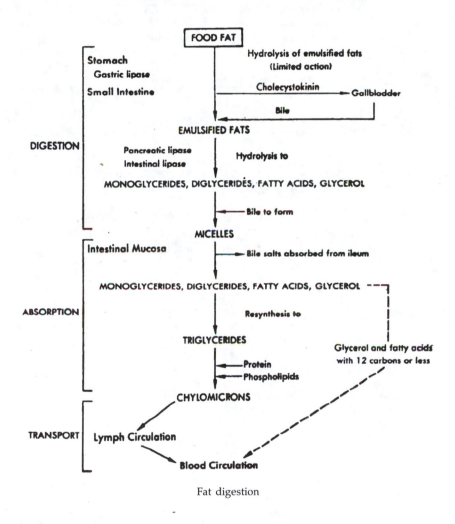

Fat digestion

fat metabolism. Fats are constantly being broken down and resynthesized, but they are at equilibrium when the caloric intake is in balance with the heat production. It does not matter from where calories come—fat, carbohydrate, or protein—an excess of caloric intake above energy expenditures will result in the accumulation of fat and a weight gain. When the caloric intake is less than the energy expended, weight is lost. Fat oxidation is the principal source of energy under most circumstances and certainly the major energy source over long periods of time. About 70% of the caloric needs of the body derive from fat oxidation. In times of emergency when a rapid burst of energy is required, the oxidation of *glucose* meets this temporary need. The oxidation of fat occurs in all tissues, but the liver and the *adipose tissue* are the principal organs of fat metabolism. The diagram shows the roles of liver and adipose tissue in fat metabolism.

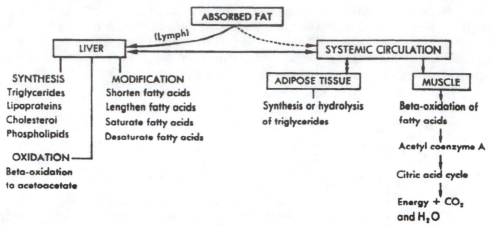

fat-soluble. Refers generally to substances that cannot be dissolved in water but can be in fats and oils, or in fat solvents such as ether or petroleum products.

fat-soluble vitamins. The fat-soluble vitamins are *retinol* (vitamin A), *vitamin D tocopherol* (vitamin E), and *vitamin* K. The table is a summary of the fat-soluble vitamins, their derivatives, functions, sources, and *Recommended Dietary Allowances* (RDA).

VITAMIN	A	D	E	K
Chemical names or active forms	Retinol retinal retinoic acid *ß-carotene*	Cholecalciferol ergocalciferol	Tocopherols (a, b, g)	Phylloquinone menadione menaquinone
Important food sources	Liver, egg yolk, butter, cream, oleo, apricots, cantaloupe, green and yellow vegetables	Enriched foods. Small amounts in butter, egg yolk, liver, salmon, sardines, tuna	Wheat germ, vegetable oil, legumes, oleo, peanuts, leafy vegetables, egg yolk	Leafy vegetables; pork liver; vegetable oils
Functions	Visual pigments, maintains bones, epithelium, skin, mucous membranes, *antioxidant*	Calcium and phosphate absorption and utilization in bone growth	Antioxidant	Essential for blood clotting
Stability	Slow loss by air, heat, drying	Very stable	Stable to food processing Unstable to ultraviolet light	Stable to heat, light & air Unstable to strong acids, alkalis & oxidizing agents
Deficiency signs	*Xerophthalmia, night blindness,* glare blindness, dry mucous membranes	*Rickets,* poor teeth, skeletal deformities	Hemolysis of erythrocytes; *Macrocytic anemia* & dermatitis in infants	Slow blood clotting time. Hemorrhagic disease of newborns
RDA	5000 IU	400 IU	30 IU	Unknown

See individual vitamins and the *Recommended Daily Allowance* (RDA) table.

fatty acid. A chemical compound often confused with *"fat."* A fatty acid is a monocarboxylic acid with a hydrocarbon residue, that may be saturated or unsaturated (containing one or more double bonds). The most abundant of the unsaturated fatty acids is *palmitic acid*, which contains 16 carbons (C_{16}), and *stearic acid*, which is next (C_{18}). Naturally occurring fatty acids up to C_{28} have been shown in animal tissues. Acetic acid (C_2) is also a fatty acid. The most abundant *unsaturated fatty acids* are *palmitoleic* (C_{16}), *oleic* (C_{18}), *linoleic* (C_{18}), and *linolenic* (C_{18}). Linoleic and linolenic are *essential fatty acids*. The table shows the fatty acid content of several common foods and the calories associated with the fatty acids.

Fatty acids in 100 g of common foods

FOOD	SATURATED FATTY ACID (SFA) (STEARIC, PALMITIC)		POLYUNSATURATED FATTY ACID (PFUA) (LINOLEIC)		MONOUNSATURATED FATTY ACID (MUFA) (OLEIC)	
	GRAMS	KCAL	GRAMS	KCAL	GRAMS	KCAL
Fats						
Butter	6	54	trace	0	4	36
Corn oil	1	9	7	63	4	36
Cottonseed oil	4	36	7	63	3	27
Oleo, soft	2	18	4	36	4	36
Oleo, firm	2	18	3	27	6	54
Olive oil	2	18	1	9	11	99
Lard	5	45	1	9	6	54
Soybean oil	2	18	7	63	3	27
Meats						
Bacon	3	27	1	9	4	36
Hamburger, lean	5	45	trace	0	4	36
Hamburger, regular	8	72	trace	0	8	72
Chicken, skinless	1	9	1	9	1	9
Lamb roast	13	117	1	9	12	108
Pork roast	9	81	2	18	10	90
Steak, broiled	13	117	1	9	12	108
Veal breast	7	63	trace	0	6	54
Salmon, pink	1	9	trace	0	1	9
Nuts						
Almonds, shelled	2	18	5	45	17	153
Peanuts, halved	5	45	7	63	10	90
Peanuts, butter	2	18	2	18	4	36
Walnuts, shelled	1	9	10	90	7	63
Other						
Avocado	7	63	5	45	17	153
Egg, large	2	18	0	0	3	27
Milk, nonfat	0	0	0	0	0	0
Milk, whole	5	45	trace	0	3	27

fatty acid synthetase. A complex of seven enzymes involved in the synthesis of fatty acids, from two carbon units, *acetyl-CoA*. Two vitamins as coenzyme derivatives are involved in these complex series of reactions. *Pantothenic acid* is a part of *coenzyme A* and part of the 4'-phosphopantetheine residue of the protein in the fatty acid synthetase complex called the acyl carrier protein (ACP). *Niacin* is a part of *nicotinamide adenine dinucleotide phosphate* (NADP), which in its reduced form, NADPH, is required as a cofactor in two steps of the synthesis. The unusual feature of this biosynthetic mechanism is that intermediate stages of the synthesis are not normally observed, and nothing is released from the enzyme complexes until a chain length of 16 carbons is attained.

favism. A food-related disease, occurring primarily in the Middle East and North Africa, mostly afflicting young males. The symptoms include fever, abdominal pain, headaches, hemolytic anemia, and, in extreme cases, coma. The fava bean contains several toxins that are suspected of being responsible for favism. There appears to be a genetic predispositon for favism that involves a red blood cell deficiency of glucose-6-phosphate dehydrogenase. The aging of fava beans decreases the toxicity.

febrile. See *fever*.

feces. The solid end-product of digestion. The quantity of feces formed varies with the quality and quantity of food digested. Feces are primarily dried digestive juices, containing about 75% water. Bacterial remains make up about 25% of the solid material. The color of feces is due to bacterial action on *urobilinogen* from *bile*, which is oxidized to urobilin and stercobilin. On an average diet, about 200 g of feces is excreted in a day. In disorders of the biliary system, feces may appear white, clay-colored, or gray. Fatty stools, usually very light in color, usually indicate a disfunction in the absorption of fatty foods. See *flatus*.

feedback control. Feedback control is the regulation of a series of biochemical reactions by the effect of an end-product of the series on one of the reaction rates at the beginning of the series of reactions. The series of reactions in the body leading to cholesterol synthesis is an example of a feedback control mechanism. Dietary cholesterol, the *bile salts* (cholesterol derivatives), and cholesterol synthesized in the body all serve to inhibit the synthesis of more cholesterol by inhibiting the beta (β)-hydroxy-beta (β)-methylglutaryl coenzyme A (*HMG Co A*)*reductase* reaction at the biosynthetic pathway. Feedback control may also involve increases in reaction rates.

fennel (*Foeniculum vulgare*). An aromatic plant belonging to the *carrot* family, native to the Mediterranean. There are three types of fennel, all of which have bright green, feathery foliage. Common fennel is a tall perennial with finely divided, feathery leaves and yellow flowers. It has a flavor reminiscent of anise. All parts of the plant can be used. The shoots are eaten raw or cooked; the leaves are used for salads and seasoning; and the seeds, which are oval, greenish, or yellowish-brown, are used as a culinary spice for cooking, candy, and liqueurs. Fennel oil is used in medicine, perfume, and soaps.

fenugreek (*Trigonella foenumgraecum*). An annual plant of the *pea* family cultivated chiefly for its aromatic seeds. The seeds are formed in a slender, beanlike pod with a beaked point. They are threshed from the pods and dried by artificial heat. They are small, irregularly shaped, and yellow-brown in color. Their flavor is pleasantly bitter, somewhat like burnt sugar. The seeds are used for curry powders, chutney, and spice blends.

fermentation. Fermentation is the result of the enzymatic reactions of microorganisms with carbohydrates, particularly *glucose*. For example, the end-product of glucose fermentation by yeast is alcohol and serves as the basis for wine production where the source of the glucose is the grape. Another example of fermentation is the souring of milk, where *lactic acid* is formed by the action of *Lactobacillus casei* on *lactose* (milk sugar). The pathways of fermentation, except for the final step, are almost identical in humans and yeast. In humans, lactic acid is formed in muscle, and the equivalent in yeast is *ethanol*. The vitamin *niacin* is important in this fermentation path, in yeast and humans, as the coenzyme *nicotinamide adenine dinucleotide* (NAD).

ferritin. An iron-containing protein with a molecular weight of 450,000. Ferritin is the form in which iron is stored in the liver, spleen, intestinal mucosa, and *reticuloendothelium* of cells. The normal male liver contains about 700 mg of iron. Once iron is inside the intestinal mucosal cell, it can be either transferred (and later released) to the tissues with the aid of a serum protein known as transferrin, or it can be stored in the mucosal cell or other body cells in the form of ferritin. Discovered in 1937, ferritin is the major form in which iron is stored in the body, representing about 10–20% of iron by weight in its molecule. The iron is in the oxidized or ferric state. No other biological substance has this great capacity to store a heavy metal.

ferrous D-gluconate. Mol. Wt. 482. The iron salt of *D-gluconic acid*, a chemical which is present naturally in the body. It is used by the pharmaceutical industry as an *iron* supplement in vitamin pills and by olive growers as an artificial coloring. D-gluconic acid is a natural product of glucose metabolism.

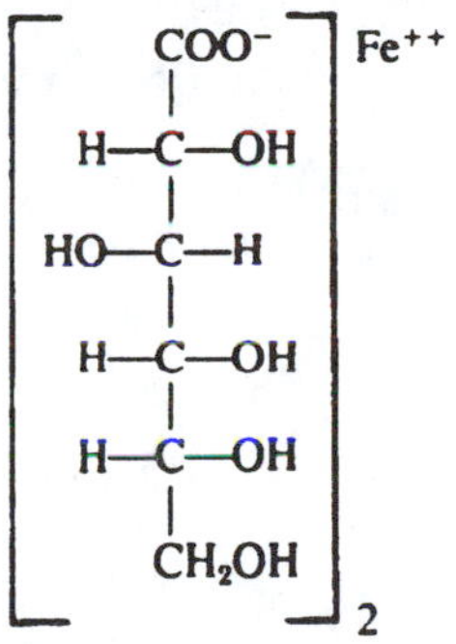

$$\left[\begin{array}{c} COO^- \\ | \\ H-C-OH \\ | \\ HO-C-H \\ | \\ H-C-OH \\ | \\ H-C-OH \\ | \\ CH_2OH \end{array} \right]_2 Fe^{++}$$

Ferrous gluconate

ferrous ion. See *iron*.

fever. Any body temperature above the normal body temperature. Normal body temperature is 98.7 °F (37 °C), although some individuals may vary slightly above or below this value. Hyperthermic fever is a fever marked by exceedingly high temperature of 105 °F (42 °C) or more. Intermittent fever is a fever that falls to normal or below during the day, but then rises again. Relapsing fever is fever that may disappear for a day or several days and then return in alternating episodes. Sustained fever is fever in which the average daily temperature remains above normal. Fevers run higher in children than in adults. Children with fevers at 102 °F (40 °C) or above should see a physician. Some children have seizures at 102 °F—usually there is no brain-damage involvement. In adults, temperatures over 99.6 °F are considered fever. Fevers not associated with any recognizable illness, such as *influenza*, warrant a visit to a physician. In an adult, a fever above 105 °F calls for hospitalization and may lead to delerium. Either *aspirin* or acetaminophen can decrease a fever in an adult. Children should be given only *acetaminophen* when they have influenza because *aspirin* under such conditions has been linked with *Reye's syndrome.*

fiber. As used in reference to therapeutic diets, this term includes indigestible organic tissue, either plant or animal. Crude fiber is made up largely of *cellulose* which is not readily soluble, and *lignin*. The fiber content is usually determined as that portion of a food sample which resists solution when boiled in dilute acid and dilute alkali.

fiber, dietary. Dietary fiber is that portion of food that is resistant to human digestive enzymes and passes through the intestine undigested. Fiber is a group of different chemical substances that make up the cell walls of plants and other nonstructured substances found in plant-starch materials. The *celluloses, hemicelluloses, gums, pectins,* and *lignins* are the major classes of fiber. Fruits, vegetables, whole-grain cereals and breads, nuts, and seeds are all good sources of fiber. Different types of fiber act in different ways, but most of them are important to health because they absorb many times their weight in water, resulting in softer and bulkier stools and lessening the chance of constipation. Because fiber swells, it gives the feeling of fullness, thus helping to control food intake and therefore to control weight. An intake of wheat bran improves bowel function in many people with chronic constipation. It is important to note, however, that a high-fiber diet must include adequate liquids. There are no Recommended Dietary Allowances (RDA) for fiber. Scientists have not yet determined how much fiber anyone should eat. Different fibers have different effects. Bran, for example, has

Dietary sources of fiber in 100 gm food

FOOD	SERVING	FIBER MG	FOOD	SERVING	FIBER MG
Breads			Cereals		
Rye	4 slices	9	All bran	1 1/2 cup	35
Whole wheat	4 slices	10	Bulgur	2/3 cup	11
Crackers			Grape Nuts	3/4 cup	11
Graham	14	14	Grits	1/2 cup	12
Rye	15	15	Shredded Wheat	4 biscuits	12
Fruit			Vegetables		
Apple	1 small	3	Kidney beans	1-1/3 cup	5
sauce	1/2 cup	1	Green beans	1 cup	2
Banana	1 medium	2	Beets	2/3 cup	2
Cantaloupe	3/4 cup	1	Broccoli	1 cup	2
Cherries, raw	14	1	Cabbage	1-1/3 cup	3
Grapefruit	1/4	1	Cauliflower	1 cup	2
Grapes, raw	26	1	Corn	2/3 cup	4
Orange	1 small	2	Kale	1/2 cup	2
Peach, raw	1 medium	2	Lentils	1/2 cup	4
canned	1/2 cup	1	Lettuce	2 cups	2
Pear, raw	1 medium	2	Peas	1-3/4 cup	5
canned	1/2 cup	1	Potato	3/4 cup	4
Plum, raw	2 small	2	Rice, brown	1-1/2 cup	2
Strawberries	1/2 cup	2	Rice, white	1-1/2 cup	1
Tangerine	1 medium	2	Spinach	4 leaves	4
			Turnip	1 cup	2

Modified from U.S. Department of Health & Human Services, Public Health Service.

a laxative effect, but some fruits and vegetables do not. While some fibers—from apples, for example—bind cholesterol derivatives and lower serum cholesterol, large amounts of fiber can also impair the body's ability to absorb certain important minerals such as *iron, zinc, copper,* and *calcium*. Experts in nutrition point out that fiber is just one part of a properly balanced diet. Adding fiber to a poor diet probably will cause more problems than it solves. More research is needed before anyone can say with certainty what the full role of fiber is in the human diet. It is estimated that the average diet in the United States contains about 20 g per day; some African tribes consume more than six times this amount.

fibrin. A whitish, insoluble protein network that forms the essential protein of a blood clot, *fibrinogen*. Fibrin derives from fibrinogen by the proteolysis of the enzyme *thrombin*. Formation of thrombin and other clotting factors depend upon *vitamin K*. See *blood clotting*.

fibrinogen. The soluble protein precursor to *fibrin*. The transformation from fibrinogen to fibrin is brought about by the *protease thrombin*, which itself is initially in the *zymogen* form, prothrombin. *Calcium* is required for the conversion of prothrombin to thrombin. *Vitamin K* is responsible for the formation of normal thrombin by participation of a carboxylation reaction. See *blood clotting*.

fibroblasts. Numerous and large flat, branching mesenchymal cells with many processes. They play a part in the formation of the *collagen* fibers. After tissue injury, these cells enlarge and become active in forming collagen fibers that fill the injured area.

fibrosis. The formation of fibrous connective *tissue* in repair processes.

fibrous proteins. Long coiled or folded chains of amino acids bound together by peptide linkages. They are found in the protective and supportive tissues of animals such as skin, hair, feathers, tendons, and the fins and scales of fish. The fibrous proteins in such tissues are very insoluble in water and for the most part indigestible. They are a valuable by-product of the food industry since gelatin and other nitrogenous substances can be extracted from them. Some fibrous proteins are *keratin*, the chief protein of hair; *collagen* of connective tissue; *fibrin* of a blood clot, and *myosin* of the muscles.

fig (*Ficus carica*). Figs are the fruit of a tree. The fruit consists of a soft pulp covered by a thin skin. There are between 600–800 varieties of figs, varying in shape from round to oblong, and in color from almost white to purple-black. Fresh figs contain moderate amounts of potassium, riboflavin, phosphorus, *calcium*, and *thiamine*. Dried figs are a source of quick food energy, high in *iron*, with good amounts of calcium and phosphorus. They supply bulk *fiber* for a natural laxative. See this item in the table under *fruits*.

filbert (*Corylus*). A *nut* which is the fruit of shrubs or small trees. It is also known as "hazelnut" or cobnut. Generally speaking, the name "filbert" is applied to the oblong nuts of two varieties of hazelnuts native to Europe, *C. ovelana pontica* and *C. maxima*; "cobnut" to another native variety, *C. avelana grandis*, which produces a large roundish nut; and "hazelnut" to the American varieties *C. americana* and *C. cornuta*, which bear small, roundish nuts. The nuts are borne in clusters and each nut is enclosed in a husk which opens as the nut ripens. Filberts are eaten dried more than almonds or walnuts. Filberts provide *fat, iron, and thiamine*.

firming agents. Substances that add firmness to processed fruits and vegetables which other-wise might become soft. They also aid in the coagulation of certain cheeses. These substances may be added to foods such as pickles, maraschino cherries, canned peas, tomatoes, potatoes, and apples. Examples of firming agents are calcium salts, aluminum sulfate, and calcium lactobionate.

fish. Fish are cold-blooded aquatic animals and, broadly speaking, include shellfish as well as the tapered, scaly animal with backbone, gills, and fins. From a nutritional viewpoint we are concerned with the edible types of fish, which are usually divided into three groups: saltwater fish such as sea bass, pompano, cod, haddock, halibut, herring, mackerel, salmon, shad, sole, sturgeon, swordfish, tuna; freshwater fish such as bass, catfish, trout, perch; and shellfish such as abalone, clams, crabs, crayfish, lobsters, mussels, oysters, scallops, and shrimps. Depending on the type, fish is a very good to excellent source of easily digested protein. Fish contains varying amounts of fluorine, *iron*, *calcium*, and *B vitamins*. Saltwater fish provides *iodine*. Fish liver oils are rich in *vitamins A* and *D*. *Roe* and livers are rich in *riboflavin* and *thiamine*. The food value of canned fish is similar to that of fresh fish, except when oil is added. *Curing* destroys much of the vitamin content of fish and sometimes increases the caloric value. The table on pages 161–162 gives the nutrient content of fish and shellfish.

fish protein. Fish protein contains a well-balanced ratio of the *essential amino acids*. Generally, there is from 18–22% protein in raw finfish muscle. In certain species, there is a notable seasonal variation in the amount of protein in the muscle tissue. When the *fat* content is high, the tendency is for the amount of protein and moisture to be lower than when the percent of fat is low. Due to loss of moisture, cooked or canned finfish muscle will contain as much as 30% protein. In fish muscle that is dried, salted, or both, there is no consistent value for protein since it is associated with the degree of dryness. In crustaceans, the amount of protein in the muscle tissue is not too different from that found in other fish products. The mollusk contains about half the amount of protein of finfish and crustaceans. The muscle alone of the whole fish can be minced, defatted, and dehydrated and then ground to make a fine, powdered material called fish protein concentrate (FPC). FPC can be used to fortify cereal products such as bread, cookies, and tortillas. The addition of 5–10% FPC to wheat or corn flour improves the nutritive value of the cereal protein to a quality equal to or better than that of *milk* protein.

fistula. A tuber-like ulcer leading from an abscess cavity or organ to the surface, or from one abscess cavity to another.

fixation. (1) Generally, it refers to the incorporation of *carbon dioxide* (CO_2) or *nitrogen* (N_2) into a biologically usable form. The incorporations are of CO_2 into *carbohydrates* by *photosynthesis* in plants and the incorporation of N_2 into more complex molecules by nitrogen-fixing bacteria. (2) The process of treating tissue in preparation for microscopic examination.

flatulence. See *flatus*.

flatus. Intestinal gas (flatus) is a natural by-product of digestion. The production of "excessive gas," flatulence, has not been studied extensively. Excessive gas is thought to arise from three causes: (1) the swallowing of air (aerophagia) while eating or drinking, (2) a decreased intestinal transit time and (3) excessive bacterial fermentation. Excessive flatus arises from decreased transit because there is not sufficient time for the absorption of gases by the colon. Flatus

Fish and Shellfish

Food and Description	Wt. GM	Approximate Measure	Food Energy CAL	Protein GM	Fat GM	Carbohydrate Total GM	Fiber GM	Water GM	Calcium μG	Phosphorus μG	Iron μG	Vitamin A I.U.	Thiamine μG	Riboflavin μG	Niacin μG	Ascorbic Acid μG
Crabs, Atlantic and Pacific, Hard shell, steamed	100	3½ ozs.	93	17	2	1		79	43	175	0.8	2,170	0.16	0.08	2.8	2
Canned, meat only	100	3½ ozs.	101	17	3	1		77	45	182	0.8		0.08	0.08	1.9	
Eels, raw, American	100	3½ ozs.	233	16	18	0	0	66	18	202	0.7	1,610	0.22	0.36	1.4	
Fish:																
Bluefish:																
Baked or broiled	100	3½ ozs.	159	26	5	0	0	68	29	287	0.7	50	0.11	0.10	1.9	
Fried	100	3½ ozs.	205	23	10	5	0	61	35	257	0.9		0.11	0.11	1.8	
Cod:																
Broiled	100	3½ ozs.	170	29	5	0	0	65	31	274	1.0	180	0.08	0.11	3.0	
Dried	100	3½ ozs.	375	82	3	0	0	12		891	3.6	0	0.08	0.45	10.9	0
Flounder, baked	100	3½ ozs.	202	30	8	0	0	58	23	344	1.4		0.07	0.08	2.5	
Haddock, fried	100	3½ ozs.	165	20	6	6	0	67	40	247	1.2		0.04	0.07	3.2	2
Halibut, broiled	100	3½ ozs.	171	25	7	0	0	67	16	248	0.8	680	0.05	0.07	8.3	
Herring:																
Atlantic, raw	100	3½ ozs.	176	17	11	0	0	69		256	1.1	110	0.02	0.15	3.6	
Pacific, raw	100	3½ ozs.	98	18	3	0	0	79		225	1.3	100	0.02	0.16	3.5	
Canned in tomato sauce	100	3½ ozs.	176	16	11	4	0	67		243				0.11	3.5	
Smoked, kippered	100	3½ ozs.	211	22	13	0	0	61	66	254	1.4	30		0.28	3.3	
Mackerel:																
Atlantic, broiled	100	3½ ozs.	236	22	16	0	0	62	6	280	1.2	530	0.15	0.27	7.6	
Pacific, canned, solids and liquid	100	3½ ozs.	180	21	10	0	0	66	260	288	2.2	30	0.03	0.33	8.8	
Salmon:																
Cooked, broiled or baked	100	3½ ozs.	182	27	7	0	0	63		414	1.2	160	0.16	0.06	9.8	
Canned: solid & liquid																
Chinook or King	100	3½ ozs.	210	20	14	0	0	65	154	289	0.9	230	0.03	0.14	7.3	
Pink or humpback	100	3½ ozs.	141	21	6	0	0	70	196	286	0.8	70	0.03	0.18	8.0	
Sockeye or red	100	3½ ozs.	171	20	9	0	0	67	259	344	1.2	230	0.04	0.16	7.3	
Smoked	100	3½ ozs.	176	22	9	0	0	59	14	245						

Food	Amount	Measure													
Sardines:															
Atlantic type, canned in oil, drained solids	100	3½ ozs.	203	24	11	0	Tr.	62	437	499	2.9	220	0.03	0.20	5.4	
Pacific type,															
In brine or mustard	100	3½ ozs.	196	19	12	2		64	303	354	5.2	30	0.01	0.30	7.4	
In tomato sauce	100	3½ ozs.	197	19	12	2		64	449	478	4.1	30	0.01	0.27	5.3	
Shad, baked	100	3½ ozs.	201	23	11	0	0	64	24	313	0.6	30	0.13	0.26	8.6	
Swordfish, broiled	100	3½ ozs.	174	28	7	0	0	65	27	275	1.3	2,050	0.04	0.05	10.9	
Tuna fish, canned in oil drained solids	100	3½ ozs.	197	29	8	0	0	61	8	234	1.9	80	0.05	0.12	11.9	0
Canned in water solids and liquid	100	3½ ozs.	127	28	1	0	0	70	16	190	1.6			0.10	13.3	
White fish, cooked baked, stuffed	100	3½ ozs.	215	15	14	6		63		246	0.5	2,000	0.11	0.11	2.3	Tr.
Lobster:															
Raw	100	3½ ozs. meat	91	17	2	1	0	79	29	183	0.6		0.40	0.05	1.5	
Canned or cooked	100	3½ ozs.	95	19	2	0	0	77	65	192	0.8		0.10	0.07		
Oysters, meat only, raw Av. Eastern	100	5–8 medium	66	8	2	3		85	94	143	5.5	310	0.14	0.18	2.5	
Oyster stew: 1 part oysters to 3 parts milk by volume	100	1/2 c. scant	86	5	5	5		84	117	109	1.4	280	0.06	0.18	0.7	
Scallops, cooked, steamed	100	3½ ozs.	112	23	1			73	115	338	3.0					
Shrimp, French fried	100	3½ ozs.	225	20	11	10		57	72	191	2.0		0.04	0.08	2.7	0
Canned, dry pack or drained	100	3½ ozs.	116	24	1	1		70	115	263	3.1	60	0.01	0.03	1.8	0

contains the following gases O_2 (oxygen), N_2 (nitrogen), H_2 (hydrogen), NH_3 (ammonia), CO_2 (carbon dioxide), and CH_4 (*methane*). The composition the flatus will vary based on the origin. The gases O_2 and N_2 are abundant in air and their presence in flatus indicates aerophagia. H_2, NH_3, CO_2, and CH_4 are not abundant in air and in flatus they indicate bacterial fermentation. Foods that produce flatus contain nutrients that are incompletely digested by human intestinal enzymes and pass on to the colon where enteric bacteria ferment them and produce gas. For example, beans contain *stachyose* and *raffinose*, polysaccharides only partially digested by humans, which pass into the colon where they produce flatus from bacterial fermentations.

flavin adenine dinucleotide (FAD). Mol. Wt. 786. A *coenzyme* that contains the vitamin *riboflavin*. FAD functions in cell respiration as a part of the *terminal respiratory chain* and in the oxidative *decarboxylations* of *pyruvic acid* and alpha (α) ketoglutaric *acid*. The enzymes and proteins which associate with FAD come under the general classification of *flavoproteins*, which in general catalyze *oxidation-reduction* reactions. See *flavin mononucleotide* (FMN).

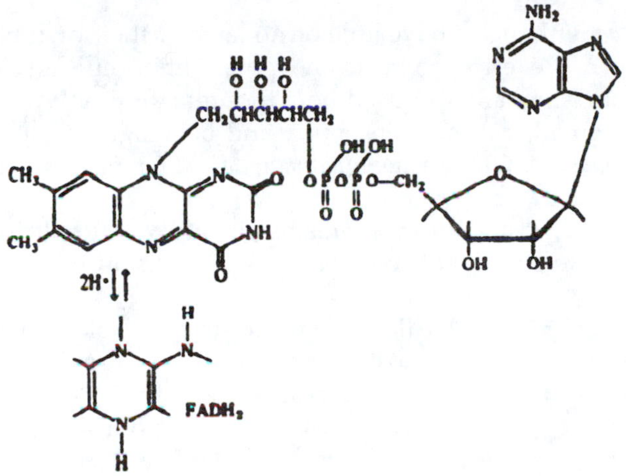

Flavin adenine dinucleotide (FAD)

flavin mononucleotide (FMN). Mol. Wt. 456. A *coenzyme* which contains the vitamin riboflavin. FMN is involved in the oxidative *deamination* of *amino acids* in kidney *mitochondria*. In general, the coenzymes FMN and FAD bind so tightly to their *apoenzymes* that they cannot be removed without causing the protein to *denature*. Since they bind so tightly, they are often referred to as prosthetic groups. See *flavin adenine dinucleotide* (FAD).

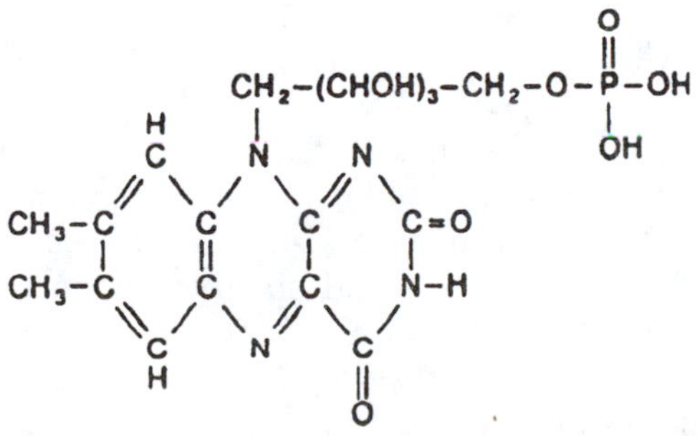

Flavin mononucleotide (FMN)

flavobacterium. Yellow- to orange-pigmented species of this genus may cause discolorations on the surface of meats and may be involved in the spoilage of shellfish, poultry, eggs, butter, and milk. Some of these organisms are able to grow at low temperatures and have been found forming on thawing vegetables.

flavor. Flavor is the result of two attributes that define flavor, *aroma* and *taste*. Aromas are the result of volatile compounds which stimulate odor receptors of the olfactory organs of the nose. Taste is the result of nonvolatile substances which stimulate the gustatory sense organs (taste buds) of the *tongue*. Both of these senses are required for what defines as flavor. See *smell* and *off-flavor*.

flavoproteins. (1) Proteins containing *riboflavin* derivatives. They are important as enzymes in the *Krebs' cycle*. (2) A conjugated protein that contains a *flavin* and is involved in tissue respiration.

flavor enhancers. *Flavor* enhancers have little or no taste of their own but amplify the flavors of other substances. They exert synergistic and potentiation effects. Potentiators were first used in meats and fish. They are also used now to intensify the flavor and cover unwanted flavors in vegetables, bread, cakes, fruits, nuts, and beverages. Common flavor enhancers are *monosodium glutamate* (MSG), *disodium guanylate*, *disodium inosinate*, and *maltol*.

flora (intestinal). The bacteria and other organisms that grow naturally in the human intestine. Some of these bacteria are sources of some of the *B vitamins* and *vitamin K*.

flounder. A large family of saltwater flatfish, including gray sole, summer flounder, winter flounder, lemon sole, and dabs. The most common flounders are dark gray on top and white on the bottom. The eyes are on top. Flounders are important food fish; the meat is lean and sweetly flavored. Their weight generally ranges from 0.5–5 pounds. Fish is a very good source of protein and contains *iron, calcium, retinol (vitamin A)*, and *B vitamins*. See this item in the table under *fish*.

flour. Generally, wheat ground to a powder. The outer layers of the wheat are generally removed as bran, and the central portion of the grain is made into flour by a process called milling. To remove more of the whole grain or bran, the flour is subjected to a series of sifting processes through finer and finer sieves. The unique properties of wheat flour that make a dough which will stick together and rise derive from the proteins *gliadin* and *glutelin*. Except for *rye*, none of the other cereal grains contains these proteins.

flu. See *influenza*.

fluid balance. *Water* and *electrolytes* (ionizable salts) are essential dietary constituents for normal cell metabolism. The tissue cell is said to be in "positive balance" with regard to fluid and electrolytes when it accumulates them, and in "negative balance" when it loses them. Proteins help to regulate the quantity of fluids in the compartments of the body and to maintain the fluid balance. To remain alive, a cell must contain a constant amount of fluid. Too much might cause it to rupture, and too little would make it unable to function. Although water can diffuse freely into and out of the cell, proteins cannot; and proteins attract water. By maintaining a store of internal proteins, the cell retains the fluid it needs. Similarly, the cells secrete proteins (and minerals) into the spaces between them to keep the fluid volume constant in those spaces. The proteins secreted into the blood cannot cross the vessel walls, and thus they maintain the blood volume in the same way. See *water regulation.*

fluoridation. The use of *fluorine*, as in water to reduce the incidence of tooth decay. Fluoridated water is a dietary control of dental decay, with the recommended concentration of 1 ppm of water. It is harmless, tasteless, odorless, and colorless. Studies indicate that fluoridated-water drinkers have fewer acid-making germs in their mouth than drinkers of nonfluoridated water. When fluoride gets into the bloodstream, it quickly incorporates into the bones and teeth. Medical studies indicate fluoride strengthens the bones and teeth that incorporate it. Dental studies show that the bloodstream also brings the fluoride to the gums. Any teeth growing there take up the fluoride by chemical action. Teeth are made up largely of living apatite crystals which contain hydroxyl ions. Fluoride in contact with apatite replaces the hydroxyl ions and becomes fluorapatite. As the tooth develops in the gum, first the crown and then the root acquire fluorapatite. The fluoride is everywhere, in the pulp, dentine, and enamel, from biting surface to root tip, strengthening the entire tooth and causing it to be more resistant to bacteria. When fluoridated water comes in contact with the surface of the teeth that are already formed and in place, it still forms fluorapatite, but only on the surface.

fluoride. See *fluoridation.*

fluorine (F). Element No. 9. At. Wt. 19. There is no known metabolic role in the body for fluorine, although it is known to activate certain enzymes and to inhibit others. The fluorine content of body tissues and foods varies widely. This trace element is present in minute amounts in nearly every human tissue but is found primarily in the skeleton and teeth. The organs contain more fluorine than do other soft tissues. Among the richer food sources of fluorine of animal origin are gelatin, the organs, and seafoods. It has been estimated that an adult may secure 0.5–1.0 mg of fluorine daily from food.

foaming agents and inhibitors. Substances used for pressure-packed whipped toppings so that they squirt whipped from their containers. Adding a foam inhibitor, such as *alginate* (seaweed derivative) adds bulk.

folacin (folic acid). Mol. Wt. 441. ($C_{19}H_{19}N_7O_6$). The generic term for *folic acid, pteroylglutamic acid*, and other compounds having the activity of folic acid is folacin. Folacin is the name officially selected to replace the term "folic acid." Folacin is a vitamin of the B-complex group necessary for the maturation of red blood cells and synthesis of nucleoproteins. Known as pteroylglutamic acid, members of this group include folacin (or pteroylglutamic acid), pteroyltriglutamic acid, pteroylheptaglutamic acid, and folinic acid or *citrovorum factor*, a derivative of folic acid which occurs in natural materials in both free and combined form. Folacin participates in the formation of complex chemical compounds known as *purines* and *pyrimidines*, components of *deoxyribonucleic acid* (DNA) and *ribonucleic acid* (RNA). The DNA is genetic material, and RNA is required for protein synthesis. The necessity of folacin in *hematopoiesis* (the manufacture of blood cells) in humans presumably resides in its function in the formation of purines and pyrimidines. Folacin stimulates the formation of blood cells in the treatment of certain *anemias*, which are characterized by oversized red cells and the accumulation in the bone marrow of immature red blood cells, called myoblasts. The bone marrow is the organ that manufactures blood cells. It cannot complete the process without folacin. *Cobalamin* (vitamin B_{12}) also is needed for the formation of blood cells and is also effective in the treatment of many anemias. The best sources include liver, dry beans, lentils, cowpeas, asparagus, broccoli, spinach, and collards. Other good sources include kidney, peanuts, filberts, walnuts, immature or young lima beans, cabbage, sweet corn, chard, turnip greens, lettuce, beet greens, and whole-wheat products. Folacin contains the pteridine group and one molecule each of *glutamic acid* and para-aminobenzoic acid. It is a yellow, crystalline substance, slightly soluble in water, relatively unstable to heat, and labile to acid and to sunlight when in solution. Folacin occurs in foods of animal and plant origin, some of it in the free form but usually as a conjugate combined with two or six additional molecules of glutamic acid. A derivative of folic acid, folinic acid, often called the citrovorum factor, leucovorum, or N_5-formyltetrahydrofolic acid, also occurs in foods usually conjugated with additional glutamic acid molecules.

Folacin (folic acid)

Folacin in μg/100 g of food

Apricots	4	Cheese		Grain, rye	34	Pepper, green	8
Avocados	30	cheddar	15	Grain, wheat	39	Pork sausage	12
Banana	10	cottage	33	Grapes	5	Potatoes	
Beans, lima	100	processed	11	Hamburger	5	peeled	8
Beans, navy	130	Chicken Liver	380	Ham, smoked	8	whole	60
Beans, snap	36	Chuck roast	15	Kidney	58	Prunes, dry	5
Beans, wax	27	Coconuts	28	Lemons	7	Pumpkin	7
Beets	13	Corn, sweet	40	Lentils, dry	99	Radishes	6
Blackberries	12	Cucumbers	7	Lettuce	29	Raspberries	5
Blueberries	8	Dates, dry	25	Limes	5	Squash,	
Bread, wheat	27	Egg, white	1	Liver, calf	290	acorn	17
Bread, white	20	Egg, yolk	13	Liver, lamb	280	crookneck	12
Broccoli	34	Egg, whole	5	Liver, pork	220	Steak, round	10
Brussel sprout	27	Figs	7	Mushrooms	16	Strawberries	4
Buttermilk	11	Filberts	67	Oats, white	45	Sweetbreads	23
Cabbage	24	Flour, cake	7	Okra	24	Sweet potato	12
Carrots	8	Flour, enriched	8	Onions	12	Tangerines	7
Cauliflower	29	Flour, whole	38	Oranges	5	Tomato	9
Celery	7	Grain, barley	50	Parsnips	23	Turnips	4
Cherries	6	Grain, rice, br.	22	Peas	20	Zucchini	11

folic acid deficiency. As iron is essential for the formation of hemoglobin, two vitamins, *folacin* (folic acid) and *cobalamin* (vitamin B_{12}), are necessary for the formation of red blood cells. They are both involved in the building of the *nucleoproteins* needed for red blood cell structure and maturation. In a deficiency of either of these vitamins, the number of red cells is markedly reduced. The red cells present in normal blood are large and filled with hemoglobin since there is no deficiency of iron. These anemias are therefore called hyperchromatic macrocytic (large-cell) *anemias*. Free folic acid does not occur naturally, but can be made synthetically and used as a medication. See *anemia, pernicious*.

follicle. A small excretory sac, cavity, or gland, for example, hair follicle, ovarian follicle.

follicle-stimulating hormone (FSH). A hormone of the adenohypophysis (anterior *pituitary gland*) that stimulates the *gonads* to produce reproductive cells (sperm or ova).

follicular hyperkeratosis. A *retinol* (vitamin A) deficiency condition in which the skin becomes dry and scaly and small pustules or hardened, pigmented, papular eruptions form around the hair follicles.

follicular keratosis. Normal human skin contains pores, which are the openings of microscopic *follicles*—small cavities or depressions. The secretions of the sebaceous and sweat-producing glands enter the follicles and reach the surface through these pores. Hairs emerge from their roots through the same follicles. In follicular keratosis, the follicles become blocked with plugs of *keratin*, a major protein of the skin, derived from their surface epithelial cells which have undergone a change to a squamous cell or flat type. The change is called a squamous metaplasia. This pathologic change is characteristic of *vitamin A* deficiency.

food. Edible material containing the nutrients from which the body derives nourishment for growth or maintenance of a nutritionally healthy condition. Food contains *fats, carbohydrates, proteins*, vitamins, and minerals necessary for good health. There are more than 40 known nutrients required for maintaining good health.

food additives. Hundreds of different substances come under the heading of intentional food additives. These are added purposely to better the product in some way or to enhance its use. Nonnutritive substances added to foods to improve their appearance, texture, flavor, and keeping qualities include stabilizers, preservatives, coloring, sweeteners, and flavoring. They perform essential functions in the production process and marketing of acceptable products. Incidental additives are those that become part of foods unintentionally. This may occur at different stages in the growing, harvesting, or marketing of foods. Residues from pesticide sprays used in the growing of vegetables are examples of undesirable incidental additives. In a broad sense, radioactive materials in the atmosphere become incidental additives to food. They are always present in the air and soil to some degree, and food and water become carriers. The table that follows lists some typical uses of intentional additives.

food allergy. Allergic reaction to specific foods may manifest in the form of allergic rhinitis, runny nose, bronchial asthma, rash, edema, dermatitis, itching, headache, labyrinthitis (ear inflammation), reddening of the eye, nausea, vomiting, diarrhea, pylorospasm, colic, constipation, bloody stool, mucous colitis, and perianal redness and itching. The incidence of food allergy depends to a great extent on age. In infants and young children, food allergy is not uncommon, but a tendency toward gradual, spontaneous disappearance or amelioration of the condition is noticeable in many individuals after the sixth year. Nevertheless, there is a higher incidence of food allergy in adults than in children. Food *allergens* are predominantly protein in nature. Any major alteration in the protein's molecular structure usually results in loss of allergic potential. Thus digestion, with the attendant splitting of the molecules into peptides and amino acids, renders the protein nonallergenic, depending on the extent of the

Technical effects of food additives

TECHNICAL EFFECT*	TYPICAL ADDITIVES IN CURRENT USE TO ACHIEVE THESE EFFECTS‡§
Anticaking agents, free-flow agents, keep seasoning salts and other mixes from turning into a solid chunk during damp weather.	Calcium stearate, cornstarch, sodium aluminosilicate, tricalcium phosphate, calcium silicate, magnesium carbonate, silica aerogel
Antigushing agents prevent the beer or other carbonated beverage from "gushing" from the container when it is first opened	None now known to be in use
Antioxidants include substances that keep edible fats and oils from turning rancid and others that prevent cut fruits and vegetables from turning brown	BHA, BHT, ascorbic acid (Vitamin C), ethoxyquin
Boiler water additives are chemicals added to boiler feed water to prevent scale from forming as a result of the hardness of the water; when steam from the boiler is used in food processing, small amounts may be carried over into the final food	Acrylamide-sodium acrylate resin, polyethylene glycol, sodium tripolyphosphate, morpholine
Clouding and crystallizing agents and inhibitors	Methyl glucoside-coconut oil ester, oxystearin
Colors, coloring adjuncts (including color stabilizers, color fixatives, color-retention agents, etc.) consist of synthetic colors, synthesized colors that also occur naturally, and other colors from natural sources	FD&C Blue No. 1, FD&C Red No. 3, and other certified synthetic colors; β-carotene; iron oxide and other exempt synthetic colors; beet powder; grape skin extract; caramel, turmeric, and other natural colors
Compounds in the manufacture of other food additives are substances that perform no function in the final food but are necessary in the manufacture of some other additive, and traces of which may survive into the final food; it is an unintentional "additive in an additive	Any common inorganic compounds, such as sodium hydroxide, sulfuric acid, food color intermediates, synthetic fatty alcohols
Curing, pickling agents preserve (cure) meats, give them desirable color and flavor, discourage the growth of microorganisms, and prevent toxin formation	Sodium nitrate, sodium nitrate, salt, sodium metaphosphate, sodium tripolyphosphate; sodium erythorbate, ascorbic acid
Dough conditioners, strengthers are both simple chemicals and also enzymes which modify the protein and cellulose in such a way as to reduce the "toughness" or "springiness" of dough and make it both easier to handle and more appealing to consume	Potassium bromate, acetone peroxide, calcium sulfate, glyceryl monostearate, ammonium sulfate, monocalcium phosphate, locust (carob) bean gum
Drying agents are intended to absorb moisture from other food components	Specially dried cornstarch, anhydrous dextrose
Emulsifiers are an important group of substances used to obtain stable mixture of liquids that otherwise would not mix or would separate quickly	Mono- and diglycerides; lecithin; propylene glycol monostearate; sorbitan monostearate; polysorbates 60, 65, and 80
Enzymes are complex proteins which promote almost all the chemical reactions that occur in all living things; some of these can be adapted to specific processing needs	Rennet for producing cheese curd, papain for tenderizing meat, pectinase for clarifying beverages
Fermentation aid, malting aid are yeast nutrients and other substances that promote rapid and proper fermentation	Gibberellic acid, potassium gibberellate, potassium bromate
Firming agents produce desirable crispness or texture	Calcium salts, aluminum sulfate, calcium lactobionate

Technical effects of food additives (*continued*)

TECHNICAL EFFECT*	TYPICAL ADDITIVES IN CURRENT USE TO ACHIEVE THESE EFFECTS‡§
Flavor enhancers do not themselves contribute significant flavors but increase the effect of certain kinds of other flavors	Soy sauce, MSG, disodium inosinate, disodium guanylate
Flavoring agents, adjuvants are the ingredients, both naturally occurring and added, which give the characteristic flavor to almost all the foods in our diet; flavor adjuvants are substances not themselves flavors, which improve the usefulness of flavors, such as solvents and fixatives	Many of the traditional spices and herbs plus nearly 1500 individual chemical entities, most of which have been identified as the constituents responsible for the flavor of natural food products
Flour-treating agents (including bleaching and maturing agents) usually both bleach and "mature" the flour; i.e., they provide the same effect as increased age. They oxidize some of the proteins and lead to better handling characteristics and larger loaf volume	Acetone peroxide, benzoyl peroxide, azodicarbonamide, potassium bromide
Formation aids cover a hodgepodge of substances which simply allow foods to be put together in a useful way with retention of quality during transportation and storage	Carrier solvents for dissolving and standardizing flavors, starch as a binder, modified starch, gum acacia, magnesium stearate, sodium caseinate, mannitol, propylene glycol, corn syrup, dextrose
Freezing agents are extremely volatile liquids—gases at ordinary temperatures and pressures—which evaporate rapidly and chill the food exposed to the cold vapor	Liquid nitrogen, dichlorodifluoromethane
Fumigants kill undesirable organisms	Methyl bromide, ethylene oxide, phostoxin
Humectants, moisture-retention agents, and antidusting agents retain the texture of food by preventing it from drying out	Sorbitol, propylene glycol, sodium tripolyphosphate
Ion-exchange resins are long, insoluble molecules (polymers) which have an affinity for certain positively or negatively charged ions, and which can be used to remove these ions from water or a solution or juice	A long list of resins, including acrylate-acrylamide resins, sulfonated copolymer of styrene and divinyl benzene, sulfonated anthracite coa, sulfite-modified cross-linked phenol-formaldehyde, etc.
Leavening agents produce light, fluffy baked goods	Yeast, monocalcium phosphate, sodium aluminum, phosphate, sodium acid phosphate, sodium carbonate, calcium carbonate and other baking powder ingredients
Lubricants, release agents allow the extrusion of foods and rapid, economical production of bread by permitting it to come cleanly out of the baking pan	Oleic acid, hydrogenated sperm oil, mineral oil
Masticatory substances for chewing gum give the bulk, plasticity, and resistance required for proper mouth feel	Chicle, rubber, paraffin, glycerol esters of rosin
Nonnutritive sweeteners having less than 2 percent of the caloric value of sucrose per equivalent unit of sweetening capacity, replace sugar or corn syrup in dietetic foods	Saccharin, cyclamate (in many countries)
Nutrient supplements restore values lost in processing or storage or insure higher nutritional value than nature may have provided	All the known essential nutrients such as vitamin A and other vitamins, iron and other trace minerals, amino acids and essential fatty acids
Nutritive sweeteners are any digestible sweeteners yielding more than 2 calories per gram	Dextrose, fructose, sucrose, corn syrup, molasses, honey

Technical effects of food additives (*continued*)

TECHNICAL EFFECT*	TYPICAL ADDITIVES IN CURRENT USE TO ACHIEVE THESE EFFECTS‡§
Oxidizing and reducing agents perform these chemical operations on food components to get rid of an undesirable component or contaminant	Peroxidase (enzyme) to destroy glucose in dried egg, so that it will store well; hydrogen peroxide added as a bleaching or antimicrobial agent
pH control agents (including buffers, acids, alkalies, neutralizing agents) reduce or increase the acidity or sourness of a food	Vinegar (acetic acid), sodium bicarbonate, hydrogen chloride, citric acid sulfuric acid, sodium citrate, sodium hydroxide, adipic acid
Preservatives, antimicrobial agents prevent bacteriological spoilage	Sodium benzoate, calcium propionate, potassium sorbate
Processing aids are added, not for the continuing effect they exert on the food, but to help make it better in the first place, for example, by aiding filtration or removing unwanted color	Charcoal, diatomaceous earth, hydrochloric acid, papain, polyvinylpolypyrrolidone, dioctyl sodium sulfosuccinate
Propellants, aerating agents, gases push the whipped cream topping from the can and make it fluffy, or exclude oxygen and prolong the shelf life and nutritional value of a packaged food	Chlorinated, fluorinated hydrocarbons; carbon dioxide; nitrous oxide; nitrogen; combustion gases
Sequestrants combine chemically with traces of metals present naturally in all foods, which if uncombined, would promote instability and off-flavors	Citric acid, *EDTA*, phosphoric acid, sodium metaphosphate
Solvents, vehicles dissolve or suspend flavors, colors, and many other ingredients in an easy-to-use form	Alcohol, propylene glycol, glycerine, triethyl citrate, triacetin, acetone
Stabilizers, thickeners give desirable viscosity and mouth feel, prevent emulsions from separating and prevent a pudding from being "sloppy"	Starch, modified food starches; natural and synthetic gums, such as guar, acacia, carrageenan, carob bean
Surface-active agents are related to the emulsifiers and permit rapid wetting of dry ingredients and better whipping of toppings; they promote foam where it is wanted or prevent it where it is not	Dioctyl sodium sulfosuccinate, sodium lauryl sulfate, lactylic esters of fatty acids, dimethyl polysiloxane
Surface-finishing agents are used on fruits, candies, and baked goods both for protection and appearance	Beeswax, carnauba wax, gum acacia, shellac wax, rice bran wax, oxidized polyethylene, rosin, polyvinylpyrrolidone
Synergists is a catch-all category of substances which produce no particular effect in themselves but help those of other additives	Citric acid, tricalcium phosphate, and other phosphates
Texturizers contribute or preserve desirable appearance or mouth feel; e.g., a smooth, slick sauce or pudding produced with normal starch is often less attractive than one with a somewhat pulpy appearance and feel produced by modified starches.	Sodium bicarbonate, glycerine, corn syrup, modified food starch
Washing-peeling aids, vegetable cleaning agents are substances that soften or dissolve the peel of a fruit or vegetable or that soften or loosen dirt; they save hand labor by making mechanical peeling and washing more effective, and they waste less food than hand processing	Sodium hydroxide (lye), sodium metasilicate, aliphatic acids, sodium hypochlorite, sodium *n*-alkylbenzene sulfonate, odorless light petroleum hydrocarbons

*R. L. Hall, "Food Additives," Nutrition Today, Vol. 8, No. 4 (Jul/Aug 1973).

‡NRC "A Comprehensive Survey of Industry on the Use of Foods General Recognized as Safe (GRAS), Table 6, PB-221 929 (Apr. 1973).

§Code of Federal Regulations, 21 Food and Drugs, Part 10 to 199, Rev. Apr. 1, 1976 (Wash. D.C. Gov. Print. Office).

hydrolytic degradation. Denaturation of many proteins by cooking also results in loss of their allergenic potential because of the attendant structural rearrangement. Although many foods may be implicated in allergy, the most common offenders are wheat, milk, eggs, seafoods, chocolate, corn, nuts, strawberries, chicken, and pork. The complete list of food allergens is larger and includes, among others, oatmeal, rye and other grains, cottonseed, the legumes, tomatoes, potatoes, beef, mustard, cucumbers, garlic, and citrus fruits. Foods that rarely if ever prove allergenic are rice, lamb, gelatin, peaches, pears, carrots, lettuce, artichokes, sesame oil, and apples.

food deterioration. See *food spoilage*.

food energy. Expressed in terms of calories per unit weight, food energy represents the energy available from its *oxidation* after deductions have been made for losses in digestion and incomplete oxidation. Energy values stated in food composition tables have been computed on the basis of the specific factor experimentally determined in a *bomb calorimeter* for the individual foods. The common factors, when applied to the total daily food intake of *protein, fat*, and *carbohydrate* from a typical American diet, provide a good estimate of the energy value of the diet. The energy in food determined by burning in a *bomb calorimeter* (heat of combustion) is higher than the energy that is available to humans. The food energy value estimates for human use are corrected for the percent of the food that is actually absorbed and the percent of complete *oxidation*. The table shows the energy values of food and the corrections for the amount of energy that is available for use. The energy value of a food can be determined with the factors in the fourth column if the weight content of the protein, fat, and carbohydrate is known. See *basal metabolism, caloric equivalent metabolism, oxidative phosphorylation, and terminal respiratory chain*.

Factor for determining the energy value of foods

FOOD	HEAT OF COMBUSTION (ΔH_C) KCAL/G FOOD	PERCENT OF ABSORPTION	CORRECTED FACTOR ENERGY AVAILABLE (ΔG) KCAL/G FOOD
Carbohydrate	4.1	98	4
Protein	5.7*	92	4
Fat	9.5	95	9

* Protein is incompletely oxidized by humans. The incomplete oxidation product is the *urea* that is excreted in the urine. The other foods are completely oxidized to CO_2, H_2O, and energy.

food exchange lists. Food exchange lists were prepared some years ago by a joint committee of the American Dietetic Association, American Diabetes Association, and Diabetes Section of the United States Public Health Service. An exchange list is a grouping of foods in which the *carbohydrate, protein*, and *fat* values are about equal for the items listed. The use of exchanges in planning meals allows for variety in the diet and enables the user to follow the guidelines of the prescribed diet under varying conditions or circumstances. An exchange has four essential characteristics: It allows choice, it specifies portion size, and it is both a caloric trade-off and a nutritional equivalent. Each item within an exchange list is interchangeable with any other item in the amount specified. Foods on different lists or from different food groups are not interchangeable. If one exchange on a food list or group is allowed on the meal plan, it means that any item on that list or in that group may be used in the amount specified. If two exchanges are allowed, it means that a double portion of any food may be used or two different items in the amount specified. A physician may prescribe the amounts of carbohydrate, protein, and fat that are to be used in measured diets. Using the values for the exchange lists, the dietitian calculates the number of exchanges to be furnished by the diet. The table gives a DIABETIC EXCHANGE LIST for Fat exchanges.

Diabetic Fat Exchange

POLYUNSATURATED FATS		SATURATED FATS	
FOOD	AMOUNT	FOOD	AMOUNT
Margarine, soft	1 tsp	Margarine, regular	1 tsp
Avocado (4" in diameter)	1/8	Butter	1 tsp
Oil: corn, cottonseed,		Bacon fat	1 tsp
safflower, soy, sunflower	1 tsp	Bacon, crisp	1 strip
Oil, olive	1 tsp	Cream, light	2 tbsp
Oil, peanut	1 tsp	Cream, sour	2 tbsp
Olives	5 small	Cream, heavy	1 tbsp
Almonds	10 whole	Cream cheese	1 tbsp
Pecans	2 large	French dressing	1 tbsp
Peanuts		Italian dressing	1 tbsp
Spanish	20 whole	Lard	1 tsp
Virginia	10 whole	Mayonnaise	1 tsp
Walnuts	6 small	Salad dressing	2 tsp
Nuts, other	6 small	Salt pork	3/4 inch

The list shows amounts of fat-containing foods to use for one Fat Exchange. For a diet low in saturated fat, select only those Exchanges that appear in the Polyunsaturated column. One Exchange of fat contains 5 g of fat and 45 calories.

food labeling. All food labels must contain at least the following: the name of the product, the net contents or net weight, and the name and place of business of the manufacturer, packer, or distributor. For most foods, the ingredients must be listed on the label and must be identified by their common or usual name. The ingredient present in the largest amount by weight must be listed first, followed by the other ingredients in descending order. Any additives must be listed. If colors and flavors are used, the Food, Drug, and Cosmetic Act permits such general language as "artificial color," "artificial flavor," or "natural flavor" to be used, but the use of Yellow No. 5 must be identified specifically because it can cause allergic reactions in some people. However, artificial colors used in butter, cheese, and ice cream do not have to be declared except, again, for Yellow No. 5. The only foods for which all ingredients may not have to be listed are those for which the Food and Drug Administration (FDA) has adopted "standards of identity," generally described as standardized foods. A standard of identity describes the ingredients the food must contain if it is to be called a particular name (ketchup, mayonnaise, etc.). Federal law does not require these mandatory ingredients to be mentioned in the ingredient list. However, most optional ingredients that a standard might permit must be shown. Jellies, jams, peanut butter, cheeses, and milk as well as ketchup and mayonnaise are examples of standardized foods. See *food labeling, nutrition.*

food labeling, cholesterol. The FDA's regulation on *cholesterol* labeling seeks to make it easier for people who are trying to limit their cholesterol for health reasons. The regulation printed in the Federal Register spells out the language about cholesterol that food companies use on their packages. In addition, this regulation makes it easier for manufacturers to put information about cholesterol and fat content on their labels. Manufacturers would have the option of using these terms on the labels of their products: (1) "Cholesterol free" can be used if the cholesterol content is less than 2 milligrams in each serving. (2) "Low cholesterol" would described products with less than 20 milligrams of cholesterol in each serving. (3) "Cholesterol reduced" or "reduced in cholesterol" would be permitted in products that have been reformulated so that cholesterol content has been reduced for at least 75% of the original product. Manufacturers would have to state what the original cholesterol content was, along with that of the cholesterol-reduced version. For foods that have less cholesterol, but not 75% less, the FDA's proposed regulation allows such language as "less cholesterol" or "lowered cholesterol." Again, the cholesterol content of both the original and reformulated products should be stated.

food labeling, grades. Some food products carry a grade on the label, such as "U.S. Grade A." Grades are set by the United States Department of Agriculture (USDA) for meat and poultry products, based on the quality levels of various characteristics of the product, such as taste, texture, and appearance. USDA grades are not based on nutritional content. The National Marine Fisheries Service grades fish products in a similar manner. Milk and milk products in most states carry a "Grade A" label. This grade is based on satisfaction of the FDA recommended sanitary standards for the production and processing of milk products, which are regulated by the states. The grade is not based on nutritional value. However, the FDA has established standards for milk and milk products, some of which require specific levels of vitamin A and others of which permit the optional addition of vitamins A and D.

food labeling, light to lite. Labeling language that suggests a food is lower in calorie content, unless some other meaning is specified or obvious. A "lite" product intended to be useful in reducing body weight or calorie intake must satisfy the Food and Drug Administration (FDA) requirements for low- or reduced-calorie foods and provide full nutrition labeling information. Product labels and nutrition-labeling should be checked carefully for calorie, fat, and sodium content. Since 1980, the FDA has required foods labeled as "low calorie" to contain no more than 40 calories in a serving and no more than 0.4 calories per gram. A "reduced-calorie" food must be at least one-third lower in calorie content than the food to which it is compared. Foods naturally low in calories cannot use these terms. Foods labeled as "diet" or "dietetic" products must meet the requirements for low- or reduced-calorie foods or must be clearly described as being useful for a special dietary purpose, other than for maintaining or reducing body weight.

food labeling, nutrition. Under the Food and Drug Administration's (FDA's) nutrition labeling regulations, the amount of each nutrient for a specified serving must be shown on the label. The label also must give the serving size (one cup, two teaspoons, etc.) and must show how many servings are in a container. *Protein, carbohydrate,* and *fat* are expressed in terms of the number of grams in a serving, and sodium is shown in milligrams. The FDA uses United States *Recommended Daily Allowances* or United States RDAs for protein and 19 vitamins and minerals. The U.S. RDA percentages in each serving must be shown for protein, five vitamins, (*vitamins A* and *C, thiamine, riboflavin,* and *niacin*), and two minerals (*calcium* and *iron*). Manufacturers are given the option of listing any of the remaining 12 nutrients if they contribute at least 2% of the U.S. RDA. If any of the 19 nutrients are added to a food or a claim is made about them, the label must include the required nutritional information about that nutrient.

Summary of nutrition labeling regulations

REQUIRED		OPTIONAL	
Name of food	Percent RDA		Percent RDA
Manufacturer or distributor	Protein	Polyunsaturated fat (g)	Vitamin D
Serving size	Vitamin A	Saturated fat (g)	Vitamin E
ounces or number of	Vitamin C	Cholesterol mg/serving	Vitamin B_6
servings per package per	Thiamine	Cholesterol mg/100 g	Folacin
package weight	Riboflavin	Sodium mg/serving	Vitamin B_{12}
	Niacin	Sodium mg/100 g	Phosphorus
	Calcium		Iodine
	Iron		Magnesium
			Zinc
			Copper
			Biotin
			Pantothenic acid

food labeling, product dating. Many consumers find product dating useful in their shopping for various foods. With only a few exceptions, such dating is not regulated by the FDA; however, there are four kinds of dating commonly used. To benefit from product dating, the consumer needs to know what kind of dating is used on the individual product and what it means.

Pack date: This is the day the food was manufactured, processed, or packaged; how old the food is. The importance of this information depends on how quickly the particular food normally spoils.

Pull or sell date: This is the last date the product would be sold, assuming it has been stored and handled properly. The pull date allows for some storage time in the home refrigerator. Cold cuts, ice cream, and milk are examples of foods with pull dates.

Expiration date: This is the last date the food should be eaten or used. Most manufacturers of infant formulas voluntarily displayed a "use by" date on their products. It was required on infant formulas after January 1986.

Freshness date: This is similar to the expiration date, although products such as baked goods can still be used for a short time after the freshness date. The food might not taste as good, but it still will be wholesome and safe.

food labeling, sodium. Since July 1, 1986, *sodium* content is included on every nutrition label. The FDA called for the addition of sodium information after studies showed an association between sodium intake and high blood pressure. Nutrition and health experts say a daily sodium intake of between 1100 and 3300 milligrams is a safe and adequate amount. The new sodium regulation permits food processors to use the following descriptive language in labeling their products: (1) *sodium free*, where the product has less than 5 milligrams in a serving; (2) *very low sodium*, 35 milligrams or less in a serving; (3) *low sodium*; 140 milligrams or less per serving; (4) *reduced sodium*, for foods where the usual level of sodium was reduced by at least 75%; (5) *unsalted* or *no salt added*, or some equivalent term for foods once processed with salt but now produced without it. A food so labeled, however, may in fact contain sodium. Salt, which is 40% sodium, is a major source of sodium in the American diet. There are, however, at least 70 sodium compounds being used in foods today. When these terms are used or whenever any sodium claim is made, the number of milligrams in a serving must be declared on the label by itself or as part of the nutritional information.

food labeling, standardized and nonstandardized foods. In 1938 Congress gave the FDA authority to adopt standards of identity of quality and of fill-of-container to protect consumers from being defrauded by cheap substitutes or deceptive packaging. Some 300 standards are in force today, covering a wide array of foods. A standard of identity spells out the mandatory ingredients of the food as well as any optional ingredients. Once a standard is set, other products that resemble it but do not conform to the standard cannot be marketed under the same name. Peanut butter, for example, is a standardized food; no product resembling it can be called peanut butter if it is made of less than 90% peanuts. There are many nonstandardized foods—those not covered by a federal standard—on the market that are perfectly acceptable and wholesome. The labels on such foods must accurately describe the food and all ingredients must be identified by their common or usual name, so that consumers know what they are buying. If a product resembles a standardized food but is nutritionally inferior to it, it must be labeled as an "imitation" of that food. If it is similar to a standardized food and is just as nutritious, it must still be described accurately on the label but need not be called an imitation food. Such provisions, which take into account the changing nature of the food industry, give manufacturers the flexibility to produce foods with different but safe ingredients and still meet FDA requirements as long as the products are appropriately labeled. Another special labeling requirement concerns packaged foods in which the main ingredient or component of a recipe is not included, as in the case of some "main dishes" or "dinners." On such foods, the common name of each ingredient must be listed in descending order by weight, for example, "noodles and tomato sauce." Identification of the food to be prepared from the package must be, for example, "for preparation of chicken casserole." A statement of ingredients must be added to complete the recipe, for example, "you must add chicken to complete the recipe."

food labeling, universal product code. Most food labels now include a small block of parallel lines of various widths, with accompanying numbers. This is the universal product code (UPC), which is not regulated by the FDA. The code on a label is unique to that product. Some stores are equipped with computerized checkout equipment that can read the code and automatically ring up the sale. In addition to making it possible for stores to automate part of their checkout work, the UPC, when used in conjunction with a computer, also can function as an automated inventory system. The computer can tell the store how much of a specific item is on hand, how fast it is being sold, and when and how much to order.

food poisoning. Any disease or toxin produced by microorganisms that are transmitted through food. Food poisoning is produced by microorganisms that are: (1) naturally occurring animal infections which can be transmitted to humans. This group of microorganisms includes *bacteria, fungi, viruses, worms*, and *protozoa*. (2) Microorganisms that may cause infections or present toxic effects in humans but are not normally present in food. The table gives some diseases produced by common microorganisms associated with food poisoning. See *food toxins*.

Food poisoning names and common sources

POISONING	FREQUENT METHOD OF SPREAD	POISONING	FREQUENT METHOD OF SPREAD
General		Meats	
Salmonella	Humans, rats, mice, cattle	Trichinosis	Pork
Staphylococcal	Man	Tape worms	Beef
Clostridial	Dust, feces, flies	Cysticercosis	Pork
Botulism	Canned foods, soil, dust	Clonorchiasis	Fish
Milk		Opisthorchiasis	Fish
Undulant fever	Cows or goats	Laragonimiasis	Crabs and crayfish
Vegetables		Diphyllobothriasis	Fish
Fasioliasis	Ruminants and pigs	Balantidiasis	Pigs

food preservatives. Food preservation methods can be divided into five major groups: (1) thermal processing, (2) dehydration, (3) freezing, (4) chemical control of the environment by additives, and (5) natural fermentation. *Thermal processing* increases the temperature of a foodstuff above the ambient temperature to prevent any chance of a food-borne disease. Heat-processing methods are highly variable, and the amount of heat determines how the food should be stored, what the shelf-life will be, and the kinds and amounts of nutrient losses that will occur. Blanching a food is done by placing it in boiling water (212 °F, 100 °C) for a short period of time. This method is used to decrease the number of microorganisms on the food's surface and to inactivate enzymes that would contribute to undesirable changes in color, flavor, or nutritive value during short-term storage. Foods are often blanched before canning or freezing because it softens the tissue and removes tissue gases, facilitating packaging of the food by decreasing its bulk. The process of pasteurization heats a food product at 160–175 °F (70–80 °C), depending on time, and inactivates part but not all of the vegetative microorganisms present. The heat treatment destroys some enzymes and nutrients present in milk, but the increased safety and shelf-life justify the decreased nutritive value. Sterilization is a term used to identify heat treatment at 212–248 °F (100–120 °C), depending on the product. The treatment is calculated to assure that *Clostridium botulinum* spores are destroyed or inactivated. The spores that may remain in commercial canned foods will not germinate under normal conditions of storage, so the food can be held as needed. *Dehydration*, or drying, of foods is a method of food preservation that decreases the water, making the food unavailable for microbial growth. Dried foods have decreased bulk, are easy to transport, and require no other conditions except dryness and absence of oxygen in order to be maintained. *Refrigeration* and *freezing* decrease the temperature of storage of foods, slowing down enzymatic reactions and microbial growth. They are particularly desirable for certain foods because they extend the shelf-life of those foods while maintaining many of the qualities the food had when fresh. *Control of chemical environment*: Substances that are put into foods during production, processing, and packaging or that are developed through microbial fermentation control the chemical environment in foods and influence their shelf-life. The substances function by reducing microbial hazards, by reducing harmful chemicals or physical spoilage that could occur in a food, or both. By minimizing spoilage, they indirectly influence the nutritive value of foods. *Fermentation* stabilizes food by the elaboration of substances by mold or bacteria that then prevent other adventitious microflora from growing. See *freeze drying* and *irradiation of foods*.

food protein, biological value. The *biological value* of food proteins depends on their amino acid composition. Proteins that do not provide all the *essential amno acids* upon digestion, or that provide some of them in suboptimal quantities, are not as valuable in supporting body protein anabolism as other proteins that can supply a full complement of the essential and nonessential amino acids. Proteins are thus classed as having a high or low biologic value primarily on the basis of their ability to supply all the amino acids required for the formation of body *tissues*, *enzymes*, and *hormones*. Other factors which influence the value of a given protein include digestibility. In the human adult, a protein must be digested completely and hydrolyzed into its component amino acids before these can be absorbed into the bloodstream and made available to the body's metabolic pool. In the event of incomplete hydrolysis of the protein, only part of the constituent amino acids become available, while others remain locked up in the nondigested protein molecules or partially hydrolyzed polypeptide fragments which are eventually excreted in the *feces* without contributing to the nutrition of the individual.

food spoilage. The spoilage or deterioration of food may be caused by natural chemical and biochemical reactions or by physical environments. Auto-oxidations represent natural chemical reactions that affect *unsaturated fatty acids*. The Maillard reaction, involving free amino and aldehyde groups, is another natural chemical reaction that effects the quality of proteins and the available of some *essential amino acids*. The crushing of cells during food processing may cause enzymatic degradations or heavy metals which contribute to the deterioration or destruction of nutrients. In addition, microorganisms and insects can contribute to food deterioration and spoilage. Among the physical environments that affect the quality of foods are storage temperature and humidity. High humidity and warm temperatures, for example, will accelerate natural chemical reactions and may also encourage the growth of microorganisms. Freezing, drying, and pressure are physical environments that can also contribute to the deterioration or the quality of foods.

The table provides a guide for the control of food spoilage as it relates to the temperature of processing and storage to inhibit spoilage.

Temperature guide for food safety

EFFECT OF TEMPERATURE ON MICROORGANISMS	TEMPERATURE	
	°F	°C
Canning temperatures for low-acid vegetable, meats, and poultry in a pressure canner	240	118
Canning temperatures of fruits, tomatoes, and pickles in a water bath canner	212	100
Cooking temperatures destroy most bacteria. Time required to kill bacteria decreases as the temperature is increased.	165	74
Warming temperatures prevent growth but allow survival of some bacteria.	140	60
Some bacterial growth may occur. Many bacteria survive.	125	52
Danger zone		
Foods held more than 2 hours in this zone are subject to rapid growth of bacteria and the production of toxins by some bacteria.	60	22
Some growth of food-poisoning bacteria may occur.	40	14
Cold temperatures permit slow growth of some bacteria that cause spoilage.	32	0
Do not store food above 10 °F for more than a few weeks.	10	-12
Freezing temperatures stop growth of bacteria, but may allow bacteria to survive.	0	-18

food storage. There are several processes that are used to store foods over time. Meats are most suceptible to food spoilage. Among the processes used are refrigeration, freezing, drying, curing, smoking, and heating. Cooling or refrigeration will perserve meats, for example, for 3–6 weeks at 32 °F (0 °C). At −4 °F (−20 °C) and 90% humidity, the shelf-life of meats is from 9–15 months. Smoking is usually associated with salting. Antioxidants and bactericidal compounds in the smoke deposit on and penetrate the meat, serving as preservatives. See *curing* and *food spoilage*.

food toxins. There occur in foods a number of compounds that are toxic or carcinogenic or have pharmacologic effects. The food toxins are grouped (1) as natural *carcinogens*, (2) as having toxic or pharmacologic effects, and (3) as nutritional inhibitors. The tables show some of the natural carcinogens in commonly eaten foods, some possible toxic or pharmacologic effects of foods, and some nutritional inhibitors naturally present in common foods.

Carcinogens in foods

SOURCE	CARCINOGEN	SOURCE	CARCINOGEN
Agricultural products	Aflatoxin	Meats, eggs, dairy products, wheat germ, leafy vegetables	Estrogens
Barbecued meats	Benzopyrene		
Teas, wines	Tannins	Orange and apple juices	Patulin
Cabbage	Thiourea	Proteins	Tryptophan
Corn	Zearalenone	Fermented products: breads, beer, wine	Ethyl carbamate
Flour	Patulin	Vegetables plus proteins (meat, fish, eggs)	Nitrates and nitrites plus 2°
Herbs	Alkaloids		amines → nitrosamines

Some possible toxic or pharmologic effects of foods

OCCURRENCE	ACTIVE AGENT	EFFECTS
Bananas and some other fruits	5-hydroxytryptamine; adrenaline; nonadrenaline	Effects on central and peripheral nervous system
Some cheeses	Tyramine	Raises blood pressure; enhanced by monoamine oxidase inhibitors
Almonds, cassava, and other plants	Cyanide	Interferes with tissue respiration
Quail	Due to consumption of hemlock	Hemlock poisoning
Mussels	Due to consumption of *Gonyaulax* (dinoflagellates)	Tingling, numbness, muscle weakness, respiratory paralysis
Cycad nuts	Methylazoxymethanol (cycasin)	Liver damage; cancer
Some fish, meat, or cheese	Nitrosamines	Liver damage; cancer
Mustard oil	Sanguinarine	Edema (epidemic dropsy)
Legumes	Hemagglutinins	Red cell and intestinal cell damage
Some beans	Vicine	Hemolytic anemia (favism)
	ß-aminopropionitrile	Interferes with collagen formation
	ß-N-oxalyl-amino-alanine	Toxic effects on nervous system Lathyrism
Ackee fruit	α-amino-ß-methylene cyclopropane propionate	Hypoglycemia, vomiting, sickness
Brassica seeds and some other Cruciferae	Glucosinolates, thiocyanate	Enlargement of thyroid gland (goiter)
Rhubarb	Oxalate	Oxalyluria
Green potatoes	Solanine; possibly other sapotoxins	Gastrointestinal upset
Many fish	Various, often confined to certain organs, or seasonal	Mainly toxic effects on nervous system
Many fungi	Various mycotoxins	Mainly toxic effects on nervous system and liver

Some nutritional inhibitors naturally present in common foods

SOURCE	INHIBITOR	ACTION	COUNTERACTION
Beans, lima, and soybeans	Antitrypsin	Prevents protein digestion	
	Hemagglutinins	Retards growth	
	Lipoxidase	Destroys vitamin A	Heat inactivation
Cabbage, kale, rutabagas	Goitrogens	Prevents synthesis of thyroxine	Additional iodine
Cereals	Unknown (niacinogen)	Binds niacin	Additional niacin or tryptophan
Corn, millet	Unknown (leucine?)	Decreases effectiveness of niacin	Additional niacin or tryptophan
Cottonseed oil	Sterculic acid	Interferes with reproduction	Heat or hydrogenation
Egg white	Ovamucoid	Prevents protein digestion	
	Avidin	Binds biotin	
	Conalbumin	Binds iron	Heat inactivation
Fish, clams	Thiaminase	Destroys thiamine	Heat inactivation
Milk, yogurt	Lactose	Diarrhea and loss of nutrients	Enzymic hydrolysis of lactose
Oatmeal	Phytin	Binds calcium	Additional calcium
		Binds iron	Additional iron
Onions	Unknown	Produces anemia	Avoid excessive intake
Peas	Nitrile compound	Interferes with sulfur metabolism (collagen formation)	Avoid excessive intake
Plant products	Molybdenum	Increases requirement for copper	Additional copper
Potatoes (immature or sprouting)	Solanine	Vomiting and diarrhea (loss of nutrients)	Avoid such potato products
Rhubarb, spinach	Oxalic acid	Binds calcium	Additional calcium
Vegetables and fruits	Ascorbic acid oxidase	Destroys vitamin C	Heat inactivation or additional vitamin C

formic acid. Mol. Wt. 46. HCOOH. The simplest organic acid. This acid is found in ants and other insects and is part of the irritant that produces itching and swelling after a bite. Formic acid derivatives occur in the body naturally and are important in protein synthesis. Transfer of the formic acid or formyl group requires the participation of the vitamin *folacin* as in the formation of *formiminoglutamic acid*.

formiminoglutamic acid (FIGLU). An intermediary product of *histidine* breakdown (*catabolism*). *Folacin* is necessary for its breakdown; the urinary excretion of FIGLU may be measured to determine the folacin status of an individual.

fortified, fortification, fortify. Adding a nutrient or nutrients to a food in amounts larger than that contained in any natural food in its class is to fortify that food. Examples are the addition of *vitamin D* to milk, fortified margarines, and fortified fruit juices and ades. Generally, no standards of identity are required when a food is labeled "fortified." See *enriched*.

fractionation. A term used by chemists when a complex of natural materials is separated in the laboratory by physical or chemical means. It is done usually to isolate or purify some specific compound present in feeds or foods.

frankfurters (weiners, hot dogs). A type of *sausage* made from beef, pork, and sometimes veal or combination of these meats. The meats are combined with seasonings and curing

Food, Approximate Measure, and Weight (in grams)		Water		Food Energy	Protein	Fat
		GRAMS	PERCENT	CALORIES	GRAMS	GRAMS

Fruits and Fruit Products

Food, Approximate Measure, and Weight (in grams)		Water grams	Water percent	Food Energy calories	Protein grams	Fat grams
Apples, raw (about 3 per lb)	1 apple	150	85	70	Trace	Trace
Apple juice, bottled or canned	1 cup	248	88	120	Trace	Trace
Applesauce, canned:						
Sweetened	1 cup	255	76	230	1	Trace
Unsweetened or artificially sweetened	1 cup	244	88	100	1	Trace
Apricots:						
Raw (about 12 per lb.)	3 apricots	114	85	55	1	Trace
Canned in heavy sirup	1 cup	259	77	220	2	Trace
Dried, uncooked (40 halves per cup).	1 cup	150	25	390	8	1
Cooked, unsweetened, fruit and liquid	1 cup	285	76	240	5	1
Apricot nectar, canned	1 cup	251	85	140	1	Trace
Avocadoes, whole fruit, raw:						
California (mid- and late-winter; diam. 3⅛ in.).	1 avocado	284	74	370	5	37
Florida (late summer, fall; diam. 3⅝ in.).	1 avocado	454	78	390	4	33
Bananas, raw, medium size.	1 banana	175	76	100	1	Trace
Banana flakes	1 cup	100	3	340	4	1
Blackberries, raw	1 cup	144	84	85	2	1
Blueberries, raw	1 cup	140	83	85	1	1
Cantaloupes, raw; medium, 5-inch diameter about 1⅔ pounds.	½ melon	385	91	60	1	Trace
Cherries, canned, red, sour, pitted, water pack.	1 cup	244	88	105	2	Trace
Cranberry juice cocktail, canned.	1 cup	250	83	165	Trace	Trace
Cranberry sauce, sweetened, canned, strained.	1 cup	277	62	405	Trace	1
Dates, pitted, cut	1 cup	178	22	490	4	1
Figs, dried, large, 2 by 1 in.	1 fig	21	23	60	1	Trace
Fruit cocktail, canned, in heavy syrup.	1 cup	256	80	195	1	Trace
Grapefruit:						
Raw, medium, 3¾-in. diam.						
White	½ grapefruit	241	89	45	1	Trace
Pink or red	½ grapefruit	241	89	50	1	Trace
Canned, syrup pack	1 cup	254	81	180	2	Trace
Grapefruit juice:						
Fresh	1 cup	246	90	95	1	Trace
Canned, white:						
Unsweetened	1 cup	247	89	100	1	Trace
Sweetened	1 cup	250	86	130	1	Trace
Frozen, concentrate, unsweetened:						
Undiluted, can, 6 fluid ounces.	1 can	207	62	300	4	1
Diluted with 3 parts water, by volume.	1 cup	247	89	100	1	Trace
Dehydrated crystals	4 oz.	113	1	410	6	1
Prepared with water (1 pound yields about 1 gallon).	1 cup	247	90	100	1	Trace
Grapes, raw:						
American type (slip skin).	1 cup	153	82	65	1	1
European type (adherent skin).	1 cup	160	81	95	1	Trace
Grapejuice:						
Canned or bottled	1 cup	253	83	165	1	Trace

| | Fatty Acids | | | | | | | | | |
| Saturated (Total) Grams | Unsaturated | | Carbo-hydrate Grams | Calcium Milli-grams | Iron Milli-grams | Vitamin A Value Interna-tional Units | Thiamine Milli-grams | Riboflavin Milli-grams | Niacin Milli-grams | Ascorbic Acid Milli-grams |
	Oleic Grams	Linoleic Grams								
—	—	—	18	8	0.4	50	0.04	0.02	0.1	3
—	—	—	30	15	1.5	—	0.02	0.05	0.2	2
—	—	—	61	10	1.3	100	0.05	0.03	0.1	3
—	—	—	26	10	1.2	100	0.05	0.02	0.1	2
—	—	—	14	18	.5	2,890	.03	.04	.7	10
—	—	—	57	28	.8	4,510	.05	.06	.9	10
—	—	—	100	100	8.2	16,350	.02	.23	4.9	19
—	—	—	62	63	5.1	8,550	.01	.13	2.8	8
—	—	—	37	23	.5	2,380	.03	.03	.5	8
7	17	5	13	22	1.3	630	.24	.43	3.5	30
7	15	4	27	30	1.8	880	.33	.61	4.9	43
—	—	—	26	10	.8	230	.06	.07	.8	12
—	—	—	89	32	2.8	760	.18	.24	2.8	7
—	—	—	19	46	1.3	290	.05	.06	.5	30
—	—	—	21	21	1.4	140	.04	.08	.6	20
—	—	—	14	27	.8	6,540	.08	.06	1.2	63
—	—	—	26	37	.7	1,660	.07	.05	.5	12
—	—	—	42	13	.8	Trace	.03	.03	.1	40
—	—	—	104	17	6	60	.03	.03	.1	6
—	—	—	130	105	5.3	90	.16	.17	3.9	0
—	—	—	15	26	.6	20	.02	.02	.1	0
—	—	—	50	23	1.0	360	.05	.03	1.3	5
—	—	—	12	19	0.5	10	0.05	0.02	0.2	44
—	—	—	13	20	0.5	540	0.05	0.02	0.2	44
—	—	—	45	33	.8	30	.08	.05	.5	76
—	—	—	23	22	.5	—	.09	.04	.4	92
—	—	—	24	20	1.0	20	.07	.04	.4	84
—	—	—	32	20	1.0	20	.07	.04	.4	78
—	—	—	72	70	.8	60	.29	.12	1.4	286
—	—	—	24	25	.2	20	.10	.04	.5	96
—	—	—	102	100	1.2	80	.40	.20	2.0	396
—	—	—	24	22	.2	20	.10	.05	.5	91
—	—	—	15	15	.4	100	.05	.03	.2	3
—	—	—	25	17	.6	140	.07	.04	.4	6
—	—	—	42	28	.8	—	.10	.05	.5	Trace

Food, Approximate Measure, And Weight (in Grams)		Water		Food Energy	Protein	Fat
		GRAMS	PERCENT	CALORIES	GRAMS	GRAMS
Grapejuice:						
Frozen concentrate, sweetened:						
Undiluted, can, 6 fluid ounces.	1 can	216	53	395	1	Trace
Diluted with 3 parts water, by volume.	1 cup	250	86	135	1	Trace
Grapejuice drink, canned	1 cup	250	86	135	Trace	Trace
Lemons, raw, 2⅛-in. diam., size 165. Used for juice.	1 lemon	110	90	20	1	Trace
Lemon juice, raw	1 cup	244	91	60	1	Trace
Lemonade concentrate:						
Frozen, 6 fl. oz. per can	1 can	219	48	430	Trace	Trace
Diluted with 4⅓ parts water, by volume.	1 cup	248	88	110	Trace	Trace
Lime juice:						
Fresh	1 cup	246*	90	65	1	Trace
Canned, unsweetened	1 cup	246	90	65	1	Trace
Limeade concentrate, frozen:						
Undiluted, can, 6 fluid ounces.	1 can	218	50	410	Trace	Trace
Diluted with 4⅓ parts water, by volume.	1 cup	247	90	100	Trace	Trace
Oranges, raw, 2⅝-in. diam., all commercial, varieties.	1 orange	180	86	65	1	Trace
Orange juice, all varieties.	1 cup	248	88	110	2	1
Canned, unsweetened	1 cup	249	87	120	2	Trace
Frozen concentrate:						
Undiluted, can, 6 fluid ounces.	1 can	213	55	360	5	Trace
Diluted with 3 parts water, by volume.	1 cup	249	87	120	2	Trace
Dehydrated crystals	4 oz.	113	1	430	6	2
Prepared with water (1 pound yields about 1 gallon).	1 cup	248	88	115	2	1
Orange-apricot juice drink	1 cup	249	87	125	1	Trace
Frozen concentrate:						
Undiluted, can, 6 fluid ounces.	1 can	210	59	330	4	1
Diluted with 3 parts water, by volume.	1 cup	248	88	110	1	Trace
Papayas, raw, ½-inch cubes.	1 cup	182	89	70	1	Trace
Peaches:						
Raw:						
Whole, medium, 2-inch diameter, about 4 per pound.	1 peach	114	89	35	1	Trace
Sliced	1 cup	168	89	65	1	Trace
Canned, yellow-fleshed, solids and liquid:						
Sirup pack, heavy: Halves or slices	1 cup	257	79	200	1	Trace
Water pack	1 cup	245	91	75	1	Trace
Dried, uncooked	1 cup	160	25	420	5	1
Cooked, unsweetened, 10–12 halves and juice.	1 cup	270	77	220	3	1
Frozen:						
Carton, 12 ounces, not thawed.	1 carton	340	76	300	1	Trace
Pears:						
Raw, 3 by 2½-inch diameter.	1 pear	182	83	100	1	1
Canned, solids and liquid.						

| Fatty Acids | | | | | | | | | | |
| Saturated (Total) Grams | Unsaturated | | Carbo-hydrate Grams | Calcium Milli-grams | Iron Milli-grams | Vitamin A Value Interna-tional Units | Thiamine Milli-grams | Riboflavin Milli-grams | Niacin Milli-grams | Ascorbic Acid Milli-grams |
	Oleic Grams	Linoleic Grams								
—	—	—	100	22	.9	40	.13	.22	1.5	—
—	—	—	33	8	.3	10	.05	.08	.5	—
—	—	—	35	8	.3	—	.03	.03	.3	—
—	—	—	6	19	.4	10	.03	.01	.1	39
—	—	—	20	17	.5	50	.07	.02	.2	112
—	—	—	112	9	.4	40	.04	.07	.7	66
—	—	—	28	2	Trace	Trace	Trace	.02	.2	17
—	—	—	22	22	.5	20	.05	.02	.2	79
—	—	—	22	22	.5	20	.05	.02	.2	52
—	—	—	108	11	.2	Trace	.02	.02	.2	26
—	—	—	27	2	Trace	Trace	Trace	Trace	Trace	5
—	—	—	16	54	.5	260	.13	.05	.5	66
—	—	—	26	27	.5	500	.22	.07	1.0	124
—	—	—	28	25	1.0	500	.17	.05	.7	100
—	—	—	87	75	.9	1,620	.68	.11	2.8	360
—	—	—	29	25	.2	550	.22	.02	1.0	120
—	—	—	100	95	1.9	1,900	.76	.24	3.3	408
—	—	—	27	25	.5	500	.20	.07	1.0	109
—	—	—	32	12	.2	1,440	.05	.02	.5	[10]40
—	—	—	78	61	0.8	800	0.48	0.06	2.3	302
—	—	—	26	20	.2	270	.16	.02	.8	102
—	—	—	18	36	.5	3,190	.07	.08	.5	102
—	—	—	10	9	.5	1,320	.02	.05	1.0	7
—	—	—	16	15	.8	2,230	.03	.08	1.6	12
—	—	—	52	10	.8	1,100	.02	.06	1.4	7
—	—	—	20	10	.7	1,100	.02	.06	1.4	7
—	—	—	109	77	9.6	6,240	.02	.31	8.5	28
—	—	—	58	41	5.1	3,290	.01	.15	4.2	6
—	—	—	77	14	1.7	2,210	.03	.14	2.4	135
—	—	—	25	13	.5	30	.04	.07	.2	7

Food, Approximate Measure, And Weight (in Grams)		Water	Food Energy	Protein	Fat
	Grams	Percent	Calories	Grams	Grams
Pineapple:					
Raw, diced	1 cup	140	85	75	1	Trace
Canned, heavy sirup pack, solids and liquid:					
Crushed	1 cup	260	80	195	1	Trace
Sliced, slices and juice.	2 small or 1 large	122	80	90	Trace	Trace
Pineapple juice, canned	1 cup	249	86	135	1	Trace
Plums, all except prunes:					
Raw, 2-inch diameter, about 2 ounces.	1 plum	60	87	25	Trace	Trace
Canned, sirup pack (Italian prunes):					
Plums (with pits) and juice.	1 cup	256	77	205	1	Trace
Prunes, dried, "softenized," medium:					
Uncooked	4 prunes	32	28	70	1	Trace
Cooked, unsweetened, 17–18 prunes and ⅓ cup liquid.	1 cup	270	66	295	2	1
Prune juice, canned or bottled.	1 cup	256	80	200	1	Trace
Raisins, seedless:					
Packaged, ½ oz. or 1½ tbsp. per pkg.	1 pkg.	14	18	40	Trace	Trace
Cup, pressed down	1 cup	165	18	480	4	Trace
Raspberries, red:					
Raw	1 cup	123	84	70	1	1
Frozen, 10-ounce carton, not thawed.	1 carton	284	74	275	2	1
Rhubarb, cooked, sugar added.	1 cup	272	63	385	1	Trace
Strawberries:					
Raw, capped	1 cup	149	90	55	1	1
Frozen, 10-ounce carton, not thawed.	1 carton	284	71	310	1	1
Tangerines, raw, medium, 2⅜-in. diam., size 176.	1 tangerine	116	87	40	1	Trace
Tangerine juice, canned, sweetened.	1 cup	249	87	125	1	1
Watermelon, raw, wedge, 4 by 8 inches (1/16 of 10 by 16-inch melon, about 2 pounds with rind).	1 wedge	925	93	115	2	1

nitrates and in some case fillers; then stuffed into casings, smoked, cooked in steam, and quickly chilled. Good source of protein, some vitamins of B group, *thiamine, riboflavin,* and *niacin.* Fair source of *calcium* and *iron.*

Nutrients in 100 g of frankfurter

Type	Calories	Protein G	Fat G	Carbohydrate G	Niacin MG	Cobalamin µG	Calcium MG
Beef	319	11	27	2	2	2	13
Beef & pork	317	11	27	2	2	1	11
Turkey	220	13	18	1	4	1	128
Chicken	255	13	19	7	4	1	75

| Fatty Acids | | | | | | | | | | |
| Saturated (Total) Grams | Unsaturated | | Carbo-hydrate Grams | Calcium Milli-grams | Iron Milli-grams | Vitamin A Value Interna-tional Units | Thiamine Milli-grams | Riboflavin Milli-grams | Niacin Milli-grams | Ascorbic Acid Milli-grams |
	Oleic Grams	Linoleic Grams								
—	—	—	19	24	7	100	.12	.04	.3	24
—	—	—	50	29	.8	120	.20	.06	.5	17
—	—	—	24	13	.4	50	.09	.03	.2	8
—	—	—	34	37	.7	120	.12	.04	.5	22
—	—	—	7	7	.3	140	.02	.02	.3	3
—	—	—	53	22	2.2	2,970	.05	.05	.9	4
—	—	—	18	14	1.1	440	.02	.04	.4	1
—	—	—	78	60	4.5	1,860	.08	.18	1.7	2
—	—	—	49	36	10.5	—	.03	.03	1.0	5
—	—	—	11	9	.5	Trace	.02	.01	.1	Trace
—	—	—	128	102	5.8	30	.18	.13	.8	2
—	—	—	17	27	1.1	160	.04	.11	1.1	31
—	—	—	70	37	1.7	200	.06	.17	1.7	59
—	—	—	98	212	1.6	220	.06	.15	.7	17
—	—	—	13	31	1.5	90	.04	.10	1.0	88
—	—	—	79	40	2.0	90	.06	.17	1.5	150
—	—	—	10	34	.3	360	.05	.02	.1	27
—	—	—	30	45	.5	1,050	.15	.05	.2	55
—	—	—	27	30	2.1	2,510	.13	.13	.7	30

freeze dry. A process of rapidly freezing a substance at an extremely low temperature and then dehydrating under vacuum. This is the most gentle method of drying food. The moisture content of the food is usually between 3–10%. See *food, preservation*.

fructose (levulose). Mol. Wt. 180. Fructose occurs in plant juices, in fruits, and especially in honey, of which it constitutes about one-half the solid matter. It results in equal quantity with *glucose* from the hydrolysis of cane sugar (*sucrose*) and in smaller proportions from some other less common sugars. Fructose is almost twice as sweet as *glucose* (dextrose); 1.7 is sweetness factor of comparison with glucose. Fructose works like glucose for the production of *glycogen*. Glucose and fructose are convertible chemically under the influence of very dilute alkalies and biochemically by an enzyme (an isomerase) that interconverts the phosphate derivatives, glucose-6-phosphate to fructose-6-phosphate. See *sugars*.

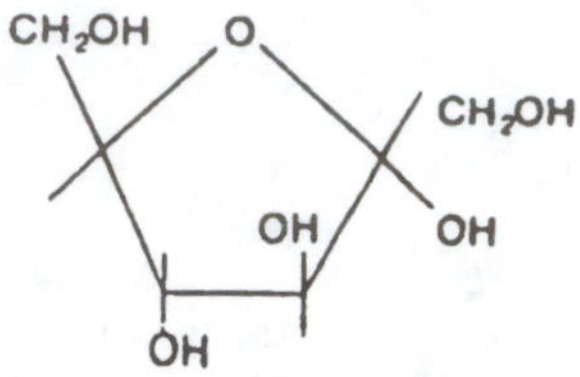

β-D-fructose (levulose)

fruit drinks. Fresh homemade drinks and many high-grade commercial preparations are good sources of *ascorbic acid*. In others, the vitamins may have been largely destroyed in the processing. Such juices have a variable energy value, depending almost entirely on their sugar content. Most natural fruit juices contain from 30–80 mmol/L of *potassium* and less than 2 mmol/L of *sodium*. They are therefore useful for individuals with edema or on diuretic therapy, which increase the renal excretion of potassium.

fruits. The edible portion of the reproductive body of the seed of a plant, which usually involves the pulp associated with the seed. In fruits, the carbohydrate is mostly in the form of the *monosaccharides, glucose,* and *fructose*. The *disaccharide, sucrose,* may be found in a few fresh fruits. The *sugar* content of fruits may vary from 6–20%, those of canteloupe and watermelon being the lowest and that of banana one of the highest. The caloric value of fruits, fresh, canned, or frozen, is determined largely by their sugar content. The table gives the nutritive content of some common fruits and fruit products.

fumaric acid (*fumarate*). Mol. Wt. 116. A solid at room temperature, inexpensive, highly acidic, and does not absorb moisture readily. A source of tartness and acidity in such products as gelatin desserts, puddings, pie fillings, candy, instant soft drinks, and leavening agents. Fumaric acid is an important metabolite in the *Krebs'* (tricarboxylic acid) *cycle* and is present in every cell of the body.

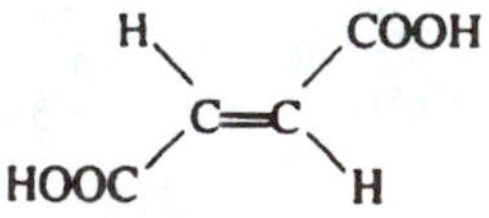

Fumaric acid

fungi. Fungi are simple plant organisms which are larger than *bacteria*. They most often attack the skin, including the hair and nails, causing such chronic infections as ringworm and athlete's foot. Infections caused by fungi are called mycotic infections and can be serious when internal organs are involved. *Mushrooms* and *yeasts* are examples of fungi. Some fungi benefit humans, such as in the production of antibiotics, cheese, and wine, while other fungi cause diseases.

furcellaran (Danish agar). A vegetable gum similar to *carrageenan* in composition and properties. It is a stabilizer and thickener in foods. This food additive is obtained from seaweed and is used by food manufacturers as a gelling agent. Puddings, cake fillings, pastry fillings, marmalades, and meat pastes commonly contain furcelleran. Furcellaran also facilitates the clarification of beer by precipitating proteins. See *stabilizers* and *thickers*.

furans. A family of compounds containing an oxygen in a five-membered ring. Some furans are lactones resulting from internal condensations of hydroxyl groups in sugars; fructose is an example. Furanones and lactones are responsible for some of the distinctive *aromas* of foods. Furanone is found in bread and coffee.

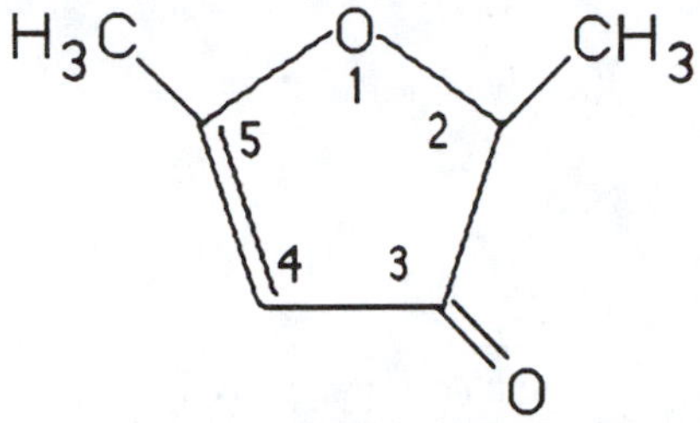

2,5-dimethyl 3 furanone

Furanones and lactones in foods

COMPOUNDS	AROMAS	SOURCES
Furanones		
4-hydroxy-5-methyl	Roasted chicory; caramel	Meat broth
4-hydroxy-2,5-dimethyl	Pineapple; caramel	Pineapple; burnt almond; meat broth; popcorn
4-methoxy-2,5-dimethyl	Sherry-like	Strawberry, raspberry
Lactones		
4-butanolide	Sweet; aromatic; butter- like	Dried mushrooms; popcorn; roasted nuts; pineapple
3-penten-4-olide	Sweet, herbaceous	White bread; soy beans; raisins
4-nonanolide	Coconut oil	Fatty foods, peaches
4-decanolide	Fruity	Fatty foods, strawberries
5-oxo-4-hexanolide	Wine-like	Wine

G

G. The alphabetic symbol for the *amino acid glycine* (Gly).

galactans. Galactans are *polysaccharides* made up of sulfonated *galactose* derivatives. They are produced by red sea weeds and are the major constituent in *carrageenans*.

galactose. Mol. Wt. 180. A natural *monosaccharide*. One of the monosaccharides in milk sugar (*lactose*). The hydrolysis of milk sugar, either by acid or by digestive enzyme, yields galactose and *glucose*. Galactose is convertible to glucose in the body. Polymeric anhydrides of galactase, known as galactans, are widely distributed in plants, and galactosides, which are compounds containing galactose in chemical combination with radicals of other than carbohydrate in nature, are constituents of the brain and nerve tissues. Galactose has also been recognized as a minor constituent of several proteins. See *galactosemia*.

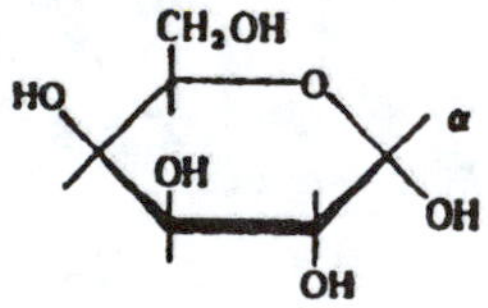

α-D-galactose

galactose-l-phosphate. An intermediate product of galactose metabolism.

galactosemia. A rare genetic disease in which galactose is not properly metabolized because an enzyme, phosphogalactose uridyl transferase, is missing. The result is an accumulation of galactose in the blood owing to a hereditary lack of this enzyme which converts galactose to *glucose*. The disease is accompanied by severe mental retardation which can be ameliorated if special diets are given immediately after birth.

gallbladder. A dark green sac shaped like a blackjack and lodged in a hollow on the underside of the liver. Its ducts join with the duct of the liver to conduct bile to the upper end of the small intestines. The main function of the gallbladder is the concentration and storage of the bile until it is needed for digestion, particularly of fats. See *bile* and *bile salts*.

gallstones. Accumulation of variable-sized stones with high *cholesterol* concentrations or *calcium* combined with *bile* in the gall bladder, ranging in size from a tiny speck to an inch or more in diameter. Cholesterol may become so concentrated in the gallbladder that it tends to crystallize out, and these crystals form gallstones. The passage through the cystic and common bile ducts often causes severe pain called gallbladder colic. Stones are especially common at ages of 50–60 years. A low-fat diet often is suggested as a treatment for gallstones, although no conclusive evidence indicates that such a diet will prevent such symptoms.

gamete. A reproductive cell; an ovum or a spermatozoon.

gamma globulins. A class of serum proteins, some of which function as *antibodies*.

ganglia (ganglion). A collection of nerve cells which form a distinct mass in the *nervous system*.

garbanzos. See *chickpeas*.

garlic (*Allium sativum*). A hardy, bulbous plant that is a member of the lily family, which also includes *leeks, chives, onions*, and *shallots*. Like the onion, the edible bulb of the plant grows beneath the ground. This compound bulb is made up of small sections or bulblets, called "cloves," which are encased in thin, papery envelopes.

gastric acid. Acid (*hydrochloric acid*) in the *stomach*.

gastric analysis. A specimen of stomach juice obtained by a stomach tube and examined chemically and microscopically as a screening test for ulcers and cancer.

gastric juice. A substance secreted by the gastric glands lining the mucous membrane of the *stomach*. It is a thin, colorless, or nearly colorless liquid containing the *digestive enzyme pepsin*, produced by the *chief cells*, and *hydrochloric acid*, produced by the *parietal cells*. The acid which is secreted by the *parietal cells* has a pH of about 0.9. In addition to salts, gastric juice also contains *glycoproteins*, one of which is the *intrinsic factor* of the antianemia principle. About 700 mL of gastric juice is secreted with each meal. See *digestive system*.

gastric ulcer. An ulcer or sore seated in the wall of the *stomach*, creating burning pain in the stomach area which is relieved by taking food, milk, or *antacids*. Pain usually occurs when stomach is empty. Vomiting may occur. See *peptic ulcer*.

gastrin. A *hormone* of the *digestive system* that stimulates the secretion of *hydrochloric acid* (HCl) by the *parietal cells* of the gastric glands. Although the secretion of gastric juice and the motility of the *stomach* are sensitive to nervous and physical influences, by far the strongest stimulus to the secretion of gastric juice comes from food in the stomach. The formation of gastrin in the pyloric glands in the pyloric region of the stomach (under the influence of food) stimulates the muscular activity of the stomach and the secretion of gastric juice.

gastritis. Inflammation of the *stomach*. It occurs in all ages, but appears more common in older people. The term often is used loosely as a catchall for any digestive complaint, particularly heartburn, belching, "sour stomach," and bloating. These symptoms more often reflect irritability rather than inflammation of the stomach. Chronic gastritis usually follows ingestion of highly spiced food or excessive amounts of alcohol over an extended period of time. See *heartburn*.

gastroenteritis. Inflammation of the *stomach* and *intestinal tract*.

gastroferrin. A protein present in normal *gastric juice*. In the small intestine, the epithelial cell lining of the intestinal wall (the mucosal cell) is the key to the mechanism of *iron* absorption. This cell lining takes in iron by regulatory procedures not fully understood. It appears that gastroferrin is involved in the regulation of the absorption of iron by the intestinal mucosal cells.

gastrointestinal. Referring to the part of the *digestive system* made up of the *stomach* and the intestines.

gastrointestinal disturbances. Digestive and eliminative processes are subject to many kinds of disorders. There are disorders of appetite and excessive eating; at the other extreme, *anorexia nervosa*, a loss of appetite so severe that it sometimes threatens life. *Gastritis*, sometimes called "nervous stomach," is marked by gastric distress and pain, occasionally with vomiting. In gastritis there is irritation of the walls of the stomach but not sharply localized injury. *Peptic ulcer* is a focal lesion of the mucous lining of stomach or duodenum, an inflamed crater that may even cause the internal loss of blood. At the eliminative end of the tract the two possibilities are chronic constipation and chronic diarrhea. The latter is usually called *colitis* (inflammation of the colon); it may be associated with chronic spasm of the smooth muscle of the colon or it may invoke ulceration of the inner walls. None of these disorders is necessarily psychogenic. Infections, metabolic disorders, glandular malfunctioning, structural defects, long-continued faulty diet, and many other conditions can cause gastrointestinal disturbances or distress.

gastrointestinal series (GI series). A series of gastrointestinal x-ray tests after swallowing barium, which is used for the diagnosis of suspected *ulcers* and *cancer* of *stomach* and *duodenum*.

gastrointestinal tract. See *digestive system*.

gastroscopy. A direct, visual examination of the *stomach* performed with the aid of a gastroscope. Especially valuable in detecting lesions, such as ulcers and tumors, not seen in an x-ray examination and for permitting a better evaluation of lesions merely suspected on the basis of x-ray examination.

gavage. Feeding through a tube passed into the *stomach* through the *esophagus*.

gelatin. A protein that swells on contact with water, dissolves in hot water, and forms a gel when cooled. The words "gelatin" and "jelly" both come form the Latin *gelatus*, meaning frozen. In cookery, gelatin is used as a thickening agent. Edible gelatin is made from animal tissues. Good gelatin is odorless and tasteless, and when dissolved gives a clear solution. There are two main types of gelatin. The alkaline type is found in unflavored gelatin and the acid type is found in flavored gelatin. Gelatin is a pure protein and is easily digested. Gelatin is also an incomplete protein. It lacks sufficient quantities of the *essential amino acids methionine, lysine, and tryptophan* to qualifiy as a useful protein supplement.

gene. The biological unit of hereditary information, self-producing and located in a definite position (locus) on a particular *chromosome*. The gene is the sequence of trinucleotide combinations (*triplet codes*) of *deoxyribonucleic acid* (DNA) in a chromosome that also contains nucleoproteins, mostly histones. It is the sequence of the triplet codes that determines the amino acid sequence of a polypeptide chain. See *genetic code*.

gene linkage. Refers to the fact that all the closely located *genes* of a given *chromosome* are inherited together.

Generally Regarded As Safe (GRAS). The Food and Drug Administration's list of food additives that have been used for relatively long periods and thus are exempt from requirements for premarket clearance.

generic drugs. The generic or official name of a drug is assigned by the producer of the drug in collaboration with the Food and Drug Administration and Council on Drugs of the American Medical Association. The generic name may be used by any interested party and is usually the name found in the United States Pharmacopoeia (USP) and the National Formulary (NF). The generic listing is usually used in the Federal Supply Catalog and in the Army Medical Department (AMEDD) pharmacies. A generic drug name is not capitalized; for example, aluminum hydroxide.

genetic. Congenital or inherited, or referring to the gene.

genetic code. The formal correspondence between the *trinucleotide* base sequence (*triplet code*) in *deoxyribonucleic acid* (DNA) and *amino acid* sequences in proteins which makes possible the synthesis of specific proteins according to hereditary information contained in the genes. Codes have been worked out for each of the amino acids. It is known exactly what combinations of *purine* and *pyrimidine* bases in the *nucleic acid* molecules instruct the *ribosomes* to attach a particular amino acid to a particular place in a growing protein or *polypeptide chain*. *Ribonucleic acids* are the messangers (*messanger RNA*, mRNA) that translate the messages from the gene to the transcription mechanisms.

genfibrozil. See *cholesterol*.

genome. The genome is the sum of all the various genes present in an organism.

genotype. The genetic makeup of individuals. Persons with the same genes have the same genotype. When persons merely show the same physical traits, they are referred to as having the same phenotype. Sometimes persons with the same genotype may differ in phenotype, as with identical twins who have developed differently because of environmental or nutritional influences. Conversely, persons with the same phenotype, showing the same physical traits, may or may not be carrying the same genes. For example, two dark-eyed persons, one of whom carried two "dark-eyed" genes, the other one carrying a dominant "dark-eye" gene plus a recessive "light-eye" gene, may appear alike, that is, they have the same phenotype but their genes are not identical. Therefore they are different genotypes.

germ. The part of a cereal seed that grows and produces new plants. Also a common name for *bacteria*.

germ plasm. The material of the germ cells, in the testes of the male or the ovaries of the female, from which the sperms or eggs with the chromosomes are fashioned.

ghee. The anglicized version of the Hindustani for *ghi*, which means "clarified butter" and is a basic ingredient in the cooking of India. Indian butter is made from buffalo's or cow's milk. To clarify it, the butter is heated until the milk solids are separated from the clear fat. Then it is strained through a cloth and poured into a container for storage. The reason for clarifying butter in a hot climate is that it will keep without refrigeration for quite a long time, depending upon the temperature.

gibberellins. A group of growth-regulating substances (hormones) for plants which are produced by certain species of fungi of the genus *Gibberella*.

gin. A simple alcoholic liquor of pure ethyl alcohol (*ethanol*, grain alcohol), plus water and flavoring. The flavor is derived by allowing the alcoholic vapors to flow over the flavoring ingredients, usually juniper berries (although orange peel, caraway seeds, and other flavoring materials are used). The principal effects of gin are produced by the alcohol and are toxic. The concentration of ethyl alcohol in beverages is expressed in proof, which is twice the percentage of the alcohol.

ginger (*Zingiber officinale*). A spice obtained from the root, or rhizome, of an erect perennial plant that grows to a height of 3 feet and has large, brilliant yellowish flowers with purple lips, which are borne in a spike. There are several hundred varieties of ginger. The pungent smell of ginger comes from an aromatic oil, the peppery taste from a substance called "gingerin." Ginger is used crystallized, preserved, or dried; whole, cracked, or ground to a powder.

ginger ale. A carbonated beverage flavored with ginger, sugar, capsicum, and other flavorings and colored with caramel. Ginger ale can also be made with an artificial sweetener rather than with sugar.

ginger beer. A clear, effervescent beverage made of ginger, sugar, and water, and fermented by yeast. It has a stronger ginger flavor than ginger ale.

gingiva. The mucous membrane and connective tissue that encircles the neck of the tooth and overlies the crowns of those teeth not as yet erupted. Commonly referred to as the gums. See *teeth*.

gingivitis. An inflammation of the gums (*gingiva*), beginning with a slight swelling along the gum margin of one or more teeth. The gum tissue in the area may have a slightly different color. As the condition grows worse, the "collar" of gum tissue loses its tight adaptation to the tooth surface, and the tissue bleeds on slight pressure. Usually, there is no pain. Gingivitis is a common symptom of vitamin deficiencies, especially *ascorbic acid* (vitamin C), which leads to scurvy.

G.I. series. See *gastrointestinal series*.

G.I. tract. See *digestive system*.

glands. Cells or groups of cells that can manufacture a secretion, a *hormone*, which is discharged and used in some other part of the body. Glands may be classified as the *exocrine*, or duct glands, which secrete into a cavity or on the body surface, the *endocrine* or ductless glands, which secrete into the tissue fluid and blood, or autocrine with hormones that exert internal effects by interacting with the surface of their own membranes.

glandular. Adjective of gland. A gland is an organ that makes and discharges a chemical substance that is used elsewhere in the body or eliminated.

gliadin. A plant protein fraction of *wheat gluten*. It belongs to a class of plant proteins called *prolamines*. It is gliadin and the protein *glutenin* in combination that give wheat *flour* its characteristic stickiness when moistened and its bonding when heated. See *bread*.

globular proteins. A classification of *proteins* based upon their shape. Globular protein molecules tend to be nearly round. The contrast of the globular proteins are the fibrous proteins, which are long and thin. Found in tissue fluids of animals and plants in which they readily disperse, either in true solution or colloidal suspension. Important globular proteins from the standpoint of nutrition are caseinogen in milk, albumin in egg white, and albumins and globulins in blood, which are not only easily digestible but which also contain in their structure a good proportion of the *essential amino acids*. See *globulin*.

globulin. A globular protein found throughout body tissues in various forms such as gamma (γ)- globulins, serum globulins, alpha (α)- and beta (β)- globulins, etc. Simple proteins insoluble in pure water but soluble in neutral salt. Examples are muscle globulin, serum globulin (blood), edestin (wheat, hemp seed, and other seeds), phaseolin (beans), legumin (beans and peas), vigin (cow peas), tuberin (potato), amandin (almonds), excelsin (Brazil nuts), and arachin and conarachin (peanuts).

glomerulonephritis (kidney disease). The most frequently occurring kidney disease is probably nephritis, or Bright's disease, characterized by inflammation of kidney tissue. Since it is the glomeruli which are first affected, this type of kidney damage is called glomerulonephritis. It usually follows a hemolytic streptococcal infection in another part of the body, or it may be precipitated by a generalized infection, or heavy metal poisoning.

glomerulus (glomerular filtration). A network of capillaries that forms a tuft at the beginning of each tubule within the kidney. It is the glomerulus and the process of glomerular filtration that is responsible for the production of *urine*. The diagram shows that the pressure developed in forcing blood through the small capillaries is greater than the opposing forces (colloidal osmotic pressure and hydrostatic pressure) by 50 mm Hg. Blood is filtered, and only small molecules can pass through the pores of the capillary walls. The pore size is estimated at 20 Å (angstroms), which is large enough to let small proteins such as myoglobin through (Mol. Wt. 17,000) but not serum albumin (Mol. Wt. 66,500). The filtered blood then passes through the tubules, where specific reabsorptions of the filtrate occurs. The glomerulus plus the tubule make up the filtration unit called the *nephron*. There are approximately one million nephrons in each kidney. See *urinary system*.

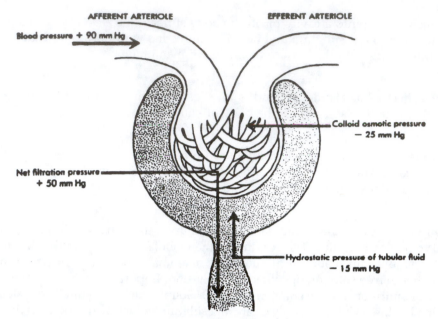

A nephron of the glomerulus

glossitis. Deficiencies of *niacin, riboflavin, cobalamin* (vitamin B_{12}), *folacin*, and *iron* all give rise to glossitis, a feature of *pellagra, sprue*, and various types of nutritional *anemias*. In acute glossitis the tongue is swollen, the papillae are usually prominent, and the color of the tongue is characteristically red. Deep, irregular fissuring is common and shallow ulcers may occur, especially in the sides or tips. The tongue is usually extremely painful, creating a problem in eating. In chronic atrophic glossitis the tongue is small, with an atrophic mucous membrane and small or absent papillae so that its surface appears smooth, moist, and abnormally clean. It is usually not painful.

glucagon. A polypeptide hormone that is functionally the opposite of *insulin*. Glucagon is synthesized in the alpha cells of the *pancreas*. Its main role is to increase the amount of *glucose* in the blood. Glucagon initiates a series of reactions in which the glycogen store of the liver is mobilized to release glucose into the blood. Also, the enzyme systems that manufacture glucose from amino acids are stimulated to synthesize glucose. Glucagon in this respect is very similar to *epinephrine*. Both glucagon and epinephrine stimulate the formation of *cyclic adenosine monophosphate* (cAMP), the so-called second messenger. Cyclic-AMP then stimulates a host of other enzymes. Insulin and glucagon work together in a seesaw mechanism to maintain the blood glucose at a required level. Glucagon increases blood glucose and insulin decreases blood glucose. Glucagon is a single chain of 29 amino acids strung end to end.

glucocorticoid hormone. A class of hormones produced by the cortex of the adrenal glands, which increases the rate of *glucose* formation, raising the concentration of liver *glycogen* and blood glucose. See *cortisol* and *cortisone*.

glucokinase. An enzyme similar to *hexokinase* found especially in the liver. Glucokinase and hexokinase catalyze the phosphorylation of *glucose* to form glucose-6-phosphate.

gluconeogenesis. The *anabolic* formation or synthesis of *glucose* and *glycogen* from the intermediate compounds of metabolism. The formation of glucose from non-carbohydrate sources. The opposite of *glycogenolysis*.

gluconic acid (gluconate). Mol. Wt. 196. Occasionally used as a component of leavening in cake mixes or as an acid in powdered gelatin and soft drink mixes. It occurs naturally in the human body as the phosphate derivative.

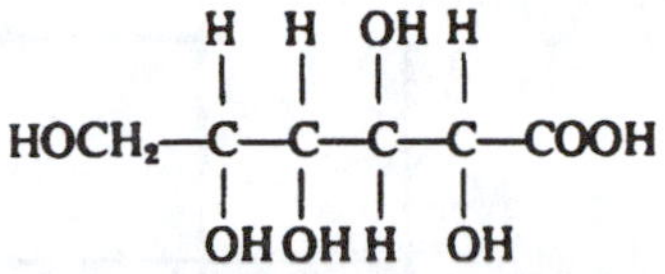

$$
\begin{array}{ccccc}
 & H & H & OH & H \\
 & | & | & | & | \\
HOCH_2 & -C & -C & -C & -C-COOH \\
 & | & | & | & | \\
 & OH & OH & H & OH
\end{array}
$$

D-Gluconic acid

glucose (dextrose). Mol. Wt. 180. A hexose (six-carbon sugar). Glucose is often called dextrose in food preparations. It is one of the important *monosaccharides* in intermediary metabolism. Glucose is the building block for *starches* and *amylopectins* in plants and for *glycogen* in animals. Glucose is a *precursor* to *ascorbic acid* (vitamin C) synthesis in plants and animals, with the exception of humans, other primates, the guinea pig, and a species of fruit bat which cannot make ascorbic acid (vitamin C). Glucose is also a source of *energy*, and under ordinary circumstances about 20% of the total energy needs derives from the oxidation of glucose. However, glucose is the major source of energy for the brain, one of a few substances that can freely cross the *blood-brain barrier* to enter brain and nerve cells. The maintenance of blood sugar (glucose) levels is an important homeostatic process since severe low blood sugar, as in the case of *insulin* overdose, will cause shock. The shock is brought on because brain cells are deprived of energy at very low blood sugar levels and the brain begins to function abnormally. The brain, which is 2% of adult body weight, utilizes 20% of the oxygen we breathe, and the utilization of oxygen by the brain is proportional to its oxidation of glucose. Glucose is also an emergency reserve in the form of liver glycogen. During emergencies, liver glycogen breaks down (*glycogenolysis*) and glucose enters the blood to meet the immediate demand for more energy. A normal blood level of glucose is 80–100 milligrams per 100 milliliters of blood. Since the body can readily synthesize glucose (gluconeogenesis), there is no dietary requirement for glucose. Glucose occurs in fruits and in chemical combinations with *fructose* and *sucrose* (table sugar). As a *carbohydrate*, glucose yields 4.0 calories per gram. The diagram shows how the blood glucose is maintained relatively constant by a balance of the sources and removal of glucose.

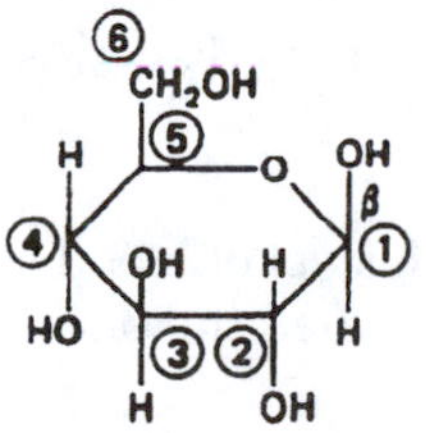

β-D-glucose (dextrose)
The numbers are conventions for carbon identification.

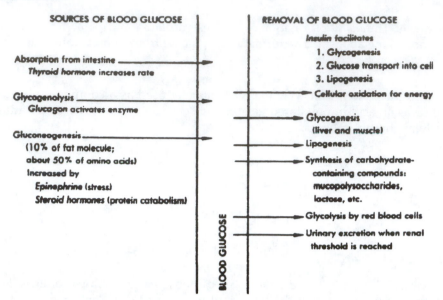

Sources and fates of blood glucose
The blood glucose is maintained within physiologic limits by replacement as rapidly as it is removed to meet metabolic needs. Glycogenesis, lipogenesis, and excretion at the renal threshold are mechanisms that prevent hyperglycemia in the normal individual.

glucose oxidase. A highly specific enzyme produced by the submerged growth of *Aspergillus niger* and other molds. It is used to remove glucose from egg white or whole eggs to facilitate drying, prevent deterioration, and improve the whipping properties (of the reconstituted dried whites). It has been also employed to extend the shelf-life of canned soft drinks by retarding the pickup of iron and the fading of color. Oxidation of the glucose by glucose oxidase forms *gluconic acid* and *hydrogen peroxide* (H_2O_2), the latter then being decomposed by the *catalase* in the same preparation. A combination of glucose oxidase and catalase is used to remove small residues of oxygen in packaged foods. Glucose oxidase is the most specific enzyme known since it can catalyze the rapid oxidation of glucose only. The high specificity of glucose oxidase and its relatively high stability for an enzyme have made it ideal for detection of glucose in urine. The test depends upon the oxidation of a dye by the hydrogen peroxide produced by glucose oxidase action on glucose.

glucose tolerance test. A test to determine how effectively an individual can remove high levels of glucose from the blood. The person being tested drinks a concentrated glucose solution and the blood glucose is subsequently measured over a period of several hours. The test is unpleasant but often necessary in the diagnosis of *diabetes mellitus* (sugar diabetes) or *hypoglycemia*.

glucostatic theory. The theory that the level of blood sugar affects cells in the hypothalamus of the brain to arouse eating behavior when the blood sugar level is low.

glucosuria. Abnormal amount of *sugar* (*glucose*) in the *urine*. It is often an indication of an abnormality in carbohydrate metabolism.

glucuronic acid. See *hyaluronic acid*.

glutamic acid (Glu, E). Mol. Wt. 147. One of the *amino acids* found in proteins. Glutamic acid contains two carboxylic acid groups in the molecule. It is therefore classified as an acidic amino acid. It is one of the few substances that can readily pass through the *blood-brain barrier*. Glutamate is a nonessential amino acid that can be synthesized by *transamination* to alpha (α)-ketoglutarate. *Pyridoxine* (vitamin B₆) participates in *transamination* as the coenzyme pyridoxamine phosphate, a *Krebs' cycle* intermediate. *Monosodium glutamate* (MSG), the *flavor enhancer*, is a sodium salt of glutamic acid.

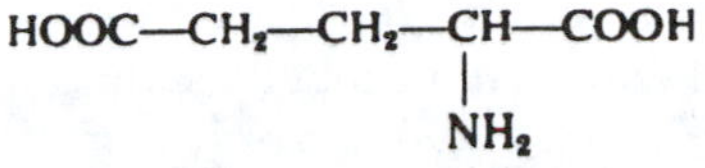

$$HOOC-CH_2-CH_2-CH-COOH$$
$$|$$
$$NH_2$$

Glutamic acid (glutamate, Glu, E)

glutamine (Gln, Glx, Q). Mol. Wt. 146. One of the nonessential amino acids found in proteins. Formed from *glutamic acid* by the addition of *ammonia* to the second carboxylic acid group to form an amide group. It is taken up by the brain in greater quantities than any other amino acid. See *blood-brain barrier*.

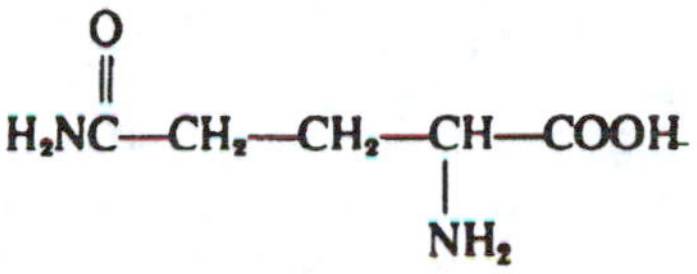

$$\overset{O}{\overset{\|}{H_2NC}}-CH_2-CH_2-CH-COOH$$
$$|$$
$$NH_2$$

Glutamine (Gln, Glx, Q)

glutaric acid. $C_5H_8O_4$. A crystalline acid used especially in organic synthesis.

glutathione. A tripeptide *coenzyme* of glutathione reductase involved in metabolism. It occurs in plant and animal tissues. It is composed of *glutamic acid, cysteine*, and *glycine*. Glutathione is an important factor in the oxidation and reduction reactions of the cell by the virtue of the sulfhydryl (−SH) group. One of its important function is to maintain the *iron of hemoglobin* in its reduce (ferrous) state.

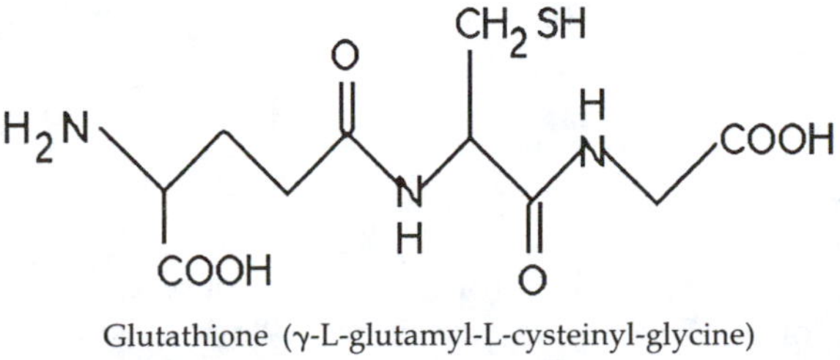

Glutathione (γ-L-glutamyl-L-cysteinyl-glycine)

glutelins. Simple plant proteins insoluble in all neutral solvents, but readily soluble in very dilute acids and alkalies. The best-known and most important members of this group are the *glutenin* from *wheat*, hordenin from barley, and oryzenin from *rice*.

gluten. A mixture of two proteins, *gliadin* and *glutenin*, found in many cereals and grains. A tough elastic substance that gives adhesiveness to dough. It is formed when the proteins in flour, especially those in *wheat* flour, absorb water. Gluten helps give shape to cooked products because it coagulates when heated. Gluten flour is higher in protein. "Hard" wheat is higher in gluten than "soft" wheat.

glutenin. A protein of the classification *glutelin* found in *wheat*. It is the combination of glutenin and *gliadin* when mixed with water that gives the characteristic stickiness and doughy consistency. Heat bonds these proteins. Rye has only a small amount of glutenin but enough to make a bread loaf. Oats, barley, rice, and millet contain too little glutenin to permit them to be used to make bread doughs.

gluten-sensitive enteropathy. A disorder characterized by the inability to digest *gluten*, a protein found in wheat, barley, oats, and rye. The presence of gluten is accompanied by damage to the mucosal villi of the digestive system, which in turn interferes with the absorption of other essential nutrients. It is commonly found in celiac disease.

glycemia. Sugar (usually glucose) in the blood.

glycemic index. A blood sugar response value of a food in relation to that of *glucose*. It is an expression of the area under the blood *glucose* response curve for each food stated as the percentage of the area after taking the same amount of *carbohydrate* as glucose.

glyceraldehyde. An aldehyde of special importance because the D-and L- configurations about asymmetric carbons of *amino acids* and *carbohydrates* are based on the mirror images of D- and L-glyceraldehydes. Separate solutions of D- and L-glyceraldehyde rotate light polarized light in equal but opposite directions.

D-Glyceraldehyde   L-Glyceraldehyde

glycerin. See *glycerol*.

glycerol (glycerin). Mol. Wt. 90.1. Glycerol is a polyalcohol containing three carbons and three *hydroxyl* ($-OH$) groups. Glycerol is a colorless, odorless, syrupy sweet liquid, a major component of neutral fat molecules and obtained by the hydrolysis of fats. Chemically, glycerol has the properties of an alcohol. When esterified with fatty acids, glycerol forms glycerides. Glycerol is added to foods to maintain moisture and to prevent them from drying out and becoming hard. Glycerol is used in marshmallows, candy fudge, and baked goods in amounts ranging from 0.5–10%. Glycerol is also used as a solvent for oily chemicals, especially flavorings that are not very soluble in water.

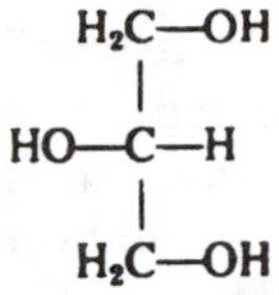

$$H_2C\text{---}OH$$
$$|$$
$$HO\text{---}C\text{---}H$$
$$|$$
$$H_2C\text{---}OH$$

D-Glycerol

glycine (Gly, G). Mol. Wt. 75. A nonessential amino acid. It is the only amino acid that does not possess an asymmetric alpha (α) carbon. Glycine can be synthesized from serine, another nonessential amino acid, with the B vitamin *folacin* acting as a coenzyme. Glycine gets its name from the Greek word meaning "sweet" and is in fact a sweet-tasting substance. During rapid growth, the demand for glycine may be enormous. It is an important precursor in many syntheses in the human body, such as those of the *purine* bases, *porphyrins*, *creatine*, and the conjugated *bile acids*. It is utilized by the liver in the elimination of toxic phenols and conjugated with the bile acid to form *bile salts*.

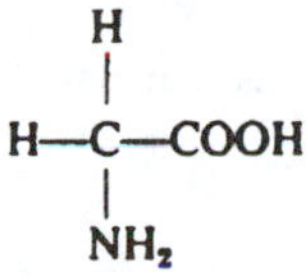

$$H$$
$$|$$
$$H\text{---}C\text{---}COOH$$
$$|$$
$$NH_2$$

Glycine (Gly, G)

glycogen (animal starch). Mol. Wt. up to 1,000,000. The name means "sugar former," given to this compound because whenever the body needs extra *glucose*, the liver glycogen can be converted back into glucose again and released into the bloodstream. Glycogen is a complex polymer of glucose. It functions as a storage form of glucose in all cells, but liver glycogen has a special role. Plants have *starch* and *amylopectin*. Although the total quantity of glycogen in the animal body is low, its role is primarily that of storing carbohydrate, similar to the role of *starch* in plant cells. It occurs in all cells and predominantly in the liver, where it is important to the mechanism that regulates the glucose level of the blood. Glycogen is a branched chain containing two types of linkages, the α 1→4 and the α 1→6. The branches occur about every 6–8 glucose units. Glucose is released from glycogen by the action of an enzyme called a phosphorylase, which yields a phosphorylated derivative, glucose-1-phosphate. Glucose-1-phosphate can then be catabolized by a series of enzymes to yield *carbon dioxide* (CO_2), water, and *energy*. These events occur in all cells and the activation of the phosphorylase to break down glycogen can be initiated with the hormones *epinephrine* or *glucagon*. Liver differs from other cells in that one of the phosphorylated derivatives of glucose, glucose-6-phosphate, can be converted to free glucose and thus leave the liver cell and enter the blood. The liver acts as a reservoir for glucose for the entire body. Tissues continually withdraw glucose from the blood for their own uses, and the glycogen in the liver must be converted to glucose to maintain blood glucose at the normal level. The amount of glycogen in the liver and muscle depends somewhat on the supply of carbohydrate in the diet. Glycogen molecules are similar in many respects to those of the branched form of plant starch (amylopectin), but glycogen has a shorter chain of glucose units and therefore a more complicated branched structure. Glycogen is well adapted to being broken into smaller units or being rebuilt as needed from smaller units in the body tissues. Only limited amounts of glycogen can be stored in the liver and other tissues, and this is used up rapidly during fasting or muscular work. Liver usually contains 1.5–5 percent glycogen by weight, while shellfish (including oysters) have 0.5–5%.

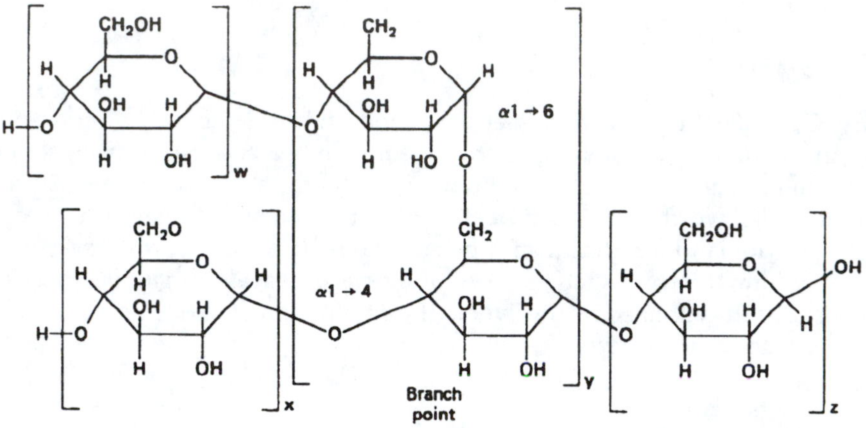

Glycogen (animal starch)

glycogenic. Related to *glycogen*.

glycogenolysis. The specific term for conversion of *glycogen* into *glucose* in the liver. Glycogenolysis is the complex series of enzymatic hydrolyses or breakdowns by which this conversion is accomplished. The hormones *epinephrine* and *glucagon* stimulate glycogenolysis. Glycogenolysis is the opposite of *gluconeogenesis*.

glycolipids. (1) Compounds of *fatty acids* which are combined with carbohydrates and nitrogen. Because they are found chiefly in brain tissue, these substances are also called cerebrosides. (2) Compounds that have the solubility properties of a *lipid* and contain one or more molecules of a sugar. Many animal glycolipids are derivatives of a class of compounds known as *ceramides*.

glycolysis. The enzymatic conversion of sugar to *pyruvic acid* and *lactic acid* (lactate), also called Embdem-Meyerhof-Parnas pathway. Glycolysis is an important part of metabolism (anaerobic metabolism). The general scheme of glycolysis is presented. The enzymatic reactions involved in human glycolysis are much the same as those in fermentations to form alcohol in beers and wines by yeast.

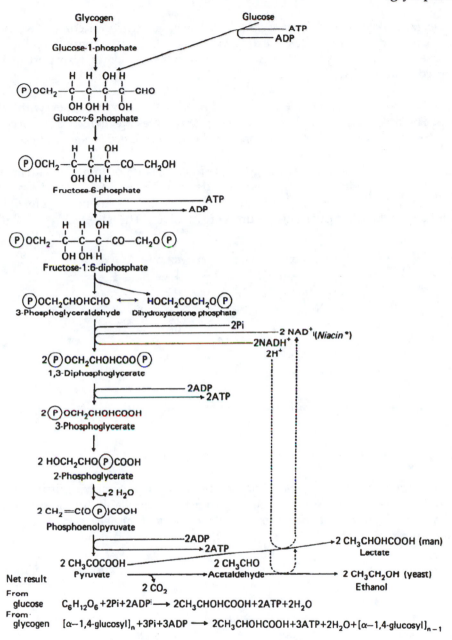

Glycolysis (Embden-Meyerhof pathway)

glycolytic. Pertaining to the breakdown of sugars.

glycoproteins. Biopolymers having proteins and sugar residues linked covalently to each other. They differ from *mucoproteins* in that they contain considerably less carbohydrate. The carbohydrate chains of glycoproteins are short, consisting of perhaps 8–10 *monosaccharide* units. The class of glycoproteins includes a large number of biologically active substances such as *enzymes, hormones,* and *immunoglobulins* as well as structural components of blood vessels and skin. Of particular interest are the glycoproteins associated with the cell-membrane surface. These cell-surface glycoproteins are likely involved in active transport of ions and intercellular communication.

glycoside. A *monosaccharide* derivative chemically linked at the carbonyl group with an alcohol (OH) group. The linkage is called a *glycosidic linkage*. Examples are *digitalis* derivatives, which are drugs essential to cardiac therapy; *steroids*; and the *hormones* of the *adrenal glands*.

glycosidic linkage. The link between the carbonyl group of a monosaccharide and an alcoholic group of another compound. Two monosaccharides can be joined in a glycosidic linkage. *Maltose* is an example in which case the glycosidic linkage is sometimes referred to as a glucosidic linkage, which indicates glucose units are involved. The α1→4 shown is a glycosidic (glucosidic) linkage.

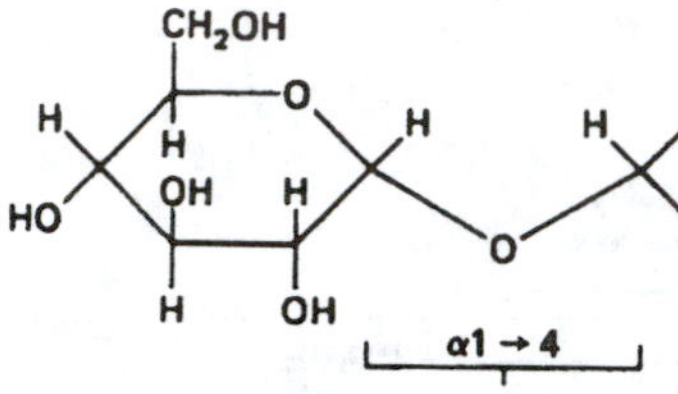

Glycosidic linkage

glycosphingolipids. A group of carbohydrates containing fatty acid derivatives of *ceramide*. See *sphingolipids*.

glycosuria. A general term for an abnormal amount of sugar in the *urine*.

goiter. The enlargement of the *thyroid gland*. Simple goiter is a complex nutritional disease, brought about in part by an insufficient supply of *iodine*. The gland enlarges in an attempt to compensate by additional glandular tissue for the shortage of necessary material (iodine) for making its internal secretion (*thyroxine*). See *thiocyanic acid* and *thiourea*.

goitrogens. A lack of *iodine* in the diet can lead to *goiter*. It is also known that eating *cabbage, cauliflower, turnips, mustard, collard greens,* and *brussels sprouts* may induce goiter formation in susceptible individuals. These plants and others of the *Cruciferae* family, including *kale, broccoli, rutabaga, kohlrabi, radish,* and *horseradish,* contain thioglucosides that under certain conditions can block the absorption of iodine. See *thiocyanic acid* and *thiourea*.

Golgi complex or apparatus. An internal structure of *cells*. Most noticeable in secreting cells, it appears as a parallel arrangement of membranes and small vacuoles, somewhat like flattened bags, lying near the centrioles. It functions in regard to concentrating the cell secretion and in the formation of cell membranes. It is also considered the site for the packaging and organization of vesicles and cell secretions.

gonad. A reproductive gland. The testicle in the male and the ovary in the female. See *sex glands*.

gonadotrophic hormone (GTH). A hormone that stimulates the *gonads* to produce hormones and reproductive cells, and regulates the female estrus cycle, such as the *follicle stimulating hormone* (FSH), luteinizing hormone (LH), and *luteotropic hormone* (prolactin) of the *pituitary gland.*

gonadotropins. Hormones from embryonic sex glands.

gooseberry (*Ribes*). A round juicy berry, a first cousin of the fresh currant. It grows on a bush. The flavor is tart yet sweet when the berries are fully ripened. Gooseberries can grow as large as 1 inch in diameter and 1½ inches in length. There are a number of varieties; red, green, white, or yellow, and smooth or hairy.

Nutrients in 100 g of gooseberries

CALORIES KCAL	PROTEIN G	FAT G	CARBOHYDRATE G	VITAMIN A IU	ASCORBATE MG	CALCIUM MG
40	1	Trace	10	300	33	18

gout. A metabolic disease, the result of a defect in the metabolism of purines, which are products of the digestion of nucleic acids. The faulty mechanism results in an elevation above normal of *uric acid* in the blood (hyperuricemia). Eventually there are deposits of the sodium salt of uric acid crystals in the joints, kidneys, cartilage of the ear, and sometimes the heart or other internal organs. Subcutaneous deposits of urate crystals are called tophi, and they appear in about one-third of those who have gout. Meats have a high *nucleic acid* content and thus a high *purine* content. A part of the treatment is a special diet. Of individuals with gout, 95% are males.

grade. The grade of a food is an indication of its general size, palatability, appearance, and maturity. The grade is not related to the nutrient value. In the United States, grading is voluntary. It is not required by law and processors and packers pay a fee for the grading service. The grading of food should not be confused with the inspection of food for its fitness to be consumed. The inspection of food passing over state lines is mandatory. Both grading and inspection are done by the United States Department of Agriculture.

grain alcohol. See *ethanol.*

grains. Edible seeds of the grass family. See *cereals.*

Nutrients in 100 g of grains

GRAIN	CALORIES KCAL	CARBOHYDRATE	PROTEIN G	FAT G	THIAMINE MG	NIACIN MG	IRON MG	CALCIUM MG
Corn	365	72	9	3	0.3	2	3	2
Millet	330	73	10	3	0.7	2	7	20
Oats	390	11	3	1	0.1	0.1	1	53
Rice	380	86	6	0.3	0.1	6	3	9
Rye	332	68	16	3	0.2	3	4	50
Wheat	334	26	13	2	0.5	4	4	40

grapefruit (*Citrus paradisi*). A member of the *citrus* family, large and round with a rind colored from pale yellow to bronze, a juicy pulp which may be yellowish-white or pink, and a slightly bitter flavor. Grapefruits can weigh from 2–12 pounds and have a diameter of 4–6 inches. Grapefruit is a good source of *ascorbic acid* (vitamin C) and is also low in calories. Fresh grapefruits or juice should be used as soon as possible as long storage or exposure to air decreases vitamin C content. See this item in the table under *fruits*.

grapes (*Vitis*). Grapes contain acid potassium *tartrate*. Acidity decreases with the age of the grape and sugar increases. The sugar is nearly all *glucose* and is more abundant than in any other fruit. *Raisins* (sweet dried grapes) contain more sugar and less water. See this item in the table under *fruits*.

GRAS. See *Generally Regarded as Safe*.

greengage (*Prunus*). A fine-quality dessert *plum*, round in shape and greenish yellow in color. The flesh is juicy and sweet, yet it has a tang. The stone is small and round and the flesh clings to it. Greengages should be tree-ripened as they do not ripen well after picking.

grits, groats. Both words refer to hulled and coarsely ground cereal grains and both mean "fragment" or "part." Grits are smaller than groats, more finely ground, usually from corn, but also from buckwheat, rye, oats, or rice. Grits ground from corn are known as *hominy* grits. Groats are most often ground from buckwheat, oats, barley, and wheat, as well as corn. Cracked wheat is another name for wheat groats or grits. Buckwheat groats are the most commonly used. They are also called *kasha*, a Russian word, and are a staple of Russia's diet.

Nutrients in 100 g of corn grits

CALORIES	PROTEIN G	FAT G	CARBOHYDRATE G	NIACIN MG
58	1	trace	13	1

grouper (*Epinephelus* **and** *Mycteroperea*). Saltwater fish which live in warm waters, at the bottom of the sea, and in rocky nooks and crevices. They resemble sea bass and are an important food fish. Groupers can grow to a great size, about 400–500 pounds. They can be cooked like sea bass or red snapper.

Nutrients in 100 g of raw grouper

CALORIES KCAL	PROTEIN G	FAT G	CARBOHYDRATE G
90	19	0.5	0

growth hormone (GH, somatotropin). (1) The only hormone of the anterior *pituitary gland* that does not exert its effect on other endocrine glands. Growth hormone or somatotropin is a protein. Unlike other hormones that influence growth, GH merely affects the rate of the process. It does not control the actual process of maturation or the development of tissues. GH also influences the level of *glucose* and *fat* in the blood. (2) GH stimulates growth, increases protein synthesis, decreases carbohydrate utilization, and increases fat *catabolism*. GH facilitates the transport of many amino acids through the cell membrane. Once in the cell, they are available for protein synthesis. As a result of the suppression of carbohydrate utilization under the influence of GH, blood glucose increases. This stimulates the secretion of *insulin*. The level of GH in plasma is normally about 2 µg/liter during the day, rising to peaks of 10–15 µg/liter during sleep. Secretion is controlled by two factors from the *hypothalamus*: (1) the growth hormone releasing factor (GRF) and (2) the growth hormone release inhibiting factor (GRIF). During protein deficiency, GH secretion increases, as it does when blood sugar level falls. Exercise increases GH secretion.

guanine. $C_5H_5N_5O$. A heterocyclic organic compound which occurs as a natural constituent of animal and vegetable *nucleic acids*. It is a *purine* that is common to both *ribonucleic acid* (RNA) and *deoxyribonucleic acid* (DNA). It is abundant in liver, muscle, and glandular tissue such as pancreas and seeds. The body is capable of synthesizing guanine. *Uric acid* is its metabolic end-point. See *guanosine triphosphate*.

guanosine triphosphate (GTP). Mol. Wt. 523. A high-energy phosphate compound equivalent in energy to *adenosine triphosphate* (ATP). The guanosine nucleotides, GTP, GDP, and GMP, are important for several specific reasons. The chemical energy of GTP is required for protein synthesis, and GDP is required in the oxidation of alpha (α)- *ketoglutaric acid* in the *Krebs'* (tricarboxylic acid) *cycle*. The GMP moiety is in all nucleic acids.

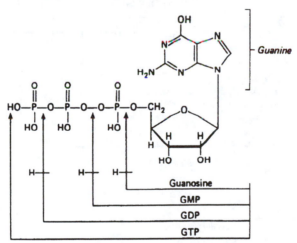

Guanosine triphosphate (GTP)

guar gum. A vegetable *gum* stabilizer which will dissolve in cold water. A guar gum solution will turn into a rubbery gel if borate is added as a cross-linking agent. It serves as a *thickening agent* in beverages, ice cream, frozen puddings, and salad dressing. Used to increase the resiliency of doughs and batters and in the production of artificial whipped cream.

gum arabic. A soluble *gum* obtained from several species of acacia tree. Used by food processors to prevent sugar crystals from forming in candy, to help citrus oils dissolve in drinks, to encapsulate flavor oils in powdered drink mixes, to stabilize foam in beer, and to improve the texture of commercial ice cream. Gum arabic is very soluble in water; solutions become very viscous only when they contain 10–20% gum.

gum ghatti. A vegetable *gum* used by food manufacturers to keep oil and water ingredients from separating out into two layers in such products as salad dressing and butter-in-syrup.

gums. Gums or *hydrophilic colloids* are polymeric materials which can be dissolved or dispersed in water to give a thickening or gelling effect. Gums are also a component in *fiber*. The table lists the commonly used gums, classified according to origin. In general, they are complex neutral or anionic *polysaccharides*, composed of *glucose, galactose,* or other sugar units commonly joined by 1→4 and 1→6 *glycosidic inkages*.

Classification of gums

NATURAL GUMS

TREE EXTRACTS	SEEDS/ROOTS	SEEDWEED EXTRACTS	OTHER
Arabic	Guar	Agar	
Ghatti	Locust bean	Algin	Gelatins
Karaya	Psyllium seed	Carrageenan	Pectins
Larch	Quince seed	Furcellan	Starches
Tragacanth			

MODIFIED GUMS

CELLULOSE DERIVATIVES	STARCH DERIVATIVES	MICROBIAL FERMENTATION	OTHER
Carbomethyl-			Carboxymethyl guar gum
Ethylhydroxymethyl-	Carboxymethyl-		Carboxymethyl locust
Hydroxypropyl-	Hydroxylethyl-	Dextran	bean
Hydroxypropylmethyl-	Hydroxypropyl-	Xanthan	Methoxyl pectin
Methyl-			Propylene glycol alginate
Microcrystalline			Triethanolamine alginate

SYNTHETIC GUMS

VINYL POLYMERS	ACRYLIC POLYMERS	OTHER
Carboxyvinyl-	Polyacrylamide	Ethylene Oxide polymers
Polyvinyl alcohol	Polyacrylic acid	
Polyvinylpyrrolidone		

H

H. The alphabetic symbol for the amino acid *histidine* (His).

haddock (*Melanogrammus aeglefinus*). A saltwater fish, an important food fish. It is closely related to the cod, but the two fish can easily be told apart. The haddock is much smaller than the cod. The flesh is firm and white, with a pleasant flavor which is on the bland side. Smoked haddock is called finnan haddie. Haddock is a very good source of protein and contains *phosphorus, potassium, niacin,* and *thiamine*. See this item in the table under *fish*.

haeme. See *heme*.

hair follicle. An invagination of the *epidermis* from which a hair develops.

hake (*Merluccius* and *Urophycis*). A saltwater food fish related to the *cod*. Hakes are slender, dark-gray fish with fins on their backs. Their average market weight is 1–4 pounds. The meat is soft and white with a delicate flavor.

Nutrients in 100 g of raw hake

CALORIES KCAL	PROTEIN G	FAT G	CARBOHYDRATE G
74	17	0.4	0

halibut (*Hippoglossus*). Cold-water fish which lives in all the seas of the world and is one of the most important food fishes. There are several varieties. The fish is flat and resembles a gigantic flounder. The flesh is white and excellent in flavor and texture. Chicken halibuts, weighing up to 10 pounds, are considered the finest. A very good source of *protein*, low in fat. Halibut liver oil is a rich source of *retinol* (vitamin A). See this item in the table under *fish*.

ham. The rear leg of a hog, from the aitchbone (hipbone) through the meaty part of the shank bone. Fresh ham is a very good to excellent source of high quality *protein* and *thiamine*, a fair to good source of *iron* and *niacin*, and a fair source of *riboflavin*.

hamburger. Ground beef prepared from the less tender cuts. Good source of protein and a variable source of *fat*, depending on the type of meat ground. See *meat*.

Nutrients in 100 g of medium fat, cooked hamburger

CALORIES	PROTEIN G	FAT G	CARBOHYDRATE G	NIACIN MG	IRON MG	CALCIUM MG
266	26	18	trace	6	4	7

haploid. Having a single set of *chromosomes*. In humans, each sperm or egg is a haploid cell, containing only one set, or 23 single chromosomes, in contrast to a developed cell with two sets. See *diploid*.

haversian canals. Vascular canals in bone or bony tissue.

hazelnut (filbert) See *filbert*.

HDL. See *high density lipoprotein*.

head cheese. A well-seasoned cold cut made of the edible parts of a calf's or a pig's head such as the cheeks, snouts, and underlips to which sometimes brains, hearts, tongues, and feet are added. The meat is boiled, stripped from the bones, skinned, cut into pieces, and seasoned with onions, herbs, and spices. Then it is put into a mold and pressed into a firm, jellied mass.

heart. The heart is a cone-shaped organ about the size of a fist. It lies in the chest, between the lungs, in a cavity called the mediastinum. The heart is essentially two pumps in a single organ. It is made up of four chambers, two atria or auricles and two ventricles. The right atrium and the right ventricle are separated completely from the left atrium and the left ventricle. Blood entering and leaving the heart is controlled by four *heart valves*, two semilunar valves, the tricuspid valve and the mitral valve. Blood with low oxygen content flows from the body tissues into the right atrium by way of large veins, the inferior and superior vena cava. The blood with the low oxygen content goes from the right atrium to the right ventricle through the atrioventricular opening. The pulmonary artery carries the blood from the right ventricle to the lungs by way of the pulmonary artery. The blood then gets oxygenated in the lungs. The oxygenated blood is returned to the heart by way of the pulmonary vein to the left atrium and then to the left ventricle. The oxygenated blood is then pumped from the left ventricle through the aorta to all parts of the body. The total volume of blood in the average man is between five and six liters. The average cardiac output is about 5.5 L/min. See *blood flow* for a table of the blood flow through various organs. The heart is a special muscle, and like other muscles it uses *phosphocreatine* as an energy reserve to form the *adenosine triphosphate* (ATP) needed for muscle contraction. The enzyme *creatine phosphokinase* (CK) is the enzyme that catalyzes the reaction forming ATP. During a myocardial infarction, heart cell tissues die and CK is released into the blood. The detection of high levels of CK activity in the blood is evidence of a heart attack. The nutrient value of heart is given in the table under *meats*. See *heart valves*.

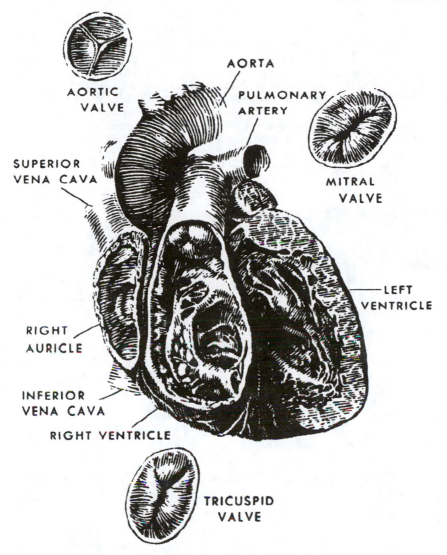

AORTIC VALVE

AORTA

PULMONARY ARTERY

SUPERIOR VENA CAVA

MITRAL VALVE

RIGHT AURICLE

LEFT VENTRICLE

INFERIOR VENA CAVA

RIGHT VENTRICLE

TRICUSPID VALVE

Section of heart showing chambers and valves

heartburn. A burning sensation under the breastbone or in the pit of the stomach is a common complaint, usually relieved by any one of the many *antacid* preparations. The most common cause is an irritable digestive tract or so-called "acid indigestion." When the junction between the *esophagus* and *stomach* is relaxed, the acid *gastric juice* flows back into the esophagus and causes irritation of its surface (esophagitis). A common cause of chronic heartburn is a rupture or weakness of the diaphragm which separates the chest from the abdomen; this weakness is called a diaphragmatic or hiatus hernia, allowing part of the upper portion of the stomach to move up into the chest. Simple measures to relieve the heartburn of diaphragmatic hernia are the use of antacids, avoiding or correcting obesity, eating smaller meals, avoiding highly seasoned foods, and sleeping with the head of the bed raised. See *gastritis*.

heart valves. The functions of the four heart valves are given in the table that follows.

VALVE	FUNCTION
Tricuspid (Between the heart chambers)	Three cusps that prevent the backflow of blood from the right ventricle into the right atrium.
Pulmonary semilunar (Base of pulmonary trunk)	Three half-moon shaped flaps that prevent the backflow of blood from the pulmonary trunk into the right ventricle.
Bicuspid (mitral) (Between the heart chambers)	The two cusps that prevent the backflow of blood from the left ventricle to the left atrium during ventricular contraction.
Aortic semilunar (Base of the aorta)	Three half-moon shaped flaps that prevent the backflow of blood from the aorta into the left ventricle during ventricular contraction.

heat labile. Changeable by heat; unstable to heat.

heat of combustion. The heat of combustion of a substance is the amount of *energy* in the substance measured in terms of the amount of heat released by its *oxidation*. By burning each of the foodstuffs in a *bomb calorimeter*, it has been found that carbohydrate has an average fuel value of 4.1; fat, 9.45; and protein, 5.65 calories per g. Differences in energy content exist in the chemical composition of the three materials. In *carbohydrates* there is enough oxygen in the molecule to combine with all the hydrogen, and only the carbon present in small proportion remains to be burned; a correspondingly small amount of heat will be produced. With *fats* which have little oxygen in the molecule, the carbon and nearly all the hydrogen are oxidized and much heat is involved. Nitrogen when burned (oxidized) has no fuel value. The heat of combustion of an average meal, that is, a mixture of foodstuffs, is usually estimated at 4.8 calories per liter of oxygen. See *energy balance*.

heat production. See *basal metabolism*.

helix. A coil or spiral; the shape assumed by some large molecules, including *proteins* and *nucleic acids*. The *alpha* (α)-*helix* is a particular conformation of protein. *Deoxyribonucleic acids* (DNA) form double helixes.

hematinic. An agent that increases the *hemoglobin* level and the number of *red blood cells*.

hematocrit. A measure of the volume of *red blood cells* in relation to the volume of *plasma*. When there has been a loss of body fluids but no cell loss, as in dehydration, the cell volume is high in proportion to the amount of liquid (plasma) in the bloodstream, that is, the hematocrit is above normal. When either hemorrhage or *anemia* has depleted the supply of cells, the blood is "thinned," and the hematocrit or cell volume is low. The normal range for the hematocrit is 38 to 54 mL per 100 mL for men and 36 to 47 mL per 100 mL for women. Hematocrit determinations are used as a screening procedure for the diagnosis of anemia, and also as a guide to treatment.

hematoma. A localized mass of blood that has escaped from injured blood vessels and has entered an organ or spaces between the cells of a tissue. The blood is often clotted or partly clotted and discolored. The discoloration is due to the breakdown products of the *heme* in *hemoglobin*.

hematopoiesis. The production and development of blood cells, normally in the bone marrow. Tissues which produce blood cells are said to be hematopoietic.

hematopoietic. Affecting the formation of blood cells. The vitamins *cobalamin* and *folacin* greatly affect the formation of blood cells.

heme (protoheme). Mol. Wt. 616. A complex heterocylcic ring structure called protoporphyrin-α containing the metal *iron* in the *ferrous* (Fe^{+2}) state. Heme is a component of *hemoglobin* and is responsible for absorption of oxygen from the blood. The heme structure is also a component of cytochrome C, and modifications of heme are present in other members of the *terminal respiratory chain*, a complex of enzymes in the *mitochondria* responsible for cell utilization of oxygen. Among the breakdown products of heme are *biliverdin*, a green bile pigment; *bilirubin*, a red bile pigment; and *urobilin*, an orange pigment. *Jaundice* is characterized as a hyperbilirubinemia.

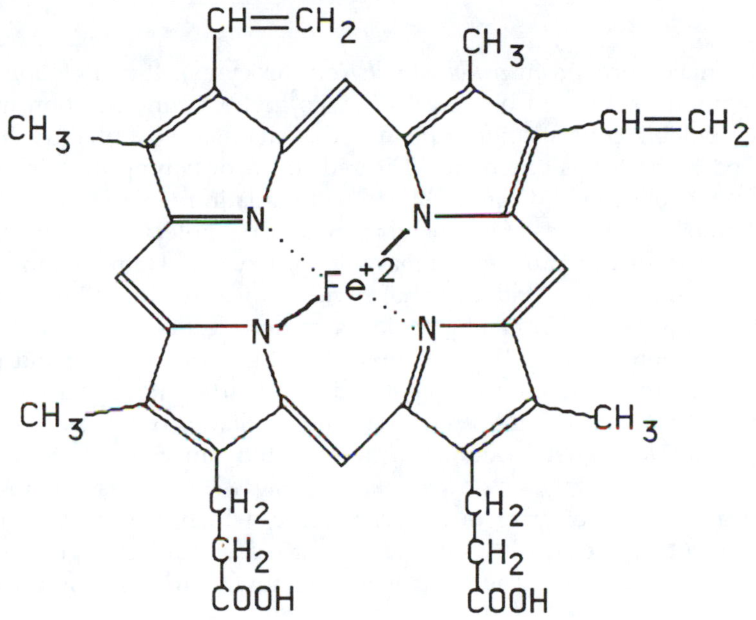

Heme

heme iron. *Iron* which is bound to *protoporphyrin* in *hemoglobin* and *myoglobin*. Unlike iron salts, the absorption by the intestinal mucosa of heme iron is not affected by phosphate or *phytic acid*, nor by *ascorbic acid* (vitamin C). The heme complex is absorbed intact into the intestinal epithelial cell and only then is the iron split off. Its absorption is more efficient than that of ionic iron, that is, iron occurring as a salt.

hemicelluloses. A heterogeneous group of *polysaccharides* closely associated with *cellulose* in plant tissues, but they can be separated by extraction with aqueous alkali. The largest chemical group are the pentosans (*pentose* polymers), xylans, and arabinoxylans; a second group consists of hexose polymers such as the *galactans*, and a third group are the acidic hemicelluloses which contain galacturonic or glucuronic acid. The hemicelluloses may also be divided into groups depending on their biochemical characteristics such as: (1) acid hemicelluloses, high in uronic acid residues; (2) polyuronide hemicelluloses, which have a high uronic acid content; (3) A hemicelluloses, which precipitate in dilute acid; (4) B hemicelluloses, which are precipitated by dilute acid treatment and subsequent addition of alcohol; (5) neutral hemicelluloses, which are not high in uronic acid residues. Together with *pectins*, the hemicelluloses form the matrix of the plant cell wall in which are enmeshed the cellulose fibers. Cell walls of annular plants contain between 15–30% of hemicellulose on a dry basis, while wood contains 20–25%. Hemicelluloses are known to take up water readily and clearly increase fecal weight. The hemicelluloses are not digested in the small intestine but are broken down by microorganisms in the colon more readily than cellulose. See *fiber*.

hemochromatosis. A disturbance of *iron* metabolism in which excessive iron storage causes a bronze discoloration of skin and viscera, liver and *pancreas* damage, and *diabetes* (bronzed diabetes). The condition is believed to be genetically transmitted by a defect occurring chiefly in males.

hemoglobin. The major protein in *red blood cells* (erythrocytes). It is a *globulin* and contains *heme*. The iron content of the red blood cells has its highest concentration in the heme or hemoglobin. Hemoglobin consists of four polypeptide chains, two alpha (α) chains, plus two beta (β) chains; each chain has one heme. The red, iron-containing protein pigment of the erythrocytes transfers oxygen and carbon dioxide and aids in regulation of pH. One red cell contains several million molecules of hemoglobin. Since one molecule of hemoglobin contains four molecules of iron, it can carry four molecules of oxygen. Hemoglobin combines with oxygen to form oxyhemoglobin. Under normal circumstances the adult body produces about 6.25 g of hemoglobin per day. Normal hemoglobin values are 14–18 g/dL (14 to 18 grams per 100 mL of blood) for men; 12–16 g/dL for women; 12–14 g% for children; and 14.5–24.5 g/dL for newborns. The entire function of hemoglobin depends upon its capacity to combine with oxygen in the lungs and then release it readily in the capillaries of the tissues. In the tissues it picks up *carbon dioxide*. Genetic variants of hemoglobin can give rise to several diseases (hemoglobinopathies), including *sickle cell anemia* and *thalassemia*. These hemoglobinopathies are the result of a mutation or error in the *genetic code*, which causes the substitution of a single amino acid out of the 574 in hemoglobin with profound changes in the ability of hemoglobin to function normally. There are over 500 known variants of normal hemoglobin.

hemolysis. The disintegration of *red blood cells* which results in the appearance of hemoglobin in the surrounding fluid.

hemolytic. Causing the destruction or lysis of the *red blood cells*.

hemolytic anemia. A type of *anemia* in which red blood cells are destroyed at rates faster than normal. Hemolytic anemia may be *congenital* or acquired, acute or chronic. In addition to symptoms common to other anemias such as fatigue and shortness of breath, hemolytic anemia usually produces some degree of *jaundice* because the destroyed red cells release their hemoglobin, which is converted into bile pigments at a rate faster than they can be removed. The increased bile pigments give the skin a yellow color, a condition known as jaundice. Some hemolytic anemias may last for years. If neglected they may lead to development of *gallstones*, and in some cases leg ulcers.

hemophilia. A hereditary blood disease characterized by greatly prolonged coagulation time. The blood fails to clot and abnormal bleeding occurs.

hemopoietic. Concerned with the formation of blood.

hemorrhage. Bleeding, particularly excessive bleeding, from blood vessels due to a break in their walls. It may be caused by a wound or disease. Hemorrhage can occur externally or internally. Bleeding in some internal areas is evidenced, however, when blood accumulates in tissues (forming a *hematoma*), or is vomited, coughed up, or excreted in urine or feces.

hemorrhoids (piles). Stretched or dilated veins, varicose veins under the mucous membrane lining of the anal and rectal area. When they occur in the wall of the rectum above the sphincter muscle, they are classified as internal; those below, in the anal canal, are called external.

hemosiderin. An insoluble iron oxide-protein compound, in which iron is stored in the liver if the amount of iron in the blood exceeds the storage capacity of *ferritin*. Such accumulation of excess iron occurs in diseases that are accompanied by rapid destruction of red blood cells (malaria, hemolytic anemia). See *hemosiderosis*.

hemosiderosis. A condition in which large amounts of the iron storage compound hemosiderin are deposited, especially in the liver and spleen. Hemosiderosis may occur as the result of excessive breakdown of red blood cells in diseases such as malaria and hemolytic anemia, or after multiple blood transfusions. See *chelate*.

heparin. The naturally occurring *anticoagulant* in blood and other tissues containing glucosamine, glucuronic acid, and varying proportions of sulfate and acetyl groups. Its structure is not entirely clear. It is produced by the *mast cells* of the connective tissue and is stored as granules within the cells. The heparin content of tissues correlates with the number of mast cells present. Heparin is secreted into the intercellular substance and functions there to prevent the *fibrinogen* that escapes from capillaries from forming *fibrin* clots. It also functions in the formation or activation of lipoprotein *lipase*, which clears *chylomicrons* from the blood plasma.

hepatic. Pertaining to the *liver*.

hepatic coma. A syndrome of progressive confusion, apathy, personality changes, muscle contractions, spasticity, and loss of consciousness, leading to eventual death. In hepatic coma, toxic nitrogenous materials from the bowel, primarily ammonia, enter the systemic circulation and reach the central nervous system without prior detoxification by a normally functioning liver. Blood ammonium-ion (NH_4^+) levels are characteristically increased in hepatic coma. A major feature of hepatic coma is ammonia intoxication of the central nervous system caused by failure of the liver to convert ammonia to nontoxic *urea*.

hepatitis. Inflammation of the liver caused primarily by food- or blood-borne infection, altering liver function and interfering with digestion. Hepatitis may lead to malnutrition.

hepatomegaly. Enlargement of the liver.

herbs. Any plants used as medicines, seasoning, or flavoring. *Mint, thyme, basil,* and *sage* are examples of herbs.

hermetic. Pertaining to food containers that do not permit gas or microorganisms to enter or escape. A properly sealed tin can is a hermetic container.

herring (*Clupea harengus*). A small saltwater fish. The *shad, alewife,* and *sardine* are related to herring. Also related to this family is a freshwater variety, lake herring, sometimes called "cisco." Herring is an important food fish. Herring have small heads; they are streamlined and covered with silvery, iridescent scales. Mature herrings measure 10 inches in length. Herring is a good source of *protein* and *fat*. Fresh herring is high in phosophorus. The caloric value of 100 g of fresh saltwater herring can vary from 98–176 calories, depending on the variety. The value of 100 g of smoked herring varies from 196–300 calories, depending upon variety and method of smoking. See this item in the table under *fish*.

heterocrine. Referring to *glands* or other tissues that secrete more than one type of substance, such as the *pancreas*, which produces both endocrine and exocrine secretions.

heterogeneous. Made up of differing ingredients or not of uniform quality throughout.

heteropolysaccharide. A *polysaccharide* containing more than one type of *monosaccharide*.

heterotrophic. Incapable of manufacturing organic compounds from inorganic raw materials, therefore requiring organic nutrients from the environment. Heterotrophic is considered the opposite of *autotrophic*. See *heterotrophs*.

heterotrophs. Organisms that require carbon in the form of carbon-hydrogen bonds in such formed organic substances as *carbohydrates, fats,* and *amino acids*. See *autotrophs*.

heterozygote. A fertilized egg or individual in which paired genes differ, because of different contributions from the two parents. A person who is heterozygous for eye color will be carrying two different "eye-color" genes, as, for instance, one "blue-eye" gene and one "brown-eye" gene. In a person who is homozygous the two "eye-color" genes would be the same.

heterozygous. Possessing dissimilar pairs of genes for any hereditary trait. See *genotype* and *phenotype*.

hexokinase. An enzyme similar to *glucokinase* found in all tissues and especially active in the liver. Glucokinase and hexokinase catalyze the phosphorylation of glucose to form glucose-6-phosphate.

hexose. A class of simple sugars (*monosaccharides*) that contain six carbon atoms. The most common members are *glucose* (dextrose), *fructose* (levulose), and *galactose*.

hiccups, hiccoughs (singultus). Short, sharp, inspiratory coughs involving spasmodic lowering of the diaphragm. May be due to indigestion, overloaded stomach, irritation under the surface of the diaphragm, alcoholism, or other causes.

high-density lipoprotein (HDL). A negative risk factor in atherosclerosis, HDLs protect against heart disease, that is, the higher the HDL level, the lower the risk. High-density lipoprotein (HDL) is synthesized mainly in the liver and then secreted into the bloodstream. Its density is high compared to the other three lipoproteins because it contains 50% protein, including apoprotein A, and A ll. Even though it contains about 20% cholesterol, HDL protects against atherosclerosis by removing cholesterol from the endothelial lining of arteries and then returning the cholesterol to the liver, where it can be stored or converted to bile salts. A level of HDL below 35 mg/dL is considered to be a high risk for cardiovascular disease. In addition to the level of HDL, LDL or cholesterol ratio is also a risk determinant. The table shows the HDL/cholesterol ratios and the associated risk. See *cholesterol*.

CARDIOVASCULAR RISK AND HDL/TOTAL CHOLESTEROL RATIO

RATIO TOTAL CHOLESTEROL HDL	ASSOCIATED RISK
3.3	Low
3.5	
4.0	Average
4.5	
5.0	
5.5	High
6.0	

histamine. Mol. Wt. 111. A nitrogenous substance found in all animal and vegetable tissues. A stimulator of the autonomic nervous system and a potent stimulant of gastric secretion. Histamine is formed by the *decarboxylation* of the essential amino acid histidine; the vitamin *pyridoxine* is involved in the biochemical reaction. Histamine is liberated from injured and dying cells. Histamine causes dilation of capillaries and arterioles and a fall in blood pressure. *Antihistamines* counteract the effects of histamine.

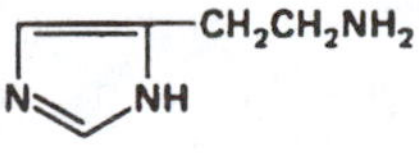

$$\text{—CH}_2\text{CH}_2\text{NH}_2$$
$$\text{N} \diagdown \text{NH}$$

Histamine

histidine (His, H). Mol. Wt. 155. An amino acid apparently essential for growth and possibly for repair of human tissue because the body is unable to make the basic ring structure of its molecule. Once provided with this structure, it can add on the amino group without difficulty. By losing its carboxyl group, histidine is converted to *histamine*, an important physiologic substance which is normally freely present in the intestine and in basophil granules in cells of the *reticuloendothelial* system. Histamine stimulates the secretion of *hydrochloric acid* (HCl) by the *stomach*.

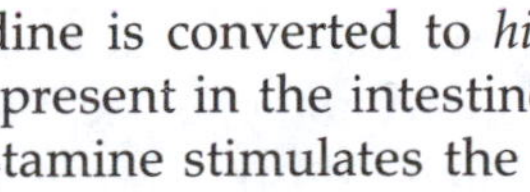

$$\text{—CH}_2\text{—CH—COOH}$$
$$\text{N} \diagdown \text{N} \qquad \text{NH}_2$$

Histidine (His, H)

histones. A class of basic proteins that are soluble in water and insoluble in very dilute ammonia. Histones often yield precipitates with solutions of other proteins and a coagulum on heating that is easily soluble in very dilute acids. On hydrolysis, histone yields several amino acids, among which the basic ones predominate. The only members of this group which may have any considerable importance in terms of food are the thymus histones and the globin of hemoglobin. Histones are also associated with the *nucleic acids*.

hives (urticaria). Raised red bumps (weals) in the skin with sharp, serpentlike borders surrounded by a red halo in the adjacent skin. The duration is no more than 8–12 hours. However, during the interval of one attack, they characteristically appear and disappear in different places on the skin. Hives cause an intense itch, stinging, or prickling as the major symptom. The typical attack of hives lasts for no more than several days and often less. Such an episode is known as acute urticaria. An attack of hives lasting for more than 6 weeks is called chronic urticaria. Acute urticaria is usually a type of allergic reaction to some environmental factor such as an insect bite, a food, or a medication, or as one part of the reaction to many different allergens.

HMG Co A reductase. The enzyme that is critical in the formation of *cholesterol* from the fatty acid intermediate HMG Co A (β-hydroxy- β-methyl glutaryl coenzyme A). It catalyzes the formation of levalonic acid, the beginning of an irreversible pathway to the formation of cholesterol. It is this step that is inhibited by cholesterol intermediates (*feedback control*) and drugs that control the synthesis of cholesterol (*cholesterol therapy*).

holoenzyme. A type of enzyme consisting of a protein portion (*apoenzyme*) and a non-amino acid part or *prosthetic group*.

homeostasis. A balanced, dynamic state or concentration of substances. Homeostasis differs from equilibrium in that no energy is required to maintain equilibrium, whereas homeostasis requires energy because the conditions, while constant, are displaced from equilibrium. Examples of homeostasis are *body temperature* and *blood pressure*.

homeostatic. Pertaining to steady states in the body, maintained by physiologic processes.

hominy. Kernels of hulled dried corn from which the germ has been removed. It is also known as "samp." Ground hominy is called *grits* or groat. Hominy is cooked in water or milk, and may then be fried, baked, or served with a sauce. Hominy is a good source of *carbohydrate*.

homogenize. A word of Greek origin, composed of *homos*, meaning "the same" and *genos*, "kin or kind." In culinary language, "to homogenize" is to reduce an emulsion to particles of the same size and to distribute them evenly. The word is most frequently used for milk, but also for salad dressings and mayonnaise. Most whole milk that has been homogenized has been put through a process that breaks up the fat into such fine particles that it remains evenly distributed in the fluid. Fats that are in small droplets in a fluid (*emulsified*), as in milk and egg yolk, are more readily digestible because the tiny droplets can be surrounded and attacked by *digestive enzymes*.

homologous chromosomes. Paired chromosomes with matching genes, one of the pair from the father, one from the mother.

homozygote. A fertilized egg or individual in which given paired genes are the same.

homozygous. Having identical pairs of genes for any given pair of hereditary traits.

honey. A sweet, sticky liquid made by honeybees from the nectar of plants. The bees suck the nectar from the flowers and store it in their honey sacs, where it undergoes certain changes. Later the bees deposit the liquid in honeycombs where, with other changes, it becomes honey. Honey is almost pure *carbohydrate*. It is a predigested sweetener, and as such is valuable in certain special diets.

Nutrients in 100 g of honey

CALORIES KCAL	PROTEIN G	FAT G	CARBOHYDRATE G	RIBOFLAVIN MG	NIACIN MG	CALCIUM MG
304	0.3	0	82	0.04	0.3	5

honeydew melon (*Cucumis*). *Melons* which belong to the muskmelon family, whose varieties include cantaloupes, honeydews, casaba, and Persian melons. Honeydews have a smooth yellowish white rind, and their flesh is sweet and green. Honeydew contains *ascorbic acid* (vitamin C).

Nutrients in 100 g of honeydew melon

CALORIES KCAL	PROTEIN G	FAT G	CARBOHYDRATE G	VITAMIN A IU	ASCORBATE MG	CALCIUM MG
33	1	0.3	8	40	23	14

hookworms. Small worms which attach themselves to the lining of the *small intestine*. The larvae of the worms generally get through the skin of the feet and lower legs and produce a "ground itch." As they pass to other parts of the body, they may produce bronchitis, big appetites, dirt-eating, constipation, headache, weakness, stupor, dropsy, and even death. Can be cured with tetrachloroethylene.

hops. See *malt* and *malt beverages*.

horehound (*Marrubium vulgare*). Horehound is a member of the *mint* family, a large family of plants including *herbs* such as *thyme*, *marjoram*, and *basil*. It shares an aromatic odor with its better-known relatives, but is very bitter in taste. Horehound also refers to the extract or candy made from the plant and used for coughs and colds.

hormones. Specific substances synthesized by specific cells or organs and secreted directly into the bloodstream to produce an effect on cellular processes in other cells or organs. Most hormones are produced in *endocrine glands* in contradistinction to *exocrine glands* which secrete substances through ducts that lead to surfaces or other ducts that are continuous with the outside of the body; for example, the *salivary glands* secrete into the *digestive system* and the prostate gland secretes into the urethra. Hormones regulate a number of familiar body functions such as growth, sexual development, and lactation (milk production). Less familiar activities regulated by hormones include control of the levels of calcium, sugar, and salt in the blood; the texture of the skin and hair; and the excretion of water by the kidneys. Over- or underproduction of a hormone makes itself apparent by changes in body functions. The glands that produce hormones are known as endocrine glands, and they include the *pituitary, thyroid, parathyroid, pancreas, adrenal, ovaries,* and *testes.* Hormones are also produced by nerve cells of the autonomic nervous system and of the hypothalamus, a portion of the brain that lies just above the pituitary gland. Each gland produces and secretes into the bloodstream a characteristic hormone or hormones. The table shows hormones that regulate secretory and motor activity of the digestive system. See *digestive hormones* and *endocrine system.*

Hormones of the digestive tract

HORMONE	WHERE PRODUCED	STIMULUS TO SECRETION	ACTION
Gastrin	Pyloric and duodenal mucosa	Food in stomach especially proteins, caffeine, spices, alcohol	Stimulates flow of gastric juices
Enterogastrone	Duodenum	Acid chyme, fats	Inhibits secretion of gastric juice; reduces motility
Cholecystokinin	Duodenum	Fat in duodenum	Contraction of gallbladder and flow of bile to duodenum
Secretin	Duodenum	Acid chyme; polypeptides	Secretion of thin, alkaline, enzyme-poor, pancreatic juice
Pancreozymin	Duodenum	Acid chyme; polypeptides	Secretion of thick, enzyme-rich, pancreatic juice
Enterocrin	Upper small intestine	Chyme	Secretion by glands of intestinal mucosa

hubbard squash (*Cucumis*). A large winter squash. See *squash.*

huckleberry (*Gaylussacia*). A dark blue to black edible *berry.* There are a number of varieties which grow in an acid soil on low or high bushes. Each huckleberry contains ten hard little seeds.

Human Immunodeficiency Virus (HIV). HIV is the virus that causes *AIDS.* HIV has a surface molecule that binds to a receptor on the T cell surface and then enters the cell. The T cells are important for the production of *antibodies.* Infection of the T cells by HIV eliminates the activation of B cells, required for the production of antibodies.

humectants. Chemicals such as *glycerol, propylene glycol,* and *sorbitol* that are added to foods to help retain moisture, fresh taste, and texture. Often used in candies, shredded coconut, and marshmallows.

hunger. A compelling need or desire for food accompanied sometimes with a painful sensation or state of weakness. Hunger differs from *appetite* in the degree of desire. Appetite is usually associated with the pleasurable sensations of food intake. With continued deprivation of food, an appetite becomes hunger. When the stomach has emptied and the food has been digested, the stomach undergoes rhythmic contractions which give rise to a sensation of hunger. These contractions are normally known as "hunger pangs." The longer the period of time following a meal, the more frequent the contractions. To a limited extent, they are controlled by the level of glucose in the blood.

hyaluronic acid. A *mucopolysaccharide* that is a component of the ground substance of intercellular material. The human *placenta*, cattle synovial fluid (*synovium*), and vitreous fluids (*eye*) are the most common sources of hyaluronic acid, but it is widely distributed and is found in most connective tissues. Its name is derived from hyaloid (vitreous) and uronic acid. Hyaluronic acid is composed of equimolar proportions of D-glucuronic acid and acetyl glucosamine occupying alternating positions in the molecule.

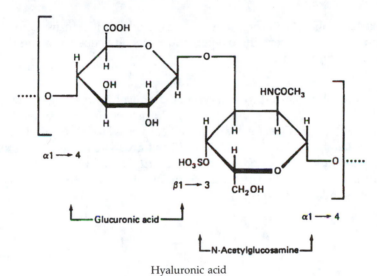

Hyaluronic acid

hydrocarbon chains. Molecular units made up solely of carbon and hydrogen atoms. See *fatty acid, oleic acid, stearic acid*.

hydrochloric acid (HCl). Mol. Wt. 36. An aqueous solution of hydrogen chloride (HCl). This normal constituent of *gastric juice* is produced by the *parietal cells* of gastric glands. The HCl concentration in the stomach is variable, depending upon several factors including rate of secretion of gastric juice and the type of food eaten. It serves the following functions: converts *pepsinogen* into *pepsin* and produces an acid medium favorable for the activity of pepsin; dissolves and disintegrates *nucleoproteins* and *collagen*; inhibits multiplication of bacteria; stimulates secretion by the *duodenum*; inhibits the action of *ptyalin*, stopping its digestive action in the *stomach*. See *chloride ions*.

hydrochlorothiazide (HCTZ). See *diuretics*.

hydrocortisone (cortisol). See *cortisol.*

hydrogen (H). Element No. 1. At. Wt. 1. Hydrogen has the smallest atomic weight. Present in *proteins, carbohydrates, fats,* and water. Hydrogen makes up approximately 10% of the human body and more than 90% of the universe.

hydrogen bonds. Weak chemical attraction between hydrogen atoms and other atoms, chiefly oxygen and nitrogen. Hydrogen bonds are important in giving *deoxynucleic acids* (DNA) and *proteins* their characteristic shapes and stability. Hydrogen bonds are one of a class of weak bonds or interactions also known as secondary valence forces. See *water.*

hydrogen ion (proton, H$^+$). The positively charged nucleus of a hydrogen atom. See *acid and base.*

hydrogen peroxide. Mol. Wt. 34. H_2O_2. A colorless liquid with an irritating odor and acrid taste. It decomposes readily, liberating oxygen and water. It is used as a commercial bleaching agent and as an oxidizing agent.

hydrogenation. Generally referred to as a type of chemical processing which adds hydrogen to unsaturated bonds of carbon or oxygen. In the *fatty acid* chains hydrogenation increases the degree of saturation of the *fat. Oils,* for example, are converted to *saturated fat* by hydrogenation. Hydrogenation prevents oxidative rancidity and thus greatly prolongs the storage life of the fat by converting *unsaturated fatty acids* to saturated fatty acids. One practice is to expose fats or oils in a continuously controlled process so that more fatty acids are not completely saturated. This process tends to convert most of the *essential fatty acid, linoleic acid,* to *oleic acid.*

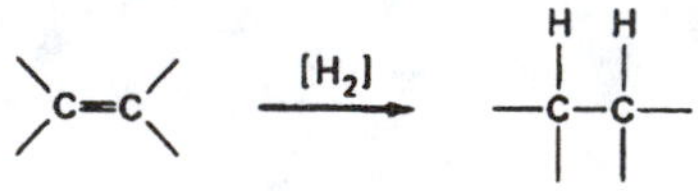

Hydrogenation

hydrolysate. The product of *hydrolysis.* For example, a *protein* hydrolysate is a mixture of the constituent *amino acids* when the protein molecule is degraded by acids, alkalies, or enzymes.

hydrolysis. A chemical or biochemical reaction in which the rupture of a chemical bond may be interpreted as the incorporation of a water molecule, resulting in the formation of two new compounds. Hydrolysis can be catalyzed by *enzymes* (proteolysis), *acids* (acid hydrolysis), or *alkalies* (alkaline hydrolysis). In all cases, the products appear to have incorporated hydrogen ion (H$^+$) in one product and hydroxyl (OH$^-$) in the other product. For example, the digestion (hydrolysis) of *proteins* or *polysaccharides* by acid, alkalies, or enzymes yields *hydrolysates* composed of amino acids or monosaccharides that are the result of a rupture of the *peptide bond* or glycolytic bond by water.

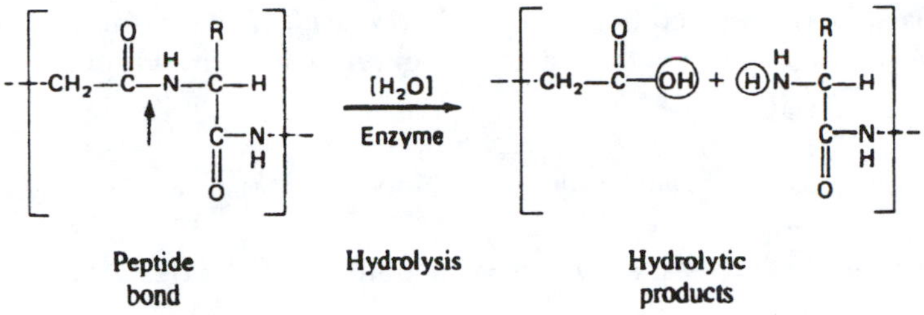

| Peptide bond | Hydrolysis | Hydrolytic products |

hydrolyzed vegetable protein (HVP). A substance used to bring out the natural flavor of food. It consists of vegetable (usually soybean) *protein* that has been chemically degraded to the *amino acids* of which it is composed. It can be found in instant soups, beef stew, frankfurters, gravy and sauce mixes, and canned chili.

hydrophilic. Soluble in water or attracting the water molecule. It is the opposite of *hydrophobic*. See *micelle*.

hydroponics. The soil-less culture of plants. The roots are immersed in a nutrient-rich aqueous medium.

hydroxocobalamine. A form of *cobalamin* (vitamin B_{12}) with a *hydroxyl group* (−OH) in place of a cyano group (−CN).

hydroxybutyric acid. See *beta (β) hydroxybutyric acid*.

hydroxyl. The univalent radical OH⁻. When combined with a metallic ion or a radical which acts as a metal, such as NH_4^+, it forms a hydroxide. Commonly called a *base* or *alkali*.

hydroxylated lecithin. A substance manufactured by treating soybean *lecithin* with peroxide. Used by the food industry as an *emulsifier* and *antioxidant* in baked goods, ice cream, and margarine.

hydroxyproline (Hyp). Mol. Wt. 131. A modified amino acid occurring abundantly in *collagen* that derives from the nonessential amino acid *proline*. The hydroxylations of proline to form hydoxyproline only occur when it is incorporated as part of a protein molecule.

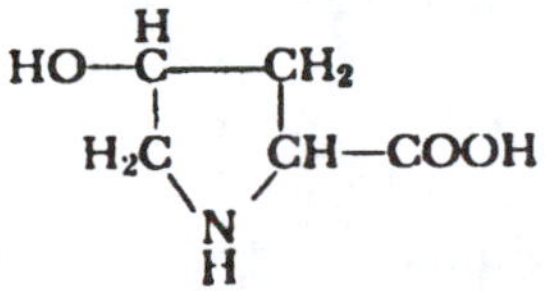

Hydroxyproline (Hyp)

hypercalcemia. An excess of *calcium* in the blood, usually due to hormone abnormality.

hypercalciuria. Abnormal calcium excretion in the urine, usually due to hormone or drug action.

hyperchlorhydria. Excessive secretion of *hydrochloric acid* in the stomach, in contrast to the opposite condition, *achlorhydria*, when acid secretion is absent. Hyperchlorhydria is often associated with *peptic ulcer*.

hypercholesteremia. Excess of *cholesterol* in the blood.

hyperchromic. Highly or excessively colored; usually used to describe blood, as in *folacin* deficiency.

hyperglycemia. An excess of sugar in the blood as occurs in uncontrolled *diabetes*.

hyperinsulinism. Excessive secretion of *insulin* by the *pancreas*, which results in *hypoglycemia*.

hyperkalemia. Excessive amounts of *potassium* (K) in blood plasma. Hyperkalemia is a serious complication of kidney (renal) failure, severe dehydration, or shock. Hyperkalemia causes the heart to dilate, and the heart rate is slowed by weakened contractions. Potassium ion (K^+) plays a vital role with ionized *sodium* (Na^+) and *calcium* (Ca^{+2}) in regulating neuromuscular stimulation, transmission of electrochemical impulses, and contraction of muscle fibers.

hyperphosphatemia. A high serum *phosphate* ion (PO_4^{-3}) concentration. Hyperphosphatemia may be caused by kidney (renal) insufficiency because the kidney cannot excrete phosphorus adequately or by hypoparathyroidism, which causes an insufficient secretion of *parathormone*, which regulates the renal excretion of phosphorus. When serum phosphate ion concentration rises, serum *calcium* ion falls, causing tetany (a muscle malfunction).

hyperplasia. An abnormal multiplication of cells with an increase in size of an organ, but without formation of a *tumor*.

hypertension (high blood pressure). Said to exist when the systolic pressure is consistently above 150 mm Hg or when the diastolic pressure exceeds 99 mm Hg. A high diastolic pressure reading that is constant, meaning that the blood vessels are under relentless pressure at all times, indicates that the person is a good candidate for heart disease or vascular disorder of some kind. Systolic hypertension may be due to increased cardiac output of blood, as in hyperthyroidism, or to loss of elasticity in the larger arteries. Diastolic hypertension is a result of a narrowing of the small arterioles that control the flow of blood out of the larger arteries. Hypertension heart disease is an increase in the blood pressure, placing an extra burden on the heart as it works harder to force the blood through the blood vessels. This brings about an increase in the size of the heart and impaired function as a result of fatigue of the heart muscle. Hypertension may result from chronic kidney infection or diseases of the arteries such as *arteriosclerosis*. It may occur without any apparent cause, having no known relationship with any other disease.

hyperthyroidism. A systemic condition resulting from overactivity of the *thyroid gland* and overproduction of the hormone thyroxine. This disorder is also known as Graves' disease, toxic goiter, and thyrotoxicosis. The result of an overactive thyroid gland is an increased *basal metabolic rate* (BMR), hyperactivity in some instances, and general weakness and weight loss in the extreme.

hypertonic dehydration. Water loss from the cell as a result of excess solutes in the blood, hence greater *osmotic pressure* in the surrounding extracellular fluid. The osmotic pressure of the extracellular fluid is higher than that of the intracellular fluid, and water moves in the direction of the higher osmotic pressure. The imbalance in osmotic pressure causes water to shift from the cell into the extracellular fluid spaces. This situation can occur from either excess water loss or water restriction.

hypertrophic. Pertaining to enlargement of an organ due to increase in size of its constituent cells.

hyperuricemia. Excess of *uric acid* in the blood; one of the characteristics of the disease *gout*.

hypervitaminosis. A pathology or toxicity due to an excess of one or more vitamins. The fat-soluble vitamins, especially *retinol* (vitamin A) and *vitamin D*, have the distinct potential to poison at high dosages because they are stored by the body. The danger of toxicity does not hold for most water-soluble vitamins, as the body eliminates any excess in the urine. See *vitamin toxicity*.

hypoalbuminemia. Abnormally low albumin content of the blood, associated with severe dietary protein deficiency. See *protein calorie malnutrition, marasmus,* and *kwashiorkor*.

hypocalcemia. Abnormally low blood calcium, usually due to hormonal or kidney abnormalities.

hypochloremic alkalosis. A condition of *alkalosis* caused by a loss of or lowered blood *chlorides*. Excessive loss of gastric acid (*hydrochloric acid*) results in loss of chlorides, with bicarbonate replacing the depleted chloride ions and hypochloremic alkalosis (a type of *metabolic alkalosis*) resulting. Such gastrointestinal disorders as excessive vomiting may lead to hypochloremic alakalosis. Prompt replacement of chloride is essential to treatment.

hypochlorhydria. Diminished secretion of *hydrochloric acid* in the stomach.

hypochromic. Pertaining to a decrease in color; usually applied to a decrease in hemoglobin content of the *red blood cells* as in *iron* deficiency.

hypoglycemia. An abnormally low level of *glucose* in the circulating blood. The person with this condition utilizes the available glucose in his or her blood to a seriously low level within a few hours after a meal or after exercise. Persons with chronic hypoglycemia are considered to be predisposed to diabetes, but the condition is relatively rare. Overdosage of *insulin* will result in hypoglycemia and in extreme cases, insulin shock. Evidence for hypoglycemia is obtained by a *glucose tolerance test*.

hypogonadism. Defective internal secretion of the gonads.

hypokalemia. Low blood potassium. Hypokalemia is a serious complication of severe diarrhea, for example, in which large amounts of potassium are lost in intestinal secretions. Hypokalemia may also result from rapid *glycogenesis* during the recovery of *metabolic acidosis*. Replacement therapy in both instances should involve added potassium.

hypoparathyroidism. Insufficient secretion of the *parathyroid glands*.

hypophosphatemia. Low serum phosphorus, which may be caused by decreased absorption of phosphorus as in intestinal diseases (*sprue, celiac disease*); or by an upset of serum *calcium to phosphorus ratio* as in bone disease (*rickets, osteomalacia*); or by excess secretion of *parathyroid hormone* with resulting excessive renal excretion of phosphorus. Hypophosphatemia can lead to bone loss or heartbeat irregularities.

hypopituitarism. A condition resulting from diminished secretion of *pituitary* hormones, especially those of the anterior lobe.

hypoproteinemia. Decrease in the normal quantity of serum protein in the blood. It can be indicative of protein deficiency. See *hypoalbuminemia, protein-calorie malnutrition, marasmus,* and *kwashiorkor*.

hypoprothrombinemia. Deficiency of *prothrombin* in the blood. Prothrombin is required for normal *blood clot* formation.

hypothalamus. A small collection of nerve cells and fibers arranged in a complicated system of nuclei in the center of the *brain* at the upper end of the brain stem. Closely related to the *pituitary gland*—many nerve fibers connect the two organs. It is essential for the regulation and control of visceral activity, body temperature, water and electrolyte balance, blood pressure, sexual and reproductive activity, and possibly body weight. It is also important in the expression of various emotions such as anger, fright, and embarrassment. The hypothalamus controls these varied activities by means of patterns of nerve impulses which are conveyed to their destinations by sympathetic and parasympathetic nerve fibers. See *nervous system*.

hypothyroidism. Underactivity of the *thyroid gland*, with a deficiency in the production of the hormone *thyroxine*. When the thyroid does not produce enough thyroxine to maintain a normal metabolic rate, hypothyroidism occurs. The effects of hypothyroidism depend on whether the condition occurs during growth or after maturity. Adult hypothyroidism is called *myxedema*. The name comes from the collection of body fluid in connective tissue (*edema*) that gives the individual a puffy, bloated appearance. Myxedema caused by an onset of thyroid insufficiency in the adult reduces the *basal metabolic rate* (BMR) by 35–40%. This results in sluggishness and chills from an inability to maintain body temperature, and reduced muscle tone. Motivation, vigor, and alertness diminish, and the individual sleeps much of the time. The central nervous system may deteriorate until the individual becomes an imbecile. Supplementary thyroxine can effect complete recovery.

I

I. The alphabetiic symbol for the *essential amino acid isoleucine* (Ile).

ibuprofen. See *acetaminophen* and *aspirin*.

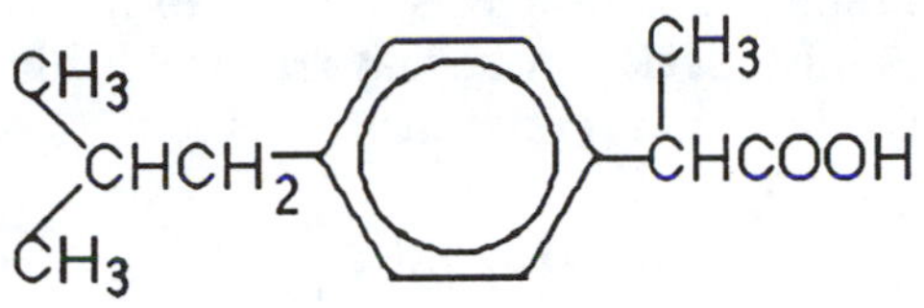

Ibuprofen

ice crystals. At temperatures low enough to freeze water, ice crystals may rupture the cell membranes or cell walls of fruits, vegetables, and meats. Generally, such ruptures do not change the nutritive value of the food, but they may have a pronounced effect on the appearance, texture, and taste. Pure water freezes at 0 °C (32 °F). The water in foods generally freezes at lower temperatures.

idiopathic. Pertaining to a disease of unknown origin.

idiopathic steatorrhea. A condition when individuals exhibit only the gastrointestinal symptoms of *sprue*, but not the complete symptomatology of the sprue syndrome, including *megaloblastic anemia*. The disorder has been called idiopathic steatorrhea after pancreatic disorders, intestinal lipodystrophy, inflammation of the lymph ducts of the small intestine, amyloidosis, and chronic inflammatory disease of the small intestine have been ruled out. In many cases of idiopathic steatorrhea, the course of the disorder is unpredictable. It is believed that a majority of cases in the adult are linked to the basic underlying *celiac disease* of childhood.

ileum. One of the sections of the *small intestine* that joins with the *cecum* (large intestine). Most of the absorption of food takes place in the ileum. The walls of the ileum are covered with extremely small, fingerlike structures called villi (*villus*) which provide a large surface for absorption. After food has been digested, it is absorbed into the capillaries of the villi. It is then carried to all parts of the body by the blood and lymph. See *digestive system*.

immunoglobulin. One of a family of closely related though not identical proteins which are capable of acting as antibodies.

impermeable. Not capable of being penetrated. It is always necessary to name the substance to which a food wrapping material is impermeable. It may be impermeable to water vapor only or to water vapor and air (or other gases).

inactivate. To suspend or terminate certain biological activities such as by heat, irradiation, or other forms of energy. See *denature*.

inborn errors of metabolism. Metabolic disorders that result from the inheritable absence or reduced presence of an *enzyme* or *cofactor* required for normal metabolism. Most inborn errors of metabolism are autosomal (not sex-linked) recessives. Some of these inherited diseases respond to nutritional therapy—*phenylketonuria* is such an example.

index of nutritive quality (INQ). Nutrient density refers to the ratio of nutrients to energy in a food. This way of evaluating foods was used as early as 1904 to express the "nutritive ratio" in rations from farm animals and it was applied to human diets in 1928. It is being used more widely as nutritionists seek precise ways of establishing criteria for comparing the nutritive value of foods. The term index of "nutritive quality" (INQ) was coined as a way of expressing nutrient density.

$$INQ = \frac{\% \text{ of the RDA for a specific nutrient supplied by a quantity of food}}{\% \text{ of the total energy requirement supplied by the same quantity of the same food}}$$

If the INQ for a nutrient in a food is greater than 1.0, that food supplies relatively more of the nutrient (compared to the amount needed) than energy (compared to the amount needed). If the INQ is less than 1.0, the nutrient density of that food is below the nutrient density needed for the total day's diet. The percentage of United States RDA values for protein and several micronutrients given on food labels can be easily used in the numerator of the INQ formula. Since there is no United States RDA value for energy, the RDA tables must be consulted for the appropriate energy value for sex and age.

indigestion. Almost any symptoms involving or related to *digestive system* distress. The term in one sense is a misnomer since digestion, the process of breaking down food into small particles for absorption, is usually normal. Acute indigestion may occur after eating irritating or spoiled food. Difficulties such as belching, gas, abdominal rumblings and gurgling, passing of gas by rectum, *heartburn*, and vague feelings of discomfort, heaviness, and unrest in the abdomen, often are termed indigestion or "gastritis." At common cause of an irritable bowel is emotional tension. The treatment for an irritable bowel includes the use of bland diet adapted to individual requirements. The production of gas by certain foods such as onions, cabbage, and beans, and the passage through the rectum of *flatus* which may have a foul odor, is due to production of gas by bacteria as they act on food in the large intestine (*colon*), together with the accumulation of swallowed air.

indirect calorimetry. The rate of metabolism or heat production is calculated from the oxygen intake or from the oxygen intake and carbon dioxide content of the expired air, as measured by a respiration apparatus. By determining either the oxygen consumed or the carbon dioxide exhaled in a given number of minutes, the caloric expenditure can be calculated. This principle may be applied to persons engaged in various types of activities or when lying at rest. A subject who is moving about has to carry the respirator with him or her. A *caloric equivalent* of 4.8 calories per liter oxygen consumed is a value used to convert oxygen utilization into heat produced. See *energy balance*.

induction. Stimulation of enzyme formation by certain lower molecular weight substances (inducers). The appearance of new stages of development during the evolution of individuals (ontogeny) of more complex organisms is also known as induction. Several hormones affect the development type of induction and affect the induction of enzyme formation.

inert gas. Gas that does not react with the materials in food. Nitrogen is an inert gas which may be used to replace air (oxygen) in packages of food to slow down the deterioration of the food.

infarction. The formation of an area of dead tissue resulting from the obstruction of blood vessels supplying the part. See *myocardial infarction*.

inflammation. The local reaction of the body to irritation or injury. It occurs in tissue that is injured but not destroyed. It is a defensive and protective effort by the body to isolate and eliminate the injuring agent and to repair the injury. A certain degree of inflammation takes place following any type of injury, including a wound made under aseptic conditions by a surgeon. *Histamine*, a derivative of the amino acid *histidine*, is responsible for some of the reactions of an inflammation.

influenza (flu, grippe). An acute infectious disease due to a virus. It is characterized by any of a number of the following: fever, headaches, nasal congestion, bronchial congestion, or gastrointestinal distress, and may involve nervous disturbances.

ingest. To eat or take in through the mouth. To take food into the body.

INH. See *isonicotinic acid hydrazide*.

inhalants. Drugs that are inhaled and absorbed through the lungs. An example is aromatic spirits of ammonia.

inhibition. The reduction or stoppage of the action of enzymes or chemical processes by substances called inhibitors. A competitive inhibitor competes with the substrate for the active site of an enzyme.

inorganic compounds. Chemical compounds that do not contain carbon. The inorganic compounds exist in cells partly as dissolved salts and partly in combination with the organic compounds. In chemical analysis of cells, the mineral elements remain either wholly or largely in the ash when the cells are incinerated; hence, they are grouped as ash constituents. Only small amounts of these elements are needed, but they are essential parts of the cells. See *minerals*.

inorganic nutrients. Mineral elements and water are sometimes called inorganic nutrients. See *minerals*.

inosine diphosphate (IDP). A *flavor enhancer*. See *inosine triphosphate*.

inosine monophosphate (IMP). See *inosine triphosphate*.

inosine triphosphate (ITP). Mol. Wt. 506. A high-energy phosphate compound equivalent to *adenosine triphosphate* (ATP) as a source of chemical energy. The pyruvate kinase reaction in *glycolysis* forms ITP from IDP. The disodium salt of IMP, disodium inosinate, and disodium guanylate are *flavor enhancers*.

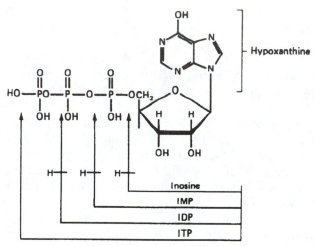

Inosine triphosphate (ITP)

inositol (myo-inositol). Mol. Wt. 180. $C_6H_6(OH)_6$. A cyclic alcohol with six hydroxyl radicals allied to the *hexoses*. It occurs in many foods, and especially in the bran of cereal grains. Inositol in combination with six phosphate molecules forms the compound *phytic acid*, which hinders intestinal absorption of *calcium* and *iron*. Like *biotin*, inositol is found in the vitamin B complex, but its role as a vitamin is not clear. It can be synthesized in the intestines of most animals. It may act in the utilization of *carbon dioxide* in certain chemical reactions within the cell. Good sources are liver, heart, yeast, and peanuts. Inositol is a colorless, water-soluble crystalline material with some carbohydrate properties. The most prevalent naturally occurring isomer of inositol is shown here.

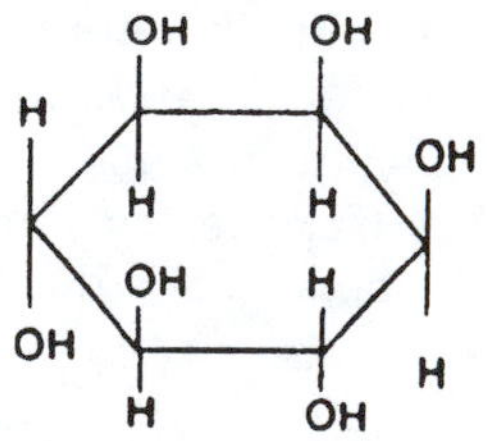

Inositol
(cis-1, 2,3,5-trans-4, 6 cyclohexanehexol)

insalivation. During the process of *mastication*, saliva is poured in large quantities into the mouth and mixed with the food to help lubricate, moisten, and reduce it to a softened mass known as a *bolus*, which can be readily swallowed.

insulin. A small protein secreted into the blood by the beta (β) cells in the islets of Langerhans of the *pancreas*. The normal stimulus to insulin secretion is the ingestion of carbohydrates and the consequent rise in blood sugar. Secretion is also stimulated by the amino acids and by the intestinal hormone *pancreozymin*. Insulin is the only known hormone that lowers blood sugar. Insulin fosters *glycogenesis* by conversion of *glucose* to *glycogen* in the liver, where the glycogen is stored. Insulin also fosters *lipogenesis*, the formation of *fat*. Glucose is converted to fat for storage in adipose tissue (*body fat*). This conversion takes place mainly in the adipose tissue itself, but some glucose is converted to fat in the liver. Insulin increases cell permeability to glucose in liver, muscle, and adipose tissues and allows glucose to pass from the extracellular fluids into the cells for oxidation to supply needed energy. It is insulin's function to direct the distribution of glucose within the body and to maintain a constant level of glucose in the blood. When insulin is secreted, it stimulates the liver to increase the uptake of glucose and to increase its synthesis of glycogen from glucose. At the same time the liver and the muscle cells react by stepping up their intake of glucose and by increasing the conversion of glucose to glycogen. Insulin seems to be important in stimulating protein synthesis in conjunction with *growth hormone*. The manufacture of large fat molecules is also enhanced by insulin. Insulin does not affect the rate of uptake of glucose in the brain. In general, insulin has an effect that opposes the effects of the "second messanger," *cyclic AMP*.

insulin shock. This type of shock is produced by an intravenous or a deep muscular injection of excessive amounts of insulin. The presence of the abnormal excess of insulin produces a *hypoglycemia* (low blood sugar) that results in vast changes in the entire physiologic reactions of the organism. The central nervous system reacts most strongly to such a condition, because *glucose* is the primary metabolic fuel of the central nervous system. In hypoglycemia, there is a profound metabolic depression which chiefly affects the brain. Those parts of the brain with the highest metabolism rates suffer first. Insulin shock was a therapy in certain mental diseases.

intake. Substances or amounts of substances which are taken in by the body, e.g., the intake of food. See *ingest*.

interferon. A protein formed during the interaction of animal cells with viruses, which is capable of conferring resistance to infection with a wide range of viruses.

intermediate metabolism. A general term that refers to any series of biochemical reactions, *anabolic* or *catabolic*, that occur with cells, tissues, or organs.

international units (IU). The measure commonly used for vitamins. The amount of the *vitamin* comprising a unit is determined by its biological activity, that is, the amount of the vitamin required to cure or prevent a disease that is associated with a deficiency of that specific vitamin. Such units are established for *retinol* (vitamin A), *ascorbic acid* (vitamin C), *vitamin D*, and *thiamine*. IUs are still used principally for vitamins A and D. There have been some recent efforts to give vitamin requirements in terms of their weights. The table gives the relationships among the weights and forms of a vitamin and the I.U. See *retinol equivalents (R.E.).*

VITAMIN	WT. EQUIVALENT OF 1 I.U. μG
Ascorbate (Vitamin C)*	50
Retinol (Vitamin A)	0.30
retinyl acetate	0.34
retinyl palmitate	0.55
ß-carotene	0.60
Thiamine hydrochloride (Vitaminl B$_1$)	3.0
Vitamin D$_2$ (ergocalciferol)	0.025
Vitamin D$_3$ (cholecalciferol)	0.025

The Food and Nutrition Board has recommended the use of retinol equivalents (R.E.) for vitamin A. The R.E. takes into account the losses of carotene during absorption and the losses in conversion to retinol: 1 R.E. for retinol is 1 μg (3.33 I.U.) 1 R.E. for b-carotene is 6 μg (10 I.U.)

interstitial. The spaces or interstices within an organ or tissue that lie between the cells. The interstitial spaces are filled with lymph fluid from the lymphatic system which bathes cells and tissues.

intestinal juice. The *mucosa* of the *small intestine* secrete a fluid termed "succus entericus" or, simply, intestinal juice. It is secreted by intestinal glands. Intestinal juice contains two enzymes; (1) *enterokinase*, which activates *trypsin*, and (2) a weak *amylase*. Intestinal juice, secreted at a rate of about 3000 mL/day, may function primarily to carry substances to be digested to the epithelial cells, where these substances are absorbed and undergo final digestion by the enzymes. See *digestive system*.

intestine, large (colon). The large intestine is about 5 feet long. The *cecum*, located on the lower right of the abdomen, is the first portion of the large intestine into which food is emptied from the *ileum*, the lower portion of the *small intestine*. The appendix extends from the lower portion of the cecum and is a blind sac. Although the appendix usually is found lying just below the cecum, by virtue of its free end, it can extend in several different directions depending upon its mobility. The colon extends along the right side of the abdomen from the cecum up to the region of the liver (ascending colon). There the colon bends (hepatic flexure) and is continuous across the upper portion of the abdomen (transverse colon) to the spleen. The colon bends again (splenic flexure) and goes down the left side of the abdomen (descending colon). The last portion makes an S-curve (sigmoid) toward the center and posterior of the abdomen and ends in the rectum. The main function of the large intestine is the recovery of water from the mass of undigested food and intestinal juices it receives from the small intestine. As the mass passes through the colon, water is absorbed and returned to the tissues. Waste materials, or feces, become more solid as they are pushed along by *peristalsis*. *Constipation* is caused by delay in movement of intestinal contents and removal of too much water from them. *Diarrhea* results when movement of the intestinal contents is so rapid that not enough water is removed. See *digestive system*.

intestine, small. The small intestine is a tube about 22 feet long. The intestine is attached to the margin of a thin band of tissue called the *mesentery*, which is a portion of the *peritoneum*, the membrane lining the abdominal cavity. The mesentery is a tissue membrane that supports the intestine and the vessels which carry blood to and from the intestine. The other edge of the mesentery is drawn together like a fan; the gathered margin is attached to the posterior wall of the abdomen. This arrangement permits the folding and coiling of the intestine so that this long organ can be packed into a small space. The small intestine is divided into three continuous parts: *duodenum, jejunum,* and *ileum*. It receives digestive juices from three accessory organs of digestion; the *pancreas, liver,* and *gallbladder*. See *digestive system*.

intracellular. Within the cell.

intracellular fluid compartment (IFC). The total water inside the body cells, which amounts to about twice that outside the *cells*. The cell is the basic unit of structure of the entire body, and cells are the sites of the vast basic metabolic activity of the body. The intracellular fluid compartment makes up about 40% of the total body weight. The water compartment outside of the cell is called the *extracellular* fluid.

intravenous. Into or from within a vein.

intrinsic factor (IF). A *glycoprotein* (transcobalamin) normally synthesized in the stomach and required for the absorption of the *extrinsic factor, cobalamin* (vitamin B_{12}), from food. Persons lacking the ability to synthesize intrinsic factor develop a condition called *pernicious anemia*.

inulin. A *polysaccharide* composed of *fructose* units and having little dietary significance. Found only in a few common foods such as onions, garlic, and artichokes. The carbohydrate inulin is only partially digested, although further breakdown by bacteria may occur in the large intestine. Storage of inulin-containing foods also affects this carbohydrate. Fresh food may have much of its carbohydrate in this unavailable inulin form; however, upon storage much of the inulin may be converted to available sugar. Although inulin is of small dietary significance, it is of interest and importance in medicine and nursing because it provides a test of kidney function. Since inulin is filtered at the *glomerulus* during the formation of *urine*, but is neither secreted nor reabsorbed by the tubule, it can be used to measure glomerular filtration rate.

invert sugar. A sugar which forms when *sucrose* is split into the two monosaccharides, *glucose* and *fructose*, by an enzyme (*invertase*) or an acid. It is called "invert" because a solution containing the 50–50 mixture and a solution containing sucrose rotate the plane of polarized light in opposite directions. A 50–50 mixture of two sugars, glucose and fructose, is used by food manufacturers because it is sweeter and more soluble and crystallizes less readily than sucrose.

invertases. Enzymes that hydrolyze *sucrose* to form the monosaccharides *glucose* and *fructose*. The product of invertase action is called *invert sugar*. Invertases are used in the confectionery industry to make invert sugar for the preparation of liqueurs and ice creams in which the crystallization of sugars from high concentrations is to be avoided. In soft-center, chocolate-coated candies, such as maraschino cherries, invertase incorporated into the center softens the fondant after it has been coated with chocolate. Invertase is added to sucrose syrups to hydrolyze that sugar and in this way prevent crystallization on standing. It also has been used in the manufacture of artificial honey.

involution. The change back to a normal condition that certain organs undergo after fulfilling their functional purposes.

iodine (I). Element No. 53. At Wt. 127. Iodine is absorbed in the inorganic form as iodide ions in the upper part of the small intestine. It may be absorbed through the skin. Estimates of the total amount in the body range from 15–30 mg, and of this small amount, about three-fifths is concentrated in the *thyroid gland*. Iodine serves but one known purpose in the body, which is to form the thyroid hormones, *thyroxine* and *triiodothyronine*. These hormones are manufactured in the thyroid gland from its stored iodide (the iodine anion, I^-) and the amino acid *tyrosine*, and they are released in small amounts into the blood. Iodide is supplied to the body by intake of foods or water and represents one of the necessary *trace elements*. Dietary iodide is absorbed from the gastrointestinal tract. Approximately 30% is removed by the thyroid gland, and the remainder is excreted in the urine. The following table gives the iodine content of some common food. See *minerals*.

Iodine content in µg/100 g of food

Bread	6	Cheese	5	Halibut	52	Potatoes	5
Butter	6	Cod fish	150	Milk	4	Salmon	34
Cabbage	5	Cod liver oil	840	Oysters	58	Spinach	20
Carrots	4	Eggs	9	Pork	5		

iodine uptake test. A radioisotope test for diagnosis of thyroid disease; done after administering a dose of radioactive iodide (I^{131})and tracing its uptake by the *thyroid gland*.

iodopsin. (1) A light-sensitive vitamin A protein complex necessary for vision in bright light. (2) Pigment found in cones of the *retina*; visual violet. See *rhodopsin*.

ion. An atom or group of atoms carrying a positive or negative charge, for example, *cations* and *anion*.

iron (Fe). Element No. 26. At. Wt. 56. About 3–5 g of iron are present in the body, most of which is in the blood as an essential component of the red protein *hemoglobin* of the red blood cells. The body guards its iron stores carefully and reuses any in the body over and over again. Only small amounts of iron lost need to be replaced, normally about 0.9 mg for males and 1.5 mg for females. The principal loss of iron in females is during *menses* and accounts for a dietary requirement of 30–90% greater than males. The average menstrual loss of blood is 35 mL, which averages to a replacement requirement. The requirements are easily established, but the amount of iron required in the diet is difficult to determine because dietary iron is not quantitatively absorbed. The form of the iron, organic or inorganic, oxidized or reduced, and the presence of other substances greatly influences the amount of iron absorbed. Large amounts of inorganic *phosphates* or oxalates that occur in spinach reduce the absorption of dietary iron by rendering it insoluble. In general, the iron obtained from foods is in organic compounds, a form less favorably absorbed than the inorganic forms. Oxidized iron (the ferric state, Fe^{+3}) is less readily absorbed than reduced iron (the ferrous state, Fe^{+2}). The variations in absorption are not understood. Iron from white bread is more readily absorbed than iron from whole wheat, and the iron in beef is readily absorbed even though it is largely in the organic compounds, chiefly in hemoglobin. Reducing agents, such as *ascorbic acid* (vitamin C), increases iron absorption. Both inorganic and some organic forms can be utilized by the body; however, hemoglobin iron from red meats (veal, beef, lamb) may be absorbed directly into the muscosal cells before the iron is released. Ferric citrate is also a highly available iron source, being converted to the ferrous form before absorption. Iron is distributed throughout the body, being a component of essential enzymes in every cell. About 65–70% is present in the blood as hemoglobin in the red blood cells. In iron deficiency, the lowered capacity to provide oxygen is largely responsible for the fatigue and apathy characteristic of iron deficiency anemia. Iron deficiency anemia occurs mainly in young children and women of childbearing age. There are many types of *anemias*. Of the nutritional anemias, iron deficiency anemia is by far the most common. The inorganic forms of iron salts are readily absorbed directly into the bloodstream, where they are transported by the protein *transferrin* rather than through the *lymphatic system*. Iron absorption occurs chiefly in the upper intestines. Absorption takes place with the iron in the ferrous form (Fe^{+2}), and therapeutically it is usually given this way as ferrous sulfate or *ferrous gluconate*. Ferric salts are reduced to ferrous salts before absorption. Absorbed iron goes to the bone marrow for red blood cell synthesis, to tissue for cellular oxidation processes, to liver, spleen, and bone marrow for storage reserve. The rate of iron absorption varies widely and is conditioned by several factors, which include the quantity of iron ingested, the body content, the rate of *erythropoiesis*, and the hemoglobin level. The table shows the iron content of some common foods.

Iron in μg/100 g of food

Almonds	5	Chocolates		Indian nuts	5	Pork	3
Bacon	4	bittersweet	5	Liverwurst	5	Sardines	3
Beans	3	semisweet	3	Livers		Scallops	4
Blackstrap		Cashews	4	beef	9	Sugar	
molasses	16	Caviar	12	calf	14	brown	3
Bran flakes	4	Clams	3	chicken	9	Syrups	
Brazil nuts	4	Dates	3	pork	29	corn	4
Breads	2	Filberts	3	Mussels	3	soybean	13
Buckwheat	3	Giblets	7	Oysters	8	Veal	3

iron deficiency anemia. See *anemia*.

irradiation. The treatment of foods with x-rays, ultraviolet rays, or the radiation from radioactive materials. The process controls the growth of certain microorganisms in some meat products. It is also used in a variety of foods besides meat. Irradiated foods must be labeled "treated by irradiation" and must show the irradiation logo. See *radiation*.

irradiation of foods. Irradiation of foods with the energy rays of radioactive materials inhibits the growth of molds or bacteria. Foods are not rendered radioactive themselves, and the changes in the character of the food are minimal.

ischemia. A local deficiency of blood caused chiefly by narrowing of the arteries or the blockage of an artery by a blood clot. See *myocardial infarction*.

Islets of Langerhans. See *insulin* and *pancreas*.

isocaloric. Containing an equal number of calories.

isoleucine (Ile, I). Mol. Wt. 131. One of the *essential amino acids* found in proteins.

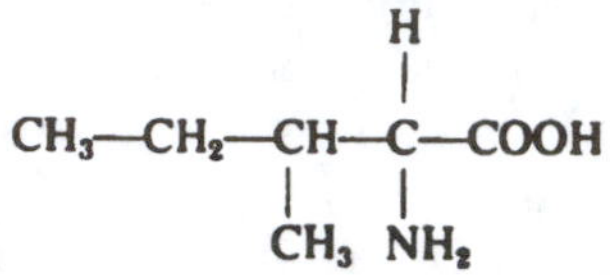

$$CH_3-CH_2-CH-\overset{\overset{\displaystyle H}{|}}{C}-COOH$$
$$\underset{CH_3}{|}\quad\underset{NH_2}{|}$$

Isoleucine (Ile, I)

isomaltose. Mol. Wt. 360. An isomer of *maltose* and a product of carbohydrate digestion. Maltose and isomaltose are both composed of two molecules of *glucose*. In maltose, the linkage between the two glucose molecules is $\alpha1\rightarrow4$, and in isomaltose the linkage is $\beta1\rightarrow6$.

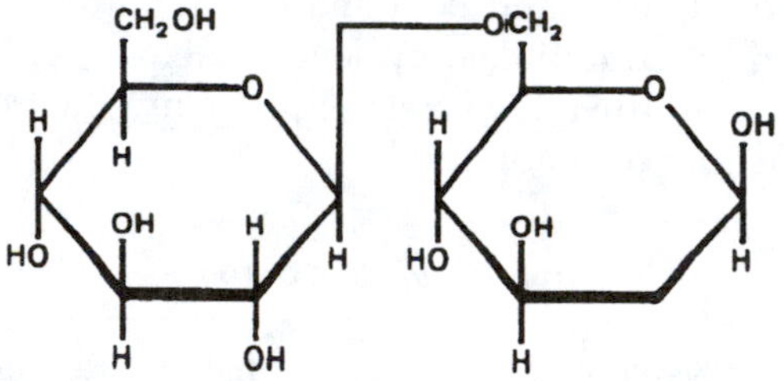

Isomaltose
(β 1$\rightarrow$6) glucopyranosyl-β-D-glucopyranose)

Isoniazid (dioxypyridoxine). Dioxypyridoxine is a chemotherapeutic drug used in the treatment of tuberculosis. It is an *antivitamin* of *pyridoxine* similar to *isonicotinic acid hydrazide*.

isonicotinic acid hydrazide (INH). INH is a chemotherapeutic drug used in the treatment of tuberculosis. It is an *antivitamin* of *pyridoxine*.

isopropyl citrate. A *chelating agent*. See *stearyl citrate*.

isozymes. Enzymes from the same source with identical catalytic properties but with slightly different chemical, physical, or kinetic properties. One of several forms in which an enzyme may exist in various tissues. Although the isoenzymes are similar in catalytic qualities, they may be separated from each other by special physical or chemical methods. Some isoenzymes are used in the diagnosis of certain diseases.

I.U. See *international units*.

J

jaundice. Jaundice is marked by a yellow tint of the skin and whites of the eyes, representing a variety of ailments which may appear at any age. The actual cause is a yellow *bile pigment* called *bilirubin*, which is normally present in a small quantity in the blood. Excessive quantities of this yellow chemical cause jaundice. Bilirubin is a breakdown product of *hemoglobin*, the oxygen-carrying red pigment in the red blood cells that is normally removed from the blood by the liver. Hepatitis is the disorder with which jaundice is associated. In this disease the liver is inflamed and can no longer perform its work of dealing with the bilirubin produced from the normal destruction of old *red blood cells*. The bilirubin content of blood is normally 0.2–0.8 mg/100 mL of plasma. Bilirubin accumulates above normal levels in the bloodstream, and jaundice appears. *Gallstones* may block the *bile duct*, causing bilirubin to back up, resulting in jaundice. In certain forms of *anemia*—for example, *hemolytic anemia*—red blood cells are destroyed at a rate that exceeds the capacity of the liver to deal with the bilirubin; the result is elevated blood bilirubin and jaundice. In all these conditions, jaundice is only a condition, not the underlying cause. Treatment is directed to the cause, not to the symptom.

jejunum. Middle portion of *small intestine*, extending from *duodenum* to *ileum*. See *digestive system*.

joule. The unit of energy is the joule (J). It is the energy expanded when 1 kilogram (kg) is moved 1 meter (m) by a force of 1 newton (N). Physiologists and nutritionists are concerned with large amounts of energy, and the convenient units are the kilojoule (kJ = 103 J) and the megajoule (MJ = 106 J). Formerly, energy was always expressed quantitatively in units of heat, the unit used being the kilocalorie (kcal). This is defined as the amount of heat required to raise the temperature of 1 kg of water from 14.5 to 15.5°C. Conversion from calories to joules is made by multiplying by 4.184.

K

K. The alphabetic symbol for the *essential amino acid lysine* (Lys).

karaya gum. A complex carbohydrate that manufacturers use as a *thickening agent* or *stabilizer* in foods. Manufacturers use karaya gum to prevent oil from separating out of whipped products and salad dressing and to prevent fat from separating from meat and juices in sausages. It improves the texture of manufactured ice cream and sherbet by preventing large ice crystals from forming.

keratin. A scleroprotein which is the principal constituent of the *epidermis*—hair, nails, horny tissues, and the organic matrix of the enamel of the teeth.

keratinization. A state in which the *epithelial cells* become dry and flattened, then gradually harden, forming rough, horny scales. The skin and the palms of the hands and the bottoms of the feet are normal keratinized tissues. This process may occur abnormally in the conjunctive cornea, the respiratory tract, the gastrointestinal tract, the genitourinary tract, or become excessive in the epidermis.

keratomalacia. Dryness and ulceration of the cornea resulting from *retinol* (vitamin A) deficiency.

keto. A prefix denoting the presence of the carbonyl group attached to two carbons. See *acetone*.

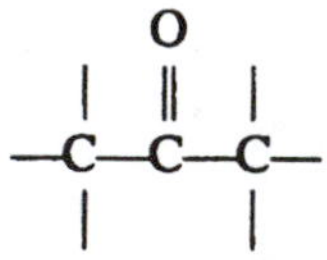

$$
\begin{array}{ccc}
 & \text{O} & \\
| & \| & | \\
-\text{C}- & \text{C} & -\text{C}- \\
| & & | \\
\end{array}
$$

Keto group

keto acid. An organic acid containing a keto group. Alpha (α) keto acid forms when *amino acids* are deaminated or transaminated and is common in intermediary metabolism. *Pyruvate* is an example of an α-keto acid; it is derived from the amino acid *alanine*.

ketogenesis. The formation of *ketone bodies* from *fatty acids* and some amino acids. See *metabolic acidosis*.

ketogenic. Capable of being converted into *ketone bodies*. Ketogenic substances in metabolism are the *fatty acids* and the amino acid *leucine*. The *amino acids lysine, phenylalanine,* and *tyrosine* are both *ketogenic* and *glucogenic*.

ketoglutaric acid. See *alpha* (α) *ketoglutaric acid*.

ketone. Any compound containing a keto group. See *acetone* and *fructose*.

ketone bodies. Substances in the blood that cause a condition called metabolic acidosis or *ketosis*. The ketone bodies are *acetone, beta* (β) *hydroxybutyric acid* and *acetoacetic acid*. The ketone bodies occur in the bloodstream as a result of incomplete oxidation of *fatty acids*.

ketosis. A condition in which there is an accumulation in the blood of *ketone bodies* (*beta* (β) *hydroxybutyric acid, acetoacetic acid*, and acetone) as a result of incomplete oxidation of fatty acids. Ketosis occurs when the amount of fat being oxidized is excessive, as with the use of ketogenic diets, in semistarvation, and in uncontrolled *diabetes mellitus*.

kidneys. The kidneys are bean-shaped organs about 4 inches long, 2 inches wide, and 1 inch thick. They lie on each side of the spinal column, against the posterior wall of the abdominal cavity, near the level of the last thoracic vertebra and the first lumbar vertebra. The right kidney is usually slightly lower than the left. Near the center of the medial side of each kidney is the central notch, or hilum, where blood vessels and nerves enter and leave and from which the ureter leaves. The kidneys are composed of an outer shell, or cortex, and an inner layer, the medulla. The cortex is made of firm, reddish-brown tissue containing millions of microscopic filtration plants called *nephrons*. Each nephron is a *urine*-forming unit made up of a *glomerulus* and a tubule. The nephron units receive and filter all the body's blood, about once every 12 minutes. Large protein molecules cannot pass through this filtering apparatus. Small molecules, small proteins, and salts are filtered through but may be actively reabsorbed by enzymes in the tubules. *Glucose* is an example of a small molecule that is filtered through the filtering apparatus, the *glomerulus*, but is reabsorbed through tubules and does not normally appear in the urine. In *diabetes mellitus* the concentration of glucose in the blood is so high that it exceeds the ability of tubules of the kidney to reabsorb it all. Glucose therefore appears in the urine during diabetes. During filtration, the *nephrons* draw off and filter the blood to

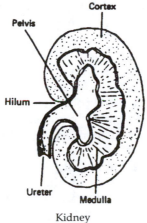

Kidney

remove wastes and to return the usable portion of the filtrate to the circulation to maintain the body's fluid balance. The final result is urine which enters the bladder by way of the collecting tubules and the ureter.

kidney stones. A kidney stone or urinary *calculus* is formed because the concentration of a particular substance in the *urine* exceeds its solubility. A low urine volume and the pH of the urine are also factors. About 95% of all kidney stones contain *calcium*. They also may contain magnesium and ammonia combined with phosphate, carbonates, and oxalates. Four percent of renal calculi consist of *uric acid,* and 1% are *cystine* stones. They vary in size from fine, gritty particles to those which fill the pelvis of the kidney, and they may form in either the kidney or the bladder. The presence of mineral deposits in the kidneys may occur in *hyperparathyroidism* (overactive *parathyroid glands*), in which oversecretion of the parathyroid hormone, *parathormone,* causes loss of calcium from the bones, resulting in a high blood level of calcium with increased secretion of calcium in the urine. Immobilization for long periods of time, *osteoporosis,* or an abnormally high intake of milk, alkalies, or *vitamin D* may also give rise to the formation of calcium phosphate stones.

kilocalorie (kC or kcal). The unit of heat used in nutrition. The amount of heat required to raise 1000 g water 1 °C (from 15.5 to 16.5 °F); also known as the large calorie.

kilogram. One thousand *grams*.

kinetic energy. The capacity to do work as a result of motion. For example, the kinetic energy of a waterfall can be used to turn a generator to make electricity.

kola. See *cola.*

Krebs' cycle (tricarboxylic acid cycle, citric acid cycle). The Krebs' or tricarboxylic acid cycle is the enzymatic pathway for the oxidation of *fatty acids, carbohydrates,* and *proteins.* The members of the cycle act in a catalytic manner in that they are regenerated, and increasing the concentration of any member of the cycle increases the rate of the entire cycle. Central to the oxidation of fatty acids, carbohydrates and proteins is their conversion to *acetyl coenzyme A* (acetyl-CoA) by catabolic processes. The acetyl-CoA, a two-carbon compound, reacts with *oxalacetic acid* of the Krebs' cycle to form *citric acid,* a tricarboxylic acid. In the progress of the cycle, oxidation and decarboxylation reactions occur. The result is that oxalacetic acid is regenerated to react with other acetyl-CoA molecules, two CO_2 molecules are produced, and several *coenzymes* are reduced. The reduced coenzymes are oxidized by the *terminal respiratory chain* via the *cytochromes.* The result of these oxidations is the formation of water. Thus, in the oxidation of acetyl-CoA, the overall action is acetyl-CoA + CO_2 = $2CO_2$ + $2H_2O$+ CoA + *energy.* The CO_2 molecules arise from the reactions of the Krebs' cycle and the H_2O and energy arise from the reactions of the terminal respiratory chain. These pathways provide for about 90% of the energy in the body. Both the tricarboxylic acid cycle and the terminal respiratory chain are contained within the subcellular particles called *mitochondria.*

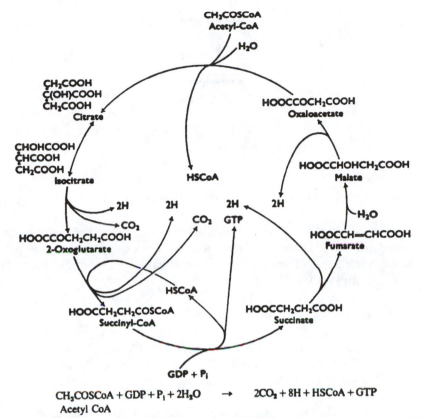

$$CH_3COSCoA + GDP + P_i + 2H_2O \quad \rightarrow \quad 2CO_2 + 8H + HSCoA + GTP$$
Acetyl CoA

Of the 8H, 3 pairs pass through NAD to the cytochrome electron transport chain·yielding 3 ATP each. 1 pair passes to FAD and hence to the electron transport system yielding 2 ATP Total—11 ATP.

$$8H + 2O_2 + 11ADP + 11P_i \quad \rightarrow \quad 4H_2O + 11H_2O + 11ATP$$

Sum Total

$$CH_3COSCoA + GDP + 11ADP + 12P_i + 2O_2 \quad \rightarrow \quad 2CO_2 + 13H_2O + GTP + 11ATP + HSCoA$$

Krebs' cycle (tricarboxylic acid cycle, citric acid cycle)

kwashiorkor. A nutritional disease described as *protein-calorie malnutrition* (PCM). The disease is caused by a low and insufficient protein intake, even though the total caloric intake may be adequate. The symptoms are *edema*, apathy, scaly and depigmented skin, and depigmented hair. The disease is usually found in the tropics and subtropics among children 1–4 years old. It is also seen in the United States among neglected and abused children. Kwashiorkor is an African word with disputed definition. It is sometimes translated as "red boy" because African children with the disease often have a characteristic red hair color. Kwashiorkor is also translated as "displaced child" since the nutritional disease has its onset when another child is born and the weanling must eat the protein-deficient diet of the community or tribe. See *marasmus*.

L

L. The alphabetic symbol for the *essential amino acid leucine* (Leu).

L. A chemical prefix that denotes a configuration around the asymmetric carbon of a compound base on the configuration of D-and L-glyceraldehyde. For example, the configuration of the alpha (α) carbon in amino acids found in proteins is always the L-configuration. The opposite configuration of D-compound series.

labile. Not fixed, unstable or easily destroyed.

lactalbumin. The albumin of milk and cheese. It is a soluble simple protein. Lactalbumin is present in higher concentration in human milk and cow's milk. When milk is heated, the lactalbumin coagulates and appears as a film on the surface of the milk.

lactase. An enzyme produced by the mucosal cells that hydrolyze the *disaccharide lactose* (milk sugar) to yield equal amounts of the *monosaccharides glucose* and *galactose* during the digestive process. If milk is absent or severely restricted in diets after weaning, the enzyme disappears in humans somewhere between infancy and adulthood, as it does in most mammals. Once lactase is lost, it cannot be recovered. The absence of lactase produces a condition called *lactose intolerance*. The symptoms of lactose intolerance are mild and are noticeable only when large amounts of milk are ingested. They include nausea, stomach cramps, and diarrhea. The majority of the adult population of the world is lactose intolerant, with the exception of some Caucasians and a few African tribes that keep cow herds and drink milk. The enthusiasm for milk as a major source of protein, worldwide or individually, should be balanced with the possibilities of an intolerance for milk.

lactate. Any salt derived from *lactic acid*.

lactation. The secretion of *milk* by the *mammary gland* is called lactation. *Progesterone* and *estrogens* inhibit prolactin (*luteotropic hormone, LTH*) and the production of milk during the pregnancy period. Following childbirth, progesterone and estrogens decrease and LTH then induces the formation of milk. Just prior to childbirth, colostrum is produced and is the newborn's first nourishment. See *oxytocin*.

lacteals. Tiny vessels in microvilli of the intestinal mucosa through which absorbed fat is transported. They are part of the *lymphatic system*. The intestinal lymphatics take up *chyle* and pass it to the lymph circulation and, by way of the thoracic duct, to the blood vascular system.

lactic acid. Mol. Wt. 90. A three-carbon acid produced in milk by bacterial fermentation of *lactose*. It is also produced during muscle contraction by anaerobic *glycolysis*. For the most part, lactic acid is produced industrially by means of homofermentative lactic acid bacteria, or bacteria resembling them. In the food industry, lactic acid is used to acidify jams, jellies, confectionery, sherbets, soft drinks, extracts, and other products. It is added to brines for pickles, olives, and horseradish, and to fish to aid in preservation. In addition, it makes milk more digestible for infants. Calcium lactate is an important ingredient of some *baking powders*.

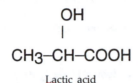

Lactic acid

lactic acid culture. The most commonly used dairy starter is the common butter or lactic starter, which normally consists of a mixture of strains of *Streptococcus lactis* and *S. cremoris* for the production of lactic acid and *Leuconostoc dextranicum* and *L. citrovorum* or *Streptococcus diacetilactis* for the production of flavor and aroma. *Leuconostoc* strains are often included in cultures for making ripened cheeses. The mixed lactic cultures are used in the manufacture of cultured buttermilk, butter, and most types of cheeses in which the curd is heated at a comparatively low temperature, for example, cottage, cream, Limburger, cheddar, blue, and brick cheeses. The aroma bacteria are especially important in flavor production in cultured buttermilk, butter, and uncured cheeses.

Lactobacillaceae. The very important food bacteria in this family are called the lactic acid bacteria, or "lactics." They ferment sugar chiefly to *lactic acid*, if they are homofermentative, plus small amounts of *acetic acid*, *carbon dioxide*, and trace products; or if they are heterofermentative, they produce appreciable amounts of volatile products, including alcohol, in addition to lactic acid. The type of lactic acid, D- or L-, produced is characteristic of the organism and the medium. The most important characteristic of the lactic acid bacteria is their ability to ferment sugars to lactic acid.

lactogenic hormone. See *luteotropic hormone (LTH)*.

lactones. Lactones are oxygen-containing heterocyclic compounds. They are usually five-membered rings having different structures and odors. Some of the lactones are added to foods for their pleasant aromas and some occur naturally. The aromas of some alcoholic beverages are in part due to lactones.

lactose (milk sugar). Mol. Wt. 342. A *disaccharide* composed of *glucose* and *galactose*. It is the form of carbohydrate in milk. Lactose occurs in the milk of all mammals, constituting usually from 6–7% of the fresh secretions in human milk and 4.5–5% in the milk of cows and goats. Lactose is less sweet and much less soluble than *sucrose*, dissolving only to the extent of about 1 part in 6 parts of water. When hydrolyzed either by heating with acid or by an enzyme such as the *lactase* of the intestinal juice, each molecule of lactose yields one molecule of glucose and one of galactose. Hence the lactose ingested is absorbed, not as such, but as a mixture of equal parts of glucose and galactose. Lactase is often lost in adults, who then become intolerant to milk.

Lactose
β (1→4) D-galactosyl-β-D-galactopyranose

lactose intolerance. The inability to digest lactose, milk, or milk products. See *lactase*.

laetrile (vitamin B$_{17}$). See *amygdalin*.

lamina propria. Connective tissue structure that supports the *epithelium* of the *intestinal mucosa*.

lard. The fat rendered from fresh, clean, sound fatty tissues of hogs at the time of slaughter. The fat tissues do not include bones, detached skin, head fat, ears, tails, organs, windpipes, large blood vessels, scrap fat, skimmings, settlings, pressings, and the like, and are reasonably free from muscle tissue and blood. Lard is used as an ingredient of margarine and cooking fats, and whenever an edible fat is required in baking. Lard contains high concentrations of *saturated fatty acids*.

lathyrism. See *lathyrogens*.

lathyrogens. A spastic paralysis of the legs, comes from *Lathyrus*, the Latin name for certain members of the pea family recognized as having toxic qualities. *Lathyrus sativa*, the chick-pea, *L. cicera*, the flat-podded vetch, and *L. clymenum*, the Spanish vetchling, are three of the more widely eaten species of *Lathyrus* from which lathyrogens can be isolated. Regular and continued consumption of chick-pea meal results in muscular weakness and spastic paralysis of the legs. It is believed that lathyrogen, β-N-oxylyl-L-α-β-diaminopropionic acid, a neurotoxic amino acid, is the substance in chick-peas and vetch responsible for lathyrism.

lauric acid (laurostearic acid). Mol. Wt. 200. $CH_3 \cdot (CH_2)_{10} \cdot COOH$. A *saturated fatty acid*. It occurs abundantly as *glyceride* in the fat of the seeds of the spice bush, and in smaller proportions in butter, coconut fat, palm oil, and some other vegetable oils.

laxative. A mild carthartic that has the action of loosening the bowels without pain or violent action.

leafy vegetables. In the amounts commonly consumed, leafy vegetables are not important energy-yielding foods; however, their less digestible carbohydrates (*hemicellulose* and *cellulose fiber*) provide an abundance of roughage, which is an important component of a normal diet. Their protein is generally of high quality, though not abundant in quantity. The value of leafy vegetables lies primarily in their vitamin and mineral content. Most vegetable leaves are rich sources of provitamin A (*carotene*) and good sources of *iron, calcium, riboflavin,* and *folacin*.

The greener the leaf, the higher the carotene content. Carotene from leafy vegetables is more readily absorbed and utilized than that from yellow ones. Fresh vegetable leaves are also good sources of *ascorbic acid* (vitamin C). Unfortunately, much of this ascorbic acid is often lost before consumption through oxidation and leaching during preparation. Though little carotene is lost in cooking, portions of the water-soluble vitamins and appreciable quantities of iron, magnesium, and phosphorus may be lost if the cooking water of vegetable leaves is discarded.

leaven. Various substances which lighten dough or batter while it is baking and make it more palatable. The word comes from the Latin *levare* which means "to raise." Though air and steam act as leavening agents to a certain extent, the oldest and best-known ingredient used for leavening is yeast. Leavening agents increase the surface area of dough through the release of gases within the dough. The expansion of these gases during baking increases the size of the finished food and gives a desirable porous structure. Of the gases created, the principal one is *carbon dioxide*; the others are air and water vapor or steam. Air is a physical means of leavening. It may be incorporated into the batter by means of an egg-white foam or to a lesser degree by creaming fat and sugar. Chiffon, angel food, sponge cakes, and soufflés are examples of air used as leavening. Steam, another physical leavening, occurs when water is exposed to high temperature. Popovers and cream puffs are leavened by steam. *Baking soda*, also known as *sodium bicarbonate* or bicarbonate of soda, is a chemical leavening agent. When the soda is heated in the presence of moisture, carbon dioxide gas is produced. When used by itself, soda leaves a disagreeable taste and produces a yellow color. To prevent this, an acid substance, such as *cream of tartar*, sour milk, or molasses, is usually used in combination with the soda. *Baking powder*, another chemical leavening agent, is in three forms. The tartrate powders, containing *cream of tartar* and *tartaric acid*, react quickly in batter or dough at room temperature. The phosphate powder, containing calcium acid phosphate, releases two-thirds of its gas at room temperature and the remainder when heat is applied. The double-acting powder contains sodium aluminum sulfate and calcium acid phosphate; it releases a small portion of gas when ingredients are combined, but the greater amount is released in the oven. Yeast is a living plant which can produce carbon dioxide under suitable environmental conditions. It is available in two forms, active dry and compressed. The metabolic processes of the yeast furnish gaseous carbon dioxide, which creates bubbles in the bread and makes it rise. Sourdough is a fermented dough which produces carbon dioxide under suitable environmental conditions. Other actively gas-forming microorganisms, such as wild yeasts, coliform bacteria, saccharolytic *clostridium* species, heterofermentative bacteria, acid bacteria, and various naturally occurring mixtures of these organisms, have been used instead of bread yeasts for leavening.

lecithin. A *phospholipid* containing *glycerol*, *fatty acids*, *phosphoric acid*, and *choline*. Any of a group of fatty substances occurring in animal and plant tissues such as soybeans, corn, and egg yolk, composed of units of choline, phosphoric acid, fatty acids, and glycerol. Because lecithin is an *emulsifying agent*, it has become widely used, especially by health food adherents, on the basis that its presence in the blood may dissolve cholesterol deposits. Lecithin, like cholesterol, also is made within the body. Food manufacturers use lecithin as an *antioxidant* and *emulsifier*. Pure lecithin is an important source of choline. The lecithin used as food additives is obtained almost exclusively from the soybean. Used primarily as an emulsifier in margarine, chocolate, ice cream, and baked goods to promote the mixing of oil (or fat) and water. The hydrocarbon chains (R, R') of the fatty acid given in the diagram vary depending upon the source of the lecithin.

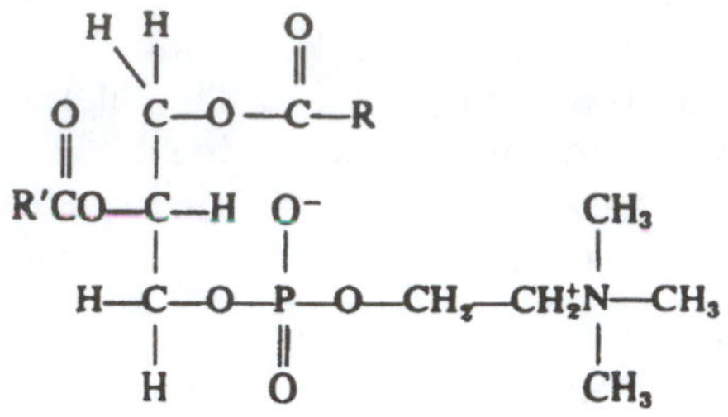

$$
\begin{array}{c}
\overset{H}{\underset{|}{\overset{H}{\diagdown}}}\,\,\,\,\,\,\,\overset{O}{\overset{\|}{}} \\
O\,\,\,\,\,\,C\!-\!O\!-\!C\!-\!R \\
\underset{\|}{\overset{\|}{}}\,\,\,\,\,\,\,| \\
R'CO\!-\!C\!-\!H\,\,\,\,O^- \,CH_3 \\
|\,\,\,\,\,\,\,\,\,\,\,\,\,\,| \\
H\!-\!C\!-\!O\!-\!P\!-\!O\!-\!CH_2\!-\!CH_2^+N\!-\!CH_3 \\
|\,\,\,\,\,\,\,\,\,\,\,\,\,\,\|\,| \\
H\,\,\,\,\,\,\,\,\,O\,CH_3
\end{array}
$$

Lecithin

leek (*Allium porrum*). The first cousin of the *onion* and *garlic* has a cylindrical stalk with a small simple bulb, and flat, juicy, compactly rolled-up leaves which are dark green at the top and white towards the bulb. Leeks have a mild onion flavor and are used as a seasoning or a vegetable. The green part has some *carotene* (vitamin A activity).

Nutrients in 100 g of leeks

CALORIES KCAL	PROTEIN G	FAT G	CARBOHYDRATE G	VITAMIN A IU	ASCORBATE MG	CALCIUM MG
52	2	0.3	11	40	17	52

legumes. Food plants which have pods that open along two seams when the seeds are ripe. Legumes are seeds and nuts, although technically they are hard-shelled fruits, similar to seeds in composition. The seeds are usually the edible part of the legume. Peas, chick-peas, beans, lima beans, soybeans, peanuts, and lentils are the best-known food legumes. There are more than 11,000 species of legumes. They are the most important food plants next to cereals. This food group resembles the grains but is characterized by almost twice as much protein as grains. The dried legumes (beans, peas, lentils, and cowpeas), because of their low moisture content, are as much as 60% carbohydrate (starch) and 22% protein. Although they are often classed as "meat substitutes," an average serving furnishes probably only about one-third as much protein as an average (l00 g) serving of meat. The quality of their protein is somewhat inferior to that of animal foods, except for the proteins of the peanut and soybean, which are of good *biological value* (BV). As a rule, most legumes are good sources of *thiamine* and contribute moderate amounts of *riboflavin* and *niacin*. They also contain significant quantities of *phosphorus* and *iron* and lesser amounts of *calcium*. Soybeans (soybean flour) have a high protein content. They are also a good source of calcium and iron and contain more fat than most other legumes.

lemon (*Citrus limon*). The lemon tree, a member of the *citrus* family, is a small tree which grows 10–20 feet in height. It has a short spine and large, fragrant, white-and-purple flowers. The light yellow fruit is small, oval, and ends in a blunt point. The pulp of the fruit is juice and acid, containing 0.5% sugar and 5% *citric acid*. An excellent source of *ascorbic acid* (vitamin

C). One lemon provides 40–80% of one day's need for vitamin C. See this item in the table under *fruits*.

lemon balm. See *balm*.

lentil (*Lens culinaris*). This *legume* is one of the first plants whose seeds were used for food. The lentil seed is small and lens-shaped. It is never used green, but is dried when it is fully ripe. The lentil is extremely nutritious, a good source of carbohydrates and incomplete protein, and a good meat, milk, cheese, and egg supplement. Lentils also contain some B vitamins and are a good source of iron, with fair amounts of calcium and *carotene* (vitamin A activity).

Nutrients in 100 g of dry, raw lentil

CALORIES KCAL	PROTEIN G	FAT G	CARBOHYDRATE G	VITAMIN A IU	THIAMINE MG	CALCIUM MG
340	25	1	60	60	370	80

lettuce (*Lactuca*). A vegetable whose nutrients are found in the part of the plant that grows above the ground. There are several hundred varieties of lettuce, all originating from a common weed of the roadsides and wastelands of southern Europe and western Asia. The most popular lettuces are: (1) Butterhead, a small, soft, loose-leafed head with its outer leaves light green and its inner leaves light yellow, with a buttery feel. It is a sweet, succulent lettuce. The most common butterhead varieties are Bibb and Boston. (2) Cos or Romaine, a long, cylindrical head with stiff leaves, dark green on the outside, becoming greenish-white near the center. (3) Crisphead, the most popular type of lettuce. The outer leaves are medium-green in color with flaring, wavy edges. The inner leaves are pale green and folded tightly. Iceberg lettuce is a variety of crisphead. (4) Lamb's tongue or field lettuce comes in small clumps of tiny, tongue-shaped leaves on delicate stems. (5) Leaf is a hardy type of lettuce with loose leaves branching from a stalk. It may have a curled or a somewhat smooth leaf of light to dark green. It has a crisp texture. (6) Stem. With an enlarged stem and no head, this lettuce has long, narrow leaves tapering to a point. The flavor is a combination of celery and lettuce. The main variety is celtuce. Lettuce has small amounts of carotene (vitamin A activity) and *ascorbic* acid (vitamin C), and *minerals*, if the outer leaves are eaten. See this item in the table under *vegetables*.

leucine (Leu, L). One of the *essential amino acids* found in proteins.

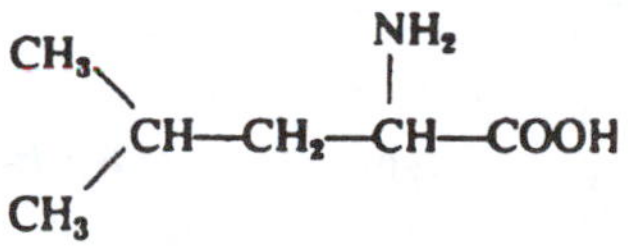

$$\begin{matrix} CH_3 & & NH_2 \\ & CH-CH_2-CH-COOH \\ CH_3 \end{matrix}$$

Leucine (Leu, L)

leukemia. A cancer of the white *blood cells*. White blood cells (leucocytes) formed in this disease are abnormal and usually increased in number. They infiltrate various parts of the body. In the bone marrow they "crowd out" the cells that produce red blood cells, normal white cells, and platelets. Since the new cells utilize the available amino acid and vitamins at a prodigious rate, the person with acute leukemia is very likely to suffer from severe debilitation and *avitaminosis*.

leukocytes, polymorphonuclear. White blood cells which are nearly twice as big as red blood cells and contain both a nucleus divided into several lobes and granules in the *protoplasm*. They are formed from primitive cells in the *lymph glands*, *spleen*, and *bone marrow*. They are concerned with the reaction of the body to infection by bacteria and to foreign material in the tissues. They can engulf bacteria and other foreign particles (*phagocytosis*), and they collect around local areas of infection or damage in very large numbers.

leukotrienes. A family of *eicosanoid hormones* that derive from the polyunsaturated fatty acid *arachidonic acid*. The other families of compounds are the *prostaglandins* and the *thromboxanes*. The leukotrienes have a variety of physiologic effects depending upon the properties of the particular leukotriene. An example of a leukotriene structure is given. See *eicosanoid hormones*, *prostaglandins*, *thromboxanes*.

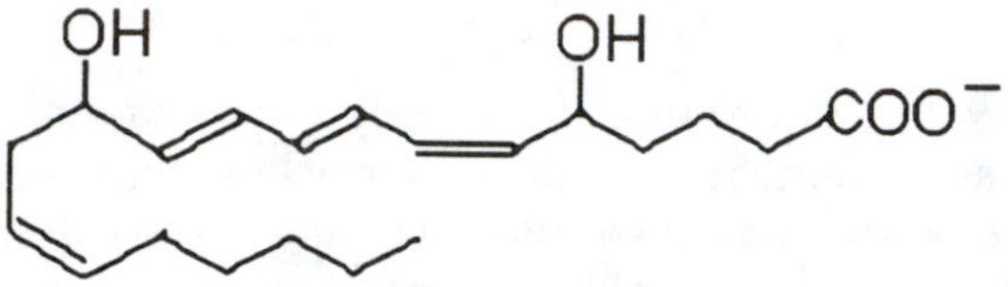

Leukotriene B_4

levulose. See fructose.

lichee. See *litchi*.

licorice (*Glycyrrhiza glabra*). A perennial *herb* of the pea family. It has long rootstocks, feathery leaves, and flowers of various colors, usually pale violet or blue. Its dried root, or an extract made from it, is used to flavor medicines, tobacco, cigars, cigarettes, soft drinks, candy, and chewing gum.

lignin. A constituent of crude *fiber*, occurring in the cell wall of plants, which is not broken down by intestinal microorganisms to any extent. Lignin is a unique compound in the plant wall. It is very insoluble and difficult to digest and thus is the major residue left after acid treatment of a cell-wall material. It is not a carbohydrate, but a small polymer whose basic units are joined by carbon-carbon bonds.

lima bean (*Phaseolus*). This round, full, slightly curved bean is an American native. Lima beans were named after Lima, Peru, where the European explorers first came across them. Fresh lima beans are higher in protein than most vegetables, with fair amounts of *carotene* (vitamin A activity) and *ascorbic acid* (vitamin C). See this item in the table under *vegetables*.

lime (*Citrus aurantifolia*). A small, bushy, and spiny tropical tree which belongs to the *citrus* family. The tree has small white flowers, and its fruit, which measures up to 2.5 inches in diameter, is small and compact and resembles the *lemon* in shape. The rind of the lime is green, with a very acid and juicy pulp, which yields a pungent juice. Oil is extracted from the rind. Limes are an excellent source of *ascorbic acid* (vitamin C). See this item in the table under *fruits*.

linoleic acid. Mol. Wt. 280. An 18-carbon *essential polyunsaturated fatty acid* containing two double bonds. The body is not able to synthesize linoleic acid. It has to be obtained in the diet for growth and general well-being. Linoleic acid occurs only in small amounts in food fats. Soybean oil, with 7%, is the highest. Linoleic acid is of central dietary importance. It is relatively more abundant in foods than *arachidonic acid* (which can be made by the body from linoleic acid) and oleic. Sources of linoleic acid include many grain oils and seed oils, which contain 50% or more. Fats and nuts, peanuts, and poultry carry 20–30%. Fats from such fruits as avocado and olive contain about 10% of linoleic acid. Those from leafy vegetables and legumes run higher, 30% or more, but the total amount of fat in greens is low.

$$CH_3 - (CH_2)_4 - CH = CH - CH_2 - CH = CH - (CH_2)_7COOH$$

Linoleic acid

lipase. Any of a class of enzymes that break down neutral fats or *triglycerides*. A small quantity of gastric lipase (lipase secreted by the gastric mucosa) acts on emulsified fats of cream and egg yolk. The major digestive lipase is pancreatic lipase, which acts upon fats in the small intestine. Intestinal lipases act within the mucosal cells. For the digestive lipases to act properly, the fat must be emulsified. *Bile salts emulsify* fat in the intestine, and it is fat in the intestine that signals the release of bile salts from the *gallbladder*. Lipases catalyze the reaction shown:

Triglyceride $\xrightarrow{\text{lipase}}$ **3 fatty acids + glycerol**

lipase

See *emulsification*, *digestive system* and *pancreatic juice*.

lipase test. An enzyme test on blood, used for the diagnosis of acute pancreatitis.

lipids. Lipids vary considerably both in composition and structure. They occur naturally in both animal and plant foods and vary widely in physical and chemical characteristics. When separated from the surrounding tissues with which they usually are associated, most natural fats and oils are found to consist of approximately 98–99% *triglycerides*; the remaining very small part is composed of *monoglycerides*, *diglycerides*, free *fatty acids*, *phospholipids*, and an unsaponifiable fraction. Neutral fat or *esters* of fatty acids and *glycerol* is a mixed glyceride containing a variety of fatty acids and glycerol. The physical characteristics of a neutral fat are affected by the size of the fat molecule and by the amount of *saturated* and *unsaturated fatty acids* it contains. In general, the more saturated the fat and the higher the molecular weight, the more solid it will be. Glycolipids or cerebrosides are compounds of fatty acids with a carbohydrate and contain nitrogen but no phosphoric acid. Cerebrosides are found in the myelin sheath of nerve fibers in connection with, and possibly in combination with, *lecithin*. *Phospholipids* or phosphatides contain both nitrogen and phosphorus. The best known are the *lecithins*, which are abundant in egg yolk and occur in brain and nerve tissues and in all the cells of the body. *Cephalins* and *spihngomyelin* are examples. *Sterols* are complex monohydroxyalcohols of high molecular weight, which are found in nature combined with fatty acids. They contain carbon, hydrogen, and oxygen. The best known is *cholesterol*, which is very widely distributed in the body, being found in the medullary coverings of nerve fibers, in the blood, in all the cells and liquids of the body, in the sebum secreted by the sebaceous glands in the skin, and in the bile. Fat substances derived from simple and compound lipids by *hydrolysis* or enzymatic breakdown are termed "derived lipids." Three important members of this group are *fatty acids, glycerides,* and *steroids*. Most digestion of fat takes place in the *small intestines*. *Bile* emulsifies the fat and puts it into a form which permits more complete hydrolysis by intestinal and pancreatic enzymes. Fats are broken down to fatty acids, glycerol, and monoglycerides. *Bile salts* and *choline* help in emulsifying these hydrolyzed compounds, producing *micelles* which are absorbed through the brush border of the intestinal mucosa. During the absorption process, the fatty acids, glycerol, and monoglycerides are resynthesized into triglycerides inside the intestinal mucosal cells. See *lipids, classification* and *digestive system.*

lipids, classification. Lipids may be classified in several ways. Two of the most common classifications are given. One classification is based upon the chemical properties and the complexity of the lipid structure. The other is based on the location of the unsaturated bond from the aliphatic end.

Lipid classifications

CLASSIFICATION BASED ON ACYL GROUP	CLASSIFICATION BASED ON POLARITY
Non-Saponifiable Simple Lipids	Polar Lipids
Carotenoids	Glycerophospholipids
Free fatty acids	Glyceroglycolipids
Sterols	Sphingophospholipid
Tocopherols	Sphingoglycolipids
Saponifiable Lipids	Neutral Lipids
Mono-, di-, tri- acyl glycerols	Carotenoids
Glycolipids	Fatty acids
Phospholipids	Mono-, di-, tri- acyl glycerols
Sterol esters	Tocopherols
Waxes	Sterols, sterol esters
	Waxes

Unsaturated fatty acid classifications

FAMILY	NAME	STRUCTURE
$\omega 9$	Oleate	$CH_3-(CH_2)_7-CH = CH-(CH_2)_7-COOH$
$\omega 6$	Arachidonate	$CH_3-(CH_2)_4-(CH = CH-CH_2)_4-(CH_2)_2-COOH$
	Linoleic (essential)	$CH_3-(CH_2)_4-(CH = CH-CH_2)_2-(CH_2)_6-COOH$
$\omega 3$	Eicosapentaenoate	$CH_3-CH_2-(CH = CH-CH_2)_5-(CH_2)_2-COOH$
	α-Linolenic (essential)	$CH_3-CH_2-(CH = CH-CH_2)_3-(CH_2)_6-COOH$

lipogenesis. The formation of *fatty acid* through biosynthetic pathways. The precursor of fatty acids is *acetyl coenzyme A.*

lipoic acid (lipoamide). Mol. Wt. 206. Lipoic acid in the amide form (lipoamide) functions as a cofactor in the oxidative decarboxylation of *pyruvic acid* and α-*ketoglutaric acid*. It functions along with the cofactor form of the B vitamin, *thiamine, thiamine pyrophosphate*. Pyruvate, a key product in *carbohydrate metabolism*, is formed in the beginning pathway of glucose oxidation. A key reaction, an oxidative decarboxylation, transforms pyruvate to *acetyl coenzyme A*, which ultimately enters the *Krebs' cycle* to produce *energy*. A quantitative requirement for lipoic acid in human nutrition has not been established. It is found in many biological materials, including yeast and liver.

Lipoic acid (lipoamide)

lipolysis. The breakdown of fat into its component *fatty acids* and *glycerol* by *hydrolysis*.

lipomas. Fatty *tumors* under the skin, which produce no pain or other symptoms. They may be no larger than a pea, feel soft, move freely under the skin, and rarely become malignant.

lipoproteins. Conjugated proteins that incorporate lipids as a part of their structure. Lipoproteins are associated with a wide variety of complexes that are significant in both the structure and function of cells. Lipoproteins appear to be of two types. Those that exist as relatively discrete and identifiable macromolecules are called "soluble types." Those that are aggregates of the complex membrane structure are called "membrane types" of structural lipoproteins. Most soluble lipoproteins circulate in the blood plasma. Some are involved in *blood clotting*. The ratio of lipid to protein in the serum lipoprotein varies widely, and these variations affect their density. Lipoproteins differ in their densities and flotation rates (Sf values), depending upon the kind and quantity of lipid associated with the protein. Lipoproteins fall into four general classifications which depend on their density. The table gives the major classifications of the lipoproteins and their general names. The HDL (*high density lipoprotein*) and LDL (*low*

Percent compositions of serum lipoproteins

CONSTITUENT	HIGH DENSITY (HDL, α*)	LOW DENSITY (LDL, β*)	VERY LOW DENSITY (VLDL, PRE-B*)	CHYLOMICRONS
Protein	49%	32%	2-13%	0.5%
Triglycerides	7	7	64-80	90
Cholesterol	17	35	8-13	6
Phospholipids	27	25	6-15	4
Density (g/mL)	1.210-1.063	1.063-1.006	1.006	<1.006
Particle size (Å)	70-100	100-300	2000	>2000

* α, pre-β*, and β refer to the relative *electrophoresis* migration rates.

density lipoprotein) levels in the serum are more sensitive indexes of coronary heart disease than total *cholesterol*. The cholesterol in LDL has a direct relationship to coronary heart disease, whereas the cholesterol in HDL has an inverse relationship. In others, it is the distribution of the total cholesterol between the LDL and HDL rather than the total blood cholesterol that better defines the risk of coronary heart disease. The general structure of lipoprotein is shown.

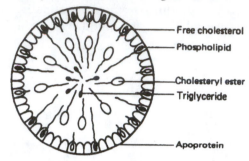

General lipoprotein structure

lipotropic. Pertaining to substances that prevent accumulation of *fat* in the liver. The lipotropic factor is an agent which has an affinity for lipids. It prevents or corrects an excess accumulation of fat in the liver. *Choline* is probably the most important of the lipotropic factors. Protein helps to prevent a fatty liver because it provides amino acids such as *methionine* that contribute to the synthesis of choline.

litchi (lichee) nut (*Litchi chinensis*). The fruit of an ornamental tropical tree, the litchi. The litchi is a very distinctive fruit. It is round and 1–2 inches in diameter. The rough shell is bright red and leathery. Inside, the shimmery, firm white flesh surrounds a single seed. It is juicy and has a pleasant mildly aromatic and slightly acid flavor.

Nutrients in 100 g of litchi nuts

CALORIES KCAL	PROTEIN G	FAT G	CARBOHYDRATE G	ASCORBATE MG	RIBOFLAVIN µG
64	1	0.3	16	42	50

lithiasis. The formation of stones (*calculus*) of any kind, for example, *gallstone* and *kidney stone* formations.

lithocholic acid. Mol. Wt. 377. One of the *bile acids* that form *bile salts* in conjugation with *taurine* or *glycine*. See *bile*.

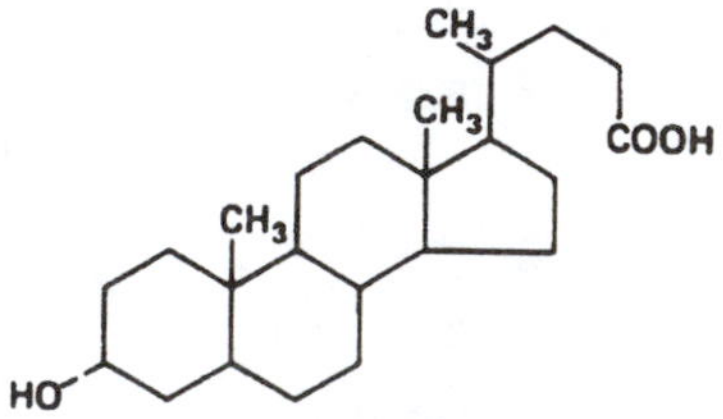

Lithocholic acid

liver. The liver is the largest organ in the body. It is located in the upper part of the abdomen with its larger (right) lobe to the right of the midline. It is just under the diaphragm and over the stomach. The liver has several important functions. One is the secretion of *bile*, which is stored in the *gallbladder* and discharged into the *small intestines* during digestion. The bile contains no enzymes but breaks up the *fat* particles by *emulsification* so that enzymes act faster. The liver performs other important functions. It is a storehouse for sugar of the body (*glycogen*), and for *iron* and the B vitamins. It plays a part in the destruction of bacteria and worn-out red blood cells. Many chemicals, such as poisons or medicines, are detoxified by the liver; others are excreted by the liver through the ducts. The liver manufactures part of the proteins of blood plasma. The blood flow in the liver is of special importance. All the blood returning from the spleen, stomach, intestines, and pancreas is detoured through the liver by the portal vein in the portal circulation, the hepatoportal circulation. Blood drains from the liver by hepatic veins which join a large vein called the inferior vena cava. The liver of animals is used as food. The liver stores more vitamin A and D than other parts of the animal. See this item in the table under *meats*.

liver spots. See *ceroid pigments*.

lobster (*Homarus*). A member of the family of crustaceans to which shrimps and crabs also belong. They lack spinal columns and have "crusty" outer skeletons or shells with jointed bodies and limbs. Live lobsters are mottled and splotched greenish blue, with touches of orange. The vivid red color characteristic of lobsters comes out in cooking. Lobster is a good source of protein and iron. It is low in fat. See this item in the table under *meats*.

locust bean gum. It comes from the endosperm of the bean of the *carob* tree. It is used in food to improve the texture and freeze-melt characteristics of ice cream; to thicken salad dressing, pie filling, and barbecue sauce; to make softer, more resilient cakes and biscuits when used as a dough additive. It also increases the palatability of *carrageenan* gels by decreasing their brittleness and melting temperature. Locust bean gum has a laxative action, indicating that it is not absorbed to any great extent by the body.

loganberry (*Rubus vursinus loganobaccus*). A *berry* resembling a blackberry in shape but its color is red and, when fully ripe, it takes on a purple tinge. In flavor it resembles the raspberry, but is more acidic.

Nutrients in 100 g of loganberries

CALORIES KCAL	PROTEIN MG	FAT G	CARBOHYDRATE G	VITAMIN A IU	ASCORBATE MG	CALCIUM MG
62	1	0.6	15	200	24	35

loquat (*Eriobotrya japonica*). A tropical evergreen tree and its fruit, that is also known as a "Japanese meddler." The loquat tree is a small, ornamental evergreen tree with broad leaves and fragrant white flowers. The fruit is small, round, downy, and yellow-orange in color, with large black seeds. The flesh is pale yellow to orange, very juicy, with a delicious, slightly acid flavor, not as rich and sweet as most tropical fruit.

Nutrients in 100 g of loquats

CALORIES KCAL	PROTEIN G	FAT G	CARBOHYDRATE G	VITAMIN A IU	CALCIUM MG
48	0.4	Trace	12	670	20

lovage (*Levisticum officinale*). A perennial *herb*, also called smellage, a member of the carrot family, to which parsley and celery also belong. Lovage is a tall plant, growing 5–7 feet, with greenish or whitish yellow flowers. Its large heavy, light-green leaves resemble those of celery, and the greens have a celerylike flavor. The root is strong in taste and smell. Fresh and dried leaves of lovage are used for flavor in cooking; the roots may be blanched and served like celery or candied. The leaves are also used as a potherb.

lovastatin. See *cholesterol therapy*.

low-acid. Low-acid foods are those that contain relatively low contents of organic acids. Meat, poultry, and vegetables, except tomatoes, are low-acid foods. Processing acid foods, such as tomatoes, in canning processes can be accomplished at boiling water-bath temperatures because the food acid aids in the destruction of spoilage organisms and prevents the growth of toxins. Processing low-acid foods requires higher temperatures than boiling water. This is usually accomplished by increasing pressures, such as in a pressure cooker.

luteinizing hormone (LH). A *gonadotrophic hormone* of the *pituitary gland* that stimulates conversion of a follicle in the *ovary* into a corpus luteum and secretion of *progesterone* by the corpus luteum. LH also stimulates secretion of sex hormones by the *testes*.

luteotropic hormone (LTH). A *gonadotropin* of the *pituitary gland*, also called the "lactogenic hormone" or prolactin. Luteotropic hormone activates the corpus luteum in the *ovary* and stimulates the production of *progesterone*. LTH may also be involved in mammary gland development.

lymph. Lymph consists of a fluid plasma containing a variable number of lymphocytes, a few granulocytes, no blood platelets, carbon dioxide, and very small quantities of oxygen. In the lymphatics of the intestine, *fat* content is high during *digestion*. Lymph is formed from tissue by the physical process of filtration. *Colloid* substances from tissue are returned to lymph capillaries rather than to the blood. Water, salts, and other substances also enter the lymph capillaries. Since the process of tissue fluid formation is continuous, lymph formation is also continuous. The *lymphatic system* supplements the *capillaries* and veins in the return of the tissue fluid to the blood. Starting as small blind ducts within the tissues, the lymphatic vessels enlarge to form lymphatic capillaries. These capillaries unite to form large lymphatic vessels, which resemble veins in structure and arrangement. Valves in lymph vessels prevent backflow. Superficial lymph vessels collect lymph from the skin and subcutaneous tissue; deep vessels collect lymph from all other parts of the body. The two largest collecting vessels are the thoracic duct and the right lymphatic duct. The thoracic duct receives lymph from all parts of the body except the upper right side. The lymph from the thoracic duct drains into the left subclavian vein, at the root of the neck on the left side. The right lymphatic duct drains into a corresponding vein on the right side. Lymph nodes occur in groups of up to a dozen or more lying along the course of lymph vessels. Although variable in size, they are usually small oval bodies composed of lymphoid tissues. Lymph nodes act as filters for removal of infective organisms from the lymph stream. Important groups of those nodes are located in the axilla, the cervical regions, the submaxillary region, the inguinal (groin) region, and the mesenteric (abdominal) region.

lymph glands. Nodules of lymphatic tissue, found along the path of a lymphatic vessel.

lymph node. A rounded body consisting of an accumulation of lymphatic tissue found at intervals in the course of lymphatic vessels.

lymphatic system. The system of lymph vessels and lymph ducts provides for a drainage system for tissue fluid and is an auxiliary part of the circulatory system, returning an important

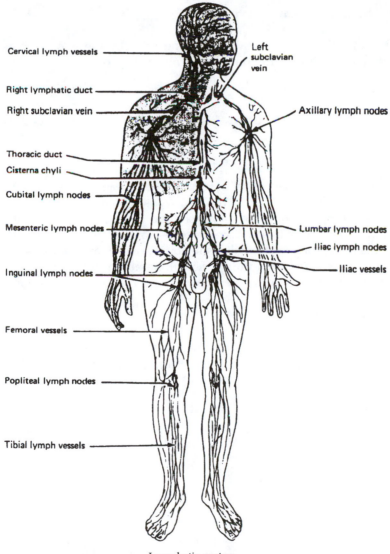

Lymphatic system

amount of tissue fluid to the bloodstream through connection with the lymphatic vessels. The *spleen* belongs in part to the lymphatic system. Unlike the cardiovascular system, the lymphatic system has no pump to move the fluid which it collects, but muscle contractions and breathing movements aid in the movement of lymph through its channels and its return to the bloodstream. A diagram of the lymphatic system is shown. The vessels in the shaded area drain into the right lymphatic duct; the rest drain into the thoracic duct.

lymphocytes. White blood cells that, upon stimulation by an antigen, give rise to plasma cells which produce *antibodies*. They normally number from 20–50% of total white cells but may increase to 90% in lymphatic *leukemia*. Lymphocytes average 10–12 micrometers in diameter but may be as large as 20 micrometers. Characterized by a deeply staining, compact nucleus taking a dark blue. The *nucleus* occupies all or most of the cell, either in the center or at one side. The *cytoplasm* is usually clear, but in some cells bright reddish violet granules are seen.

lyophilization. See *freeze drying*.

lysine (Lys, K). Mol. Wt. 146. It is a basic amino acid. Lysine is one of the *essential amino acids* that is often in low concentration in proteins of plant origin.

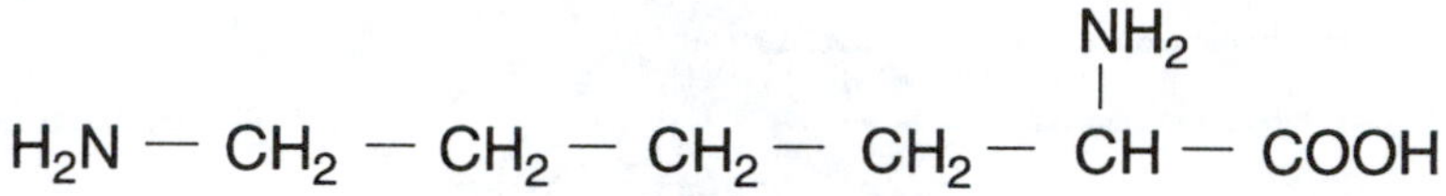

$$H_2N - CH_2 - CH_2 - CH_2 - CH_2 - \overset{\displaystyle \overset{NH_2}{|}}{CH} - COOH$$

Lysine (Lys, K)

lysosomes. Structures (*organelles*) of cell *cytoplasm* that contain degradative enzymes. Seen as "droplets" within the cell which are of different consistency from the rest of the *cytoplasm*. Separation of these droplets from the cytoplasm and chemical analysis indicate that various degradative enzymes are contained within the lysosomal membrane at the edge of the "droplet"—thus cytoplasm is protected from digestion by these enzymes. At the same time, ingested nutrients coming into contact with the lysosomal membrane are engulfed and acted on. In this way, the larger molecules are broken down to smaller ones which the cell can use. See *cells*.

lysozyme. An enzyme that *hydrolyzes* complex *polysaccharides*. It is found in high concentrations in egg white and in human tears. In human tears, lysozyme protects the eyes by hydrolyzing the cell walls of airborne bacteria and thus preventing infection of the *cornea*. It was the first protein for which the complete three-dimensional structure was determined.

M. The alphabetic symbol for the *essential amino acid methionine* (Met).

macaroni. A food paste made from a mixture of semolina and water, and dried in the form of slender tubes or fancy shapes—elbow macaroni and macaroni shells, for example. The *semolina* used is the purified middlings (medium-size particles of ground grain) of durum or other hard *wheat*. Primarily a source of carbohydrate with small quantities of B vitamins.

Nutrients in 100 g of macaroni

CALORIES KCAL	PROTEIN G	FAT G	CARBOHYDRATE G	THIAMINE MG	NIACIN MG	CALCIUM MG
120	4	0.4	25	0.3	3	45

mace. An aromatic *spice* made from the arillode, or false aril, which covers the seed of the *nutmeg*. The nutmeg, a tropical evergreen tree, bears a golden pear-shaped fruit which, when its external covering is removed, reveals a red arillode over its hard kernel (the nutmeg itself). This arillode is dried, becoming yellowish orange and, either whole or powdered, is the mace available.

mackerel (*Scomber scombrus*). A long, slender, saltwater fish, averaging a length of 1 foot and weighing 1–2 pounds. Mackerel scales are small and smooth, its back steely blue or greenish, its belly silvery white. The flesh is firm and fatty with a distinctive flavor and a savory taste. See this item in the table under *meat*.

macrobiotic. Pertaining to a diet based on whole *grains*.

macrocyte. An abnormally large *red blood cell*. The vitamin deficiency disease *pernicious anemia* is characterized by the appearance of macrocytes and a condition called *megaloblastic anemia*. See *folacin (folic acid) deficiency*.

macromolecules. Large molecules made from many smaller units or building blocks by synthesis in living organisms. *Proteins, nucleic acids,* and *polysaccharides* are examples of macromolecules that have *amino acids, nucleotides,* and *monosaccharides*, respectively, as building blocks. Their spatial structure and function are determined by the number and sequence of their smaller units.

macrophage. Cells of the *reticuloendothilium* that can phagocytose particulate substances and colloidal substances.

magnesium (Mg). Element No. 12. At. Wt. 24. Of the total magnesium, about 0.5 mg/kg fat-free tissue, roughly 60%, is located in *bone*. The function of magnesium in hard tissues is not known. One-third of it is in combination with phosphate, and the remainder appears to be absorbed loosely on the surface of the mineral structure of bone. A small amount of magnesium is dissolved in the extracellular fluid and is easily exchanged with that absorbed at the bone surface. Within the cells of soft tissue, the concentration of magnesium is greater than any other mineral except potassium. Loss of magnesium from the body is usually associated with tissue breakdown and cell destruction. Magnesium is required for cellular respiration, specifically in *oxidative phosphorylation* leading to formation of *adenosine triphosphate* (ATP). Magnesium is the activator for many enzymatic reactions, and all reactions where ATP is formed. Magnesium is present in foods from both animal and plant sources. Meats, milk, and cereal grains have more magnesium than other foods. In a diet, most magnesium comes from milk (23%), vegetables including potatoes (20%), cereal products and flour (18%), meat and eggs (13%), coffee and cocoa (9%), fruit (6%), and dry beans, nuts, and legumes (11%). The precise magnesium requirements of humans have not been determined, but diets supplying 250–300 mg per day keep healthy adults in balance.

Magnesium in mg/100 g of food

Grains		Nuts		Meats		Miscellaneous	
bread, white	37	almonds	270	bacon	25	chocolate	131
bread, whole wheat	23	Brazil	225	beef	23	table salt	290
Graham crackers	47	hazel	184	chicken	27	peanut butter	360
oat cereals	112	peanuts	206	lamb	24	Molasses	
oatmeal, dry	144	walnuts	131	pork	25	light	46
Fruits		Vegetables		turkey	28	medium	81
bananas	33	lima beans	48	veal	23	blackstrap	258
blackberries	30	parsnips	33	Fish			
cantaloupe	20	spinach	59	shell fish	28		
raisins	35	Swiss chard	65	shrimp	34		

magnesium trisilicate ($Mg_2O_8Si_3$). A compound salt used as a gastric *antacid*. See *aluminum hydroxide*.

Maillard reaction. The Maillard reaction is the interaction of the ε-amino group with reducing sugars such as *glucose*. The reaction is not enzyme-catalyzed and occurs slowly but spontaneously. It is this reaction that is responsible for the glucosyl forms of hemogloblins in uncompensated *diabetes*.

maize. See *corn*.

malabsorption syndrome. A term used to grossly describe such conditions as the *sprues*; *celiac disease*, and idiopathic *steatorrhea*, which have in common the failure to absorb various nutrients such as fats, calcium, and other minerals, as well as certain vitamins, notably the fat-soluble ones: *retinol* (vitamin A), *vitamin D*, *tocopherol* (vitamin E), and *vitamin K*.

malic acid (malate). Mol. Wt. 134. A substance occuring in large amounts in apples, with other fruits containing smaller amounts. The change in flavor that occurs as a fruit ripens is due partly to a decrease in malic acid content and to an increase in sugar content. Malic acid is an important metabolite and is present in all living cells. Used by the food industry as an *acidulant* and *flavoring agent* in fruit-flavored drinks, candy, lemon-flavored ice tea, ice cream, and preservatives. Two forms of malic acid exist, the D-form and the L-form.

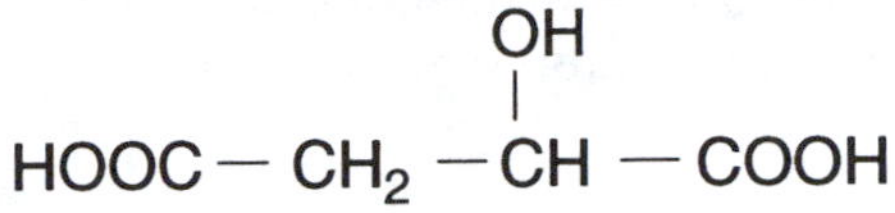

$$HOOC - CH_2 - \overset{\displaystyle OH}{\overset{\displaystyle |}{CH}} - COOH$$

Malic acid

malignant. Occurring in severe degree, frequently fatal. In tumors it refers to uncontrolled growth, as in *cancer*.

malnutrition. A state of impaired functional ability or development caused by an inadequate or excessive intake of essential nutrients or calories to provide for long-term needs. When any of the vitamins is inadequate, the condition is described generally as an *avitaminosis*. Some of the well-defined avitaminoses are given in the table. Most conditions that lead to malnutrition involve the deficiencies of more than a single essential nutrient and the disease symptoms are usually very complex and vary greatly among individuals. Malnutrition may also result from insufficient intake of certain essential *minerals*. Some well-defined mineral deficiencies are given in the table. Malnutrition resulting from insufficient protein and calorie intake results in disease states described as *protein energy malnutrition* (PEM) or protein-calorie malnutrition (PCM). The disease primarily associated with insufficient protein intake is *kwashiorkor*; and with insufficient calories and protein, *marasmus*. The precise nutritional needs for an individual vary with age, sex (and in the case of women, pregnancy), and energy expenditure, among other factors. Severe malnutrition in children leads to retarded growth and mental development,—all patients suffer from impaired healing, impaired resistance to infection, and impaired ability to withstand stress.

VITAMIN DEFICIENCY	NUTRITIONAL DISEASE OR SYMPTOM
Vitamin A (retinol)	Nyctalopia (Night blindness)
Vitamin B$_1$ (thiamine)	Beri-beri
Niacin (nicotinamide)	Pellagra
Vitamin C (ascorbic acid)	Scurvy
Vitamin D	Rickets (children)
	Osteomalacia (adults)

MINERAL DEFICIENCY	NUTRITIONAL DISEASE OR SYMPTOM
Calcium	Osteomalacia
Iron	Anemia
Iodine	Goiter

malonyl coenzyme A. An intermediate compound in the biosynthesis of *fatty acids*.

malt. A substance made by sprouting or germinating grains, generally barley, but occasionally corn, rye, and oats. After sprouting, the grains are dried and ground. During the process, various enzymes, among them diastase, are formed, partially converting the starch to sugar and changing proteins to amino acids. This makes the formerly hard, raw grain into a mellow, crisp, sweet-tasting malt. When grain is malted, it contributes carbohydrates and proteins to the diet. Malt is used in brewing, distilling, yeast making, vinegar making, and as an additive to milk.

maltase. An enzyme in the *intestinal juices* that splits *maltose* by enzymatic *hydrolysis* into two molecules of *glucose*. See *digestion*.

malt beverages. Beer and ale are the principal malt beverages, made of malt, hops, yeast, water, and malt adjuncts. Malt is prepared from barley grains which have been germinated and dried, and then had the sprouts or germs removed. Hops are the dried flowers of the hop plant. The malt adjuncts are starch- or sugar-containing materials added to the carbohydrates. Starch adjuncts include corn and corn products, rice, wheat, barley, sorghum, grain, soy beans, cassava, potatoes, etc., with corn and rice used most frequently.

maltol, ethyl maltol. A substance used by food manufacturers to enhance the flavor and aroma of fruit-, vanilla-, and chocolate-flavored foods and beverages. Small amounts of maltol occur naturally in bread crust, coffee, and chicory and as a degradation product in heated milk, cellulose, and starch. Used in gelatin deserts, soft drinks, ice cream, and other foods that are high in carbohydrates. Levels used range from 15–250 ppm for maltol and 1–50 ppm for ethyl maltol. Ethyl maltol can be used in diet foods to mask the bitter aftertaste of *saccharin* and in ordinary foods to permit a lower sugar content.

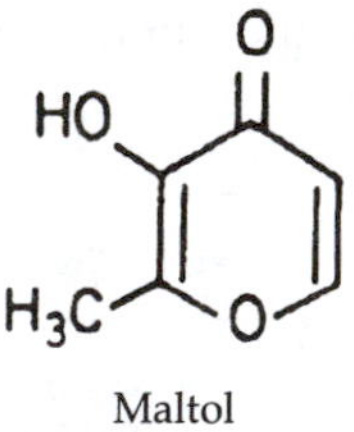

Maltol
3-Hydrooxy-2-methylpryan-4-one

maltose. Mol. Wt. 360. A *disaccharide* resulting from starch hydrolysis. Maltose yields two molecules of *glucose* on hydrolysis. It forms from starch by the action of enzymes (*amylases*). Malt and malt products are important constituents of germinating cereals. It is also formed as an intermediate product when starch is digested in the human or other animal body or hydrolyzed by boiling with dilute mineral acid as in the manufacture of commercial glucose. Maltose is also readily and completely hydrolyzed by boiling with dilute mineral acids or by the enzyme *maltase* during *digestion*. In either case each molecule of maltose yields two molecules of *glucose*.

CH₂OH   CH₂OH

Maltose
α(1→4) glucopyranosyl-β-D-glucopyranose

mammary glands. Mammary glands are present in females and in males in a rudimentary state. When pregnancy occurs, the mammary glands undergo marked changes. *Estrogens* induce the growth and development of the duct system. *Progesterone* induces the development of the alveoli and other presecretory changes. Prolactin (*luteotropic hormone, LTH*) from the *pituitary gland* induces the active secretion of milk. Near the end of a pregnancy, a clear watery fluid called *colostrum* is produced. Milk is produced about the fourth day after delivery. After *lactation*, all of the mammary gland secreting elements undergo an involution. After menopause, there is a further reduction in size.

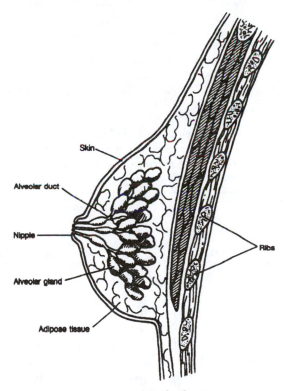

Mammary gland
(van de Graaff, K.M., and Rhees, R.W., *Human Anatomy and Physiology*, 1987. Reproduced with permission of McGraw-Hill.)

manganese (Mn). Element No. 25. At. Wt. 55. A *trace element* that can be toxic at high concentrations and cause symptoms of neurologic trouble similar to those found in Parkinson's disease. Manganese has many essential functions in each cell of the body. High concentrations are in the *pituitary gland*, lactating *mammary glands*, *liver*, *pancreas*, *kidney*, *intestinal wall*, and *bone*. The entire adult human body contains about 20 mg manganese. The highest concentration is in the bones, where it is found both in inorganic salts and in the cells of the organic matrix. Absorption of manganese by the body is rather poor and is adversely affected by large amounts of dietary calcium and phosphorus. Excretion is considerable in the *feces*, but urinary losses are very small. The mineral is transported through the body in the plasma, bound to a protein called transmanganin. Manganese is most plentiful in wheat germ, meat, whole buckwheat, barley seed, grapenuts (a cereal), pecans, almonds, and Brazil nuts, dry green split peas, fresh turnip greens, fresh spinach, and fresh brussels sprouts. See *minerals*.

Manganese in µg/100 g of food

Bananas	640	Flour, wheat	4300	Peas, dried	1990
Beans, dried	1500	Kale	590	Prunes	436
Beans, green	325	Lettuce	1240	Rice, white	1010
Beets	575	Liver	390	Rye, whole	3065
Corn, whole	680	Oatmeal, dry	4945	Spinach	825
Flour, white	710	Onions	363	Sweet potato	405

mango (*Mangifera indica*). A tropical fruit of the mango tree. The fruit is oblong in shape and about the size of a large pear. It is green in color, turning orange-yellow when ripe, and has a delicious, pleasantly acid pulp. Mangoes are eaten fresh or may be made into jams or jellies or such desserts as ice cream. Mangoes are rich in β-*carotene* (vitamin A activity), *ascorbic acid* (vitamin C), and *vitamin D*.

Nutrients in 100 g of mango

CALORIES KCAL	PROTEIN G	FAT G	CARBOHYDRATE G	VITAMIN A IU	ASCORBATE MG	CALCIUM MG
140	1	1	34	4000	30	10

manioc (*Manihot*). A tropical plant, also known as cassava, mandioc, or yucca. The roots yield a tuber which is a staple food in Central and South America. The word comes from the language of the Tupi and Guarani, South American Indian tribes. The manioc or cassava plant is a shrubby perennial that grows to a height of 9 feet, with large parted leaves and roots that end in very large tubers. The tubers produce a flour with an extremely high starch content, which varies from 15–30 percent in contrast to 15–20 percent for potato flour. The flour has very little taste and is used in place of wheat flour. It is either made into nonsweet, thin cakes used like wheat bread, or sprinkled over rice and beans to make them more filling. There are many varieties of manioc; the two most widely grown for their starchy content are the bitter manioc (*Manioc utilissima* or *esculenta*) and the sweet (*Manioc dulcis*, variety *Aipi*). *Tapioca* is made from properly treated manioc flour. After the juice has been extracted from the pulp, the pulp is heated over a slow fire until it forms grains which harden in cooking. The roots of the sweet manioc contain no poisonous juices. They are usually roasted under hot ashes and eaten plain or with butter. Their flavor resembles that of the chestnut and they are very high in starch.

manna. The dried sap of certain species of ash, tamarisk, and other trees that grow in the Sinai Desert.

mannitol. Mol. Wt. 182. A versatile substance occurring naturally in the *manna* ash tree. It is made by hydrogenation or reduction of *mannose* and *galactose* in the same manner as *sorbitol* is made from *glucose*. Commercial quantities are made by synthesis from sugar. Mannitol has a variety of industrial uses in the manufacture of foods. It is used as a "dust" in chewing gum, to prevent gum from absorbing moisture and becoming sticky. Mannitol is about two-thirds as sweet as *sucrose*. Since only about 50% is used by the body it only generates half as many calories as an equal weight of sugar. Mannitol is frequently used as a sweetening agent in noncalorigenic chewing gum because bacteria in the mouth have an even harder time digesting it than do humans.

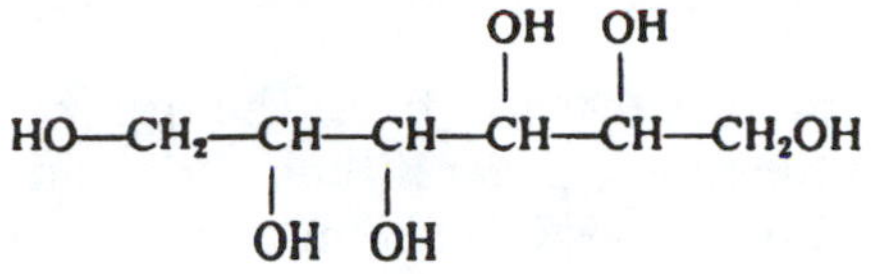

$$HO-CH_2-CH-CH-CH-CH-CH_2OH$$

with OH groups at positions as shown

Mannitol

mannose. Mol. Wt. 180. A hexose of more interest to sugar chemists than nutritionists. Small amounts are found in certain foods such as *manna*, from which it takes its name.

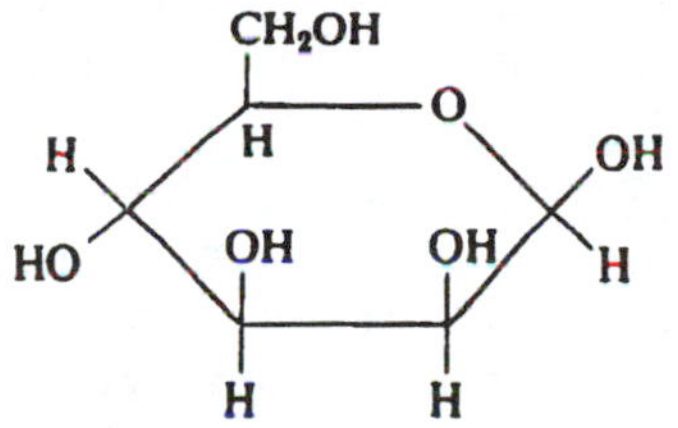

Mannose
β-D-mannopyranose

maple (*Acer*). A tree native to the north temperate zone. There are 13 species of maple native to the American continent. The sugar, or rock maple (*A. saccharum*) is highly valued as a timber and shade tree and is the chief source of maple sugar. All maples have a sweet sap, but only the sugar maple and the black maple are tapped to make maple syrup. When the syrup is boiled to the density of strained honey, it is called maple honey. Maple cream or maple butter is syrup boiled to the soft-sugar stage, cooled, and then stirred smooth. Maple sugar is syrup boiled to the hard-sugar stage and then stirred to prevent the individual crystals of sugar from hardening together. Maple syrup can be used on hot cereals, pancakes, waffles, and other quick breads; to sweeten milk, custards, bread puddings, and applesauce and other fruits. A good source of *sucrose* with some *invert sugar* and *ash*.

marasmus. A *protein-calorie malnutrition* (PCM) disease. In marasmus, both protein and calories are deficient. It is most common in children under 2 years old. There is no *edema* but there is emaciation and diarrhea is common. There is no depigmentation of the skin or dermatosis. See *kwashiorkor*.

margarine. A smooth-textured *fat* used as a spread and in cooking. It may be prepared from animal or vegetable fats or a combination of them in amounts specified by law. The fats may or may not be *hydrogenated*. The fat ingredients are mixed with pasteurized cream, milk, skim milk, or nonfat dry milk, or any combination of these. When the fat source is vegetable, the fat may be mixed with ground soybeans and water. Optional ingredients such as coloring, flavoring, preservatives, *retinol* (vitamin A activity) and *vitamin D, emulsifiers*, butter, and salt may be added. Differences in ingredients affect the flavor, texture, color, spreadability, baking quality, and nutritive value of the finished product. Margarine contributes calories and vitamins A and D.

marjoram (*Majorana hortensis*). A culinary *herb*, a member of the mint family, known better as sweet marjoram or knotted marjoram. Its downy light-green oval leaves, up to 1 inch long, have a mild sagelike flavor, although less strong than *sage*.

marmalade. A preserve of fruit, usually *citrus* fruit. The fruits are cut into thin slices with the peel, and cooked in water until tender. Sugar is then added and the mixture is cooked again until the solids are suspended in a clear, jellylike mixture. The word marmalade comes from the Portuguese *marmelada*, derived from the Latin *melimelum* meaning "honey apple," which in turn can be traced to the Greek *melimelon*, from *meli*, "honey," and *melon*, "apple."

marrow, beef. The fatty filling of beef bones, which is prized for its rich and delicate taste and which is also one of the lightest and most digestible of *fats*. Marrow is used to enrich dishes, or by itself as a spread, or baked or broiled in the bone. It is very rich in fat with very small amounts of protein. It has the same caloric value as beef fat.

marrow, vegetable (*Cucurbita pepo*). A squash-like edible gourd shaped like a long egg. These gourds can grow to a very large size, but it is the smaller marrows which are best for eating. They are peeled, cut into halves, and seeds removed from the center; they are cooked as any firm *squash* is cooked. Marrow is similar to squash in food and caloric value.

marshmallow. An American confection made of sugar, unflavored gelatin, corn syrup, and flavoring. The mixture is whipped until very light, poured into a pan lined with sugar and cornstarch, and allowed to stand until firm. Then the marshmallows are cut into squares and rolled in additional sugar and cornstarch. A 100 g serving of marshmallows contains about 135 calories.

mast cells. Loose connective tissue cells. They are most numerous along blood vessel beds. They form the *anticoagulant heparin*. *Histamine* is also liberated from those cells in allergic and inflammatory reactions.

mastication. The act of chewing. The function of the mouth, as far as alimentation is concerned, is the ingestion of food, the reduction in its size by the action of the teeth, the mixing of particles with *saliva*, and then the passage of the food into the pharynx in order to be swallowed. Saliva contains an enzyme—*ptyalin*, or *salivary amylase*—that initiates the digestion of at least one of the foodstuffs, namely, carbohydrates.

maté. A beverage made from the leaves of various species of holly, chiefly, *Ilex paraguensis*, which is also known as yerba maté or Paraguay tea. The plant is an evergreen shrub or small tree. Maté is a relatively inexpensive drink popular in most South American countries. It is greenish in color, has an agreeable aroma, and a slightly bitter taste, which is different from that of tea and less astringent. It is a stimulant, containing up to 5% *caffeine*. Maté is usually drunk as is, but can be flavored in any way. It can be bought in specialty and health-food stores, and prepared and served like tea.

matrix. The groundwork in which something is cast; for example, protein in the bone matrix into which mineral salts are deposited.

mayonnaise. A cold sauce of French origin made with egg yolks, oil, and seasonings, which are blended into an emulsion. It is used as a spread; a sauce for fish, meat, and vegetables; and a salad dressing. One tablespoon contains 110 calories, and 100 g contains 718 calories.

mead. An ancient drink made of water and honey, fermented with malt, yeast, and other ingredients. The word is connected with the Greek *methy*, "wine," and the Sanskrit *madhu*, "sweet," "honey," or "mead."

meat. The meat group includes beef, veal, mutton, lamb, pork, poultry, and fish. It is essentially the flesh of any animal, of which more than 100 species are regularly eaten by humans. Mammalian lean meat contains about 20% protein and 5% fat. Lean fish contains about 10% protein and less than 1% fat. Fat fish contain from 8–15% fat. Shellfish, lobsters, crayfish, crabs, shrimp, and other crustaceans have very little fat but are rich in *cholesterol*. Meat ranks as high nutritionally as it does in popularity. It forms the basis for one of the four major food groups required for a balanced diet (the others are the milk, bread-cereal, and vegetable-fruit groups). Meat is essentially protein and the word comes from the Greek word meaning "first" or "of primary importance." In general, meat contains about 20–23% protein, a variable amount of fat and lesser constituents, and about 60% water. The amount of fat in meats varies with the nutritional state of the animal and the extent of trimming and method of preparation. In addition to protein, muscle meat contributes moderate amounts of *thiamine* and *riboflavin*, moderate amounts of *iron*, and generous quantities of *niacin* and *phosphorus*. The organ meats, particularly *liver* and *kidney*, furnish proteins of a very high quality, generous quantities of practically all the B-complex vitamins, iron, phosphorus, *copper*, and other *trace minerals*, and small amounts of *ascorbic acid* (vitamin C). In addition, liver contains very large quantities of *retinol* (vitamin A). Besides the muscle of animals, almost any part of the animal organs is a good source of high-quality protein and *biological value*, having a good supply of all of the *essential amino acids*. Liver and kidney have been mentioned, but heart, tongue, brain, thymus and pancreas (sweetbreads), tripe (ox or sheep stomach), calves and pig feet, maws (pig stomach), and chitterlings (pig intestines) are a few examples of organ meats which are used as food. It is all of good nutritional value. The table gives the nutritional content of some of the common meats and organ foods.

medium-chain triglycerides. Medium-chain triglycerides are used in treating various aspects of malabsorption syndromes, such as *sprue* and *steatorrhea*. It is known that medium chain esters are absorbed from the gastrointestinal tract by pathways different from conventional fats. The absorption rate and metabolism of medium-chain triglycerides is rapid. They have a low tendency to be deposited in the depot fat. It has been shown that chain lengths of 12 carbons (C_{12}) and above tend to be deposited as depot fat, but chain lengths of C_{10} and below do not have this tendency. Medium-chain triglycerides are saturated in nature, but they lower

Meat and Organ Foods	Wt. GM	Approximate Measure	Food Energy CAL	Protein GM	Fat GM	Carbohydrate Total GM	Fiber GM	Water GM	Calcium μG	Phosphorus μG	Iron μG	Vitamin A I.U.	Thiamine μG	Riboflavin μG	Niacin μG	Ascorbic Acid μG
Brains, all kinds, raw	100	3½ ozs.	125	10	9	1	0	79	10	312	2.4	0	0.23	0.26	4.4	18
Crabs, Atlantic and Pacific, hard shell, steamed	100	3½ ozs.	93	17	2	1		79	43	175	0.8	2,170	0.16	0.08	2.8	2
Canned, meat only	100	3½ ozs.	101	17	3	1		77	45	182	0.8		0.08	0.08	1.9	
Duck, domestic raw, flesh only	100	3½ ozs.	165	21	8	0	0	69	12	203	1.3		0.10	0.12	7.7	
Eels, raw, American	100	3½ ozs.	233	16	18	0	0	66	18	202	0.7	1,610	0.22	0.36	1.4	
Fish:																
Bluefish:																
Baked or broiled	100	3½ ozs.	159	26	5	0	0	68	29	287	0.7	50	0.11	0.10	1.9	
Fried	100	3½ ozs.	205	23	10	5	0	61	35	257	0.9		0.11	0.11	1.8	
Cod:																
Broiled	100	3½ ozs.	170	29	5	0	0	65	31	274	1.0	180	0.08	0.11	3.0	
Dried	100	3½ ozs.	375	82	3	0	0	12		891	3.6	0	0.08	0.45	10.9	0
Flounder, baked	100	3½ ozs.	202	30	8	0	0	58	23	344	1.4		0.07	0.08	2.5	
Haddock, fried	100	3½ ozs.	165	20	6	6	0	67	40	247	1.2		0.04	0.07	3.2	
Halibut, broiled	100	3½ ozs.	171	25	7	0	0	67	16	248	0.8	680	0.05	0.07	8.3	2
Herring:																
Atlantic, raw	100	3½ ozs.	176	17	11	0	0	69		256	1.1	110	0.02	0.15	3.6	
Pacific, raw	100	3½ ozs.	98	18	3	0	0	79		225	1.3	100	0.02	0.16	3.5	
Canned in tomato sauce	100	3½ ozs.	176	16	11	4	0	67		243				0.11	3.5	
Smoked, kippered	100	3½ ozs.	211	22	13	0	0	61	66	254	1.4	30		0.28	3.3	
Mackerel:																
Atlantic, broiled	100	3½ ozs.	236	22	16	0	0	62	6	280	1.2	530	0.15	0.27	7.6	
Pacific, canned, solids and liquid	100	3½ ozs.	180	21	10	0	0	66	260	288	2.2	30	0.03	0.33	8.8	
Salmon																
Cooked, broiled or baked	100	3½ ozs.	182	27	7	0	0	63		414	1.2	160	0.16	0.06	9.8	
Canned: solid & liquid																
Chinook or King	100	3½ ozs.	210	20	14	0	0	65	154	289	0.9	230	0.03	0.14	7.3	

Food	Measure														
Pink or humpback	100 3½ ozs.	141	21	6	0	0	70	196	286	0.8	70	0.03	0.18	8.0	
Sockeye or red	100 3½ ozs.	171	20	9	0	0	67	259	344	1.2	230	0.04	0.16	7.3	
Smoked	100 3½ ozs.	176	22	9	0	0	59	14	245						
Sardines:															
Atlantic type, canned in oil drained solids	100 3½ ozs.	203	24	11	0	Tr.	62	437	499	2.9	220	0.03	0.20	5.4	
Pacific type,															
In brine or mustard	100 3½ ozs.	196	19	12	2		64	303	354	5.2	30	0.01	0.30	7.4	
In tomato sauce	100 3½ ozs.	197	19	12	2		64	449	478	4.1	30	0.01	0.27	5.3	
Shad, baked	100 3½ ozs.	201	23	11	0	0	64	24	313	0.6	30	0.13	0.26	8.6	
Swordfish, broiled	100 3½ ozs.	174	28	7	0	0	65	27	275	1.3	2,050	0.04	0.05	10.9	
Tuna fish, canned in oil drained solids	100 3½ ozs.	197	29	8	0	0	61	8	234	1.9	80	0.05	0.12	11.9	0
Canned in water solids and liquid	100 3½ ozs.	127	28	1	0	0	70	16	190	1.6			0.10	13.3	
White fish, cooked baked, stuffed	100 3½ ozs.	215	15	14	6		63		246	0.5	2,000	0.11	0.11	2.3	Tr.
Frog legs, raw	100 3½ ozs.	73	16	Tr.	0	0	82	18	147	1.5	0	0.14	0.25	1.2	
Heart:															
Beef, lean, braised	100 3½ ozs.	188	31	6	1	0	61	6	181	5.9	30	0.25	1.22	7.6	1
Chicken cooked	100 3½ ozs.	173	25	7	Tr.	0	67	4	107	3.6	30	0.06	0.92	5.3	4
Pork, cooked	100 3½ ozs.	195	31	7	Tr.	0	61	4	121	4.9	40	0.20	1.72	6.7	1
Kidneys, raw:															
Beef	100 3½ ozs.	130	15	7	1	0	76	11	219	7.4	690	0.36	2.55	6.4	15
Lamb	100 3½ ozs.	105	17	3	1	0	78	13	218	7.6	690	0.51	2.42	7.4	15
Pork	100 3½ ozs.	106	16	4	1	0	78	11	218	6.7	130	0.58	1.73	9.8	12
Lamb, trimmed to retail basis cooked:															
Chop, thick, broiled															
Lean and fat	100 3½ ozs.	359	22	29	0	0	47	9	172	1.3		0.12	0.23	5.0	
Lean only (from above serving)	66 2.4 ozs.	125	19	5	0	0	41	8	145	1.3		0.10	0.18	4.1	
Leg, roasted															
Lean and fat	100 3½ ozs.	266	26	17	0	0	55	11	212	1.8		0.15	0.27	5.6	
Lean only (from above serving)	85 3 ozs.	121	19	4	0	0	41	8	157	1.5		0.11	0.20	4.1	

Meat and Organ Foods	Wt. GM	Approximate Measure	Food Energy CAL	Protein GM	Fat GM	Carbohydrate Total GM	Fiber GM	Water GM	Calcium μG	Phosphorus μG	Iron μG	Vitamin A I.U.	Thiamine μG	Riboflavin μG	Niacin μG	Ascorbic Acid μG
Shoulder, roasted																
Lean and fat	100	3½ ozs.	338	22	27	0	0	50	10	172	1.2		0.13	0.23	4.7	
Lean only (from above serving)	74	2.7 ozs.	150	20	7	0	0	46	9	162	1.4		0.11	0.21	4.3	
Liver:																
Beef:																
Raw	100	3½ ozs.	140	20	4	5	0	70	8	352	6.5	43,900	0.25	3.26	13.6	31
Fried	100	3½ ozs.	229	26	11	5	0	56	11	476	8.8	53,400	0.26	4.19	15.6	27
Calf, fried	100	3½ ozs.	261	30	13	4	0	51	13	537	14.2	32,700	0.24	4.17	16.5	37
Chicken, simmered	100	3½ ozs.	165	27	4	3	0	65	11	159	8.5	12,300	0.17	2.69	11.7	16
Lamb, broiled	100	3½ ozs.	261	32	12	3	0	50	16	572	17.9	74,500	0.49	5.11	24.9	36
Pork, fried	100	3½ ozs.	241	30	12	3	0	54	15	539	29.1	14,900	0.34	4.36	22.3	22
Lobster:																
Raw	100	3½ ozs. meat	91	17	2	1	0	79	29	183	0.6		0.40	0.05	1.5	
Canned or cooked	100	3½ ozs.	95	19	2	Tr.	0	77	65	192	0.8		0.10	0.07		
Luncheon meat:																
Canned, ham or pork	100	3½ oz. slice	294	15	25	1	0	55	9	108	2.2	0	0.31	0.21	3.0	
Oysters, meat only, raw																
Av. Eastern	100	5–8 medium	66	8	2	3		85	94	143	5.5	310	0.14	0.18	2.5	
Oyster stew:																
1 part oysters to 3 parts milk by volume	100	½ c. scant	86	5	5	5		84	117	109	1.4	280	0.06	0.18	0.7	
Pork, fresh, trimmed to retail basis, cooked:																
Chop, thick:																
Lean and fat	100	1 large chop 3½ ozs.	391	25	32	0	0	42	12	268	3.4	0	0.96	0.28	5.6	
Lean only from 1 chop	72	2.6 ozs.	195	22	11	0	0	38	9	248	2.7	0	0.82	0.24	4.9	
Roast, loin or shoulder	100	3½ ozs.	373	23	31	0	0	45	10	232	2.9	0	0.50	0.23	4.9	

Food	g	Measure													
Lean only from above serving	77	2.9 ozs.	182	22	10	0	0	44	9	226	2.8	0	0.46	0.22	4.2
Picnic cut simmered															
Lean and fat	100	3½ ozs.	374	23	31	0	0	46	10	139	3.0	0	0.54	0.25	4.8
Lean only from above serving	74	2.6 ozs.	157	21	7	0	0	45	9	130	2.7	0	0.49	0.22	4.4
Pork, smoked ham															
Ham, cooked															
Lean and fat	100	3½ ozs.	289	21	22	0	0	54	9	172	2.6	0	0.47	0.18	3.6
Lean only from above serving	84	3 ozs.	157	21	7	0	0	52	9	170	2.7	0	0.49	0.19	3.8
Ham, canned	100	3½ ozs.	193	18	12	1	0	65	11	156	2.7	0	0.53	0.19	3.8
Pork, fat, salted raw	100	3½ ozs.	783	4	85	0	0	8	Tr.	Tr.	0.6	0	0.18	0.04	0.9
Shrimp, French fried	100	3½ ozs.	225	20	11	10		57	72	191	2.0		0.04	0.08	2.7
Canned, dry pack or drained	100	3½ ozs.	116	24	1	1	0	70	115	263	3.1	60	0.01	0.03	1.8
Sausage:															
Bologna	100	3½ ozs.	304	12	28	1	0	56	7	128	1.8		0.16	0.22	2.6
Frankfurter, cooked	100	2 medium	309	13	28	2	0	56	7	133	1.9		0.16	0.20	2.7
Liver, liverwurst	100	3½ ozs.	307	16	26	2	0	54	9	238	5.4	6,350	0.20	1.30	5.7
Pork, links or bulk, cooked	100	3½ ozs.	476	18	44	0	0	35	7	162	2.4	0	0.79	0.34	3.7
Pork, bulk, canned	100	3½ ozs.	381	18	33	0	0	43	11	210	2.8	0	0.20	0.24	3.0
Vienna sausage, canned	100	3½ ozs.	240	14	20	0	0	63	8	153	2.1	0	0.08	0.13	2.6
Scallops, cooked, steamed	100	3½ ozs.	112	23	1	Tr.	0	73	115	338	3.0				
Tongue beef, canned	100	3½ ozs.	267	19	20	0	0	57	10	180	2.5	0	0.05	0.22	2.5
Turkey, total edible roasted	100	3½ ozs.	263	27	16	0	0	55				Tr.	0.09	0.14	8.0
Flesh only, roasted	100	3½ ozs.	190	32	6	0	0	61	8	251	1.8		0.05	0.18	7.7
Veal, cooked:															
Cutlet, broiled	100	3½ ozs.	234	26	13	0	0	59	11	225	3.2	0	0.07	0.25	5.4
Roast, medium fat, rib 82 percent lean	100	3½ ozs.	269	27	17	0	0	55	12	248	3.4	0	0.13	0.31	7.8
Stew meat without bone medium fat, cooked	100	3½ ozs.	303	26	21	0	0	52	12	138	3.3	0	0.05	0.24	4.6

serum *cholesterol* levels much like the polyunsaturated oils. In animal studies, the medium-chain triglycerides demonstrate a low order of deposition of cholesterol in liver, arteries, and heart, in contrast to the conventional fats and oils, saturated and unsaturated.

megakaryocyte. Large *bone marrow* cells with large or multiple nuclei.

megaloblast. Primitive *red blood cells* of large size with large nuclei; present in blood when there is a deficiency of *cobalamin* (vitamin B_{12}) and/or *folacin*. See anemia, *pernicious*.

megaloblastic anemia. *Anemia* marked by the presence of oversize nucleated red blood cells in bone marrow (megaloblasts). *Megaloblasts* are large-size nucleated abnormal red blood corpuscles from 11–20 microns in diameter, oval and slightly irregular. The condition is found in cases of *cobalamin* (vitamin B_{12}) and *folacin* deficiency.

megavitamin doses. The ingestion of vitamins at levels many times the *Recommended Dietary Allowances* (RDA). Except when recommended by a physician as a specific therapy, there is no clear evidence that any of the vitamins taken in excess of the RDA has an added beneficial effect. High ingestion levels of *retinol* (vitamin A) and *vitamin D* have in fact led to *vitamin toxicity* (*hypervitaminosis*). Even the water-soluble vitamins, though not generally considered as toxic, can cause toxic symptoms in some individuals when taken for prolonged periods at high levels. The toxicity level for vitamins appears to vary considerably among individuals, and may vary by factors as high as 100.

meiosis. (1) The process whereby a germ cell, with two of each *chromosome*, gives rise to sperm, or eggs, each with only one of every pair of chromosomes. (2) The mechanism underlying the process that produces sex cells. As for genetics, the most important consequence of meiosis is that it results in cells that contain only one complete set of genes. Since genes are located on chromosomes, this means that cells produced by meiosis contain only half the chromosome number that other cells have, the *haploid* number as compared with the *diploid* number. *Mitosis* results in two cells identical to one another and to the parent cell that divided to produce them. All have the diploid number of chromosomes. In human beings, meiosis produces cells with 23 chromosomes in the nucleus of sperm and eggs, and mitosis produces cells with 46.

melanin. The dark, amorphous pigment of the skin, hair, and certain other tissues. The amino acid *tyrosine* is a precursor to melanin. An inborn error of tyrosine metabolism called albinism causes a generalized lack of pigment in the skin, eyes, and hair. Exposure to sunlight stimulates melanin production. It is present in some cancers such as melanoma.

melanocyte-stimulating hormone (MSH). The smallest part of the *pituitary gland* is the median lobe which produces just one hormone, melanocyte-stimulating hormone (MSH). Melanocytes are cells in the skin which contain the dark pigment melanin. In the presence of MSH, these cells become more prominent and so make the skin darker. There are also indications that MSH can affect the excitability of the central nervous system. Like all pituitary hormones, MSH is made up of *peptides*. Compared with other hormones, MSH is really quite a small peptide.

melatonin. A hormone of the *pineal gland* that inhibits the output of sex hormones. Evidence suggests that melatonin influences the *biological clock*.

melon. A fruit of a number of annual trailing plants which grow from seed and belong to the gourd family, *Cucurbitaceae*. The word "melon" comes from the Greek *meleopepon*, a combination of *melon* meaning "apple" and *pepon*, a kind of edible gourd. The two best-known groups of edible melons are *Cucumis melo*, the *muskmelons*, and *Citrullus vulgaris*, the *watermelons*. Muskmelons are divided into two principal varieties: the net-skinned, *C. melo cantalupensis*, of which *cantaloupes* and Persian melons are the most familiar; and the smooth-skinned, *C. melo inodorus*, to which group *honeydews* and *casabas* belong. There are many varieties of these two types of muskmelons, including Crenshaw, honeyball, and Christmas melons.

membrane. A thin layer of cells forming a pliable tissue that serves as a covering or envelope of a part, a lining of a cavity, a partition (septum), or a connection between structures. Certain membranes are combined layers of *tissues* that form partitions, lining envelopes, or capsules. They reinforce and support body organs and cavities. Others are a combination of connective tissue only (examples: mucous, pleural, pericardial, and peritoneal membranes). Connective tissue membranes are combinations of connective tissue only (examples: meninges, fascia, periosteum, and synovia). Different kinds of membranes are associated with different body systems (examples: pleural membranes with the respiratory system; pericardial membranes with the *circulatory system*; peritoneal membranes with the *digestive system*; meningeal membranes with the nervous system; fascial membranes with the muscular system; and periosteal and synovial membranes with the skeletal system).

membrane, mucous. A mucous membrane is usually composed of three layers of tissue: the *epithelium*, a supporting lamina propria, and a thin, usually double layer of smooth muscle. The mucous membranes are attached to the parts beneath them by loose connective tissue, called submucous connective tissue. The functions of the mucous membranes are protection, support of blood vessels and lymphatics, and provision of a large surface for secretion and absorption.

membranes, serous. Thin, transparent, strong, and elastic membranes whose surfaces are moistened by a self-secreted serous fluid. They consist of simple squamous *epithelium* and a layer of areolar connective tissues which serve as a base. Serous membranes are found lining the body cavities and covering the organs which lie in them, and forming the fascia bulbi and part of the membranous labyrinth of the ear. The functions of the membranes are mainly protective, such as secreting serum which covers their surfaces, and supplying the lubrication for organs as they move over each other. See *tissues*.

membranes, synovial. Membranes associated with the bones and muscles. They consist of an outer layer of fibrous *tissue* and an inner layer of areolar connective tissue with loosely arranged collagenous and elastic fibers, connective tissue cells, and fat cells. Synovial membranes secrete synovia, a viscid fluid that resembles the white of egg and contains *hyaluronic acid*. They are divided into three classes: articular marosae, mucous sheaths, and bursae mucosae. The function of synovial membrane is mainly protective, such as providing secretory serum which covers its surface, and supplying the lubrication for organs as they move over each other.

menadione. Mol. Wt. 172. A synthetic compound, having greater *vitamin K* activity than the naturally occurring vitamin; used as a reference standard for biological assays of vitamin K.

In large doses, this form of synthetic vitamin K has produced toxic effects; consequently, a dose in excess of 5 mg should be avoided.

menhaden oil (*Brevoortia tyrannus*). The menhaden is a food fish found in very large quantities off the eastern coasts of North America. The flesh of the fish contains about 14% *oil*. The color varies with the quality of the oil and the care and speed that have been secured in its production.

Menkes' syndrome. A rare, genetically determined failure of *copper* (Cu) absorption, leading to progressive mental retardation; failure to keratinize hair, which becomes kinky; hypothermia; low concentrations of Cu in plasma and liver; skeletal changes, and degenerative changes in the elastic membrane.

menopause. A permanent cessation of menses.

menses. A physiologic hemorrhage in females that occurs at approximately 4-week intervals. The source of the hemorrhage is the uterine membrane. Under normal circumstances, hemorrhage is preceded by ovulation.

menstrual. Pertaining to the *menses*.

mercury (Hg). Element No. 80. At. Wt. 201. A silver-white, heavy liquid metal, slightly volatile. Though naturally occurring in small amounts, mercury has increased in concentration because of industrial wastes. It has been found to be close to toxic levels in some samples of seafoods. The highest permissible level in American foods is 0.5 ppm. Mercury is readily absorbed by intact skin and the respiratory and gastrointestinal tracts.

mesentery. A peritoneal fold encircling the greater part of the *small intestine* and connecting the intestine to the posterior abdominal wall.

messenger RNA (mRNA). A *ribonucleic acid* (RNA) that carries the code (translation) for a particular protein or peptide sequence from the nuclear *deoxyribonucleid acid* (DNA) to a *ribosome* in the cytoplasm and acts as a template for the assembly of that protein from amino acids attached to a transfer ribonucleic acid (tRNA).

metabolic acidosis. Metabolic acidosis is a blood pH value below 7.4 as a result of acid substances caused by metabolic processes. Metabolic acidosis occurs in circumstances and diseases such as *ketosis* in uncompensated diabetes, starvation, chronic renal failure, or the loss of bicarbonate in severe diarrhea.

metabolic alkalosis. A result of faulty intake or output of *bases*. Metabolic alkalosis occurs where there is an abnormally high loss of *hydrochloric acid* (HCl). Loss of HCl occurs as a result of vomiting. Metabolic alkalosis can also occur by the ingestion of large amounts of alkaline salts such as bicarbonates.

metabolic disorders. Any disorders of metabolism of acquired or genetic origin. See *inborn errors of metabolism*.

metabolic pool. The assortment of nutrients available within the body at any given moment for the metabolic activities of the body, for example, amino acid pool, calcium pool. A reference to metabolic pools may be considered from the cellular level to the whole animal.

metabolism. A general term used to cover all the chemical changes that go on in the tissues of the body. It includes both synthetic (*anabolic*) and degradative (*catabolic*) pathways. Metabolism = anabolism + catabolism. Under *energy metabolism* are included the chemical changes by which *fats, carbohydrates,* and *proteins* (and alcohol) are broken down and gradually oxidized to release energy as heat, or by which they may be synthesized into compounds such as *adenosine triphosphate* (ATP), chemical energy used for work and biosynthetic processes. Metabolism includes only chemical changes within tissue cells; it does not include those changes that occur in digestion of foods. The diagram greatly simplifies the metabolism of the foodstuffs protein, fat, and carbohydrates. Anabolism includes the chemical changes whereby simple substances are combined to form more complex substances with the net result that new cellular materials are produced and energy may be stored. This is necessary for growth and for maintenance and repair of body tissues. Catabolism includes those processes concerned with the breaking down of the complex substances into simpler constituents for energy production or excretion. These processes occur constantly and simultaneously in the body. When anabolism exceeds catabolism, the breakdown is faster than the build-up process, making the body lose substance and weight. In health, a balance is maintained between these two constantly operating opposing processes so that body weight and tissue substances are maintained in adults.

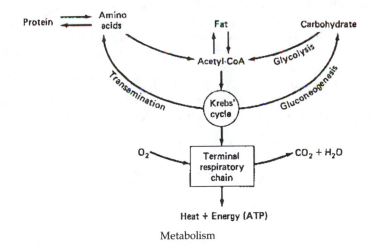

Metabolism

metabolite. A nutrient or compound used in normal biological processes, especially in intermediary metabolism.

metastasis. The establishment of malignant tumors or malignant neoplasm or cancers at sites distant from the primary site of development. Malignant cells migrate from the initial or primary site and establish growth sites at distant sites or organs. Benign tumors grow but do not metastasize.

methanol (wood alcohol). Mol. Wt. 32. CH_3OH. An *alcohol* derived from wood. It is poisonous and cannot be treated to make it nonpoisonous. It is not to be confused with *ethanol* (CH_3CH_2OH).

methemoglobin. When the iron in hemoglobin becomes oxidized to the ferric (Fe^{+3}) state the result is methemoglobin, which lacks the ability to combine with oxygen. Methemoglobin formation can be caused by phenacetin, nitrites, nitrates, and acetanilid.

methionine (Met, M). Mol. Wt. 149. An *essential amino acid*. The body can make *cysteine* from methionine but not vice versa, so methionine is the dietary essential. Methionine is concerned with the important process of transmethylation. The chief dietary sources of methyl ($-CH_3$) groups appear to be methionine and betaine. They are called methyl donors. Methionine gives up the −CH3 group attached to its sulfur atom.

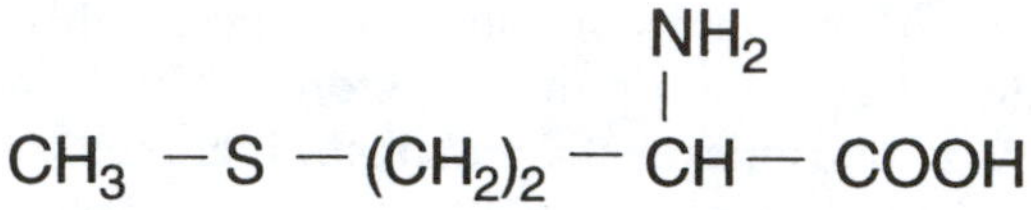

$$CH_3 - S - (CH_2)_2 - \overset{\overset{\displaystyle NH_2}{|}}{CH} - COOH$$

Methionine (Met, M)

methotrexate. See *aminopterin*.

methycellulose. A chemical derivative of *cellulose* that is used as a thickening agent and as an emulsifier. Mehtylcellulose has no caloric or nutritive value.

methyl malonic acid. Mol. Wt. 118. As a Co-enzyme A derivative (methyl malonyl- CoA) it is an important intermediate in the synthesis of *fatty acids*. It is one of the few reactions in which carbon dioxide is incorporated into an intermediate in animals. It is required to convert methyl malonate to succinate. In certain genetic diseases relating to *cobalamin* deficiency, methyl-malonuria results because it cannot be converted to succinate. The determination of methyl malonate in urine can be used to determine cobalamin (vitamin B_{12}) status.

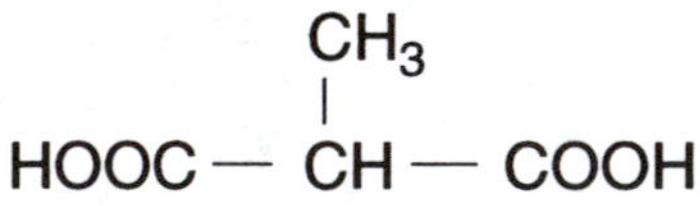

$$HOOC - \overset{\overset{\displaystyle CH_3}{|}}{CH} - COOH$$

Methyl malonic acid

methyl malonyl coenzyme A. An intermediate in fatty-acid synthesis and a derivative of *methyl malonic acid*.

micellar bile-fat complex. A *micelle* is a microscopic particle formed by an aggregate of molecules. In the micellar *bile-fat complex*, the particle is formed by the combination of *bile salts* with fat substances (*fatty acids* and *triglycerides*) to achieve the absorption of fat across the intestinal mucosa. Bile salts act as detergents to emulsify *lipids* for digestion and absorption.

micelle. A dispersion of particles to form an emulsion of a two-phase lipid-water complex of macromolecular dimensions by the detergent action or soap effect of a dispersing agent.

Common dispersing agents (*emulsifiers*) in the body are *phospholipids*, such as *lecithin*, and the *bile salts*. The dispersing agents have two distinct solubility properties in a single molecule. One part of the molecule is fat-soluble (*hydrophobic*) and the other part is water-soluble (*hydrophilic*). The center of micelles contain lipid material dissolved or held together by the hydrophobic forces of the molecule. The hydrophilic part of the molecule is either positively (+) or negatively (−) charged and is on the surface of the micelle. The hydrophilic part interacts with water and holds the particles in suspension in water to form an *emulsion*. Micelle formation is important in the digestion of fats and lipids, and in the transport of fat as *chylomicrons*. See *emulsification*.

microbiological. Pertaining to microorganisms (microscopic plants or animals).

microgram (μg). One thousandth of a milligram, one millionth of a gram.

micronutrients. Nutrients present in very small amounts of food. As applied to mineral elements, the term usually refers to those present in the body in amounts less than that of *iron*. See *minerals*.

milk. Distinguished by the high quality of its proteins and its high content of *calcium* and *phosphorus*. It is a good source of *riboflavin* and *retinol* (vitamin A) and supplies generous quantities of *lactose* and readily digested milk fat. The major protein of milk is *casein*; lesser amounts of lactalbumin and lactoglobulin are also present. Milk is a fluid secreted by female mammals as food for their young. Human milk is the sole natural food for the human infant. Cow's milk is the usual substitute for human milk, but milk from other mammals is substituted in many parts of the world. Cow's milk is much higher in protein, 35 g/liter, than human milk, 15 g/liter of protein. Human milk is usually richer in *retinol* (vitamin A) and *ascorbic acid* (vitamin C) than cow's milk. All milks are poor sources of *iron* and of *vitamin D*. Cow's milk cannot be fed to human infants directly. It must be processed first by diluting to reduce the protein concentration, then adding sugar to bring the carbohydrate level up to that of human milk; and finally the milk is pasteurized to protect it from *pathogens*. An infant's normal requirement for milk is about 160 mL/kg/day (2.5 oz/lb/day). Milk is a valuable food for children. From ages 1–5 about 500 mL (about 6 oz) of milk per day, and about half that amount until growth ceases, are ample amounts. Casein is the major protein of milk and has a high biological value. The major carbohydrate is *lactose* (milk sugar). The casein found in milk of most warm-blooded animals is similar; the lactalbumin and lactoglobulin are, however, species-specific and differ in the composition and immunologic properties. The retinol (vitamin A) content of milk varies with the feed of the cow; the vitamin D content of nonenriched milk varies with the availability of sunlight and is greater in the summer months. Much of the nutritional excellence of fresh, whole fluid milk is also found in evaporated and powdered milk. Fat-free skimmed milk is as desirable, and skimmed milk powder is the most economic source of good protein, calcium, and phosphorus. Cheese contains all the casein and some of the albumin and minerals of the whole milk, from which it is derived. When made from whole milk it also contains the original butterfat.

milk products. Many products derive from milk and are staples in many diets, countries, and cultures. Some of the more important of these milk products are listed:
   Pasteurized milk: Milk that has been heated to kill any harmful bacteria and then cooled immediately to 10 °C (50 °F) or lower. It is heated at 85 °C (185 °F) for 2 seconds or at about

Table of Food Composition

Milk, Cheese, Cream, Imitation Cream; Related Products		Grams	Water Percent	Food Energy Calories	Protein Grams	Fat Grams
Milk:						
Fluid:						
Whole, 3.5% fat	1 cup	244	87	160	9	9
Nonfat (skim)	1 cup	245	90	90	9	Trace
Partly skimmed, 2% nonfat milk solids added.	1 cup	246	87	145	10	5
Canned, concentrated, undiluted:						
Evaporated, unsweetened.	1 cup	252	74	345	18	20
Condensed, sweetened.	1 cup	306	27	980	25	27
Dry, nonfat instant:						
Low-density (1⅞ cups needed for reconstitution to 1 qt.).	1 cup	68	4	245	24	Trace
High-density ⅞ cup needed for reconstitution to 1 qt.).	1 cup	104	4	375	37	1
Buttermilk:						
Fluid, cultured, made from skim milk.	1 cup	245	90	90	9	Trace
Dried, packaged	1 cup	120	3	465	41	6
Cheese:						
Natural:						
Blue or Roquefort type:						
Ounce	1 oz.	28	40	105	6	9
Cubic inch	1 cu. in.	17	40	65	4	5
Camembert, packaged in 4-oz. pkg. with 3 wedges per pkg.	1 wedge	38	52	115	7	9
Cheddar:						
Ounce	1 oz.	28	37	115	7	9
Cubic inch	1 cu. in.	17	37	70	4	6
Cottage, large or small curd:						
Creamed:						
Package of 12-oz., net wt.	1 pkg.	340	78	360	46	14
Cup, curd pressed down.	1 cup	245	78	260	33	10
Uncreamed:						
Package of 12-oz., net wt.	1 pkg.	340	79	290	58	1
Cup, curd pressed down	1 cup	200	79	170	34	1
Cream:						
Package of 8-oz., net wt.	1 pkg.	227	51	850	18	86
Package of 3-oz., net wt.	1 pkg.	85	51	320	7	32
Cubic inch	1 cu. in.	16	51	60	1	6
Parmesan, grated:						
Cup, pressed down	1 cup	140	17	655	60	43
Tablespoon	1 tbsp.	5	17	25	2	2
Ounce	1 oz.	28	17	130	12	9
Swiss:						
Ounce	1 oz.	28	39	105	8	8
Cubic inch	1 cu. in.	15	39	55	4	4
Pasteurized processed cheese:						
American:						
Ounce	1 oz.	28	40	105	7	9
Cubic inch	1 cu. in.	18	40	65	4	5

| Fatty Acids | | | | | | | | | | |
| Saturated (Total) Grams | Unsaturated | | Carbo-hydrate Grams | Calcium Milli-grams | Iron Milli-grams | Vitamin A Value Interna-tional Units | Thiamine Milli-grams | Riboflavin Milli-grams | Niacin Milli-grams | Ascorbic Acid Milli-grams |
	Oleic Grams	Linoleic Grams								
5	3	Trace	12	288	0.1	350	0.07	0.41	0.2	2
—	—	—	12	296	.1	10	.09	.44	.2	2
3	2	Trace	15	352	.1	200	.10	.52	.2	2
11	7	1	24	635	.3	810	.10	.86	.5	3
15	9	1	166	802	.3	1,100	.24	1.16	6	3
—	—	—	35	879	.4	[1]20	.24	1.21	.6	5
—	—	—	54	1,345	.6	[1]30	.36	1.85	.9	7
—	—	—	12	296	.1	10	10	.44	.2	2
3	2	Trace	60	1,498	.7	260	.31	2.06	1.1	—
5	3	Trace	1	89	.1	350	.01	.17	.3	0
3	2	Trace	Trace	54	.1	210	.01	.11	.2	0
5	3	Trace	1	40	0.2	380	0.02	0.29	0.3	0
5	3	Trace	1	213	.3	370	.01	.13	Trace	0
3	2	Trace	Trace	129	.2	230	.01	.08	Trace	0
8	5	Trace	10	320	1.0	580	.10	.85	.3	0
6	3	Trace	7	230	.7	420	.07	.61	.2	0
1	Trace	Trace	9	306	1.4	30	.10	.95	.3	0
Trace	Trace	Trace	5	180	.8	20	06	.56	.2	0
48	28	3	5	141	.5	3,500	.05	.54	.2	0
18	11	1	2	53	.2	1,310	.02	.20	.1	0
3	2	Trace	Trace	10	Trace	250	Trace	.04	Trace	0
24	14	1	5	1,893	.7	1,760	.03	1.22	.3	0
1	Trace	Trace	Trace	68	Trace	60	Trace	.04	Trace	0
5	3	Trace	1	383	.1	360	.01	.25	.1	0
4	3	Trace	1	262	.3	320	Trace	.11	Trace	0
2	1	Trace	Trace	139	.1	170	Trace	.06	Trace	0
5	3	Trace	1	198	.3	350	.01	.12	Trace	0
3	2	Trace	Trace	122	.2	210	Trace	.07	Trace	0

Milk, Cheese, Cream, Imitation Cream, Related Products		Water Percent	Food Energy Calories	Protein Grams	Fat Grams
	Grams				
Pasteurized processed cheese:					
Swiss:					
Ounce	1 oz.	28	40	100	8	8
Cubic inch	1 cu. in.	18	40	65	5	5
Pasteurized process cheese food,					
American:					
Tablespoon	1 tbsp.	14	43	45	3	3
Cubic inch	1 cu. in.	18	43	60	4	4
Pasteurized process cheese spread, American.	1 oz.	28	49	80	5	6
Cream:					
Half-and-half (cream and milk).	1 cup	242	80	325	8	28
	1 tbsp.	15	80	20	1	2
Light, coffee or table	1 cup	240	72	505	7	49
	1 tbsp.	15	72	30	1	3
Sour	1 cup	230	72	485	7	47
	1 tbsp.	12	72	25	Trace	2
Whipped topping (pressurized)	1 cup	60	62	155	2	14
	1 tbsp.	3	62	10	Trace	1
Whipping, unwhipped (volume about double when whipped):					
Light	1 cup	239	62	715	6	75
	1 tbsp.	15	62	45	Trace	5
Heavy	1 cup	238	57	840	5	90
	1 tbsp.	15	57	55	Trace	6
Imitation cream products (made with vegetable fat):					
Creamers:					
Powdered	1 cup	94	2	505	4	33
	1 tsp.	2	2	10	Trace	1
Liquid (frozen)	1 cup	245	77	345	3	27
	1 tbsp.	15	77	20	Trace	2
Sour dressing (imitation sour cream) made with nonfat dry milk.	1 cup	235	72	440	9	38
	1 tbsp.	12	72	20	Trace	2
Whipped topping:					
Pressurized	1 cup	70	61	190	1	17
	1 tbsp.	4	61	10	Trace	1
Frozen	1 cup	75	52	230	1	20
	1 tbsp.	4	52	10	Trace	1
Powdered, made with whole milk.	1 cup	75	58	175	3	12
	1 tbsp.	4	58	10	Trace	1
Milk beverages:					
Cocoa, homemade	1 cup	250	79	245	10	12
Chocolate-flavored drink made with skim milk and 2% added butterfat.	1 cup	250	83	190	8	6
Malted milk:					
Dry powder, approx. 3 heaping teaspoons per ounce.	1 oz.	28	3	115	4	2
Beverage	1 cup	235	78	245	11	10

Saturated (Total) Grams	Oleic Grams	Linoleic Grams	Carbohydrate Grams	Calcium Milligrams	Iron Milligrams	Vitamin A Value International Units	Thiamine Milligrams	Riboflavin Milligrams	Niacin Milligrams	Ascorbic Acid Milligrams
Fatty Acids										
	Unsaturated									
4	3	Trace	1	251	.3	310	Trace	.11	Trace	0
3	2	Trace	Trace	159	.2	200	Trace	.07	Trace	0
2	1	Trace	1	80	.1	140	Trace	.08	Trace	0
2	1	Trace	1	100	.1	170	Trace	.10	Trace	0
3	2	Trace	2	160	.2	250	Trace	.15	Trace	0
15	9	1	11	261	.1	1,160	.07	.39	.1	2
1	1	Trace	1	16	Trace	70	Trace	.02	Trace	Trace
27	16	1	10	245	.1	2,020	.07	.36	.1	2
2	1	Trace	1	15	Trace	130	Trace	.02	Trace	Trace
26	16	1	10	235	.1	1,930	.07	.35	.1	2
1	1	Trace	1	12	Trace	100	Trace	.02	Trace	Trace
8	5	Trace	6	67	—	570	—	.04	—	—
Trace	Trace	Trace	Trace	3	—	30	—	Trace	—	—
41	25	2	9	203	.1	3,060	.05	.29	.1	2
3	2	Trace	1	13	Trace	190	Trace	.02	Trace	Trace
50	30	3	7	179	.1	3,670	.05	.26	.1	2
3	2	Trace	1	11	Trace	230	Trace	.02	Trace	Trace
31	1	0	52	21	.6	[2]200	—	—	Trace	—
Trace	Trace	0	1	1	Trace	[2]Trace	—	—	—	—
25	1	0	25	29	—	[2]100	0	0	—	—
1	Trace	0	2	2	—	[2]10	0	0	—	—
35	1	Trace	17	277	.1	10	.07	.38	.2	1
2	Trace	Trace	1	14	Trace	Trace	Trace	Trace	Trace	Trace
15	1	0	9	5	—	[2]340	—	0	—	—
1	Trace	0	Trace	Trace	—	[2]20	—	0	—	—
18	Trace	0	15	5	—	[2]560	—	0	—	—
1	Trace	0	1	Trace	—	[2]30	—	0	—	—
10	1	Trace	15	62	Trace	[2]330	.02	.08	.1	Trace
1	Trace	Trace	1	3	Trace	[2]20	Trace	Trace	Trace	Trace
7	4	Trace	27	295	1.0	400	.10	.45	.5	3
3	2	Trace	27	270	.5	210	.10	.40	.3	3
—	—	—	20	82	.6	290	.09	.15	.1	0
—	—	—	28	317	.7	590	.14	.49	.2	2

Milk, Cheese, Cream, Imitation Cream; Related Products		Grams	Water Percent	Food Energy Calories	Protein Grams	Fat Grams
Milk desserts:						
Custard, baked	1 cup	265	77	305	14	15
Ice Cream:						
Regular (approx. 10% fat).	½ gal.	1,064	63	2,055	48	113
	1 cup	133	63	255	6	14
	3 fl. oz. cup	50	63	95	2	5
Rich (approx. 16% fat).	½ gal.	1,188	63	2,635	31	191
	1 cup	148	63	330	4	24
Ice milk:						
Hardened	½ gal.	1,048	67	1,595	50	53
	1 cup	131	67	200	6	7
Soft-serve	1 cup	175	67	265	8	9
Yogurt:						
Made from partially skimmed milk.	1 cup	245	89	125	8	4
Made from whole milk	1 cup	245	88	150	7	8

73 °C (165 °F) for 15 to 40 seconds (the flash process) or at about 63 °C (146 °F) for 30 minutes followed by cooling.

Sterilized Milk: Milk that is heated in autoclaves (under steam pressure) at about 115 °C (237 °F) for about 15 minutes followed by cooling.

Homogenized milk: Pasteurized milk in which the particles have been broken down and evenly distributed throughout the milk by a mechanical process. In homogenized milk the cream does not rise to the top of the container as it does in nonhomogenized milk. Homogenized milk forms a softer curd in the stomach and is more easily digested.

Fortified milk: Pasteurized milk containing added amounts of one or more of the essential nutrients present in milk. The most common addition is *vitamin D*.

Low-sodium milk: Milk used for special low-salt diets. It is milk from which 90% of the sodium has been removed and replaced with potassium. Part of the B vitamins and calcium are lost in the process. Low-sodium milk is also in powdered form.

Chocolate milk: Pasteurized milk to which chocolate syrup or cocoa is added. Vanilla, salt, sugar, and a stabilizer may also be added to keep the drink well mixed.

Evaporated milk: Homogenized whole milk from which about 60% of the water has been removed by heating. Vitamin D is added to provide 400 International Units per pint of evaporated milk. When diluted with an equal amount of water, it has about the same food value as a fresh whole milk.

Condensed milk: Milk made by evaporating a mixture of whole milk and sugar. It differs from the unsweetened evaporated milk only in the addition of the sugar, which accounts for 40–45 percent of the final product.

Skim milk: Fresh milk from which some fat has been removed; available as fluid skim milk, buttermilk, fortified skim milk, and flavored milk drinks.

Fluid skim milk: Made of whole milk from which some fat has been removed. The milk fat remaining usually varies from 1–2 percent.

Saturated (total) grams	Oleic grams	Linoleic grams	Carbohydrate grams	Calcium milligrams	Iron milligrams	Vitamin A Value International Units	Thiamine milligrams	Riboflavin milligrams	Niacin milligrams	Ascorbic acid milligrams
7	5	1	29	297	1.1	930	.11	.50	.3	1
62	37	3	221	1,553	.5	4,680	.43	2.23	1.1	11
8	5	Trace	28	194	.1	590	.05	.28	.1	1
3	2	Trace	10	73	Trace	220	.02	.11	.1	1
105	63	6	214	927	.2	7,840	.24	1.31	1.2	12
13	8	1	27	115	Trace	980	.03	.16	.1	1
29	17	2	235	1,635	1.0	2,200	.52	2.31	1.0	10
4	2	Trace	29	204	.1	280	.07	.29	.1	1
5	3	Trace	—	—	—	—	—	—	—	—
2	1	Trace	13	294	.1	170	.10	.44	.2	2
5	3	Trace	12	272	.1	340	.07	.39	.2	2

The Fatty Acids (Unsaturated) heading spans the Oleic and Linoleic columns.

Buttermilk: Milk to which a lactic-acid-producing culture is added. Generally, the milk used is skim, although buttermilk may occasionally be produced from whole milk, concentrated fluid milk, or reconstituted nonfat dry milk. Butter granules may be added to enhance the flavor.

Acidophilus milk is a form of buttermilk used for special diets and available in fluid form.

Fortified skim milk: Skim milk to which vitamins, including *ascorbic acid* (vitamin C), and minerals are added. Each quart usually contains the minimum daily vitamin and mineral requirements for health.

Cream: The milk fat that separates from whole milk. It contains almost all of the fat, about one-third the concentration of protein, and about one-third the concentration of lactose in milk.

Butter: An emulsion of milk-fat globules, air, and water produced by churning cream or whole milk. The liquid that remains after the churning is called *buttermilk*.

Rennet: Commercial preparation of *renin* which causes milk protein to precipitate. It is the first step in cheese-making.

Whey: The fluid from the precipitated protein in the formation of curds. It contains lactose, little protein, and little fat.

Cheese: Cheese is made from clotted milk. The clotting of the milk is effected by adding *rennet*. The clot or curd is separated from the liquid (whey), salted, and pressed to form a cake. Bacteria and molds then ferment and ripen the cheese cake. The characteristic flavor, color, and texture of cheese depends upon the source of milk (cow, sheep, goat, etc.), the kind and combination of bacteria and mold, and the conditions of the ripening process. Cheeses are very nutritious foods containing 25–35% of a protein of high biological value, and are rich in calcium, retinol (vitamin A), and riboflavin. The fat content varies widely, from 16–40%, depending upon the type of cheese. Cheeses should be avoided when certain antidepressant drugs are prescribed. Some antidepressants inhibit an enzyme, *monoamine oxidase*, which ordinarily destroys *tyramine*, a product of the amino acid *tyrosine*. Tyramine stimulates the sympathetic nervous system and may cause headaches, nausea, dizziness, and a rise in blood pressure. The caution applies to any other food, drink, or medicine which contains amines.

Fermented milk sources: Various bacteria are used to sour or curdle milk. All of these bacteria break down lactose to *glucose* and *galactose* which are eventually converted to *lactic acid*, which may be as high as 3%. Sour or fermented milks are usually hygienically safe when there may be doubt about dairy hygiene because the initial steps involve boiling the milk to reduce the volume. After cooling, the boiled milk is usually inoculated with a small quantity of sour milk and allowed to stand for 24 hours. *Acidophilus milk* is obtained by inoculating milk with *Lactobacillus acidophilus*, which will grow so profusely in milk that growth of a pathogenic contaminant is greatly diminished. *L. acidolphilus* is also found naturally in the alimentary tract of human adults.

Yogurt is milk that has been greatly concentrated by boiling various bacteria which are inoculated for the souring (lactic acid). In some countries, yeast fermentation produces alcohol in addition. Soured and fermented milks contain all fat, protein, calcium, and vitamins that occur in the original milk. These milk products are therefore nutritious foods, but there is no evidence that they possess any special properties beyond that. The table gives the nutrient values of some milks and milk products.

millet (*Panicum miliaceum*). Any of a large number of small seeded cereal *grains* and forage grasses, or the grain or seed of these grasses. It is generally grown as a cereal in Asia and Africa, providing a diet staple for one-third of the world's population. In North America it is used mostly as forage. High in carbohydrates and proteins. See this item in the table under *grains*.

milligram (mg). One thousandth of a gram or 1/28000 of an ounce (weight).

milliliter (mL). On thousandth of a liter or 1/30 of an ounce (volume).

minerals. "Inorganic elements." The following are known to be present in body tissue: calcium, cobalt, chlorine, fluorine, iodine, iron, magnesium, manganese, molybdenum, phosphorus, potassium, selenium, silicon, sodium, sulfur, and zinc. Although mineral elements constitute but a small proportion (4% by weight) of the body tissue, they are essential as structural components and in many vital processes. Mineral constituents obtained from food aid in the regulation of the *acid-base balance* of body fluids and of *osmotic pressure*, in addition to the specific functions of individual elements in the body. Some minerals are present in the body largely in organic combinations, as iron in *hemoglobin* and *iodine* in *thyroxine*. Others occur in the body in inorganic form, such as calcium salts in *bone* and sodium *chloride* in blood. The terms "minerals" and "inorganic elements" do not imply that the elements occur in inorganic form in food or body tissue. Minerals that are electropositive are known as *cations* and those include the metallic-element minerals such as calcium, magnesium, potassium, and sodium ions. The electronegative minerals are known as *anions* and include chlorine, fluorine, iodine, and, in their ionic forms, phosphorus as phosphate and sulfur as sulfate. Combinations of these positive and negative elements lead to formation of salts such as sodium chloride, calcium phosphate, and potassium sulfate. In body fluids, the salts dissociate completely in their respective *anion* and *cation* forms. In foods, minerals are present in various forms mixed or combined with proteins, fats and carbohydrates. Some processed or refined foods, such as fats, oils, sugar, and cornstarch, contain almost no minerals. The total mineral content of a food is determined by burning the organic or combustible part of a known amount of food and weighing the resulting ash. The ash is then analyzed for individual mineral elements. Most foods have been analyzed for 10 or more minerals, but in dietary practice the figures most commonly used are those for calcium, phosphorus, and iron, and for therapeutic purposes, sodium, potassium, and magnesium. The elements concerned in the mineral metabolism may exist in the body and take part in its functions in at least three ways. (1) As a constituent of the bones and teeth, giving rigidity and relative permanence to the skeletal tissues. (2) As essential elements of the organic compounds which are the chief solid constituents of the soft tissues (muscles, blood cells, enzymes, etc.). (3) As soluble salts (electrolytes) held in solution in the fluid of the body, giving these fluids their characteristic influence upon the elasticity and irritability of muscle and nerve. They supply the material for the acidity or alkalinity of the *digestive juices* and other secretions, and yet maintain the approximate neutrality of the body's fluids as well as their *osmotic pressure* and solvent power. Minerals found in the human body may be grouped according to whether they are present in large amounts (major minerals) or are present in small amounts and have a known function (trace minerals), or are present in small amounts but their function is not understood. There are seven minerals contributing from 60–80% of all the inorganic material in the body. The tables on pages 282–285 show the minerals, their functions, their sources in food, and the *Recommended Dietary Allowances* (RDA).

mineral oil. A specific hydrocarbon fraction that has use in cosmetics and as a *laxative*.

mineral waters. Mineral waters contain small quantities of sodium chloride, sodium carbonate and bicarbonate, and salts of calcium and magnesium and sometimes iron or hydrogen sulfide. They are usually mildly alkaline. The total mineral content is seldom as high as 8 g/liter and is often much less. Many of these waters are naturally aerated with *carbon dioxide*. Soda water is simply water from any wholesome source with carbon dioxide forced into it under pressure and has no medicinal properties.

mint (*Mentha*). A fragrant *herb* of which there are over 30 species. Among the most popular varieties of this upright plant with red-veined stems and sharply aromatic leaves are *peppermint* and *spearmint*, as well as American apple mint, bergamot mint, curly mint, and red mint. The names indicate the difference either in flavor or in shape of the mint leaves.

miscible. Pertaining to a liquid capable of being dissolved in another liquid at any ratio.

mitochondrion. The "powerhouse of the cell" responsible for transforming chemical bond energy of nutrients into higher-energy phosphate bonds of *adenosine triphosphate* (ATP). There may be 50–2500 of these organs of respiration in a single cell, each containing 500–10,000 complete sets of oxidative enzymes. Each enzyme assembly contains 15 or more active molecules in a highly ordered arrangement, which is an integral part of the organelle structure. The mitochondria contain the *Krebs'* (tricarboxylic acid) *cycle* and the *terminal respiratory chain*. The mitochondria are, in general, about the size of bacteria, but size and shape can vary markedly depending on the cell type and physiologic state. A schematic presentation of a mitochondrion is given. Most of the activity of the cell that is necessary for survival is completely dependent upon the ability of the mitochondria to release the energy in a nutrient molecule and transduce that energy into a form of cellular work: osmotic, mechanical, electric, chemical. The major source of chemical energy for cellular processes is the compound *adenosine*

Group I Major Minerals

Minerals	Functions in the Body	Metabolism	Food Sources	Daily Allowances
Calcium	Hardness of bones, teeth Transmission of nerve impulse Muscle contraction Normal heart rhythm Activate enzymes Increase cell permeability Catalyze thrombin formation	*Absorption:* about—40 percent, according to body need; aided by gastric acidity, vitamin D, lactose; excess phosphate, fat, phytate, oxalic acid interfere *Storage:* trabeculae of bones; easily mobilized *Utilization:* needs parathyroid hormone, vitamin D *Excretion:* 60–85 percent of diet intake in feces; small urinary excretion; high protein intake increases urinary excretion *Deficiency:* retarded bone mineralization; fragile bones; stunted growth; rickets; osteomalacia; osteoporosis	Milk, hard cheese Ice cream, cottage cheese Greens: turnip, collards, kale, mustard, broccoli Oysters, shrimp, salmon, clams	Infants: 360–540 mg Children: 800 mg Teen-agerse: 1200 mg Adults: 800 mg Pregnancy: 1200 mg Lactation: 1200 mg
Phosphorus	Structure of bones, teeth Cell permeability Metabolism of fats and carbohydrates: storage and release of ATP Sugar-phosphate linkage in DNA and RNA Phospholipids in transport of fats Buffer salts in acid-base balance	*Absorption:* about 70 percent; aided by vitamin D *Utilization:* about 85 percent in bones; controlled by vitamin D, parathormone *Excretion:* about one third of diet in feces; metabolic products chiefly in urine *Deficiency:* poor bone mineralization; poor growth; rickets	Milk, cheese Eggs, meat, fish, poultry Legumes, nuts Whole-grain cereals	Infants: 200 to 400 mg Children: 800 mg Adults: 800 mg Pregnancy: 1200 mg Lactation: 1200 mg
Magnesium	Constitutes of bones, teeth Activates enzymes in carbohydrate metabolism Muscle and nerve irritability	*Absorption:* parallels that of calcium; competes with calcium for carriers *Utilization:* slowly mobilized from bone *Excretion:* chiefly by kidney *Deficiency:* seen in alcoholism, severe renal disease; hypomagnesemia, tremor	Whole-grain cereals Nuts; legumes Meat Milk Green leafy vegetables	Infants: 60 to 70 mg Children: 150 to 250 mg Women: 300 mg Men: 350 mg Pregnancy and lactation: 450 mg

Sulfur	Constituent of proteins, especially cartilage, hair, nails Constituent of melanin, glutathione, thiamin, biotin, coenzyme A, insulin High-energy sulfur bonds Detoxication reactions	Absorbed chiefly as sulfur-containing amino acids Excreted as inorganic sulfate in urine in proportion to nitrogen loss	Protein foods rich in sulfur-amino acids Eggs Meat Milk, cheese Nuts, legumes	Not established Diet adequate in protein meets need
Sodium	Principal cation of extracellular fluid Osmotic pressure; water balance Acid-base balance Regulate nerve irritability and muscle contraction "Pump" for glucose transport	*Absorption:* rapid and almost complete *Excretion:* chiefly in urine; some by skin and in feces; parallels intake; controlled by aldosterone *Deficiency:* rare; occurs with excessive perspiration and poor diet intake; nausea, diarrhea, abdominal cramps, muscle cramps	Table salt Milk Meat, fish, poultry Egg white	Not established Probably about 500 mg except with excessive perspiration Diets supply substantial excess
Potassium	Principal cation of intracellular fluid Osmotic pressure; water balance; acid-base balance Nerve irritability and muscle contraction, regular heart rhythm Synthesis of protein Glycogenesis	*Absorption:* readily absorbed *Excretion:* chiefly in urine; increased with aldosterone secretion *Deficiency:* following starvation, correction of diabetic acidosis, adrenal tumors; muscle weakness, nausea, tachycardia, glycogen depletion, heart failure	Widely distributed in foods Meat, fish, fowl Cereals Fruits, vegetables	Not established Diet adequate in calories supplies ample amounts
Chlorine	Chief anion of extracellular fluid Constituent of gastric juice Acid-base balance: chloride-bicarbonate shift in red cells	*Absorption:* rapid, almost complete *Excretion:* chiefly in urine; parallels intake *Deficiency:* with prolonged vomiting, drainage from fistula, diarrhea	Table salt	Not established Daily diet contains 3 to 9 gm, far in excess of need

Trace Minerals

Minerals	Functions in the Body	Metabolism	Food Sources	Daily Allowances
Iron	Constituent of hemoglobin, myoglobin, and oxidative enzymes: catalase, cytochrome, xanthine oxidase	*Absorption:* about 5 to 10 percent; regulated according to body need; aided by gastric acidity, ascorbic acid *Transport:* bound to protein, transferrin *Storage:* as ferritin in liver, bone marrow, spleen *Utilization:* chiefly in hemoglobin; daily turnover about 27 to 28 mg; iron used over and over again *Excretion:* men, about 1 mg; women, 1 to 2 mg; in urine, perspiration, menstrual flow; fecal excretion is from unabsorbed diet *Deficiency:* anemia; frequent in infants, preschool children, teenage girls, pregnant women	Liver, organ meats Meat, poultry Egg yolk Enriched and whole-grain breads, cereals Dark-green vegetables Legumes Molasses, dark Peaches, apricots, prunes, raisins Diets supply about 6 mg per 1000 kcal	Infants: 10 to 15 mg Children: 10 to 15 mg Teen-agers: 18 mg Men: 10 mg Women: 18 mg Pregnancy: 18+ mg Lactation: 18 mg
Manganese	Activation of many enzymes; oxidation of carbohydrates, urea formation, protein hydrolysis Bone formation	*Absorption:* limited *Excretion:* chiefly in feces *Deficiency:* not known	Legumes, nuts Whole-grain cereals	Not established
Copper	Aids absorption and use of iron in synthesis of hemoglobin Electron transport Melanin formation Myelin sheath of nerves Purine metabolism Metabolism of ascorbic acid	*Transport:* chiefly as protein, ceruloplasmin *Storage:* liver, central nervous system *Excretion:* bile into intestine *Deficiency:* rare; occurs in severe malnutrition Abnormal storage in Wilson's disease	Liver, shellfish Meats Nuts, legumes Whole-grain cereals Typical diet provides 2 to 5 mg	Infants and children: 0.08 mg per kg Adults: 2 mg
Cobalt	A constituent of cobalamin no other role known.	*Absorption:* as a cobalamin-protein (intrinsic factor) complex; about 2–3 μg daily. Maximum about 5 to 10 percent. *Transport:* bound to a protein, transcobalamin.	Meats, poultry Fish, eggs. Not present in plants. Typical diet provides about 10 μg.	Infants: 0.3 μg Children: 1–2 μg Adults: 2–3 μg

Mineral	Functions / Metabolism	Food Sources	Recommended Daily Amount
	Storage: liver mainly; small amount in bone marrow. *Utilization:* as a constituent of cobalamin; 2–5 μg is enough for 3–5 years. *Excretion:* almost completely reabsorbed. *Deficiency:* megaloblastic anemia; pernicious anemia; rare.		
Iodine	Constituent of diiodotyrosine, triiodothyronine, thyroxine; regulate rate of energy metabolism. *Absorption:* controlled by blood level of protein-bound iodine. *Storage:* thyroid gland; activity regulated by thyroid-stimulating hormone. *Excretion:* in urine. *Deficiency:* simple goiter; if severe, cretinism—rarely seen in U.S.	Iodized salt is most reliable source; Seafood; Foods grown in non-goitrous coastal areas	Infants: 35–45 mcg; Children: 60–110 mcg; Teen-agers: 115–150 mcg; Men: 130 mcg; Women: 100 mcg; Pregnancy: 125 mcg; Lactation: 150 mcg
Zinc	Constituent of enzymes: carbonic anhydrase, carboxypeptidase, lactic dehydrogenase. *Absorption:* limited; competes with calcium for absorption sites. *Storage:* liver, muscles, bones, organs. *Excretion:* chiefly by intestine. *Deficiency:* only in severe malnutrition	Seafoods; Liver and other organ meats; Meats, fish; Wheat germ; Yeast; Plant foods are generally low; Usual diet supplies 10 to 15 mg	Infants: 3–5 mg; Children: 10 mg; Teen-agers: 15 mg; Adults: 15 mg; Pregnancy: 20 mg; Lactation: 25 mg
Fluorine	Increases resistance of teeth to decay; most effective in young children. Moderate levels in bone may reduce osteoporosis. *Storage:* bones and teeth. *Excretion:* urine. Excess leads to mottling of teeth.	Fluoridated water; 1 ppm	Not established
Molybdenum	Cofactor for flavoprotein enzymes; present in xanthine oxidase. Absorbed as molybdate. Stored in liver, adrenal, kidney. Related to metabolism of copper and sulfur	Organ meats; Legumes; Whole-grain cereals	Not established
Selenium	Antioxidant. Constituent of glutathione oxidase. Stored especially in liver, kidney. Spares vitamin E	Meat and seafoods; Cereal foods	Not established
Chromium	Efficient use of insulin in glucose uptake; conversion of glucose to fat, glucose, oxidation, protein synthesis. Activation of enzymes. Usable form in organic compound: glucose tolerance factor	Liver, meat; Cheese; Whole-grain cereals	Not established

There is an additional group of trace minerals that occurs in food for which no functions are known. These minerals are as follows: lithium; lead; mercury; boron; aluminum; arsenic; tin; nickel; and silicon.

triphosphate (ATP). The major source of ATP comes from the mitochondria. The mitochondria contain the *Krebs' cycle* and *terminal respiratory chain* that are instrumental in the oxidation of foodstuffs to carbon dioxide (CO_2), water (H_2O), and *energy* (ATP + heat). More than 90% of the oxygen (O_2) used by the cells can be accounted for by the oxidation processes in mitochondria. Mitochondria also produce *citric acid*, which provides acetyl *coenzyme A*, the building block for the synthesis of *fatty acids* in the *cytoplasm*. The major functions of mitochondria are oxidative, and in that sense they are degradative processes, but mitochondria are also involved in the elongation of fatty acids, a process also peformed by the *microsomes* in the cytoplasm.

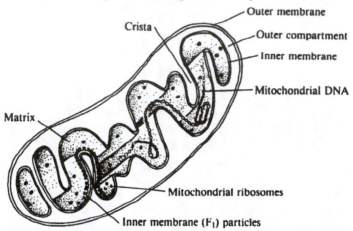

Mitochondrion
(Kuchel, P.W., and Ralston, G.B., *Biochemistry*, 1988. Reproduced with permission of McGraw-Hill.)

Mitochondrial compartments

OUTER MEMBRANE	INTERMEMBRANE SPACE	INNER MEMBRANE	MATRIX
Monoamine oxidase Phospholipase A_2 Kynurenine 3-monoxygenase NADH dehydrogenase;	Adenylate kinase Nucleoside diphosphokinase	NADH dehydrogenase Terminal respiratory chain Carnitine acyltransferase ATPase Glutamate dehydrogenase ß-Hydroxybutyrate dehydrogenase	Krebs' (tricarboxylic acid) cycle Aspartate transaminase Fatty acid oxidation enzymes

mitosis. The process whereby cells divide and multiply, each cell forming two daughter cells which contain replicas of all the original chromosomes.

moisture. See *water content*.

molasses. The thick brown syrup that is separated from raw sugar during the various stages of refinement. The sugar cane is cut close to the ground because the lowest ends are the richest in sugar. The stalks are torn into small pieces and passed through three sets of rollers to extract a dark-grayish, sweet juice. The juice is boiled down to a thick syrupy mass which includes crystals of sugar. This heavy syrup is then put into containers with holes through which the liquid drips, leaving the crystallized sugar behind. The liquid is molasses. The best grade of molasses is obtained by crude milling processes, as the syrup contains more sugar at this point. If the syrup is boiled more than once, the first boiling produces a darker, thicker, less sweet product which is used in cakes and candies. *Blackstrap molasses*, a cattle food and industrial product as well as a popular health food, is the result of a third boiling. The word molasses comes from the Portuguese *melaco* derived from the Latin root *mel*, which means "honey," and *aceus*, which means "resembling." Sorghum molasses is the syrup from the stalk of a group of grains which look much like corn. This syrup is a pure product from which no sugar is extracted. It has the consistency, color, and taste of molasses. A fair source of iron and calcium.

molecule. A group of atoms held together by chemical bonds. The identifiable units of chemical structure. A chemical combination of two or more atoms that form a specific substance. For example, the combination of an atom of sodium and an atom of chlorine makes a molecule of sodium chloride, or table salt. There are also large, complex molecules such as hemoglobin. Proteins and starches are examples of even larger and very complex molecules containing many atoms.

molybdenum (Mo). Element No. 42. At. Wt. 96. The molybdenum content of tissues of all animal species is very low. In adult humans, the liver contains about 3.2 ppm and kidneys about 1.6 ppm. Molybdenum content of muscle, brain, lung, and spleen ranges from 0.14–0.20 ppm. Molybdenum is a component of the enzymes xanthine oxidase and aldehyde oxidase. Both enzymes contain *flavin adenine dinucleotide* (FAD) as well as molybdenum, and both function in the *terminal respiratory chain*. There is little concrete evidence establishing the quantitative requirement for molybdenum in humans. Among the food sources of available or enzyme-producing molybdenum, those containing 0.6 ppm weight include legumes, cereal grains, some of the dark-green leafy vegetables, and animal organs. Fruits and most root and stem vegetables contain less than 0.1 ppm. The element plays a role in the activity of several *flavoproteins* and is thought to facilitate the linkage of flavin nucleotide to protein. Xanthine oxidase contains one atom of molybdenum. Parts of the body containing comparatively large amounts of the element are the liver, kidneys, and bones.

monilial vaginitis. An inflammation of the vagina caused by *Candida albicans*, a member of the *yeast* family that thrives in warm, moist places. The condition is often seen in uncontrolled *diabetes mellitus* because the sugar from urine provides an excellent medium for the growth of the yeast.

monoamine oxidase (MAO). An enzyme responsible for intracellular degradations of the *catecholamines, tyramine, epinephrin*, and *norepinephrin*. Inhibitors of MAO are found in many foods. Inhibition of MAO can produce an increase in blood pressure by causing release of norepinephrine at the presynaptic neuron. *Tyramine*, a product of the amino acid *tyrosine*, is usually metabolized by intestinal and hepatic MAO. When a person is taking a monoamine oxidase inhibitor (MAOI) or has a genetic deficiency of MAO, the tyramine escapes degradation and is able to provoke an acute rise in blood pressure. As little as 6 mg of tyramine is deleterious, and 25 mg may be dangerous. A severe pounding headache comes within 1–2 hours after ingestion of tyramine-containing food and can create a hypertensive crisis. It is often accompanied by arrhythmia, tachycardia, anxiety, tremors, chest pain, flushing, hyperpyrexia, and vertigo. Several of the antidepressants are monoamine oxidase inhibitors. Foods with significant tyramine content are beer, cheddar cheese, pickled herring, meat extracts, dried sausage, Chianti wines, yeast extracts, and chicken liver.

monocytes. Monocytes are twice as big as the polymorphonuclear *leukocytes* but they have a single large nucleus and no granules. They have similar functions to the polymorphonuclear leukocytes but they can engulf many more bacteria and a greater amount of dead tissue. They contain enzymes which attack the fatty walls of certain bacteria like the tuberculosis bacillus. In general, monocytes are more prominent in the reaction to chronic infections and in the later stages of acute infections.

monoglyceride. The *glycerol* molecule with a single *fatty acid* attached through an *ester* bond.

monosaccharides. Simple sugars, containing one sugar group, expressible by the general formula $C_n(H_2O)_n$. Monosaccharides are polyhydric, that is they contain several $-OH$ groups, which account for their sweet taste and their solubility. Monosaccharides are classified according to the number of carbons in the molecule. For example, *glucose* has six carbons and is therefore a hexose, and according to whether the molecule contains an aldehyde group, an aldose, or a keto- group, a ketose. Glucose is an aldose, and *fructose* is a ketose. The classifications of several naturally occurring monosaccharides are given in the table. Monosaccharides are soluble and can be absorbed into the body fluids without further change. They are the units from which the more complex carbohydrates are formed. Glucose or dextrose is found in fruits, especially the grape, and in body fluids; fructose or levulose is found with glucose in fruits; *galactose* is obtained by hydrolysis of *lactose* (milk sugar) and certain gums. The monosaccharides are important in nutrition because they are the units of complex lipids and proteins in addition to their use as a source of energy. The monosaccharides in *honey* arise largely from the breakdown of *sucrose*, which contains one glucose and one fructose unit. Fruits and certain fresh vegetables are the richest sources of monosaccharides eaten.

Classification of monosaccharides

CLASSIFICATION	ALDOSES	KETOSES
Trioses	Glyceraldehyde	Dihydroxyacetone
Tetroses	Erythrose	Erythrulose
	Threose	
Pentoses	Xylose	Xylulose
	Ribose	Ribulose
	Arabinose	
Hexoses	Glucose (dextrose)	Fructose (levulose)
	Galactose	Sorbose
	Mannose	
Heptoses		Sedoheptulose

monosodium glutamate (MSG). Mol. Wt. 159. A sodium salt of *glutamic acid*. A widely used *flavor enhancer*. Monosodium glutamate imparts no flavor of its own in the concentration allowed in foods. The detailed chemical and biological action of flavor enhancers is only partially understood. In 1908 a Japanese chemist, Dr. Kidunae Ikdea, discovered the flavor-enhancing properties. He discovered that the ingredient in the seaweed *Laminaria japonica* that had an unusual ability to enhance or intensify the flavor of many high-protein foods was monosodium glutamate. Monosodium glutamate is added to meats and fish and their products, sauces, soups, and other foods to accentuate their flavor. Other flavor enhancers are sodium *guanylate* and disodium *inosinate*.

$$NH_2$$
$$HOOC-CH_2-CH_2-CH-COO^- \ Na^+$$

Monosodium glutamate (MSG)

monounsaturated. Having a single double bond as in a *fatty acid*, for example, *oleic acid*.

mucilage. A vegetable preparation used in pharmaceuticals. A gelatinous substance, especially from seaweeds, that contains protein and *polysaccharides*. It is similar to plant gums.

mucin. A *glycoprotein* or *mucopolysaccharide* found in *mucus*, secreted by globlet cells of the intestine and other glandular cells such as the salivary glands. It is also found in bile, in the skin, and in connective tissue, tendon, and cartilage. It is formed from mucigen and in water forms a slimy solution.

mucopolysaccharides. Heteropolysaccharides that occur in combination with protein in both body secretions and structures. Many tend to be highly viscous and are responsible for the viscosity of body mucous secretions. They are generally components of the extracellular, amorphous ground substances that surround the *collagen* and *elastin* fibers and the cells of connective tissue, and may be involved in the induction of calcification; the control of metabolites, ions, and water; and the healing of wounds. Mucopolysaccharides, along with *glycoproteins* and *glycolipids*, also form the cell coat that is present in most animal cells. Mucopolysaccharides contain amino sugars, either *D-glucosamine* or D-galactosamine, together with uronic acids, either *D-glucuronic acid* or L-induronic acid. In addition, they may contain acetyl or sulfate groups.

mucoprotein. A conjugated protein containing a carbohydrate group such as chondroitin sulfuric acid.

mucosa. The cells that make up the *mucous* membrane lining of passages and cavities, as in the gastrointestinal, respiratory, and genitourinary tracts.

mucous membrane. See *membrane, mucous*.

mucus. A viscous fluid secreted by mucous membranes and glands, consisting mainly of mucin (a *glycoprotein*), inorganic salts, and water. Mucus serves to lubricate the gastrointestinal mucosa and thus helps move food along the digestive tract, and protects linings and cavities generally.

mulberry (*Morus*). A tree and its edible berrylike fruit. There are three principal varieties: black, red, and white. The leaves of the white mulberry, *Morus alba*, are used in silkworm cultivation. Mulberries resemble blackberries in shape and structure, ranging in color from white through red to black. The fruit is soft and bland in taste and can be eaten raw. Cooked it is used in making desserts, preserves, and wine.

mullet. The name is used to describe several families of important food fish. The best known are the gray mullets of the family *Mugilidae*, which include the genera known as striped and white mullets; and the red mullets, including striped red mullet, surmullet, and goatfish, of the family *Mullidae*. Mullets are of moderate size, from a half to five pounds in weight. Their flesh is tender, white, and firm-textured with a sweet, delicate taste. The flesh contains a clear yellow oil with a mild nutlike flavor.

mung bean. Small green beans grown mainly in India. Popular with health food devotees for cultivating sprouts.

Nutrients in 100 g of mung bean sprouts, raw

CALORIES KCAL	PROTEIN G	FAT G	CARBOHYDRATE G	VITAMIN A IU	CALICUM MG	SODIUM MG
35	4	trace	6	20	19	5

muscat, muscatel (*Vinifera*). Muscat is the name of several varieties of grapes, cultivated especially for making raisins and wine. The muscat is a white or black grape with a sweet and musty flavor. Muscatel, the wine made from the muscat grape, is a sweet dessert wine which can vary in color from golden or russet-amber to light red. It is a sweet, rich, and fruity wine with the typical aroma and flavor of the grape.

muscle. The muscles of the body include three types: the smooth muscle in the walls of internal organs; the cardiac muscle in the walls of the heart; and the skeletal muscle attached to and causing movements of bones. The cells of muscles can contract, and it is this power of muscle contraction that produces body movement. Muscle tissue is made up of cells that are specialized for changing shape, which they accomplish by shortening their elongated form. When muscle cells are attached to one another and to other tissues of the body, they are organized into muscles. Muscles are made up of muscle cells (for contraction), connective tissue (to hold the cells together), and vascular or blood vessel tissue (to nourish the other cells). Muscles are organs made up of several kinds of specialized tissue. The major protein component of skeletal muscle filaments is *myosin*. Myosin and another protein, actin, interact with one another during the process of contraction. *Calcium* is intimately involved in the complex contraction mechanism also. The energy for contraction derives from *adenosine triphosphate* (ATP) by a mechanism that is not definitively understood, although mechanisms have been proposed that accommodate what is known about the details of contraction. Contractions result in the hydrolysis of ATP to *adenosine diphosphate* (ADP), inorganic phosphate salt, and heat. Since muscle requires sustained levels of energy for work, the ATP is supplied by *glycolysis* and by enzymes that will convert ADP back to ATP. One of these enzymes is adenylate kinase (2 ADP → ATP + AMP) and another is creatine phosphokinase (CPK). The CPK uses a storage form of chemical energy that is almost exclusively in muscle, *creatine phosphate* (CP). The conversion of CP to ATP by CPK is as follows: CP + ADP → creatine + ATP. *Creatine* can either be rephosphorylated at some later time during rest or be converted into *creatinine* and excreted in the *urine*. The major skeletal muscles in humans are shown in the diagram.

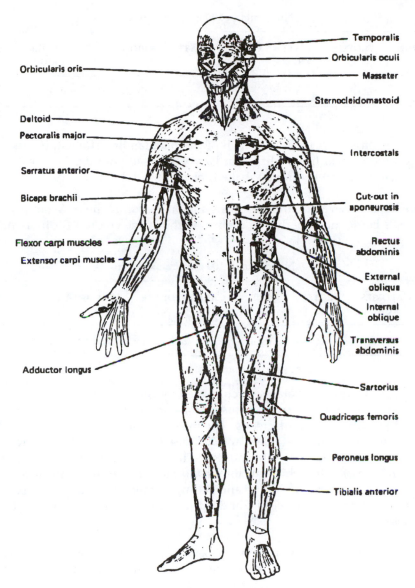

Principal anterior muscles

mushroom. Mushrooms are fungi, members of the enormous and varied group of living things which are responsible for decay. They belong to the *Basidiomycetes* class, together with such organisms as smuts and rusts. Like most other fungi, mushrooms lack chlorophyll, which means that, unlike green plants, they cannot manufacture their own food but must obtain nourishment from others, living or dead. When the mycelium is mature enough to reproduce, a sudden rain or a damp night provides the needed stimulus and the fruit springs up. Mushrooms can be bland or peppery, nutty or sweet, resemble veal cutlet, breast of chicken, steak, sweetbreads, kidneys, or oysters. The aroma runs the gamut from delightful to a stink like rotten fish. Although about 50 of the species growing wild in America are edible, experts urge those interested to concentrate on the few that are easy to identify. First is the morel, then the shaggymane, the sulfur shell, and the puffball.

Nutrients in 100 g of mushroom

CALORIES KCAL	PROTEIN G	FAT G	CARBOHYDRATE G	RIBOFLAVIN MG	CALCIUM MG	ASCORBATE MG
28	3	1	4	460	6	3

muskellunge or **musky**. A freshwater fish of the pike family. The fish is greenish brown in color, spotted with black. In weight it can vary from 7–40 pounds. The flesh is lean, white, firm, and delicious. It can be broiled, baked, or pan-fried.

muskmelon. One of several varieties of the melon Cucumis melo. Vitamin A content will vary from I.U., being much higher in melons with orange-colored flesh; ascorbic acid, mg. See *melon*.

Nutrients in 100 g of muskmelon

CALORIES KCAL	PROTEIN G	FAT G	CARBOHYDRATE G	VITAMIN A IU	ASCORBATE MG
30	1	Trace	8	280 to 3400	33

mustard (*Brassica*). Any of several *herbs* cultivated for their pungent seeds and/or leaves. The seeds are used to make the various forms of mustard seasonings; the leaves are used as a vegetable and known as mustard greens. The mustard plant belongs to a large family which includes many well-known vegetables: *broccoli*, *brussels sprouts*, Chinese *cabbage*, collards, *kale*, kohlrabi, red cabbage, rutabaga, and *turnips*. The word mustard is derived from the Old French *mostarde* or *moustard*, which meant a condiment made from mustard seed and must, the juice of grapes or other fruit before and during fermentation. Excellent source of *carotene* (vitamin A activity), *thiamine*, *riboflavin*, and *ascorbic acid* (vitamin C). See this item in the table under *vegetables*.

mutagens. (1) Agents inducing mutation, for example, short-wave radiation and certain chemicals. (2) Any force or influence, radiation, a chemical or other factor, which can cause mutation to occur in genes. Most mutagens are also *carcinogens*.

mutation. A change in the genetic material, the *deoxyribonucleic acid* (DNA) of the organism, which involves changes in the *deoxyribonucleotide* sequences (changes of type or number). This may result in proteins with altered structures and/or functions. Many mutations occur spontaneously in the normal course of events. It has been found possible to increase the frequency of mutations by exposing organisms to radiation and to chemical agents called *mutagens*. Not all mutations are harmful. There are more than 500 variants of the human hemogloblin molecule but only a few are associated with a dysfunction.

mycoses. Infections caused by *fungi*. Members of the vegetable kingdom of which molds that grow on bread or cheese are representative. Fungi contain no chlorophyll. There are many varieties, including yeastlike forms and molds that produce penicillin.

mycotoxins in foods. Ergotism is probably the oldest known disease caused by toxic substances which are produced by fungi growing in food. Poisoning occurs because of ingestion of the powerful alkaloid *ergot*. This substance is found in the fruiting body of fungus that is ground up and disseminated into flour during milling. Ingestion of bread made from the unmixed, undiluted flour may result in severe and even fatal symptoms pertaining to the circulatory or central nervous systems. Symptoms are due to the powerful vasoconstrictive action of the alkaloid and its induction of severe muscular contractions. Molds are often encountered on bread, fruit, or dairy products in the home. They usually belong to the genera *Aspergillus, Penicillium, Mucor*, and *Rhizopus*. There have been reports of toxic reactions (usually vomiting and gastritis) after ingestion of foods heavily overgrown with common food molds. Some of these are known to be harmless, such as the fungus responsible for the flavor and texture of camembert cheese. In contrast, a grave and frequently fatal reaction or "aleukia" (inhibition of blood-platelet synthesis) is associated with the ingestion of grain on which fungi which grow at cold temperatures have proliferated (or of foods prepared from such grain). *Fusarium sporotrichioides* and other fungi are implicated in this toxicosis, which is characterized by reduced platelet and white blood cell synthesis by the bone marrow, causing hemorrhages in a variety of tissues and organs, or eventually fatal secondary bacterial infections. Significant attention has also been focused on *aflatoxin*, a potent toxin produced by the ubiquitous fungus *Aspergillus flavus*, present in a variety of food crops when they are permitted to mold, particularly in peanuts. See *food toxins*.

myocardial infarction. Development of an infarct (an area of dead tissue) in the myocardium, usually the result of myocardial ischemia (oxygen deprivation) following occlusion of a coronary artery.

myocardium. The heart muscle.

myoglobin. An iron-protein complex in muscles that transports oxygen. Myoglobin combines with oxygen more firmly than hemoglobin. Myoglobin is a major protein component of red muscle.

myosin. A protein in muscle; the contractile element in *muscle* that combines with actin to form actomyosin, an enzyme that catalyzes the dephosphorylation of *adenosine triphosphate* (ATP) during muscle contraction.

myristic acid. Mol. Wt. 228. $CH_3(CH_2)_{12}COOH$. A long-chain *saturated fatty acid* obtained from nutmeg butter, coconut oil, butter, lard, and many other *fats*, as well as from spermaceti (a wax) and wool wax.

myxedema. A condition which results from a deficiency of *thyroxine* secretion by the *thyroid gland* in an adult. Myxedema is characterized by a low *basal metabolic rate* and decreased heat production. Myxedema in adults presents a picture almost the exact opposite of *hyperthyroidism*. All functions are markedly reduced. Inertia, exhaustion, apathy, and lack of initiative are the outstanding traits. The individual in advanced cases thinks slowly and inefficiently. As the condition progresses, the intellectual deterioration becomes more marked, together with a notable lack of imagination. The general picture is that of an advanced schizoid state. While psychosis is rare in this condition, a syndrome resembling the depressed phase of manic-depressive psychosis or of paranoid schizophrenia may occur. These states may be characterized by a great variety of illusions, hallucinations, confusion, and delirium.

N

N. The alphabetic symbol for the amino acid *asparagine* (Asn, Asx).

NAD (NADH). See *nicotinamide adenine dinucleotide*.

NADP (NADPH). See *nicotinamide adenine dinucleotide phosphate*.

natural foods. A vaguely used term, usually is taken to mean foods that have a minimum of refining (e.g., whole-grain cereals), and no additives or preservatives. Sometimes it is used to include foods grown without chemical fertilizers, hormones, or pesticides. The so-called *organic foods*.

natural toxins. Some foods contain active substances which can cause a druglike effect or which can interact with a drug to produce an unexpected or side effect. *Licorice* extracted from natural sources contains a substance which, when consumed regularly in excessive amounts, may cause an elevation in blood pressure. Licorice is an ingredient used in candy and as a flavoring for some pharmaceuticals. Continued regular use of products containing natural licorice extract could aggravate high blood pressure or counteract the effect of medication for high blood pressure. Some foods, such as soybeans, rutabagas, brussels sprouts, turnips, cabbage, and kale, contain substances known as goitrogens which inhibit production of the *thyroid hormone* binding *iodine* and thus can produce *goiter*. Scientists suggest caution in eating these foods when taking thyroid medications. Perhaps the most hazardous food-drug interaction is the one between *monamine oxidase* (*MAO*) inhibitors, drugs often prescribed for depression and high blood pressure, and such foods as aged cheese, Chianti wine, and chicken livers. MAO inhibitors can react with a substance called *tyramine* in these foods and force the blood pressure to dangerous levels, sometimes causing severe headaches, brain hemorrhage, and in extreme cases, death. See *food toxins*.

natural vitamins. Vitamins derived from natural foods, in contrast to synthetic vitamins.

necrosis. Death of areas of tissue or bone surrounded by healthy parts, as distinguished from necrobiosis, which is gradual degeneration. The dead part in bone is called sequestrum; in soft tissue it is called a slough or sphacelus. The term is applied to small areas of bone or tissue destruction, while "gangrene" is generally applied to the destruction of specific parts or larger areas. Necrosis may arise from insufficient blood supply, physical agents such as trauma, radiant energy (infrared, ultraviolet, roentgen, and radium rays), or chemical agents acting locally following absorption or topical application.

nectarine. A delicate variety of peach, smaller in size, roundish, and with a smooth skin that ranges in color from orange-yellow to red, sometimes mixed with green. The flesh is very juicy and may be red, yellow, or white in color. The fruit contains a pit. It is a fair source of *carotene* (vitamin A activity) and *ascorbic acid* (vitamin C).

Nutrients in 100 g of nectarine

CALORIES KCAL	PROTEIN G	FAT G	CARBOHYDRATE G	VITAMIN A IU	ASCORBATE MG
64	1	1	17	1650	13

negative nitrogen balance. See *nitrogen balance*.

neonatal. Pertaining to the newborn.

neoplasm. A neoplasm is any new growth, usually rapid and uncontrolled, such as a tumor or a *carcinoma*.

nephritis. Sometimes called "Bright's disease," refers to a general inflammation and resulting degeneration of the cells of the *kidney*. Classified as a noninfectious disease. Two specific diseases are classified under the general heading, *glomerulonephritis* and *nephrosclerosis*. Glomerulonephritis may be acute or chronic.

nephron. The functional unit of the *kidney*, consisting of a tuft of capillaries known as the *glomerulus* attached to the renal tubule. Blood flows through afferent arterioles into the glomerulus, where the filtration of blood occurs, and leaves by way of efferent arterioles. The filtered blood, containing low-molecular-weight substances, only passes from the glomerulus to the tubules. About 1.2 liters of blood are filtered each minute. The tubules have three functions: (1) The selective reabsorption of small molecules and ions in the filtrate such as water, sodium ion, bicarbonate, *amino acids*, and *glucose*. If these materials and others were not reabsorbed, within half an hour the body would have lost all of the substances. (2) The secretion of substances concerns primarily the *acid-base balance* maintenance. This balance, the maintenance of the pH at 7.4, is accomplished as positive ions such as sodium (Na^+) are absorbed from the filtrate by the cells lining the tubule, and hydrogen ion (H^+) replaces Na^+ in the filtrate. The H^+ is then neutralized by ammonia (NH_3) to form ammonium ion (NH_4^+). The kidneys thus excrete ammonia to balance the charge and the acid in the exchange of the Na^+ from the filtrate into the cells. The NH_3 is generated from the amino acid *glutamine*. After the selective absorption and secretion functions are complete, what remains is *urine*. (3) The third function is the conversion of *vitamin D* derivative, 1-hydroxy-cholecalciferol (formed in the liver) to the very active vitamin D form 1,25-dihydroxycholecalciferol. The diagram shows the nephron within the *kidney*. See *vitamin D*.

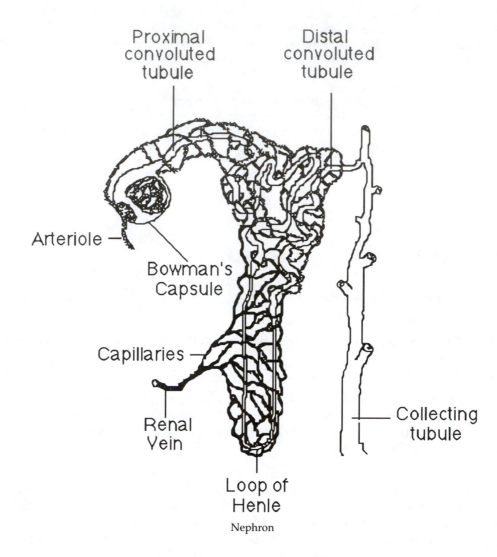

Nephron

nephrosclerosis. A kidney disease that occurs among older people, usually the result of *atherosclerosis* and essential *hypertension* of long standing. The blood supply to the kidney decreases gradually because of the thickening of the wall and the narrowing of the lumen of the blood vessels. Usually this is accompanied by increased blood pressure and is characterized by urea nitrogen retention in the blood. Disorder may run a prolonged benign course or an acute malignant one.

nephrotic syndrome. Those cases of renal disease which, regardless of underlying etiology, exhibit *albuminuria*, *hypoalbuminemia*, and massive *edema*. There is no concomitant hypertension or nitrogen retention. This syndrome may be seen during the nephrotic stage of chronic *glomerulonephritis*, in syphilitic nephritis, lipoid *nephrosis*, renal amyloidosis, and other disorders. In this condition, large amounts of protein may be lost daily in the urine. The kidney is able to retain plasma globulins to some extent, but plasma albumins leak out into the urine passively. The total blood proteins may be reduced from 7–4.5 g per 100 mL or less because of the massive albumin loss. In the nephrotic syndrome, the kidneys are also often unable to excrete salt normally, and salt retention, and consequently edema, compounds the effects of the prevailing *hypoalbuminemia*.

nervous system. The nervous system is composed of the brain, spinal cord, *ganglia*, nerve fibers, and their sensory and motor terminals. It is an integrated system that separates into the somatic and the autonomic systems that are based on function for the most part. The autonomic system is further divided into the sympathetic and parasympathetic, again based on function. Generally, the sympathetic and parasympathetic divisions have opposing effects when stimulated. The diagram is a schematic presentation that illustrates the basic relationships among the parts of the nervous system.

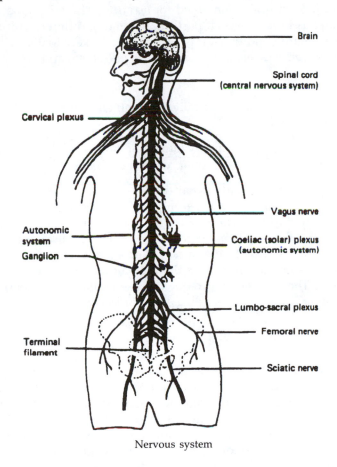

Nervous system

net dietary protein calories percent (NDpCal%). A value denoting the quality and quantity of a protein in a given diet, but also accounting for the percent of the total calories that derive from protein. A given diet may be of high-quality protein but of an insufficient percentage of the diet, a condition which might lead to *marasmus*, a disease of *protein-calorie malnutrition* (PCM). The NDpCal% is defined as

$$\text{NDp Cal \%} = \frac{\text{protein calories} \times \text{NPU} \times 100}{\text{net dietary calories}}$$

The NDPCal% allows comparisons of the qualities of various types of diets, particularly among different cultures. The value is obtained under specific standard conditions. See *NDPV*, *biological value*, *chemical score*, *net dietary protein value*, and *net protein utilization*.

net dietary protein value (NDpV). A value denoting the quantity and the quality of proteins in diets. It is defined as

$$\text{NDpV} = \text{dietary nitrogen intake} \times 6.25 \times \text{NPUop}$$

where NPUop is net protein utilization stand for *operative*. The NDpV permits comparisons of the qualities of various types of diets, particularly among different cultures. This value is not obtained under standard conditions. It is a value that is likely to derive from field studies. See *NDPCal%*, *biological value*, *chemical score*, *net protein utilization*, and *net dietary protein calories percent*.

net protein utilization (NPU). A biologically determined value to indicate the quality of proteins. The value is defined as

$$\text{NPU} = \frac{\text{dietary nitrogen retained} \times 100}{\text{dietary nitrogen intake}}$$

It differs from the *biological value* (BV) in that the losses due to the process of digestion are taken into account in the NPU value, since only the retained nitrogen is considered in the determination. The method for determining the NPU may vary, but in general most proteins are tested by either their ability to promote growth in young animals or their ability to maintain *nitrogen balance*. The NPU is usually measured at or slightly below the maintenance level required of proteins. Values determined for all other conditions are called operative and are designated as NPUop. The NPUop is a frequently used value in comparisons of diets. See *net dietary value*, *net dietary protein calories percent*, and *chemical score*.

neuritic. Pertaining to inflammation of a nerve.

neurons. Cells specialized to carry on the rapid communications required for coordinated function both within the organism and between the organism and its environment. The exploitation of two characteristics of protoplasm, irritability and conductivity, permits these cells to react to various stimuli in a fraction of a second and to transmit the excitation to another location. A typical neuron consists of a nucleated cell body with protoplasmic branches of processes. The size and distribution of these processes vary greatly at different sites and in cells with different functions, but two main kinds are found, the axon and the dendrite. The dendrites normally conduct impulses toward the cell body and the axons conduct away from it. The overall size of the neuron structure varies from a millimeter or so in the spinal cord to over a meter in length in the leg. The neurons that carry nerve impulses from the tissues of the body into the central nervous system are called afferent. The diagram depicts a typical neuron.

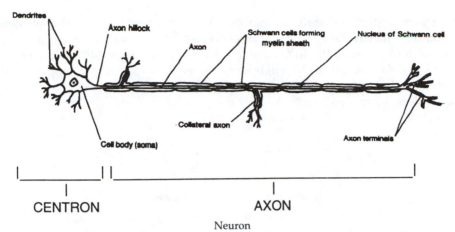

Neuron

(van de Graaff, K.M., and Rhees, R.W., *Human Anatomy and Physiology*, 1987. Reprinted with permission of McGraw-Hill.)

neuropathy. Disease of the nervous system.

neutral fats. *Esters* of *fatty acids* with *glycerol*, in the ratio of three fatty acids to each glycerol base. They are therefore called *triglycerides*. See *fat*.

niacin (nicotinic acid, nicotinamide). Mol. Wt. 123. A water-soluble, heat-stable vitamin of the B complex. Functionally active as the *niacin coenzymes, nicotinamide adenine dinucleotide* (NAD) and *nicotinamide adenine dinucleotide phosphate* (NADP). These coenzymes are essential to cell respiration, carbohydrate and protein metabolism, and lipid synthesis. Deficiency results in skin lesions and gastrointestinal and cerebral manifestations which characterize the neural disease *pellagra*. Dietary sources include preformed niacin and the precursor to *niacin equivalents* (*tryptophan*) and are related to caloric consumption. The actual requirement for niacin varies with the nature of the diet; approximately 1 mg of niacin may be expected to be formed for each 60 mg of tryptophan in the diet. Because niacin can be formed in the body if tryptophan is furnished, the amount of preformed niacin in foods that comprise the diet is not necessarily a measure of the total quantity available to the body. Milk, for example, is much more effective in preventing pellagra than would be expected from its niacin content, because milk proteins have a very high tryptophan content. It is not entirely clear whether humans themselves or bacterial flora convert tryptophan to niacin. In general, animal products contain the vitamin as nicotinamide, while in plants most of it is present as nicotinic acid. Both the acid and the amide are equally effective. Most foods that are good sources of the B vitamins *thiamine* and *riboflavin* are also high in niacin content, such as liver, lean meats, whole grains, nuts, yeast, and legumes. The tables show the niacin content of several common foods and the nicotinic acid (niacin) equivalents in foods with high concentrations of tryptophan but sometimes low concentrations of niacin itself. Niacin functions in *glycolysis* and tissue respiration. The coenzyme forms of niacin, NAD and NADP, function in many important enzyme systems which are necessary for cell respiration. Along with flavine coenzyme, *flavin adenine dinucleotide* (FAD), they act as hydrogen acceptors and donors in a series of *oxidation-reduction* reactions concerned with the release of energy from food. Niacin, riboflavin (the vitamin precursor of FAD), and other members of the vitamin B complex are also involved in the oxidation of *glucose* and the synthesis and oxidation of the *fatty aids*. Recent studies indicate that very high doses of niacin may be effective in lowering blood cholesterol levels by some unknown mechanisms. The niacin levels required for such an effect are about 1.5 g per day, more than 18 times the RDA. The RDA for the average adult male and female are 18 and 13 mg per day, respectively. High levels of niacin intake are accompanied by a side effect—a very unpleasant flushing and burning sensation that may be lessened by aspirin. See *cholesterol therapy*.

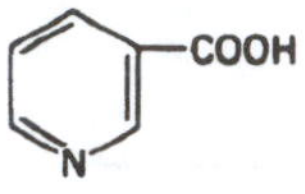

Nicotinic acid 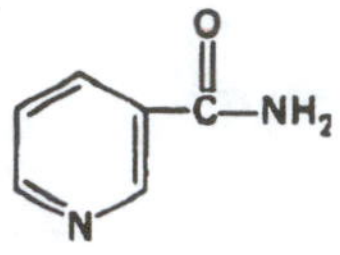   Nicotinamide

Niacin

Niacin in mg/100 g of food

GOOD SOURCES		MODERATE SOURCES	
Beef, lamb, pork	5	Cashews	2
Brewer's yeast	65	Chocolate	1
Fish	4	Cocoa	1
Liver, kidney	12	Corn	2
Meat extract	70	Fruit, dried	1
Millet	3	Legumes	2
Rice, brown	4	Oatmeal	1
Sorghum	3	Rice, white	1
Wheat bran	35		
Wheat, whole	5		
Wheat germ	5		

niacinamide (nicotinamide). See *niacin*.

niacin equivalent. The total niacin available from the diet, including preformed niacin plus that derived from the metabolism of tryptophan; 60 mg *tryptophan* = 1 mg niacin.

nickel (Ni). Element No. 28. At. Wt. 59. Nickel is known to activate several enzyme systems, although whether this is a specific function is not known. It is present in high levels in *ribonucleic acids* for reasons that are not yet clear. Nickel is widely distributed in foods, especially plant foods. A normal diet would supply about 0.3–0.6 mg per day.

nicotinamide. See niacin.

nicotinamide adenine dinucleotide (NAD, NADH). Mol. Wt. 663. A *coenzyme* form of the vitamin *niacin* used for a number of enzymes, chiefly the *dehydrogenases*, that function to exchange hydrogen atoms with substrate molecules. NAD is necessary for tissue respiration, through its association with the dehydrogenases. *Lactate dehydrogenase*, malate dehydrogenase, and beta (β)-hydroxybutyrate dehydrogenase are examples of enzymes that require NAD or NADH as a coenzyme. *Oxidation-reduction reactions* are associated with the reactions in which NAD participates. It is the oxidation of NADH by the *terminal respiratory chain* that accounts for the major conversion of oxidation energy to chemical energy, *adenosine triphosphate* (ATP). See *glycolysis, mitochondrion,* and *oxidative phosphorylation.*

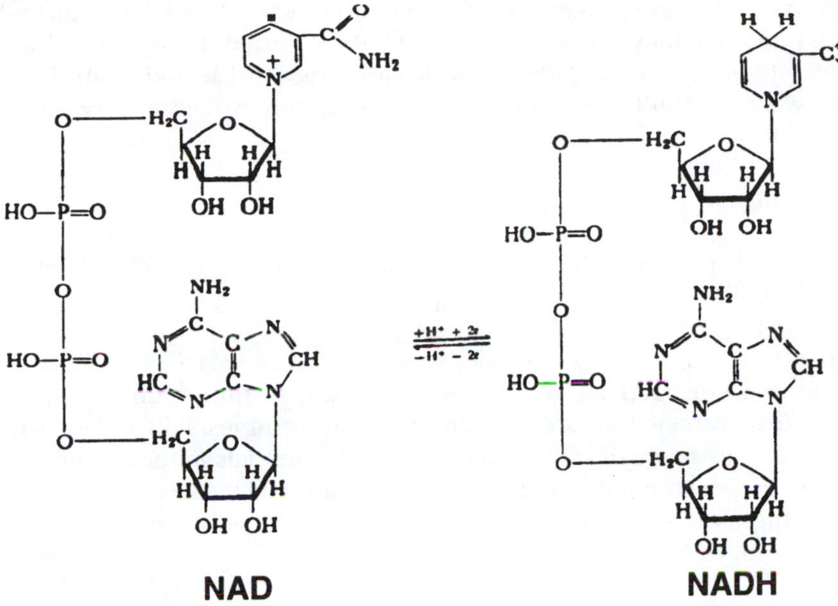

NAD   **NADH**

Nicotinamide adenine dinucleotide

nicotinamide adenine dinucleotide phosphate (NADP, NADPH). Mol. Wt. 743. A *coenzyme* form of the vitamin *niacin* used for a number of enzymes, chiefly the dehydrogenases. The oxidized (NADP) and reduced (NADPH) forms are equivalent structurally to the oxidized and reduced forms of NAD AND NADH (*nicotinamide adenine dinucleotide*). The NADP and

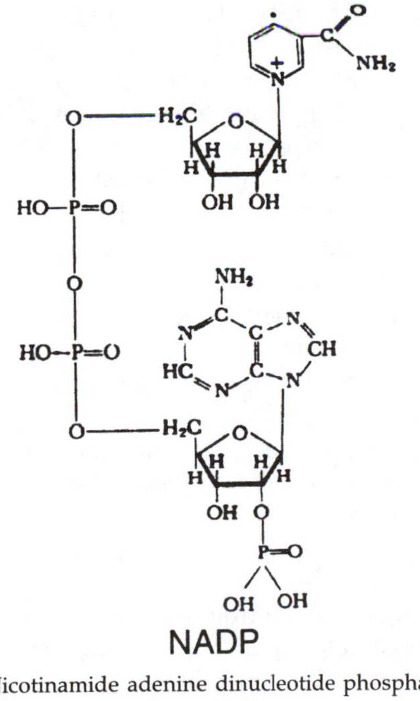

NADP

Nicotinamide adenine dinucleotide phosphate

NADPH also function with *dehydrogenases* and are associated with oxidation and reduction reactions. As a broad generalization, it can be stated that oxidation-reduction reactions that involve NADP and NADPH are generally anabolic (synthetic) and those reactions that involve NAD and NADH are generally catabolic (degradative). An example of these separate roles for the niacin derivatives is *fatty acid synthesis* and *fatty acid oxidation* (degradation). The fatty acid synthetic pathway uses NADPH oxidation-reduction reactions, while the fatty acid oxidation pathway uses NAD.

nicotinic acid. See *niacin*.

ninhydrin. A chemical compound that gives color with *peptides*, *proteins*, and *amino acids*. It is used to quantify amino acids and to identify peptides.

nitrites and nitrates. Commonly used to refer to sodium nitrite ($NaNO_2$). Nitrites are food additives used to prevent bacterial growth. At high temperatures, nitrite combines with secondary amines from protein breakdown to produce nitrosamines. Nitrosamines have been found to produce diverse types of tumors in experimental animals, although no evidence of direct link between these compounds and tumors in humans has been reported. Nitrates play a role in nitrosamine formation because they are readily reduced to nitrites under certain conditions. See *nutrient additives*.

nitrogen (N). Element No. 7. At. Wt. 14. A chemical element essential to life. Some plants can use nitrogen compounds directly from the soil, and nitrogen-fixing bacteria can use nitrogen directly from the air. They ultimately reduce nitrogen to synthesize amino acids for protein foods.

nitrogen balance. Nitrogen balance means that the amount of nitrogen ingested is equal to the amount of nitrogen excreted. To determine the extent of protein metabolism, the nitrogen balance is studied. The amount of nitrogen is an accurate index of the amount of protein involved. The amount of nitrogen that goes into the body in food and the amount that leaves the body in the excreta are determined, and what has been used by the body can be calculated. If the nitrogen intake and nitrogen output are equal, the individual is in nitrogen balance or equilibrium. Should the intake of nitrogen be greater than the amount excreted in the urine and feces, the individual is in a state of positive balance. That is, the buildup (anabolism) or synthesis of tissue proteins is greater than the breakdown (catabolism) actives. An example of a positive nitrogen balance would be the case of a growing child or animal where the nitrogen goes into new tissue and material during growth. Should the intake of nitrogen, however, be less than the amount excreted, a negative balance exists. A negative nitrogen balance inevitably occurs when the protein intake is reduced below the amount required for maintenance of body tissues. Negative nitrogen balance may occur temporarily when the levels of protein intake are decreased. Negative nitrogen balance may occur at levels of protein intake that are above the minimum requirement, if the body is forced to burn protein because the diet furnishes too little carbohydrate and fat to meet the energy requirement. The equation is an expression for the nitrogen balance

$$\textbf{Nitrogen balance (N}_b\textbf{)} = N_i - N_u - N_f - N_s = 0$$

where N_i is total nitrogen intake, N_u is the nitrogen exceted in urine, N_f is the nitrogen excreted in feces, and N_s is the nitrogen excreted in sweat. The amount of nitrogen excreted depends upon the amount of nitrogen intake. A person on a high-nitrogen intake will excrete more than one on a low-nitrogen intake and both could be in nitrogen balance. The table shows how the urine nitrogen excretion profiles might differ for a high- and a low-nitrogen diet.

Nitrogen excreted in the urine

FORM OF NITROGEN	HIGH-NITROGEN DIET	LOW-NITROGEN DIET
Urea	12	3
Creatinine	0.5	0.5
Ammonia	0.5	0.5
Uric acid	1	0.5
Undetermined	1	0.5
Total nitrogen intake	**15**	**5**

nitrogenous. A substance containing nitrogen is referred to as nitrogenous. Proteins contain nitrogen, as do the chemical components of protein, amino acids. Protein decomposition products containing nitrogen are called nitrogenous extractives. They are found in well-ripened meat and contribute to the flavor of meat.

nitrosamine. A class of organic nitrogen compounds with the general structure $R_2C=N=O$. Nitrosamines are mutagenic and can arise from heating *nitrites* added to foods as antibacterial agents.

norepinephrine (noradrenaline). A *hormone* produced by the *adrenal medulla*, similar in chemical and pharmacologic properties to *epinephrine* but chiefly a vasoconstrictor with little effect on cardiac output.

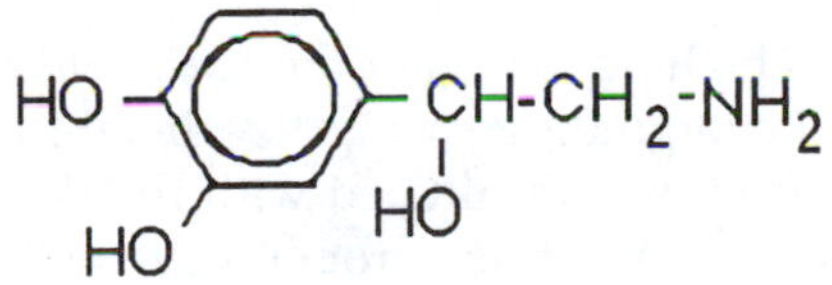

Norepinepherine (noradrenaline)

normal saline. See physiologic saline.

nuclease. A *nucleic acid*-splitting enzyme which results in the production of *nucleotides* from *deoxyribonucleic acid* or *ribonucleic acid*, depending on the specificity of the enzyme. They are termed DNases and RNases, respectively.

nucleic acid. Nucleic acids are complex, high-molecular-weight molecules containing nitrogenous bases (*purines* and *pyrimidines*), five-carbon sugars (*ribose* or *deoxyribose*), and phosphate. The nucleic acids are divided into two major groups which relate to their structure, the *deoxyribonucleic acids* (DNA) and the *ribonucleic acids* (RNA). The DNA molecule contains as major constituents *cytosine, thymine, adenine,* and *guanine* as the nitrogenous bases, and deoxyribose as the five-carbon sugar. The RNA molecule contains as major constituents cytosine, *uracil*, adenine, and guanine as the nitrogenous bases, and ribose as the *pentose*.

Nucleic acids are found in all living cells, with the exception of the red blood cells of humans, and the structures of these compounds are directly related to the characteristics of the individual cell and the organism itself. The almost infinite variety of possible structures for nucleic acids allows information in coded form to be recorded in giant DNA molecules. Such stored information controls the inherited characteristics, as well as many of the ongoing live processes of the organism. DNA is found primarily in the *nucleus* of the cell and is identified as the gene or genetic material. RNA is found mainly in the cytoplasm the and functions prominently in protein synthesis by translating the genetic code through *messenger* or *mRNA* and bringing the individual amino acids to the site of protein synthesis by *transfer* or *tRNA* on the *ribosomes*.

nucleolus. A spherical body found within the cell *nucleus*, it is rich in *ribonucleic acid* and believed to be the site of synthesis for *nucleoproteins*.

nucleoprotein. Conjugated protein found in cell nuclei that results from the combination of a protein with nucleic acid. Nucleoproteins are essential for cell division and reproduction though their roles are not entirely understood.

nucleotide. A molecule composed of a phosphate group, a five-carbon sugar—*ribose* or *deoxyribose*—and a nitrogenous base, a *flavin*, *purine*, *pyrimidine*, or *pyridine*. *Flavin adenine dinucleotide*, *adenosine triphosphate*, *cytosine triphosphate*, and *nicotinamide adenine diphosphate* are respective examples of nucleotides.

nucleus. A formed element in cytoplasm that separates itself by a nuclear membrane. The *nucleus* contains the genetic materials, *deoxyribonucleic acids*, and much of the apparatus for cell division. It contains the *chromosomes*. Somatic *tissues* are *diploid*, containing a pair of chromosomes. The sperm and egg contain half the chromosome number of the somatic cells in their nuclei.

nutmeg (*Myristica fragrans*). The hard kernel of the apricot like fruit of the different varieties of the nutmeg tree, a tropical evergreen growing to a height of 20–40 feet. In appearance it resembles the pear tree. The fruit is intermingled with the flowers and carefully split in half to expose the hard seed, which is the nutmeg proper, covered by a false aril which is carefully removed, dried, and used to make *mace*, sister spice of nutmeg. The nutmeg itself is also dried in the sun or over charcoal fires. It is oval in shape, gray-brown in color, and contains fat, volatile oil, acid, and starch. It is an aromatic spice, used a great deal in cooking.

Nutrasweet®. An artificial sweetener containing *aspartame*.

nutrient. A general term for any substance which can be used in the metabolic processes of the body. Scientists have identified about 50 different elements or chemical substances in food. These substances are grouped into six major classes called "nutrients." The basic six are *proteins, carbohydrates, vitamins, minerals, fats*, and *water*. The real bulk of all foods are proteins, carbohydrates, fats, and water. Many of the minerals and vitamins are only needed in minute amounts in a balanced diet. In digestion, nutrients are reduced to their simplest forms in preparation for absorption. In human nutrition, there are about 40 nutrients that are required for growth in children and the maintenance of health in the normal adult. The tables list what are considered nutrients, though some of the evidence that a substance is a nutrient in humans is not well documented. Some of the assignments as a nutrient are based on animal rather than human studies. Requirements in the table are only approximate. For more detailed information, see the individual nutrient.

nutrient additives. One class of food additives is nutrients added to improve or maintain the nutritional value of foods. Included among these are the four nutrients added to refined grains to enrich them, the iodine added to salt, vitamins A and D added to dairy products, and the nutrients added to fortified breakfast cereals. Nutrients are sometimes also added for other purposes. Vitamins C and E are examples. Both are antioxidants and are added to foods to help keep them from spoiling. Vitamin E is now added to bacon because it prevents *nitrosamine* formation from *nitrites* while not interfering with the antibotulinal activity of nitrite. See *botulism*.

nutrient density. The relation of the concentration of specific nutrients in a food (vitamins, minerals, proteins) to the caloric value of that food. The enrichment and fortification of selected foods (e.g., cereals, flour, bread, and milk) represent efforts to provide a good nutrient density in popular foods. In the case of packaged foods, including convenience-packaged meals and liquid meals, the responsibility falls directly on the producer to provide appropriate nutrient densities.

nutrition. The combination of processes by which the living organism receives and utilizes the materials necessary for the maintenance of its functions and for the growth and renewal of its components. Normal nutrition is a condition of the body resulting from the efficient utilization of sufficient amounts of the essential nutrients provided in the food intake.

nutritional anemia. See *anemia*.

nutritional antagonist. A compound whose structure is so similar to a specific nutrient (an *antimetabolite*) that it can substitute for the nutrient in certain enzyme systems for which the specific nutrient is necessary, thus leading to at least partial inactivity of these systems. Hence, an effect similar to a deficiency is produced in a short time. True nutritional antagonism, or inhibition, can be overcome by high enough levels of the nutrient in question. See *antivitamins*.

nutriture. The condition of well-being of the body as related to the consumption and utilization of food for growth, maintenance, and repair. Nutriture, or nutritional status, may be appraised by such methods as clinical examination of the condition of the skin, eyes, mouth, tongue, gums, and muscles; determination of overweight or underweight; often, measurement of blood pressure and pulse rate; biochemical tests on the blood for various constituents associated with health; and urinalysis.

nuts. A large number of dry fruits which generally consist of a single kernel enclosed in a woody shell. Acorns, filberts, and hazelnuts are examples of true nuts. The Brazil nut represents another type of dry fruit popularly classed as a nut; some nuts are, botanically speaking, *legumes*. The peanut, for instance, is the pod of a vine of the pea family. Some fruits whose kernels are not dry are called nuts because of their nutlike shells. The litchi nut, for example, is a fleshy raisinlike fruit enclosed in a shell. But not all the shells of true nuts are hard. The almond and pecan, for instance, come in more than one variety. Some have hard shells, some have soft ones, and some have paper-thin shells. The edible portion is the kernel. Most edible nuts contain less carbohydrate than legumes and are rich in protein and very rich in fat. They

nutrients (1)

NUTRIENT	REQUIREMENT	MAJOR FUNCTION(S)	BEST FOOD SOURCE
Water	2.4 L/day	The solvent and suspending fluid for tissue substances.	Directly and from foods generally
Carbohydrates	Not essential; about 55% of caloric intake	Supplies food energy. Spares the need for the essential amino acids. Allows the oxidation of fat to be more efficient.	Starchy vegetables, breads, grains, sugars
Fats	30% of caloric intake	Supplies most of the food energy. Spares the need for the essential amino acids.	Saturated fats derive from animal tissues and hydrogenated oils
Essential fatty acids			
Linoleic acid	Requirements unknown	The essential fatty acids are required for the synthesis of hormone-like substances— prostaglandins, prostacyclins,	Unsaturated fats derive from fish and vegetable oils
Linolenic acid	Requirements unknown	and thromboxanes —which regulate physiologic processes. The essential fatty acids are highly unsaturated.	
Proteins	About 15% of caloric intake or 0.8 g/kg of body wt./day	Supplies the amino acids for the formation of new tissues, hormones, nitrogenous compounds, and energy.	Meats, fish, eggs, cheese, beans, milk, legumes
Essential amino acids			
Histidine	The ratio of	All of the essential amino acids are	
Isoleucine	essential amino	required for nitrogen balance and	
Leucine	acids determines	some are required for special	
Lysine	biological value	synthetic processes, such as	
Methionine	(BV) of proteins.	hormones. Histidine is required	
Phenylalanine	Egg protein is the	for infants.	
Threonine	standard		
Tryptophan			
Valine			
Fat-soluble vitamins			
Vitamin A Retinol	900 RE	Essential for night vision. Maintains epithelial tissues. Normal bone and tooth development in children. Toxic in large quantities.	Occurs in plant foods as the provitamin carotene; yellow and dark-green vegetables, organ meats, egg yolk, peaches, apricots, cantaloupes
Vitamin D Calciferol	300 I.U. 7.5 µg	Essential for normal bone and tooth formation. Affects phosphorus and calcium absorption. Prevents rickets in children and osteomalacia in adults. Toxic in large quantities.	Sunlight exposure, irradiated foods, vitamin D milk, liver, egg yolk, fish liver oils
Vitamin E Tocopherols	9 alpha-TE	A powerful antioxidant. Protects red blood cells from hemolysis. Maintains the cell membrane integrity. Prevents the oxidation of unsaturated fatty acids and vitamin A. Interrelated with selenium metabolism.	Wheat germ, green leafy vegetables, vegetable oils, egg yolk, nuts

continued

NUTRIENT	REQUIREMENT	MAJOR FUNCTION(S)	BEST FOOD SOURCE
Vitamin K Phylloquinone	Unknown	Required for normal blood clotting. Essential for the rapid conversion of several blood clotting factors to their active forms — such as prothromin to thrombin.	Liver, vegetable oils, wheat bran, green-leafy vegetables, synthesized by enteric bacteria
Water-soluble vitamins Thiamine Vitamin B_1	0.5 mg/1000 kc 1.4 mg/day	Dietary deficiency leads to beriberi. Essential for growth, normal appetite, normal nerve function, and normal muscle tone. One of the coenzymes involved in conversion of the energy in food into chemical energy through tissue respiration. Coenzyme form is thiamine pyrophosphate (TPP).	Liver and organ meats, legumes, enriched cereals and breads, nuts, whole grains, synthesized by enteric bacteria
Riboflavin Vitamin B_2	0.6 mg/1000 kc 1.5 mg/day	Essential for normal growth. One of the coenzymes involved in conversion of the energy in food into chemical energy. Coenzyme forms are FMN and FAD.	Milk, dairy foods, organ meats, green-leafy vegetables, enriched cereals, breads, eggs, synthesized by enteric bacteria
Niacin Nicotinamide Nicotinic acid	6.6 NE/1000 kc 17 mg/day	Dietary deficiency leads to pellagra. Important for cell respiration. One of the coenzymes involved in the conversion of the energy in food into chemical energy. Coenzyme forms are NAD and NADP.	Organ meats, lean meats, nuts, poultry, fish, eggs, cheese; synthesized by enteric bacteria
Vitamin B_6 Pyridoxine	21 mg/day	Essential for normal growth. Important for the metabolism of amino acids. Important for the formation of blood cells. Maintains normal nerve function. The coenzyme forms are pyridoxal and pyridoxamine.	Rice, wheat germ, fish, meats, organ meats, poultry, synthesized by enteric bacteria
Folacin Folic acid	0.4 mg/day	Important in the synthesis of nucleic acids. Required for the formation of blood cells and hemoglobin. The coenzyme form is tetrahydrofolic acid. Interacts with vitamin B_{12}.	Green-leafy vegetables, meats, organ meats, eggs, fish, whole wheat; synthesized by enteric bacteria
Vitamin B_{12} Cobalamin	3 µg/day	Required for normal red blood cell formation. Essential for normal nerve function. Interacts with folacin. Inability to absorb cobalamin leads to pernicious anemia. Coenzyme forms are coenzyme B_{12} and cobalamin.	Meats, organ meats, milk, dairy foods, eggs, no known plant sources
Biotin	Estimated as 4–7 mg/day	Essential for fatty acid metabolism. Involved in carbon dioxide and amino acid metabolism. Interrelated with folacin, panthothenic acid, and vitamin B_{12}.	Organ meats, meats, eggs, most vegetables, some fruits, synthesized by enteric bacteria

continued

NUTRIENT	REQUIREMENT	MAJOR FUNCTION(S)	BEST FOOD SOURCE
Pantothenic acid	Estimate 0.2 mg/day	An integral part of coenzyme A. Involved in many metabolic pathways of carbohydrates, fats, and proteins.	Available in most animal and plant foods; possibly synthesized by enteric bacteria
Vitamin C Ascorbic acid	60 mg/day	Dietary deficiency leads to scurvy. Required to maintain connective and elastic tissues. Important for normal collagen synthesis. Involved in amino acid metabolism.	Citrus fruits, peppers, potatoes, green-leafy vegetables, melons, tomato, pineapple
Macroelements			
Calcium	0.8–1.2 g/day	Bone and teeth formation. Nerve transmission. Enzyme activations. Muscle activity. Blood clotting. Cell permeability. 99% is in bones and teeth.	Milk, milk products, nuts, soft fish bones, green-leafy vegetables
Sodium	1–3 g/day	Maintenance of water balance outside the cell. The major extracellular cation. Muscle and nerve functions. pH regulation. 40% is in bone.	Table salt, most foods except fresh vegetables, fruits
Potassium	0.2–0.5 g/day	The major intracellular cation. Water balance. pH regulation. Membrane transfer. Muscle function. Protein and carbohydrate metabolism. Insulin secretion.	Fruits, milk, legumes, meats, cereals, nuts, vegetables
Magnesium	0.3 g/day	About 50% in bone and 50% inside cells. An activator of many enzymes. Complexes with ATP.	Cereals, meats, milk, nuts, legumes, green vegetables
Chlorine	0.2–0.5 g/day	Water and acid-base balance. An extracellular anion (85%). A component the of gastric juice (HCl). An enzyme activator.	Table salt, milk, meats, eggs
Phosphorus	0.8–1.2 g/day	Bone and tooth formation. A component of nucleic acids, sugars, and proteins. 80% is in bones and teeth. pH regulation.	Milk, milk products, rice, wheat bran, meats, fish, seafood, nuts, grains, protein foods
Sulfur	Supplied by amino acids—cysteine, methinoine	Mostly in the sulfur-containing amino acids. Oxidation-reduction reactions.	
Microelements			
Chromium	0.02 0.2 mg/day	Enhances insulin activity. An enzyme activator.	Animal meats, wheat bran, seafoods, liver, butter, margarine, corn oil, molasses
Copper	0.6 mg/day	Hemoglobin formation. Iron absorption and release. Component of proteins. Bone formation	Liver, meats, nuts, molasses, wheat bran, legumes, dark-green vegetables
Iron	10–18 mg/day	Hemoglobin formation. Cellular oxidations.	Organ meats, wheat bran, dark-green vegetables, nuts, legumes

continued

NUTRIENT	REQUIREMENT	MAJOR FUNCTION(S)	BEST FOOD SOURCE
Manganese	2–5 mg/day	Bone and connective tissue formation. Blood clotting. Insulin activity. Enzyme activations.	Cereals, whole grains, nuts, fruits, vegetables
Molybdenum	0.5 mg/day	Tooth enamel. A component of enzymes metabolizing fats, proteins, and carbohydrates.	Legumes, leafy vegetables, organ meats, yeast, whole grains
Selenium	0.1 mg/day	Interrelated with vitamin E. Associated with the maintenance of red blood cells. Associated with antioxidant activity.	Beer, yeast, seafoods, molasses, whole grains
Zinc	15 mg/day	Normal skin, hair, and bone. Component of many enzymes. Energy metabolism/protein synthesis	Meats, liver, seafoods, whole grains, eggs, milk
Fluoride	1–3 mg/day	Sound bones and teeth.	Fluoridated water, seafoods
Iodine	0.15 mg/day	Essential component of the hormone thyroxin.	Iodized salt, seafoods, kelp, vegetables grown in iodine-rich soil

ULTRATRACE ELEMENTS	REQUIREMENTS EXTRAPOLATED FROM ANIMAL STUDIES	POSSIBLE FUNCTIONS
Arsenic	Unknown	Appears to be essential for normal growth and for fertility. May play a role in the urea cycle.
Bromine	Unknown	Evidence that it is essential for good health is very weak.
Boron	Unknown	Growth and bone development. Involved in mineral metabolism. Evidence for essentiality is weak.
Cadmium	Unknown	Evidence that it is essential for good health is very weak.
Cobalt	Unknown	Essential as a component of vitamin B_{12}.
Lead	Unknown	Facilitates iron absorption.
Lithium	Unknown	Regulation of the endocrine system. May be involved in the maintenance of fertility.
Nickel	< 1 µg/day	Component of metalloenzymes involved with iron metabolism.
Silicon	Unknown	Essential for normal connective tissues structures and bone calcification and healing.
Tin	< 1 µg/day	Associated with wound healing and tissue growth.
Vanadium	200 µg	High concentrations in teeth. May have a role in lipid metabolism.

contain fair to generous amounts of *thiamine, riboflavin,* and *niacin* and represent good sources of iron and phosphorus. The proteins of nuts have a biologic value similar to the legumes (soybeans excepted). The digestibility of nuts is rather low, primarily because of their compact physical state.

nyctalopia. Night blindness due to a vitamin A deficiency. See *retinal, retinol, rhodopsin,* and *rod vision*.

oat, oatmeal (Avena). Oats are the grains of a cereal grass plant, or the plant itself. Like the rest of the grains, oats consist of a soft inner part surrounded by a husk which is removed before being eaten by humans. Some varieties of oats, however, are hull-less. The grain is used to make rolled oats and oatmeal and as feed for livestock. Most cultivated varieties of oats have a smooth-surfaced hull, although some varieties are hairy. To produce rolled oats, the husked, sterilized grains are flattened by heated rolls into the flakes. To make oatmeal, the groats (edible portion of the oats with the hull removed) are steel-cut in three sizes and ground in grades from coarse to extra-fine. Oats are the most nutritious of cereals, containing a good amount of fat, proteins, fiber, and minerals. Good source of *niacin*, fair source of *thiamine* and *tocopherol* (vitamin E). See this item in the table under *fiber, dietary* and *grains*.

obesity. The accumulation of excess fat. Obesity is usually determined by comparing an individual's weight to tables of standard weights. Overweight is then determined by the percent above the norm for a given height. Sometimes a body frame may not fit the norm and a person with a large frame and a large musculature can be more than 20% above the standard weight and not be obese. For a normal young man about 12% *body weight* is standard, and for young women the value is about 25%. Measurement of body fat is difficult, but a simple, reasonable reflection of obesity can be obtained by the skinfold test. An instrument called "skin calipers" measures the thickness of skin folds at four sites, the biceps and triceps muscles, over the iliac crest bone, and under the scapula bone. Obesity arises only when the intake of food or calories is in excess of the physiologic caloric need. While genetics may play a role in obesity, the influence of heredity is a difficult one to separate from the environment. Occasionally, individuals are obese because of some glandular disorders, *hypothyrodism, Cushing's syndrome, hypopituitarism,* and *hypogonadism,* but such instances are very rare and are not an essential feature of these conditions. The overwhelming majority of obese individuals show no clinical evidence of glandular disorders. The basal metabolic rates of obese individuals are within normal limits. The obese individual appears to have biochemical patterns with respect to fat and carbohydrate metabolism that differ from the nonobese person. The obese person does not develop *ketosis* readily and *glucose* appears to be oxidized at a slower rate. These observations appear to be a consequence of obesity and not the cause since all of the biochemical patterns become normal when the obese individual reaches normal weight. Many complications appear to accompany obesity. They include an association with high levels of *cholesterol,* an increased incidence of *diabetes mellitus,* increased tendency towards heart disease, increased incidence of varicose veins, and decreased life expectancy. See *muscle* and *skeleton* diagrams.

odor. See *aroma* and *taste*.

oedema. See *edema*.

offal. The word derives from "off-fall," the parts of an animal removed in the dressing process. Offal includes the brains, sweetbreads, stomach, and intestines of as well as the organ meats. See the items in the table under *meat* for nutrient contents.

off-flavors. Off-flavors is a term that describes the presence of an strange taste or aroma that is not normally associated with the food. Off-flavors can arise during food processing or storage. The causes of off-flavors are many. Bacterial or fungal contaminations, photo-oxidations, and photolysis are among the common causes of off-flavors. See *aroma*, *flavor*, and *taste*.

oil. The nutrient oil is a liquid, digestible *fat*. An oil differs from a fat by its liquid state at ordinary temperatures. Chemically, oils differ from fats in that they contain a great number of unsaturated bonds in the *fatty acids* esterified to *glycerols*. Fat and oils belong to the same class of food, neutral fats. Processed fatty oils are hydrogenated oils, stearines, oleins, segregated oils, interesterified oils, products of fractional crystallization (e.g., certain cocoa butter substitutes), margarines, butter, and cooking fats. Refined fatty oils are products prepared from the crude fatty oils by neutralization, bleaching, and deodorization. Oil is also used to describe a class of nondigestible, hydrocarbon chemicals unrelated to nutrition.

okra (*Hibisucus esculentus*). A tall annual plant of the mallow family which yields an edible pod with a gooey, mucilaginous quality. Okra should be eaten when very tender. Okra is used to flavor and thicken gumbos or soup-stews. Fair source of carotene (vitamin A activity) and *ascorbic acid*. A good source of the *fiber* which lowers serum *cholesterol*. See this item in the table under *vegetables*.

oleic acid (oleate). Mol. Wt. 282. An *unsaturated fatty acid*. Oleic acid is a liquid *oil* at room temperature, a property of most unsaturated fatty acids. The transisomer of oleic acid, elaidic acid, is a solid at room temperature. The difference in the physical properties is related to the ease of association of molecules in the transisomer. In high concentrations in olive oil, oleic acid has been shown to lower serum *cholesterol* when substituted for *saturated fats*. See *cis-* and *trans-* isomerism.

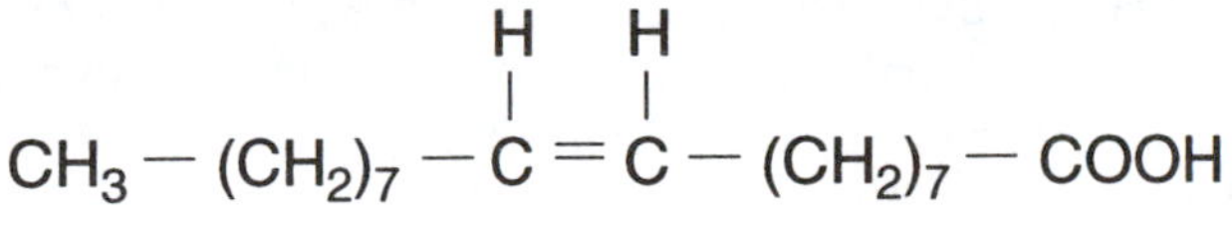

$$CH_3 - (CH_2)_7 - \overset{\overset{\displaystyle H}{|}}{C} = \overset{\overset{\displaystyle H}{|}}{C} - (CH_2)_7 - COOH$$

Oleic acid

$$CH_3 - (CH_2)_7 - \overset{\overset{\displaystyle H}{|}}{\underset{\underset{\displaystyle H}{|}}{C}} = C - (CH_2)_7 - COOH$$

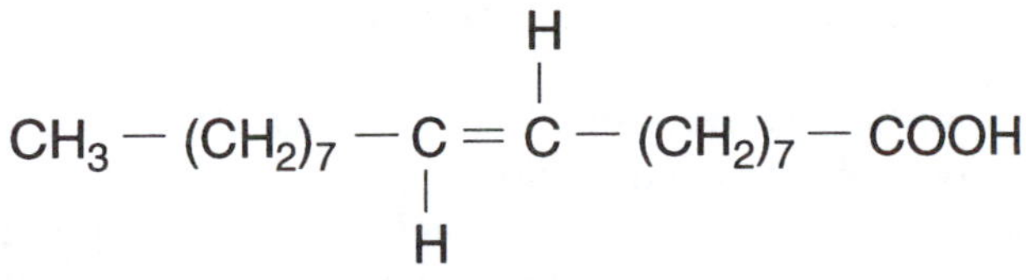

Elaidic acid

oleomargarine. A smooth-textured fat used as a spread and in cooking. The name comes from *elo-*, a combining form meaning "oil" and from margaric acid, a constituent of animal fat. See *margarine*.

olfactory nerve. The nerve that receives and transmits impulses associated with the sense of *smell*. Cell bodies of the bipolar neurons of this nerve are located in the olfactory mucosa of the superiormost portion of the nasal cavity. The sense of smell is a necessity for a discriminating sense of *taste*. See *aroma* and *flavor*.

oligosaccharides. A general term to express the linkage of several *monosaccharides* in a single molecule. The general class of oligosaccharides includes sugars containing any number from three to as many as ten monosaccharide units joined together. More than ten monosaccharide units is generally classified as a *polysaccharide*, but there is no definite division between the classifications. This bonding is the *glycosidic linkage* common to the *disaccharides*, oligosaccharides, and polysaccharides.

olive (*Olea europaea*). The fruit of a 25- to 40-foot subtropical evergreen tree. Olives, as they grow on the tree, are pale green. When they begin to turn straw-colored, they are picked and prepared in various ways for eating. Fresh olives are very bitter. The bitterness is removed in the preparation. Green fermented olives, the well-known Spanish-style olives, are soaked in lye for a short time, washed, and then kept in barrels of salt solution for 6–12 months. This causes a lactic-acid fermentation and gives them their astringent taste. Sugar is added from time to time to keep fermentation going. When the olives are properly fermented, they are packed in a weak salt brine and bottled. As the olive becomes riper it develops more oil. Ripe olives are either green or black. The "black" color of the "ripe" olive is developed during the lye treatments. Between treatments they are exposed to the air to develop the characteristic dark color.

Nutrients in 100 g of green olives

CALORIES KCAL	PROTEIN G	FAT G	CARBOHYDRATE G	VITAMIN A IU	CALCIUM MG
116	1	13	1	300	62

olive oil. A product obtained by crushing tree-ripened olives, then extracting the liquid by pressing the pulp or by centrifugal separators. The first "crude olive oil" is obtained from this liquid by settling and skimming or by "washing" by a continuous flow of clear water. Refining produces the clear oil used for salads and cooking.

omega (ω)-3-fatty acid. See *unsaturated fatty acids* and *eicospentaenoic acid*.

onion (*Allium cepa*). An underground bulb. There are many kinds of onions with different-colored skins, and in size they vary from the very small bulbets of the spring or green onions, also known as scallions, to the huge round red Italian onions. A pungent, volatile oil, rich in sulfur, is the cause of the onion's strong smell and flavor. Onions are a member of the lily family which includes such flowers as the tulip, hyacinth, and lily-of-the-valley as well as the edible leek, garlic, chive, and shallot. All have a bulb growing under the ground and a stalk, leaves, and flowers above. The word "onion" comes through French from Latin, probably from the Latin word *unus*, meaning "one," perhaps because the onion is a single bulb with a spherical shape. Onions contain some *ascorbic acid* (vitamin C) with small amounts of other vitamins and minerals. Green parts of the onion yield some *carotene* (vitamin A activity). See this item in the table under *vegetables*.

opsin. A protein compound which combines with *cis*-11 *retinal*, vitamin A aldehyde, to form rhodopsin, visual purple. Visual purple is necessary for night vision via the rods in the retina. A vitamin A deficiency will lead to night blindness because rhodopsin is not formed at normal levels. See *retinal*, *retinol*, and *rhodopsin*.

orange (*Citrus*). There are many varieties of oranges, but the three principal species are the sweet, common, or China orange, *C. sinensis*; the loose-skinned orange, *C. nobilis*; and the sour, bitter Seville orange, *C. Aurantium*. The best known sweet oranges are the golden-yellow Valencia, or Spanish, heavy and juicy, with large coarse-grained fruit; Mediterranean oranges which have a fine-grained fruit; blood oranges with a red or red-and-white streaked pulp; and the seedless navel or Washington navel oranges. Oranges are excellent sources of *ascorbic acid* (vitamin C) and some *carotene* (vitamin A activity). Once juices are squeezed or canned juices are opened, vitamin C combines with air and forms a new compound which has no vitamin value. After 24 hours in a refrigerator, 20% of vitamin C is lost; after 24 hours at room temperature, 60% of vitamin C is lost. See this item in the table under *fruits*.

Nutrients in 100 g of orange

CALORIES KCAL	PROTEIN G	FAT G	CARBOHYDRATE G	VITAMIN A IU	ASCORBATE MG	CALCIUM MG
54	1	0.2	12	200	115	41

oregano (*Origanum vulgare*). Also called wild *marjoram*, a beautiful *herb* which grows in clumps with purplish, pink, lilac, or white flowers. It is the dark-green leaf, shaped like a roundish egg, that is used as a culinary herb. Leaves may be used fresh or dried. The tops of the plant may also be used. The flavor is similar to that of sweet marjoram or thyme, all belonging to the mint family. Oregano is considerably more bitter and pungent and should be used with discretion. Vegetable juice cocktails and bean, beef, game, or tomato soups may be flavored with oregano. Oregano is often used as a seasoning in Mexican and Italian dishes.

organ. A member of a system, composed of cells and tissues associated in performing some special function for which it is especially adapted. Systems are made up of organs, such as the *nervous system*, with a corresponding division of labor and special adaptation of the organ to its particular share of the work of the whole system.

organelles. Organelles are various formed structures within the cell. Some examples of formed elements of the cell are the *mitochondria*, the *Golgi complex* or apparatus, the *endoplasmic reticulum*, the *ribosomes*, and *lysosomes*. Some of the functions of the organelles are given in the table. See *cells*.

Functions of organelles

ORGANELLE	FUNCTIONS
Plasma membrane	Protects cell. Regulates the entry and exit of materials.
Nucleus	The control center of cell activity. Contains DNA.
Ribosomes	The site of protein synthesis.
Endoplasmic recticulum (ER)	Rough ER: contains ribosomes. Site of protein synthesis.
	Smooth ER: Detoxifications. Steroid synthesis. Transport apparatus.
Golgi apparatus	Secretory vesicles. Formation of lysosomes. Packaging of large complex molecules, e.g. glycoproteins.
Lysosomes	Degradation of worn cell components. Digestion of engulfed materials.
Mitochondria	Oxidative processes. Krebs' cycle. ATP synthesis.
Vesicles	Storage of secretory materials.
Granules	Storage of cellular materials, e.g. glycogen.
Fat droplets	Storage of fat and lipids.
Microtubules	Cell infrastructure. Orients movement of materials within the cell.
Microfilaments	Cell infrastructure. Involved in cellular movements.
Centrioles	Involve in cell division, contractile activity, and cilia activity.

organic. A group of chemical compounds that contain carbon.

organic acids. The acid group of organic acids contains only carbon, hydrogen, and oxygen and is called carboxylic acid group ($COOH^-$); in solution it releases protons (H^+). They are generally weak acids because they release their protons with more resistance than most inorganic acids, which are generally strong acids. Organic acids and their salts form *buffers*. Among the better known is *citric acid* which occurs in high concentrations in citrus fruits. Another is *acetic acid*—the major acid in *vinegar*. Aerobically the organic acids may be oxidized completely to carbon dioxide and water. In the body, long-chain *fatty acids* are degraded two carbons at a time by way of acetic acid derivatives. See *oxidation*.

organic foods. A somewhat loosely used term most generally taken to mean foods grown by "organic gardening" methods, with no chemical fertilizers or pesticides. Sometimes the term is used more broadly and interchangeably with "natural foods," to include foods not only "organically" grown but containing no chemical additives, such as preservatives, hormones, dyes, and antibiotics, and which have undergone only a minimum of refining to preserve original nutrients.

organic salts. Organic salts are formed when they are neutralized by a base. The resulting salt is identified by the suffix "-ate." For examples, the salt forms of citric acid and acetic acid are called cit*rate* and *acetate*, respectively. An organic acid and its salt in solution is a *buffer*.

orgeat. A syrup used in France, Spain, Italy, and Latin American countries as a refreshing drink when mixed with water or as a flavoring for frostings and fillings. The syrup is usually made from an emulsion of almonds and sugar with a little rosewater or orange-flower water added.

ornithine. Mol. Wt. 132. A nonessential *amino acid* of the *urea cycle* formed from *arginine* when urea is split off. Ornithine and *citrulline* are the two amino acids that do not occur in proteins.

$$NH_2$$
$$H_2N-CH_2-CH_2-CH_2-CH-COOH$$

Ornithine

osmole. An osmole is a standard unit of osmotic pressure. It is proportional to the gram molecular weight of a substance divided by the number of ions or particles into which the substance dissociates in solution.

osmosis. The word osmosis comes from the Greek word *osmos* meaning "to push" or "to thrust." Osmosis is the passage of solvent molecules from the lesser to the greater concentration of solute when two solutions are separated by a membrane which selectively prevents the passage of solute molecules but is permeable to the solvent.

osmotic pressures. The force that a dissolved substance exerts on a membrane that allows solvent to pass through but not the solute, when solutions of differing solute concentrations are separated by a semipermeable membrane. The tendency is for solvent to pass the higher concentration until the concentrations of solute on both sides of the semipermeable membrane are equal. Osmotic pressure is a measure of the force of that tendency for water to pass across the semipermeable membrane from the less-concentrated to the more-concentrated solution until the concentrations of dissolved particles on both sides are equal. Net exchanges of water between the various fluid compartments of the body occur as a result of osmotic pressure, due chiefly to differences in the concentrations of electrolytes. Osmotic pressure in the cellular fluid is regulated mainly by the concentration of *potassium* ions and in the extracellular fluid by the concentration of *sodium* ions. Plasma proteins also play important roles in maintaining osmotic equilibria in the extracellular fluid compartments by remaining in the plasma. Because they are not permeable to cell membrane, the plasma proteins prevent the net exchange of water from plasma into the *interstitial* space. An excess of fluid in the interstitial space is known as *edema* and results from lowered osmotic pressure in the plasma relative to the interstitial space.

ossification. The process of forming *bone* is ossification. *Cartilage* is made into bone by the process of ossification. The minerals, calcium and phosphorus are deposited in the cartilage matrix, changing it into bone.

osteoarthritis. A common type of arthritis in which there is a gradual degeneration of the joint rather than an *acute* inflammatory type of process. It rarely leads to crippling. Most persons suffering from this disease are over 40 years of age and have only mild pain and stiffness of the joints. The joints of the fingers are often affected.

osteoblasts. Bone-forming cells.

osteoclasts. Giant multinuclear cells found in depressions on bone surfaces, which cause resorption of bone tissue and the formation of canals.

osteomalacia. A nutritional disease. Prolonged deficiencies of dietary calcium and *vitamin D* or sunlight may result in osteomalacia, sometimes called adult *rickets*. This condition is characterized by poor calcification of the bones with increasing softness, so that they become flexible, leading to deformities in the spine, thorax, or pelvis. These bone changes may be accompanied by rheumatic pains and exhaustion.

osteoporosis. A condition of abnormal porousness or "thinning" of bone due to insufficient production of the protein matrix in which calcium salts are deposited, and/or deposition of other minerals in the matrix. It occurs principally in women after middle age and in elderly men and women. When calcium enters the body, it is absorbed into the bloodstream. If there is any excess, it is deposited in bone where it is stored until the body needs to tap this reserve. When the calcium supply is deficient, the blood must take it back from the bones. If calcium remains inadequate over a longer period of time, the bones eventually become porous and weak. That postmenopausal women tend to get osteoporosis suggests a hormonal disorder, as *estrogens* in women of this age fall off sharply. This disease most frequently affects the spinal column, causing backaches and rounded spines. In severe cases the bone becomes as porous as a sponge and can collapse as a result. The etiology of osteoporosis is not clear. Osteoporosis is a condition distinct from the nutritional condition *osteomalacia*, resulting from a dietary deficit of *calcium*.

ovaries. They appear as two almond-shaped glands, one on either side of the abdomino-pelvic cavity. They produce female germ cells, ova, and female hormones, *estrogen* and *progesterone*. These hormones maintain the normal menstrual cycle. An *ovum* is expelled from the surface of an ovary in a process called ovulation, which generally occurs about halfway between each menstrual period. An expelled ovum is picked up by the free end of a fallopian tube for transportation to the uterus.

ovum. The female reproductive or germ cell. A cell that is capable of developing into a new organism of the same species after fertilization with a sperm cell.

oxaloacetic acid (oxalacetate). Mol. Wt. 132. An intermediate in the *Krebs'* (tricarboxylic acid) *cycle*. The reaction of oxalacetate with acetyl coenzyme A to form *citric acid* is considered the first step in the Krebs' cycle. Oxalacetate is the α-keto acid equivalent of the nonessential amino acid *aspartic acid* which can be formed by *transamination*.

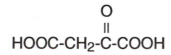

Oxaloacetic acid

oxalic acid (oxalate). Mol. Wt. 90. HOOC–COOH. A dicarboxylic acid which occurs as a result of metabolic processes in the body and is found in certain foods, especially cocoa, rhubarb, spinach, and some other greens. Oxalic acid forms insoluble salts with calcium, magnesium, and iron, and acts to prevent these minerals from being absorbed during digestion.

oxidation. Oxidation may be interpreted in several ways. The addition of oxygen to a molecule is one form of oxidation. The oxidation of hydrogen to form water is an other example. Every oxidation must also be accompanied by the opposite reaction, a *reduction*, and in this example oxygen is reduced. In the oxidation of food, the overall products are carbon dioxide, water, and *energy*. The carbons and hydrogens of food are oxidized and the oxygen is reduced. Oxidations do not need to involve oxygen and may be interpreted as a removal of hydrogens. For example, the oxidation of a *saturated fatty acid* to an *unsaturated fatty acid* results when hydrogens are removed.

$$CH_3-CH_2-CH_2-COOH + FAD \longrightarrow CH_3-CH=CH-CH-COOH + FADH_2$$

saturated fatty acid $\qquad\qquad\qquad\qquad$ unsaturated fatty acid

Oxidation of a saturated fatty acid

This reaction takes place during the oxidation of fatty acids (except that the fatty acid is a *coenzyme A* derivative). The fatty acid is oxidized by the removal of two hydrogens, and the FAD (*flavin adenine dinucleotide*) undergoes reduction by the addition of hydrogens. A more general interpretation of oxidation and reduction reactions is based on the removal of electrons (oxidation) and the addition of electrons (reduction) to atoms in the molecule. This interpretation of oxidation-reduction reactions covers all cases and types of oxidation, but it is often not so clear or so graphic as the interpretations above. Oxidations and reduction are essential in utilization of food to provide energy. The oxidation of foodstuffs, *fats, carbohydrates*, and *proteins* takes place in a stepwise manner with one carbon being oxidized to carbon dioxide at a time. The oxidation of the carbons occurs mainly through the *Krebs' cycle*, the oxidation of hydrogen mainly through *oxidative phosphorylation* in the *terminal respiratory chain*, where chemical energy, *adenosine triphosphate* (ATP), is produced. Both the Krebs' cycle and oxidative phosphorylation occur in the *organelles* called *mitochondria*. Mitochondria account for more than 90% of the oxygen we use to oxidize foods to carbon dioxide, water, and energy.

oxidation of food. Biological oxidation yields the same energy as that obtained by burning food in a *bomb calorimeter*. The difference is that all of the energy dissipates as heat when food is burned and a part of the energy is conserved as chemical energy when food is biologically oxidized. The chemical conservation of energy in biological systems is in the form of *adenosine triphosphate* (ATP) through the process of *oxidative phosphorylation*. The energy in ATP is used for muscle contractions and biosynthetic processes. An example of the oxidation of a food is given using glucose oxidation as an example.

glucose $\qquad\qquad\qquad\qquad$ **carbon dioxide** $\qquad\qquad$ **ENERGY**

$$C_6H_{12}O_6 + 6\,O_2 \longrightarrow 6\,CO_2 + H_2O + 665\ kcal/mol$$

$\qquad\qquad$ **oxygen** $\qquad\qquad\qquad\qquad\qquad\qquad$ **water**

Oxidation of food

The table shows the amount of heat that can be derived from the three foods, carbohydrates, proteins, and fats. The amount of energy as heat that can be derived by the direct burning of foods is larger than the amount that derives from biological systems. There are two downward correction factors that must be applied to biological systems. The first is that not all of the food that is ingested is absorbed by the gastrointestinal tract—some is excreted through the feces. The second correction applies to proteins because proteins are not completely oxidized to carbon dioxide and water, as are carbohydrates and fats. The table shows these corrections. The name given the energy that is available for work is *free energy* and is symbolized by ΔG.

The amount of energy that is obtained as heat from direct burning of food is called *heat of combustion* and is symbolized by ΔH_c.

Energy available from the oxidation of food

FOOD	HEAT OF COMBUSTION ΔH_C KCAL/G	PERCENT ABSORPTION	FREE ENERGY ΔG KCAL/G
Carbohydrate	4.11	98%	4[b]
Fat	9.45	95%	9
Protein	5.65 (4.4)[a]	92%	4

[a] In the parenthesis is a correction for the incomplete combustion of protein in humans. The incomplete combustion of protein carbon is excreted in the *urine* as *urea*.

[b] These are the rounded-off values that are generally used in the calculation of the amount of energy in given food type.

It should also be recognized that the energy values assigned to each of the foodstuffs are also approximations derived from the average composition of a meal. For example, individual carbohydrates have different ΔG values. The value of 4 kcal/g of carbohydrate is an average of the type of carbohydrate that is likely to occur in a meal. The table shows the different ΔG values for different carbohydrates. The same circumstance applies to fats and to proteins.

ΔG kcal/g for different types of carbohydrate

GLUCOSE	SUCROSE	STARCH
3.69	3.96	4.12

oxidative phosphorylation. The cellular process responsible for the conversion of the energy in foods into chemical energy. The process is called "oxidative" because the hydrogens of foods (metabolites) are oxidized to water (see *oxidation*), and "phosphorylation" because the addition of phosphate to *adenosine diphosphate* (ADP) is coupled to the oxidation process. The result is the formation of the principal form of chemical energy in the cell, *adenosine triphosphate* (ATP). The enzymatic complex involved with oxidative phosphorylation reactions is called the *terminal respiratory chain*. The terminal respiratory chain is contained within *mitochondria*. The process of oxidative phosphorylation has a theoretic efficiency of about 40%. That means that in the oxidation of foodstuffs about 60% of the energy is converted to heat and the remainder is converted to ATP. The ATP can then be used for work or converted to other forms of energy, such as muscular work or electric energy or synthetic or chemical energy. The conversion of ATP to other forms of energy is again accompanied by a conversion of a part of the energy to heat. Overall, the efficiency of extracting the energy in foods into chemical, osmotic, electric, and kinetic end-products is between 25%–30%. The remainder of the energy is converted to heat, a necessary energy form for the environment (body). The apparatus in the mitochondria consists of the enzymes from the Krebs' cycle that produce the reduce cofactors NADH and FADH$_2$. These hydrogens are ultimately oxidized by the addition of oxygen to form water. In the complex process that involves the stepwise *oxidation-*

reduction of *cytochromes*, ATP is formed from ADP and inorganic phosphate along the pathway, thus conserving some of the oxidation energy. See *food energy*.

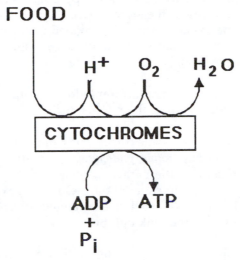

Synthesis of ATP from food oxidations

oxycalorimeter. An instrument that measures the amount of oxygen consumed. In the indirect measurement of heat (*indirect calorimetry*) the amount of oxygen required to burn a weighed sample of food or used by a living system is measured. The energy yield of the food is then obtained using standard factors established with the *bomb calorimeter* to convert the known volume of oxygen to calories. The dried sample, a single food or a mixture of foods, is ignited and burned in a stream of nearly pure oxygen in a closed circuit. In the measurements involving living systems, the utilization of oxygen for a given period of time is measured.

oxygen (O). Element No. 8. At. Wt. 16. Oxygen is the final acceptor of electrons in aerobic life systems. The result of the reduction of oxygen to O^{-2} is the immediate formation of water (H_2O). The details of the mechanism of reduction of oxygen are not known. In the passage of electrons to oxygen, several *oxidation-reduction* processes occur, and in some processes the energy of oxidation is conserved as chemical energy. Thus, in the maintenance of aerobic life, electrons flow from foodstuffs to oxygen. This flow of electrons and conservation of energy occur in each cell, the oxygen being carried to the cells by the hemoglobin in the *red blood cells*. In anaerobic life systems, the processes are similar except that the final electron acceptor is not oxygen. See *oxidative phosphorylation* and the *terminal respiratory chain*.

oxygen debt. A term that accounts for the continued hyperventilation and the increased metabolic and physiologic rates that follow the cessation of exercise, particularly vigorous exercise. An explanation for the phenomenon is related to *glycolysis* and the accumulation of *lactic acid*. During vigorous exercise, *energy* is required. The immediate source of energy is the metabolism of *glucose* which is increased to accommodate the sudden demand. Glucose via *glycolysis* is degraded to *pyruvic acid* at a rate faster than the pyruvate can be oxidized. During glycolysis, *adenosine triphosphate* (ATP), a form of chemical energy required for muscle contraction and some biosynthetic processes, is produced. The accumulating *pyruvate* is converted to a reduced form, *lactic acid*, which accumulates as muscle activity continues. In other words, the muscle has received a part of its energy under *anaerobic* conditions. When muscle activity ceases, the lactic acid can be oxidized back to pyruvate, since the pyruvate formation from glycolysis diminishes. However, the store of lactic acid and its conversion to pyruvate mean that the oxidation mechanisms are still being flooded with pyruvate. As a consequence, the oxygen demand for pyruvate oxidation remains above resting rates and continues until lactic acid concentrations are at resting levels.

oxystearin. A modified fatty acid that manufacturers add in amounts up to 0.125% of vegetable oils to prevent them from clouding up in the refrigerator.

oxytocin. A hormone that stimulates uterine contractions and lactation in females. A polypeptide with eight amino acids: *tyrosine, proline, glutamic acid, aspartic acid, glycine, cystine, leucine, and isoleucine*. It is formed mostly in the paraventricular nuclei of the *hypothalamus*. It is so named because it causes vigorous contractions of the uterus, thus expelling the fetus. Oxytocin also causes contraction of the myoepithelial cells arranged around the mammary ducts in such a way that contraction forces the milk out. See *lactation*.

oyster. Shellfish eaten raw or cooked. When eaten raw or partially cooked, oysters may be source of infectious hepatitis virus. See this item in the table under *fish*.

P

P. The alphabetic symbol for the amino acid *proline* (Pro).

PABA. See *para-aminobenzoic acid*.

palatability. The quality characteristic (such as color, flavor, and texture) of a food product that makes an impression on the organs of touch, *taste*, *smell*, or sight and has significance in determining the acceptability of the food produced to the user. See *aroma* and *tongue*.

palm oil. The palm *oil* bears a great number of nutlike fruits and oil that is expressed from both the pulp and the kernel. The oil from the kernel is palm oil, an important source of margarine, and is used in cooking in many parts of the tropics. It contains a large amount of *saturated fatty acids* even though it is a vegetable oil.

palmitic acid. Mol. Wt. 254. A 16-carbon *saturated fatty acid* widespread in foods. The difference in consistency of various fats at room temperature is due to differences in the kinds and amounts of fatty acids that enter into their composition. Palmitic and *stearic acids* enter largely into the compounds of solid fats. They are called saturated fatty acids because they cannot take up any more hydrogen.

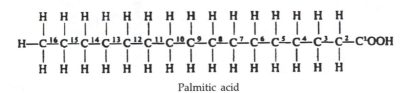

Palmitic acid

pancreas. A long, tapering organ lying behind the stomach. The head of the gland lies in the curve of the small intestine near the pyloric valve. The body of the pancreas extends to the left toward the spleen. The pancreas secretes a *digestive juice* which acts on all types of foods. Several proteolytic enzymes in pancreatic juice digest proteins. Other glycolytic enzymes digest starches into sugars, and *lipases* digest fats into their simplest forms. The pancreas has another important function, the production of the hormones *insulin* in the β cells or *islets of Langerhans* and of *glucagon* by the *alpha cells*. See *digestion, digestive system*.

pancreatic juice. Pancreatic juice contains at least four classes of enzymes: (1) *proteases*, (2) *amylases*, (3) *lipases*, and (4) *nucleases*. In addition, the pancreatic secretion contains a considerable quantity of bicarbonate ion, which makes it alkaline and which functions to neutralize the highly acid *gastric juice*. Sodium, potassium, calcium, and magnesium concentrations in pancreatic juice reflect the concentrations of these cations in the plasma. The pancreas secretes trypsinogen. When trypsinogen reaches the intestinal tract, it is converted into trypsin by trypsin already present and by enterokinase. Trypsin is a proteolytic enzyme. Pancreatic amylases are enzymes that speed the conversion of carbohydrates to simple sugars. *Ptyalin* is the salivary amylase that initiates this process. The pancreatic amylases continue the work so that intermediary sugars, *maltose* and *isomaltose*, are formed. The pancreatic juice also contains amylases which act specifically on the intermediary sugars maltose, sucrose, and lactose to convert them to the simple sugars glucose, fructose, and galactose. Pancreatic lipase catalyzes the conversion of the fat molecules into component fatty acids and glycerol. The bile salts make it possible for the lipase to act on fat and to bring about this conversion. *Nucleases* break down *nucleic acids* to component parts. See *digestive system*.

pancreatitis. An inflammation of the *pancreas*. It may be acute or chronic in nature and frequently accompanies obstruction of the pancreatic duct due to gallstones or the backflow of *bile* into the pancreatic duct.

pancreozymin. A hormone produced in the mucosa of the duodenum (small intestine) that stimulates secretion of enzymes from the pancreas.

pangamic acid (vitamin B$_{15}$). Mol. Wt. 281. Isolated from apricot kernels, rice bran, seeds, brewer's yeast, oxblood, and liver. Appears to be found wherever the B-complex vitamins are found. There is no clear evidence of its effectiveness or function in humans, but it was proposed for treatment of cardiovascular and rheumatic diseases in the past.

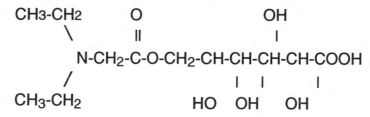

D-Gluconic acid 6-[bis(methylethyl)] amino acetate

panocha. A candy made of brown sugar, milk, butter, and nuts. Also a coarse sugar made in Mexico.

pantothenic acid. Mol. Wt. 291. The biochemical role of pantothenic acid is primarily as a part of *coenzyme A*, one of the most important substances in body metabolism. As part of coenzyme A, pantothenic acid is essential for the intermediary metabolism of carbohydrates, fats, and proteins for their synthesis, breakdown, and release of energy. It functions primarily by affecting the removal or acceptance of important chemical groups with two, three, four (or more) carbon atoms at a time. Coenzyme A is also needed for the formation of such important sterols as cholesterol and the adrenocortical hormones. Pantothenic acid functions also as a component of the enzyme *fatty acid synthase* involved in fatty acid synthesis in the body. Pantothenic acid exists in all cells of living tissues and therefore is present in all natural foods. Foods especially rich are yeast, heart, salmon, liver, eggs, wheat and rice germ or bran, peanuts, and peas. Moderate to good amounts are contained in such foods as milk, poultry, whole grains, broccoli, mushrooms, and sweet potatoes. Most vegetables, fruits, and refined foods contain lesser amounts. Losses of up to 50% can occur in frozen vegetables and meat and in many canned food products. The quantitative requirement for pantothenic acid in humans has not been established. In animals, pantothenic acid supplements have been shown to increase fertility and longevity. Pantothenic acid is fairly stable in neutral solutions but is destroyed by acid and alkali and by prolonged dry heat. The calcium salt of the vitamin is the form in which it is used generally. Calcium pantothenate is odorless and slightly bitter in taste. Pantothenic acid in pure form is a pale yellow, viscous oil.

$$HO-CH_2-\underset{\underset{CH_3}{|}}{\overset{\overset{CH_3}{|}}{C}}-\underset{\overset{OH}{|}}{CH}-\overset{\overset{O}{||}}{C}-\underset{\overset{H}{|}}{N}-CH_2-CH_2-COOH$$

Pantothenic acid

Pantothenic acid in µg/100 g of foods

Bananas	300	Lamb	600	Pork, bacon	600
Beans, dried lima	830	Lamb, kidney	4300	Pork, ham	500
Beef, brain	2500	Milk, whole	290	Pork, kidney	3100
Beef, heart	2300	Mushrooms	1700	Pork, liver	6600
Beef, kidney	3400	Oats	1300	Pork, muscle	1000
Beef, liver	7000	Onions	140	Potatoes, Irish	500
Beef, muscle	1100	Oranges	340	Potatoes, sweet	950
Bread, whole wheat	570	Oysters	490	Salmon	900
Bread, white	400	Peaches	140	Soybeans	1800
Broccoli	1400	Peanuts, roasted	2500	Tomatoes	310
Cauliflower	920	Pears	70	Veal chop	200
Cheese	655	Peas, fresh	800	Wheat, whole	1300
Chicken	700	Peas, dried	2800	Wheat, germ	2000
Eggs	2700	Pineapple	170	Wheat, bran	2400

papain. A *proteolytic enzyme* with a low specificity (a broad range) from papaya. It is used in medicine and in meat tenderizers. Papain is used medically as an aid for stomach disorders and sold in health food stores as a digestant.

papaw or pawpaw (*Asimina triloba*). A North American fruit of the custard family, varying from 2–6 inches in length and shaped like a short, fat banana, dark brown to blackish in color, with a soft creamy flesh in which many seeds are embedded. It is sweet, rich, custardlike, and slightly aromatic.

papaya (*Carica papaya*). A small tropical tree with a large, fleshy fruit which grows on the stalk from the trunk, just below the leaves. The fruit, which resembles a melon, has a rind and a juicy flesh that is orange in color. It has a delicious, sweet-tart, musky taste. The fruit is the source of the proteolytic enzyme *papain*.

paprika. The Hungarian name given to a spice or condiment made by grinding the ripe dried pods of red capsicum or bell peppers.

para-aminobenzoic acid. Mol. Wt. 137. A part of pteroylglutamic acid, one of the forms of the vitamin *folacin*. Para-aminobenzoic acid is a growth factor for bacteria which can use it to synthesize folacin. The fact that para-aminobenzoic acid (PABA) is a unit in the structure of folacin may have been a reason for its past status as a vitamin. It is no longer considered as such for human beings, since it is now known to function solely as a component of pteroylglutamic acid. It also is not a necessary constituent in the human diet. Clinically PABA has been used to treat some rickettsial (bacterial) diseases. It is effective because it acts as an antimetabolite to a material essential to the growth of the *rickettsiae*.

Para-aminobenzoic acid

parabens. Nickname for methyl, propyl, and heptyl esters of parahydrobenzoic acid. Used as a preservative, closely related to *sodium benzoate*. Parabens can prevent bacteria and mold from growing in almost all foods.

parasitic worms. Some parasitic worms can be seen with the unaided eye, but others have to be identified only with a microscope. The smallest are roughly the size of pinheads, while a tapeworm can grow to a 30-foot length. Many parasites, including the flukes (one of two types of flatworms), are more prevalent in the tropics. The other type of flatworm, the tapeworm, is found in the United States and is acquired by eating beef, pork, or fish containing the parasite. Inside the intestine, the tapeworm attaches itself to the intestinal wall and proceeds to grow. Some roundworms common in this country include the pinworm, intestinal roundworm, and hookworm. Another roundworm, found in pork, causes trichinosis, a disease in which the parasites eventually penetrate muscles.

parasympathetic nervous system. A divison of the *autonomic nervous system*. The autonomic nerve fibers which originate from cell bodies lying in the brain stem and in the sacral part of the spinal cord. Preganglionic nerve fibers arising from cells in the midbrain level out with the third nerve fibers to the ciliary *ganglia*, which give rise to postganglionic fibers supplying the pupil, iris, and ciliary muscles. Other preganglionic fibers arise from nerve cells in the medulla and travel with the nerve fibers of the seventh and ninth cranial nerves to innervate the salivary and other glands of the head and neck. Other cell bodies in the medulla give rise to the largest autonomic nerve in the body, the vagus nerve (tenth nerve), which contains all the preganglionic fibers to the many ganglia lying in or near the viscera of the chest or upper abdomen. Short postganglionic nerve fibers run from these ganglia to supply the heart, intestines, pancreas, and spleen. Ninety percent of all the parasympathetic nerve fibers in the body travel in the vagus nerve. The remainder of the parasympathetic nervous system consists of preganglionic fibers arising in the sacral region of the spinal cord and eventually terminating in pelvic ganglia, from which postganglionic fibers travel to the smooth muscle of the bladder, rectum, and genitalia.

parathormone (parathyroid hormone, PTH). A hormone of the *parathyroid glands* which controls calcium and phosphorus metabolism in three ways: (1) It stimulates the intestinal mucosa to increase calcium absorption; (2) it mobilizes calcium rapidly from bone; and (3) it causes renal excretion of phosphate. All of these responses act together and are needed to regulate the circulating amounts of calcium and phosphorus to maintain them within normal levels.

parathyroid glands. The parathyroid glands, usually four in number, are located in the posterior surfaces of the lobe of the *thyroid gland*. These glands produce the hormone *parathormone*, which helps to regulate the amount of *calcium* and *phosphorus* in the blood. Calcium normally stored in the bones is released into the blood as required for normal nerve and muscle-tissue function. When there is too little calcium in the blood, a type of muscle twitching called *tetany* develops. Calcium is given by intravenous infusion to relieve the symptoms of tetany.

parathyroid hormone. See *parathormone*.

parboiled rice (converted rice). Rice that has been specially treated with heat and water before the husks are removed so that the nutrients in the outer layers of the kernel are driven inward to the kernel. This reduces the loss of nutrients when the outer layers are removed in milling. See *rice*.

parenchyma. Functional tissue of an organ or gland as distinct from its supporting framework.

parenteral. The entrance of a substance into the body by means other than through the gastrointestinal tract. For example, the introduction of nutrients by way of veins or into subcutaneous tissues.

parfait. French parfait is an ice made of a single flavor frozen in a plain mold. American parfait consists of ice cream served with whipped cream in a tall narrow glass called a parfait glass. The ice cream is layered into the glass with the cream (or fruit or sauce).

parietal cells. Cells of the gastric glands in the fundus of the stomach which produce hydrochloric acid for the purpose of digestion. See *gastric juice*.

parsley (*Petroselinum crispum*). A hardy biennial herb plant widely used for flavoring and as a garnish. The parsley family, or *Umbelliferae*, includes many herbs and spices such as anise, dill, angelica, chervil, caraway, coriander, cumin, fennel, lovage, sweet cicely, and the common vegetables celery and carrots. Parsley is a small green plant of which there are more than 30 varieties, distinguished by the shape of their foliage; curled, moss-curled, double-curled, or fern-leafed, for example; and plain or common parsley. Bunches of parsley leaves are used whole as a garnish or in a bouquet garni. Chopped, either fresh or dried, parsley is used to flavor soups, meat dishes, fish stuffings, cream or cheese sauces, eggs, breads, flavored butter, marinades, and most vegetables and salads. See this item in the table under *vegetables*.

part per million (ppm). A way of expressing amounts, especially of trace minerals or contamistnants in diets or foods. Examples of how small a part per million is: It is equal to 1 pound in 500 tons, 1 inch in about 16 miles, or 1 cent in $10,000.

passion fruit (*Passiflora*). The edible fruit of the passion flower, a vine with solitary, spectacular flowers which is a native of tropical Brazil. The fruit is also known as granadilla. It has a sweet-acid flavor and is used as a table fruit, as well as for making sherbets, candy, and refreshing beverages.

Nutrients in 100 g of passion fruit

CALORIES KCAL	PROTEIN G	FAT G	CARBOHYDRATE G	VITAMIN A IU	CALCIUM MG	ASCORBATE MG
90	2	1	21	700	13	30

pasta. The Italian word for "paste," which in culinary usage describes an alimentary paste made from *semolina* (wheat) and water. Semolina is the purified middlings of hard wheat. There are over 100 varieties of pasta, some shaped like lasagna, others in small decorative shapes such as stars, hearts, animals, and letters.

pasteurization. A heat treatment that kills part but not all of the microorganisms present in a substance and usually involves the application of temperatures below 100°C (212°F). The heating may be by means of steam, hot water, dry heat, or electric currents, and the products are cooled promptly after the heat treatment. Pasteurization is used (1) when more rigorous heat treatment would harm the quality of the product, as with milk; (2) when one aim is to kill pathogens; (3) when the main spoilage organisms are not very heat resistant, like the yeasts in fruit juices; (4) when any surviving spoilage organisms will be taken care of by additional preservative methods, as is done in the chilling of market milk; and (5) when competing organisms are to be killed, allowing a desired fermentation by specific microorganisms, usually by added starter organisms, as in cheese making, for example. See *pasturized milk* and *sterilized milk* under *milk*.

pastrami. A preserved meat of eastern European origin, made from plate brisket or round of beef dry-cured with salt and saltpeter, *sodium nitrate*. The beef is then rinsed and rubbed with a paste or garlic powder, ground cumin seed and pepper, cinnamon cloves, and allspice, then smoked and cooked.

paté. A meat or fish paste, or a pie or patty with a filling such as meat or fish paste. The most famous is the paté de foie gras, or goose liver paté.

pathogen. A microorganism that causes a disease or pathologic condition.

pavlova. A dessert of Australian origin which consists of a meringue topped with whipped cream and berries, or whipped cream, passion fruit, and banana slices.

pawpaw. See *papaw*.

PBI. See *protein-bound iodine of serum*.

pea (*Pisum sativum*). The seed and plant of a cool-season hardy annual. Chief among the many varieties are the garden or green pea and the field or stock pea, *P. Sativum* var. *arvense*. The seeds of garden peas can be classified as smooth-skinned or wrinkled. Field peas, which have a small, hard seed, are used chiefly for making yellow split peas and as livestock fodder. See this item in the table under *vegetables*.

peach (*Prunus perica*). A rounded fruit with a fuzzy, velvety skin, creamy yellow when ripe. The flesh may be white or yellow with a pitted or furrowed stone of the free or cling type. See this item in the table under *fruits*.

peanut (*Arachis hypogaea*). A spreading annual plant related to peas and beans. Peanuts are often called groundnuts, monkey nuts, and earthnuts. The pods of the peanut vary. They may grow from 1–2 inches in length, with one, two, or three seeds. The seed has a thin, papery coat which may be any color from white to purple. The most common colors are mahogany, red, rose, and salmon.

Nutrients in 100 g of raw peanuts

CALORIES KCAL	PROTEIN G	FAT G	CARBOHYDRATE G	CALCIUM MG	NIACIN MG	THIAMINE µG
560	27	47	18	50	19	900

peanut butter. A blend of peanuts which have been shelled, roasted, blanched, and then ground to a paste. Small amounts of salt, emulsifier, and hydrogenated vegetable oil are added.

Nutrients in 100 g of peanut butter

CALORIES KCAL	PROTEIN G	FAT G	CARBOHYDRATE G	CALCIUM MG
581	28	49	19	63

peanut flour. Flour made from ground peanuts from which the greatest part of the oil has been extracted.

peanut oil. Oil obtained by the cold pressing of peanuts. When filtered it is sweet, nearly colorless, and used both for table use and in cooking.

pear (*Pyrus communis*). A tree and its fruit cultivated in temperate zones. The pear tree belongs to the rose family, whose varieties include apples, plums, apricots, raspberries, and strawberries. The fruit may be roundish or bell-shaped, symmetric or uneven. It may have a long or short neck. The stem is attached to the fruit. The skin ranges in color from green, to yellow with a red tinge, to russet. Flesh is fine-grained and juicy. Taste may be sweet to buttery, spicy to acid. See this item in the table under *fruits*.

pecan (*Carya illinoensis*). A native American nut of the pecan tree. Pecans have very thin shells and the meat has a fat content of over 70%, which is higher than that of any other vegetable product.

Nutrients in 100 g of pecan

CALORIES KCAL	PROTEIN G	FAT G	CARBOHYDRATE G	VITAMIN A IU	CALCIUM MG	ASCORBATE MG
696	9	73	13	50	74	2

pectic substances. A class of polymers of galacturonic acid, a derivative of *galactose*, found in fruit. See *pectins*.

pectinases. Enzymes that hydrolyze pectin, a carbohydrate in fruits that causes the juice to jell. See *pectins*.

pectins. Nondigestible polysaccharides that are polymers of galacturonic methyl esters (oxidized forms of *galactose*). Pectins are common in all cell walls and are also present in the intercellular layers. Pectins constitute 1%–4% percent of the total cell wall polysaccharides, and in some plants are more abundant in seeds or skins. The rind of citrus fruit contains 30% pectin; apple peel, 15%, and onion skins 11%–12% percent. Between 0.5%–1% of the total fresh fruit of an apple is pectin. As a group, pectins are biochemically less well defined than the other polysaccharides, but in general are smaller with molecular weights in the region of 60,000–90,000 daltons. Pectins are often used as a base for fruits and jellies because they gel or solidify in the presence of the sugar and acid in fruit juices. This property of solidifying into a gel also makes them useful in cosmetics and drugs. See *fiber, dietary*.

pectolytic bacteria. Some bacterial species of *Erwinia*, *Bacillus*, and *Clostridium* contain pectolytic *enzymes* which are responsible for the softening of plant tissue and the loss of the gelling power of fruit juices. Most authorities agree that two enzymes, pectinesterase and polygalacturonase, are chiefly involved in the *hydrolysis* of *pectin*, which prevents gel formation. The pectolytic enzymes or pectinases are used in the food industry for clarification of fruit juices, wines, vinegars, syrups, and jellies which contain suspended particles of pectin. Pectinases also help prevent the gelling of fruit-juice concentrates. Pectinases are extracted from bacteria or plant materials for these uses.

pellagra. A vitamin deficiency disease caused by lack of *niacin* (nicotinic acid, nicotinamide) in the diet. The disease is rare in Europe and North America, although several decades ago high incidences occurred among the poor in the southern United States. The earliest symptom of pellagra is *glossitis*, a burning sensation of the tongue. Advanced stages of the disease are characterized by the 4 D's: diarrhea, dermatitis, dementia, and death. The dermatitis is precipitated by exposure to the sun, heat, or friction and appears only on areas of the body subjected to those conditions. The disease is closely associated with cultures or conditions that are nutritionally poor but have a high consumption of corn. Corn or maize is not deficient in niacin, but it appears to be bound in some form that makes niacin unavailable. Corn is also very low in the amino acid *tryptophan*, which has niacin activity. Pellagra is almost unknown in Mexico, though it has a corn culture. However, during the preparation of tortillas, the maize (corn) is treated with lime water and the bound form of niacin is apparently released by treatment with alkali. See *niacin*.

pemmican. A North American Indian cake made of dried and powdered meat mixed with melted fat, various berries, and herb seasoning.

penicillin. One of a group of antibiotics biosynthesized by several species of molds, especially *Penicillium notatum*, and *P. chrysogenum*. There are many different penicillins, including synthetic ones, and their effectiveness varies for different organisms.

pentose. A class of simple sugar (*monosaccharide*) containing five carbon atoms, as for example, *ribose*, arabinose, and *xylose*. Pentoses are synthesized by all types of animals as well as humans from *glucose* and are not essential in the diet. Pentose sugars most commonly present in human foods are L-arabinose and D-xylose, which are widely distributed in fruits and root vegetables. The pentoses, *deoxyribose* and ribose, are components of *deoxyribonucleic acid* (DNA) and *ribonucleic acid* (RNA). The pentoses are normally found in human urine in small amounts, related to the dietary intake.

penuche. A candy made from brown sugar which is cooked to a soft-ball stage, cooled to lukewarm, and then beaten until smooth and creamy.

pepper. A spice that is used as a condiment, stimulant, and colorant. Red peppers are the ground products derived from cayenne peppers and long peppers of the cayenne group, such as the long red cayenne. Cayennes are used to add flavor to meat, fish, and egg dishes, sauces, etc. Peppers generally have a high carotene (vitamin A activity) content.

Nutrients in 100 g of sweet green pepper

CALORIES KCAL	PROTEIN G	FAT G	CARBOHYDRATE G	VITAMIN A IU	CALCIUM MG	ASCORBATE MG
22	1	trace	5	420	9	128

peppergrass (*Lepidium*). Garden cress and shepherd's purse are other names for this annual spring herb. The flavor is similar to watercress, and like watercress it is used as a garnish or in salads.

peppermint (*Mentha piperita*). An aromatic perennial *herb*, with a cool, refreshing flavor. Its leaves are used for flavoring and oil. The oil is made by steam distillation after the crop, in full blossom, is dried, and it is used widely for gum, candy, dentifrices, and other pharmaceutical preparations.

pepperone. A highly spiced dry *sausage* of Italian origin. It is made from coarsely ground beef and pork mixed with salt, coarsely ground black pepper, cayenne, and garlic. The mixture is cured and stuffed into casings and linked in pieces 10–12 inches long. The sausage is then air-dried at moderate room temperatures for 3–4 weeks.

pepsin. A substance formed in the *pyloric glands* and the *chief cells* of the gastric glands in the stomach. It is present in these cells in the form of a *zymogen*, an antecedent inactive substance called propepsin, or pepsinogen, which is quickly changed to active pepsin by the action of hydrochloric acid. Pepsin (gastric protease) is a proteolytic enzyme requiring an acid medium in which to function. It has the property of hydrolyzing proteins through several stages into polypeptides, with hydrolysis taking place preferentially at the amino acid residues *tryptophan*, *phenylalanine, tyrosine, methionine*, and *leucine*.

peptic ulcer. An ulcer is a circumscribed defect of varying depth in the lining of the stomach or duodenum. If deep enough, it may extend through the wall of the digestive tract and perforate, causing *peritonitis*; or it may erode into a blood vessel, producing bleeding. A primary cause of many peptic ulcers is bacteria. *Hydrochloric acid* (HCl) plays an important role in ulcer development and is important in the production of ulcer pain. The continuous neutralization of acid promotes the healing of ulcers. The term "peptic" ulcer relates to the enzyme pepsin which, together with hydrochloric acid, is believed to contribute to the digestive action of stomach contents upon the surface of the stomach or duodenum, presumably impairing the integrity of localized areas and thus leading to the formation of peptic ulcer.

peptidases. See *proteases*.

peptide. The linkage of amino acids together by *peptide linkage* or amide bonds in a chainlike molecule. Prefixes indicate the number of amino acid units involved, for example, a dipeptide consists of two amino acids joined together, and a polypeptide contains a large but unspecified number of amino acids. Peptides are intermediate products of the enzymatic hydrolysis of protein. See *peptide linkage*.

peptide linkage (peptide bond). The amide linkage of two *amino acids* by condensation of the amino group of one amino acid with the *carboxyl group* of another amino acid.

Peptide linkage

peptization. Colloidal dispersions are sometimes prepared by adding a third substance to the system. This substance acts upon the particles and reduces them to colloidal dimensions. Such a substance is called a peptizing agent and the process is known as peptization. Certain of the digestive processes of animals involve peptization. See *emulsifiers*.

peptones. Intermediate products of the enzymatic hydrolysis of protein. The term is seldom used today; polypeptide is used in its stead. One of the soluble forms that results from the action of gastric juice upon proteins. Peptones are a stage in protein digestion prior to the formation of amino acid. Soluble in water, not coagulable by heat, and not precipitated by saturating their solutions with ammonium sulfate or zinc sulfate. These represent an advanced stage of cleavage to small polypeptides.

perch (*Perca fluviatilis*). A widely distributed, spiny-finned freshwater food fish. Known also as the yellow, barred, or ring perch, they are carnivorous, voracious, and prolific. Perch grow to a large size in still, brackish waters of bays and inlets. They are distinctively colored with an olive back lightening along the sides to golden yellow. The pike-perch is a genus closely related to the perch family, but showing some resemblance to the pike in the elongated body shape. One of the best-known species of this group is the wall-eyed pike, a famous game fish. The name "perch" is also widely applied to many other spiny-finned fish, including some saltwater varieties. Among the latter are the so-called "ocean perch" which belong to the sea bass and rockfish family. Perch is a mild fish, with firm, white, coarse flesh and a delicate flavor. Perch are a good source of protein.

percomorph. Fish of the perch family. Percomorph oil, prepared from the livers of such fish, is a concentrated source of *vitamin D*.

periosteum. The membrane covering bone surfaces. See *bone*.

peristalsis. The rhythmic motion of the *gastrointestinal tract*. The esophagus is composed chiefly of muscles which contract in wavelike fashion along the length of the tube and the entire digestive tract. These are called peristaltic waves or movements. The term peristalsis means "clasping and compressing" and describes the contraction of one part of the tube, then contraction below it and relaxation of the originally constricted segment, etc. Many tubes composed of smooth muscle exhibit peristalsis. It is peristalsis that moves the *bolus* and *chyme* along the gastrointestinal tract.

peritoneum. The serous membrane covering the viscera and lining the abdominal cavity. Parietal peritoneum is the peritoneum lining the abdominal and pelvic walls and the undersurface of the diaphragm. Visceral peritoneum is the peritoneum that surrounds the abdominal organs. The peritoneum holds the viscera in position by its folds. Peritonitis is inflammation of the peritoneum.

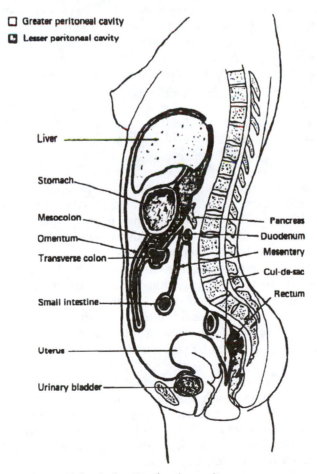

Abdominal cavity showing peritoneum.

peritonitis. An inflammation of the peritoneum, the membrane covering the intestine. It usually occurs when one of the organs it encloses ruptures or is perforated so that the organ's contents (including bacteria) are spilled into the abdominal cavity. The most common cause is rupture of the appendix following appendicitis. Symptoms are nausea, vomiting, and severe abdominal pain. The abdominal muscles become very rigid and are tender to pressure.

pernicious anemia. See *anemia, pernicious*.

peroxidase. An enzyme that catalyzes the oxidation of certain organic compounds with hydrogen peroxide. The general reaction is shown.

$$R - CH_2 - CH_2OH + H_2O_2 \longrightarrow R - CH_2 - CH_2 - COOH + H_2O$$

Peroxidase

The enzyme is very active in plant tissue and a small amount of this activity is found in kidney, liver, milk, and leukocytes. The enzyme contains iron. See *catalase*.

peroxidation. Unsaturated fats and fatty acids not stable in food because they are readily oxidized to hydroperoxides by a nonenzymatic process. The peroxidations result in a number of volatile and nonvolatile compounds. The volatile compounds are exceptionally odorous and can be detected in very small quantities. These odors are often referred to as stale, rancid, fishy, or metallic. Some of the peroxidation products are carcinogens that are believed to result from the free radical and aldehyde products. In general, heavy metals promote peroxidation, which includes molecules containing *heme*.

peroxisomes. Organelles within the cytoplasm that contain several oxidative enzymes. Among their contents are *catalase* and D-amino acid oxidase. The *organelle* is about 0.5 microns in diameter.

persimmon (*Diospyros*). A warm-weather fruit of which there are two species of importance. One of them is the common or American persimmon, *D. virginiana*. This species produces a small, pulpy fruit which can vary in size from a half to two inches in diameter, is yellow or orange with a reddish cheek, and has large seeds embedded in its soft flesh. The second species, *D. kaki*, is known as the Oriental or Japanese persimmon. The tree can reach 40 or more feet in height; its fruit grows to some three inches in diameter. Some varieties have large seeds in the semitransparent pulp; other varieties are seedless. When ripe the fruit somewhat resembles a tomato in size and surface texture, and is reddish orange in color. The taste is deliciously sweet, with a faint acid tinge, but persimmons must be ripe to be edible. Persimmons are eaten out-of-hand and used in salads and puddings. Persimmons contain fair quantities of *ascorbic acid* (vitamin C) and *carotene* (vitamin A activity).

pH. The pH is an expression of the *hydrogen ion* (H^+) concentration in water solutions. The generally used scale is from 0–14, where 0 is equivalent to a concentration of 1 molar hydrogen ion and 14 is 10^{-14} (0.00000000000001 molar). The pH scale has an exceptional function. The "p" comes from the German word *potenz*, which means power in the sense of an exponent, for example, a^2 is a to the second power. The pH is exactly neutral with equal quantities of H^+ and OH^- ions in solution, as in water. A deviation from 7–14 indicates increasing alkalinity, whereas a deviation from 7 toward 1 indicates increasing acidity. Blood, at pH 7.4, is slightly alkaline. Urine varies from strongly acid, pH 5, to strongly alkaline, pH 8. Very small changes in the numeric value of pH represent large changes in acidity or alkalinity; for example, a change in pH 7–6 represents a tenfold increase in acidity. The acidity or alkalinity of a solution is referred to as its reaction, and in physiology the reaction of body fluids is usually expressed in terms of pH. The reaction of blood, for example, is pH 7.4, which is slightly alkaline. See *acid, acid and base.*

phagocyte. A cell which can ingest and destroy particulate substances such as bacteria, protozoa, cells and cell debris, dust particles, and colloids. An example is macrophage (leukocytes) in the blood and in the lymph nodes and other organs. See *phagocytosis.*

phagocytosis. The engulfing of microorganisms and cells by *phagocytes,* usually white blood cells (leukocytes) or other related cells. Phagocytes are present in the blood and lymph and also in the lungs, liver, and spleen.

pharmacology. The science of drugs, especially the actions of drugs on the body. No drug can introduce a new action in the body. Drugs modify actions which are already there and can either increase or decrease the actions or functions of the cell.

pharynx. The pharynx, or throat, connects the nose and mouth with the lower air passages and *esophagus.* It is divided into three parts; the nasopharynx, the oropharynx, and the laryngopharynx. It is continued as the esophagus. Both air and food pass through the pharynx. It carries air from the nose to the larynx, food from the mouth to the *esophagus.* The walls of the pharynx contain masses of lymphoid tissues called adenoids and tonsils.

phenacetin. A white crystalline analgesic that is used to ease pain or fever. See *acetaminophen, aspirin,* and *ibuprofen.*

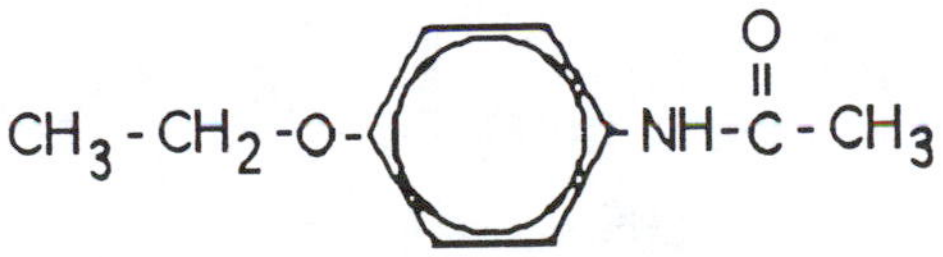

$$CH_3-CH_2-O-\langle\bigcirc\rangle-NH-\overset{\overset{\textstyle O}{\|}}{C}-CH_3$$

Phenacetin

phenol. Phenols are relatively strong aromatic acids that occur in very low concentrations in foods and contribute to their characteristic smells and tastes. Among the foods that contain phenol or phenol derivatives are coffee, beer, sherry, milk, peanuts, asparagus, and tomatoes.

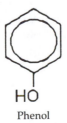

HO

Phenol

phenotype. The physical appearance of an individual. Some phenotypes, such as the blood groups, are completely determined by heredity, while others, such as stature, are readily altered by environmental agents. See *genotype*.

phenylalanine (Phe, F). Mol. Wt. 165. An *essential amino acid*. The nonessential amino acids *tyrosine* and cystine are an intermediate class between amino acids that can easily be formed from a number of precursors and those that cannot be made at all. Tyrosine can be made only from the essential amino acid phenylalanine by addition of one hydroxyl (−OH) group, and the reverse reaction (removal of the OH from the *tyrosine* to form phenylalanine) does not take place. Part of the need for phenylalanine in the body is to form tyrosine if the latter is not included in the diet. Thus the presence of tyrosine will reduce or spare the amount of phenylalanine required in the diet. Phenylalanine is a precursor to several important metabolites in addition to tyrosine. They include the skin pigment *melanin* and the hormones *epinephrine*, *norepinephrine*, and *thyroxine*.

$$\text{—CH}_2\text{—}\overset{\displaystyle \text{H}}{\underset{\displaystyle \text{NH}_2}{\text{C}}}\text{—COOH}$$

Phenylalanine

phenylketonuria (PKU). The excretion of phenylpyruvic acid and other phenyl compounds in the urine, resulting from the hereditary lack of an enzyme necessary for conversion of the amino acid *phenylalanine* to *tyrosine*. Phenylalanine derivatives accumulate in blood and tissues, and mental retardation occurs in infants.

phenylpyruvic acid. Mol. Wt. 164. An intermediate metabolic product of the essential amino acid phenylalanine.

$$\text{CH}_2\overset{\displaystyle}{\underset{\displaystyle \text{O}}{\text{C}}}\text{—COOH}$$

Phenylpyruvic acid

phosphates. Salts of phosphoric acid, important in maintenance of acid-base balance of the blood, the principal ones being monosodium and disodium phosphate. The former is acid-forming, the latter alkaline-forming. In the blood, because of their low concentration, they exert a minor buffering action. In the formation of urine, by altering the proportions of acid and alkaline phosphates, acid urine is formed and the body's sodium and potassium, magnesium, and calcium are conserved. Decreased phosphate excretion in urine occurs when alkaline reserves are high as in nephritis, tetany (*hypoparathyroidism*), adrenal cortical insufficiency, and certain bone diseases. Increased phosphate excretion in urine occurs when *alkali reserve* is low as in starvation, hyperparathyroidism, high-protein diet, and heavy muscular exercise.

phosphatides. A class of *phospholipids* found in all tissues, especially in brain and nerve tissues. Phosphatides are composed of a glycerol, two fatty acids, phosphate and an organic base.

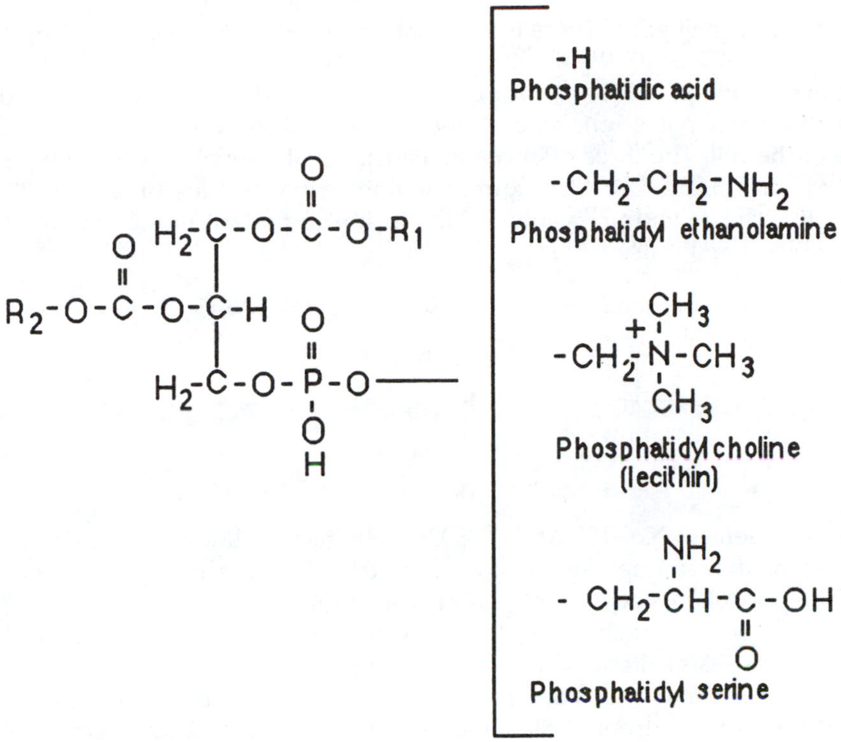

$$
\begin{array}{c}
\qquad\qquad\qquad O \\
\qquad\qquad\qquad \parallel \\
O \quad H_2\text{-}C\text{-}O\text{-}C\text{-}O\text{-}R_1 \\
\parallel \qquad\quad | \\
R_2\text{-}O\text{-}C\text{-}O\text{-}C\text{-}H \quad O \\
\qquad\qquad | \qquad \parallel \\
\qquad H_2\text{-}C\text{-}O\text{-}P\text{-}O\text{——} \\
\qquad\qquad\qquad | \\
\qquad\qquad\qquad O \\
\qquad\qquad\qquad H
\end{array}
$$

-H
Phosphatidic acid

$-CH_2\text{-}CH_2\text{-}NH_2$
Phosphatidyl ethanolamine

$$
\begin{array}{c}
\qquad\qquad CH_3 \\
\qquad + | \\
-CH_2\text{-}N\text{-}CH_3 \\
\qquad\qquad | \\
\qquad\qquad CH_3
\end{array}
$$
**Phosphatidyl choline
(lecithin)**

$$
\begin{array}{c}
\qquad\qquad NH_2 \\
\qquad\qquad | \\
-CH_2\text{-}CH\text{-}C\text{-}OH \\
\qquad\qquad\quad \parallel \\
\qquad\qquad\quad O
\end{array}
$$
Phosphatidyl serine

Phosphatides
R1 and R2 are saturated or unsaturated fatty acid side chains.

phosphocreatine (creatine phosphate). Mol. Wt. 211. A chemical form of energy stored primarily in muscle tissues. It is the energetic equivalent of *adenosine triphosphate* (ATP) and acts to provide energy for muscle contraction. The end-product of phosphocreatine is *creatinine*, which is excreted in the urine.

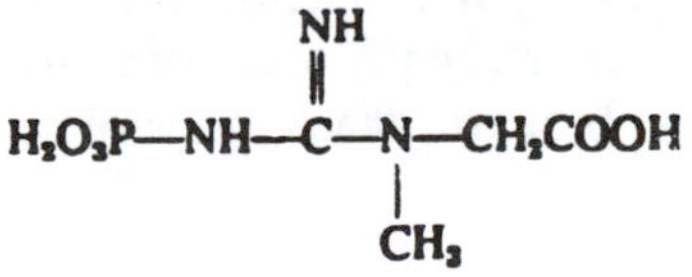

$$
\begin{array}{c}
\qquad\qquad\qquad NH \\
\qquad\qquad\qquad \parallel \\
H_2O_3P\text{—}NH\text{—}C\text{—}N\text{—}CH_2COOH \\
\qquad\qquad\qquad\qquad | \\
\qquad\qquad\qquad\qquad CH_3
\end{array}
$$

Phosphocreatine

phosphokinase. Kinases are enzymes that catalyze the transfer of phosphate from ATP (*adenosine triphosphate*) to an acceptor.

phospholipids. Compounds consisting of *glycerol*, two *fatty acids*, and a phosphate group. Phospholipids have the useful property of attracting both water-soluble and fat-soluble substances due to the hydrophilic (water-attracting) phosphoryl grouping and the hydrophobic (water-repelling) fatty acids in the molecule. They act as *emulsifiers* in the body and during *digestion*. In combination with protein, they are constituents of cell membranes and membranes of subcellular particles where they serve as liaisons between fat-soluble and water-soluble materials that must penetrate the membrane. Examples of phospholipids are *lecithin* and *phosphatidic acid*, the precursor to other phospholipids.

phosphoprotein. A conjugated protein that contains phosphorus, as for example, *casein*.

phosphoric acid. Mol. Wt. 101. A strong acid capable of dissociating three hydrogen ions (H^+). The sodium and potassium salts of phosphoric acid serve as important buffers within and outside of the cell. The three dissociation constants of phosphoric acid are $7.25 \times 10^{-3}M$, $6.31 \times 10^{-8}M$, and $3.98 \times 10^{-13}M$, corresponding to pK' values of 2.14, 7.20, and 12.4, respectively. It is the second pK' value, 7.20, which is important in maintaining the *acid-base balance* of the blood and cells.

$$
\begin{array}{c}
\text{O} \\
\parallel \\
\text{HO}-\text{P}-\text{OH} \\
\mid \\
\text{OH}
\end{array}
$$

Phosphoric acid

phosphorus (P). Element No. 15. At. Wt. 30.97. The human body contains roughly 12 g/kg fat-free tissue; of this amount about 85% is contained in the inorganic phase of skeletal structures. The phosphorus content of plasma is about 3.5 mg/100 mL plasma. Organic phosphates are a part of the structure of all body cells and are intimately involved in cellular functions, and phosphate salts act as important *buffers*. Phosphorus is a constituent of the high-energy compound ATP and thus is necessary for energy transductions, which are necessary for all cellular activity. Rich sources of phosphorus in the diet are meats (especially organs), fish and poultry, cheeses and milk, eggs, nuts, legumes, and all foods made from grains. Fruits (especially dried ones) and vegetables contribute lesser amounts of phosphorus to the diet. In general, edible roots, stems, and flowerlets of plants contain similar amounts of both calcium and phosphorus. The intake of phosphorus is considered sufficient if the diet is adequate in *calcium*.

phosphorus absorption. Normally about 70% of the phosphorus ingested in foods is absorbed. Most favorable absorption takes place when calcium and phosphorus are ingested in approximately equal amounts. As with *calcium*, the presence of *vitamin D* increases absorption. Simple phosphates such as calcium phosphate or potassium sodium phosphate are absorbed as such in the small intestine.

phosphorus test. A chemical test on blood; used in diagnosis of certain diseases of the kidney and metabolism.

phosphorylation. The chemical combination of phosphoric acid or the phosphate moiety with an organic compound. An example of phosphorylation in the metabolic processing of carbohydrates is the formation of glucose-6-phosphate, the initial step in the cellular oxidation of glucose. Generally, *adenosine triphosphate* (ATP) is involved in intracellular phosphorylations, though other triphosphates have a similar function. A phosphate group from ATP is transferred to glucose to form glucose-6-phosphate, a reaction catalyzed by either *glucokinase* or *hexokinase*. Once a compound is phosphorylated, it cannot cross the cell membrane.

photolysis. The splitting of a molecule under the action of light; for example, the cleavage of water in photosynthesis by the radiant energy absorbed by chlorophyll.

photosynthesis. The metabolic process that makes possible the capture and utilization of the energy in sunlight. The process by which plants and bacteria containing chlorophyll are able to manufacture carbohydrates by combining carbon dioxide (carbon dioxide *fixation*) from the air and water from the soil. Sunlight is the energy source and chlorophyll the catalyst driving the reactions. See *photolysis*.

phylloquinone. A compound used as a prothrombogenic agent. See *vitamin K*.

physical activity energy requirements. The amount of energy required to maintain human life is the sum total of the calories needed to satisfy the requirements for *basal metabolism* and the specific dynamic or thermogenic action of food, as well as for growth, repair, and physical activity. Even minor physical activity adds to the caloric expenditure above the basal requirement; this includes postural effort. It has been estimated that the total caloric requirement of a sitting adult is about 15% higher than his or her maintenance energy expenditure when supine; assuming a standing position adds another 15% to the caloric requirements. The act of walking on level ground at 2.5 mph requires an expenditure of about 180 kcal/hr on the part of the average adult; walking uphill on a 5% grade requires 270 kcal/hr and on a 15% grade, 490 kcal/hr. See *energy requirements* and *energy reserves*.

physiologic saline. A solution of sodium chloride isotonic (having the same osmotic pressure) as blood. The isotonic concentration of physiologic saline is 0.154 N (normal) or about a 0.9% solution.

phytic acid. Mol. Wt. 660. Inositol hexaphosphonic acid. It is a phosphoric acid ester of *inositol*; occurring in nuts, legumes, and outer layers of cereal grains. The insoluble calcium magnesium salt is called phytin. Because phytic acid forms insoluble salts with calcium, iron, and magnesium, it interferes with the intestinal absorption of these minerals. Phytic acid is associated with *fiber*.

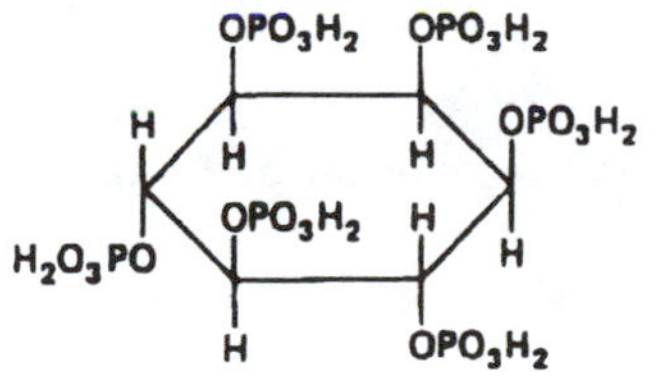

Phytic acid

piccalilli. A pickle relish made with chopped green tomatoes, red and green peppers, onions, sugar, vinegar, pickling spices, and often cabbage. It originated in the East Indies.

pigeon pea (*Cajanus cajan*). A tropical legume, widely grown in India where it is known as red gram; also popular in the West Indies.

pigment. Any of the coloring materials in the cells and tissues of plants and animals. In fruit and vegetables, the green pigment is chlorophyll; orange-to-red pigments are carotenoids; red-to-blue colors are anthocyanins; light-yellow pigments are flavones and flavonols. In humans, the dark skin pigment is *melanin*, a derivative of the essential amino acid *phenylalanine*. In meat, the chief pigment producing the pink or red color is *myoglobin*.

pignolia. The edible seed of the cones of a nut pine (*Pinus*).

Nutrition in 100 g pignolia

CALORIES KCAL	PROTEIN G	FAT G	CARBOHYDRATE G	VITAMIN A IU	THIAMINE μG
552	31	47	12	230	1000

pike (*Esox lucius*). An important family of American freshwater food and game fish which includes the pike, the smaller pickerel, and the larger muskellunge. All have long bodies, heads with sharp points, jaws that look like a duck's bill, and vicious teeth. The common or Great Lakes pike is grayish blue or green with many whitish or yellowish spots. Their average weight is about 10 pounds. Pickerels average 2–3 pounds, and muskellunges average 5–6 feet in length and often weigh over 60 pounds. Pike have a good texture and flavor, and are a good source of protein.

pilaf. A rice dish basic to the cuisines of Greece, the Near East, and southern Asia. The dish is usually made of well-seasoned long-grained rice sauteed in oil or butter, then boiled in bouillon or broth. A pilaf can contain meats, fish, seafood, vegetables, and any herbs or spices.

pilchards. Fully grown sardines, smaller than herrings. They are usually canned in oil, brine, or tomato sauce.

pili nut (*Cananium ovatum*). An edible seed of the Philippine burseraceous tree. The seed tastes like a sweet almond.

Nutrients in 100 g of pili nut

CALORIES KCAL	PROTEIN G	FAT G	CARBOHYDRATE G	VITAMIN A IU	THIAMINE μG	CALCIUM MG	IRON MG
669	11	71	8	40	1000	140	3

pimento. The sweet red pepper, the kind from which *paprika* is made.

pineal gland. Shaped somewhat like a pine cone (hence the name), it is connected to the thalamus of the brain by a hollow stalk. The pineal gland excretes *melanocyte-stimulating hormone* (MSH).

pineapple (*Ananas comosus*). A hardy perennial herbaceous plant native to northern South America. The plant grows about knee-high and has a short stem and a round head of stiff, grayish, striped leaves with spiny tips and prickly edges. Lavender-blue flowers grow in these heads, and the golden-yellow fruit emerges from the leaves. Pineapples weigh from 1–20 pounds; the average weight is 3–6 pounds. Pineapple is a fair source of *ascorbic acid* (vitamin C) and has small amounts of *carotene* (vitamin A). See this item in the table under *fruits*.

pine nut (*Pinus*). The edible seed of several varieties of pines; the seed develops in the pine cone, which is heated in order to spread its scales and make the seed easy to dislodge. Some pine nuts come from native American trees and are known as Indian nuts, pignons, or piñons. Others come from the Mediterranean stone pine. Pine nuts are the size of a small bean, with a thin, light-brown shell. The meat is white or cream-colored. The texture is soft and the flavor mild. Pine nuts contain some protein and are high in fat. Imported, 100 g = 552 calories; domestic, 100 g = 635 calories.

pinocytosis. Proteins and fats sometimes enter cells by the process of pinocytosis. The word means "cell drinking." It does not mean the cell itself is engulfed. Rather, as these large molecules become attached to the cell's outer surface, the cell membrane forms a pocket and encircles them. This creates an invagination on the cell surface that is engulfed material which eventually is released into the cell cytoplasm. This is the mechanism by which fat, for example, is absorbed from the small intestine.

pinto beans. Speckled, pink beans related to the kidney bean and common in Mexico and the southwestern United States.

pirogi. A Russian dish of savory and plump turnovers made from dough filled with a meat, fish, or vegetable mixture. Served with borscht or a meat broth.

pistachio (*Pistacia vera*). The edible seed of a small evergreen tree. Cashew and sumac trees are members of the same family. The fruits of the pistachio tree grow in clusters. Each fruit is about the size of an olive, about one-half to one inch long, with a thin, hard, brownish red shell. Within it is found a seed, the pistachio nut, which is pale green to creamy white in color, a single solid piece. It has a fine texture and a mild, pleasing flavor. The nutmeats are used for coloring and flavoring ice cream, cakes, and confectionery. They are also eaten out of the shell as is or salted. The color of the nut is so distinctive that its name has been given to a special shade of light green. Pistachios contain some protein and niacin and are rich in calcium, phosphorus, iron, *carotene* (vitamin A), and *thiamine*.

pituitary gland. The pituitary gland, located deep within the skull, is also called the hypophysis. This small gland has two lobes, the adenohypophysis (the anterior lobe) and the neurohypophysis (the posterior lobe), each producing distinctive hormones. The hormones produced by the adenohypophysis of the pituitary have names with the suffix "trophin," meaning nourishing. (1) *Somatotropin* (STH) means body-nourishing. This hormone influences skeletal and soft-tissue growth. (2) *Adrenocorticotropic hormone* (ACTH) stimulates the cortex and the *adrenal gland* to produce its hormone, *thyroxine*, an *iodine* derivative of the amino acid *tyrosine*. The posterior lobe, the neurohypophysis, produces the hormone oxytocin, which stimulates the contraction of the smooth muscle of the uterus, so it is important in childbirth. Another posterior-lobe hormone which helps prevent excessive water excretion from the kidneys is called the *antidiuretic hormone* (ADH).

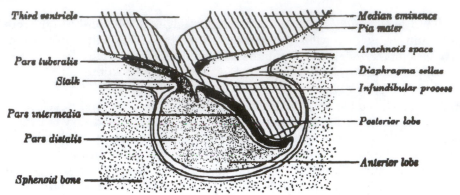

Diagrammatic median sagital section of the hypophysis cerebri or pituitary gland

Hormonal secretions of the pituitary gland

ANTERIOR LOBE	POSTERIOR LOBE
Growth hormone (STH, somatotropic hormone)	*Vasopressin* (pitressin)
Thyroid-stimulating hormone (TSH, thyrotropic hormone)	*Antidiuretic hormone* (ADH)
Follicle-stimulating hormone (FSH)	*Oxytocin*
Luteinizing hormone, (LH)	
Lactogenic hormone (prolactin)	
Adrenocorticotropic hormone (ACTH)	

pizza. A savory open pie of Italian origin. The word "pizza" in Italian means "pie"— any kind of pie—and the particular pie known in the United States as pizza is pizza alla Napoletana, a dish typical of Naples. A pizza consists of a thin layer of yeast dough, rolled or patted to fit a large cookie sheet or special pizza pan, topped with tomatoes, tomato paste, herbs, and slices of mozzarella cheese. The variations are endless; anchovies, sausages, vegetables, olives—anything can go into the sauce. The pizza is then baked until the cheese is bubbly and the crust edge is golden brown.

placenta. An organ within the uterus of the mother which connects to the developing fetus. The fetus obtains food and oxygen from the mother through the placenta. The blood vessels of the mother are in close contact with the blood vessels of the fetus so that interchanges of fetal blood substances and oxygen diffuse from maternal blood vessels into fetal blood vessels. Waste products and carbon dioxide diffuse fetal blood vessels into maternal blood vessels. The fetus is connected to the placenta by the umbilical cord. The health status and development of the fetus depend upon the condition of the placenta.

plantain (*Musa paradisiaca*). The fruit of a large-treelike tropical herb. The plantain belongs to the same family as the common eating banana, but plantains are larger, starchier, and less sweet; they must be cooked to be palatable. When boiled, baked, fried, or made into flour they are excellent and very digestible. Plantain is an important food plant in the tropics, occupying the same position of an essential staple as does the potato in the temperate zones. Plantain is high in carbohydrates and a fair source of *carotene* (vitamin A activity) and vitamin B.

plaque. Patches of unnatural formations on tissues such as tooth surfaces and inner arterial walls. The plaque on teeth surfaces is mineral deposits and predisposes to tooth decay. The plaque found in walls of arteries, called atheroma, contains *cholesterol, oleic acid, neutral fat,* and some connective or scar tissue of protein origin. Formation is related to fat and cholesterol metabolism. Plaque contributes to stiffening of blood-vessel walls, closing of arteries, choking circulation, and rupturing arteries. See *atherosclerosis*.

plasma. Making up more than one-half of the total volume of blood, plasma is the liquid carrier for blood cells, carbon dioxide, dissolved wastes, and nutrients. It brings hormones and antibodies (protective substances) to the tissues. Other components of plasma are water, oxygen, nitrogen, fat, carbohydrates, and proteins. Fibrinogen, one of the plasma proteins, helps blood clotting. When blood clots, the liquid portion that remains is *serum*. Blood serum contains no blood cells.

plasma cells. Round or irregularly shaped white blood cells found in greatest numbers in all connective tissues but especially in the connective tissue of the alimentary mucous membrane and great omentum. Plasma cells derive from lymphocytes and are the actual formers of circulating *antibodies*.

plasmalogens. A class of fats, which are phosphoglycerides. Ethanolamine ($NH_2-CH_2-CH_2-OH$) is the most common polar group.

plasma proteins. Plasma proteins consist mainly of the proteins *albumin* and *globulin*, which influence the shift of water from one compartment to another. Proteins are colloids and form colloidal solutions. Such solutions are mixtures of large, gelatinous particles or molecules which do not readily pass through separating membranes. Therefore, they normally remain in the blood vessels, where they exert a *colloidal osmotic pressure* (COP), which maintains the integrity of the blood volume in the vascular compartment.

Plasma proteins in g/L blood

Total Protein	58–78	Globulins	16–31
Albumin	35–56	Fibrinogen	2–4

platelet count. A microscopy test on blood; used in the diagnosis of persons having a tendency to hemorrhage.

platelets. One type of *white blood cell*. Tiny, granular corpuscles about 2 μ in diameter which are formed from special bone-marrow cells called megakaryocytes and are concerned in the control of bleeding after injury. There are usually 250,000–750,000 in every milliliter of blood, and their presence is essential for the normal retraction of blood clots which expresses the serum. The platelets break up in areas of damage to the blood vessels and liberate a compound called serotonin which causes small blood vessels to contract strongly, tending to reduce bleeding after injury.

plum (*Prunus*). The tree and edible fruit of many species. A large family which also includes almonds, apricots, cherries, and peaches. The fruits grow in clusters, and have a smooth skin and a flattened pit. Plums may be round or oval, with a skin in various shades of purple, red, blue, yellow, or green. The flesh is thick and juicy and it may be sweet or tart. Plums are delicious in the natural state, stewed, or made into sauce. Most important among the many plum varieties are the common, or European plum, *domestica*; the oriental, or Japanese plum, *P. salicina*; the native American wild plums including *P. americana* and *P. nigra*; and the beach plum, *P. maritima*. See this item in the table under *fruits*.

plumcot. A cross between an apricot and a Japanese plum. The fruits are characteristically large, resembling the apricot externally. The color may range from bright yellow to mottled red, with the flesh having similar variations.

plum pudding. A sweet pudding made with currants, raisins, citrus peel, and spices, either steamed or boiled. Served for dessert with hard sauces or other preferred sauces.

poi. A staple food in the Pacific islands, made from the edible root of the *taro*. The taro is a plant of the subtropics and tropics, grown for its large underground tuber, which has a high starch content and is extremely digestible. The taro root is too acrid to eat raw. To make poi, the root is cooked, pounded, and kneaded until smooth, then mixed with water. It is either strained and served immediately, or more commonly allowed to ferment for a few days.

poisons. Any substances which may cause death, serious illness, or some other harmful effect when introduced into the body in a relatively small quantity. The effects of poisons may be local or remote; some poisons have both effects. Local effect means direct action on the part to which the poison is applied, such as corrosion or irritation of the skin. Remote effect means that the action of the poison is in some organ removed from the seat of application or point of introduction. Acute poisoning is the condition brought about by taking an overdose of poison. Chronic poisoning is the condition brought on by taking repeated doses of a poison or as a result of the absorption of poison over a longer period. Some occupational groups are subject to chronic poisoning such as phosphorus, mercury, lead, arsenic, etc. See *food poisoning* and *food toxins*.

pollack or pollock (*Pollachius virens*). A saltwater fish which resembles the cod. Also known as the coalfish, found in the Atlantic from Norway to the Mediterranean. A closely related species, the Alaska pollack, is plentiful in the Bering Sea and north Pacific waters. The flesh is white, firm, and lean, with a pleasant, delicate flavor. A good source of protein.

polyalcohol. See *polyhydric alcohols*.

polycythemia. A condition characterized by excess *red blood cells* that contain a high concentration of *hemoglobin*. There are several types of polycythemia. One type may be caused by an excess of cobalt. Cobalt is the core of *cobalamin* (vitamin B_{12}), which is an essential factor in red blood cell formation.

polyglycerol esters. Polyglycerol esters are available in a number of colors, odors, tastes, and consistencies and have many uses, particularly in the role of *emulsifiers* in foods. They are unique in offering a broad and flexible range of properties, from complete water solubility to complete oil solubility. They can be solids or liquids, saturated or unsaturated, low molecular weight or high, all depending on the polymer chain length of the polyglycerol, and the type and number of fatty acids used in the esterification of the polyglycerol backbone. Polyglycerol esters are usually prepared by direct esterification with the appropriate type and amount of the fatty acids desired and by a transesterification reaction where a given kind and amount of oil can be arranged within a specific polyglycerol. The variations in molar ratios and of the fatty acid or oil will determine the formulation of the specific reaction product. The polyglycerol partial esters look like fat, taste like fat, but are really hybrid fats. Their mono- and diesters range from 6.04–9.15 kcal/g as compared to 9.2 kcal for conventional fats. By using polyglycerol esters in place of fat, one can lower the caloric content by perhaps 20–25%.

Caloric value constants of polyglycerol esters

| | CALORIC VALUE EXPRESSED IN KCAL/GM MOLECULAR WEIGHT | | | |
GLYCEROL TYPE	NO ESTER	MONOESTER	DIESTER	TRIESTER
Glycerine	4.28	8.49	9.15	9.43
Diglycerol	4.65	8.22	9.01	9.34
Triglycerol	4.93	7.77	8.73	9.21
Tetraglycerol	5.00	7.43	8.41	8.93
Pentaglycerol	5.04	7.17	8.14	8.61
Hexaglycerol	5.07	6.97	7.92	8.39
Heptaglycerol	5.10	6.82	7.72	8.21
Octaglycerol	5.12	6.67	7.56	8.06
Monoglycerol	5.13	6.55	7.43	7.90
Decaglycerol	5.15	6.46	7.24	7.77
Triacontaglycerol	5.24	5.65	6.04	6.35

polyhydric alcohols. Organic chemists classify as polyhydric alcohols such substances as glycerine (glycerol), mannitol, sorbitol, and propylene glycol, which have one thing in common: They have more than one hydroxyl or OH group. All polyhydric alcohols have in common the ability to readily absorb and retain water (in chemical terms they are hydroscopic) and are sometimes added to foods to keep them moist. They are *sweet* to the *taste*. Polyhydric alcohols are allowed in foods as *humectants* (water retainers), sweetness controllers, dietary agents, and softening agents. Their action is based on their multiplying of hydroxyl groups that *hydrogen bond* to water. This holds water in the food, softens it, and keeps it from drying out. An added feature of polyhydric alcohol is its sweetness. Polyalcohols are not readily metabolized by humans or bacteria. Polyalcohols added to sweeten sugarless chewing gum are *mannitol*, *sorbitol*, and *xylitol*.

polymorphism. The existence in a population of multiple genetic forms of a given characteristic.

polyneuritis. A term applied to any condition in which there is symmetric involvement of the peripheral nerves and which is usually believed to be the result of some nutritional, toxic, or metabolic disturbance, but may be inflammatory in nature. Polyneuropathy may result from a deficiency of any one of three B vitamins: *thiamine*, *pyridoxine* (vitamin B_6), or *pantothenic acid*. This polyneuritis resulting from a vitamin deficiency is exhibited occasionally by alcoholics, and is sometimes associated with stomach and liver symptoms. There has been considerable evidence that polyneuritis is due to disturbances in the enzyme system of the peripheral nerves.

polyneuropathy. A disease which involves many nerves and affects the peripheral nerves. Symptoms similar to *beriberi*, usually relieved by *thiamine* or vitamin-B complex therapy. Chief symptoms are weaknesses, numbness, partial paralysis, and pain in the legs. Motor, reflex, and sensory reactions are lost in most cases. Recovery is a slow process involving weeks or months, and a year may pass before an individual is able to walk unaided. See *polyneuritis*.

polynucleotide. Composed of two or more *nucleotides*.

polyols. Chemically, polyols or polyalcohols are sugar alcohols or reduced carbohydrates. Because of their desirable sensory and functional properties and slower absorption rate, sweet-tasting polyols are replacements for sugar in special dietary foods for diabetics. Of the various sugar alcohols in the table only sorbitol, mannitol, malitol, and xylitol are considered of industrial importance as sugar substitutes. Many sweet-tasting polyols are natural metabolic intermediates and are widely distributed in plants and animals. In the plant kingdom, berries

Representative sugars and their polyalcohol derivates

SUGAR	POLYALCOHOL DERIVATIVE
Xylose	Xylitol
Glucose	Sorbitol
Mannose	Mannitol
Galactose	Galactitol (dulcitol)
Maltose	Malitol

of the mountain ash, the service tree, and the whitehorn are rich sources of sorbitol. Red algae and the fruit of rosaceae (apples, apricots, pears, cherries, peaches, plums, greengages) also contain a high percentage of sorbitol. Xylitol is found in a number of fruits, vegetables, cereals, mushrooms, lichens, seaweed, and microorganisms. In general, the polyols are phosphorylated or are oxidized to the corresponding sugar derivatives and then converted to energy. See *polyhydric alcohols*.

polypeptide. A compound consisting of more than three amino acids joined together by *peptide linkages*. See *protein*.

polypeptide chains. Macromolecules consisting of amino acids joined by *peptide linkage*. The term polypeptide is often used in the same sense as the term protein, but the concept of protein includes additional characteristics. See *protein*.

polysaccharides. (1) The prefix poly- means "many," and polysaccharides are complex carbohydrates composed of many simple sugar building blocks (monosaccharides) bonded together in long chains. They are synthesized by exactly the same kind of condensation reactions as the disaccharides, and like disaccharides they can be broken down to their constituent monosaccharides by hydrolyses. *Starches* are polysaccharides and are the principal carbohydrate storage products of higher plants; they are composed of many glucose units bonded together. *Glycogen* is a polysaccharide and is the principal carbohydrate storage product in animals. Glycogen is sometimes called "animal starch." *Cellulose* is a highly insoluble polysaccharide occurring widely in plants. Cellulose is the most abundant product of life in the world. (2) The polysaccharides are complex compounds of high molecular weight composed of varying numbers of monosaccharide molecules linked together in long chains. The characteristics of a polysaccharide are determined by the number and kind of monosaccharide units it contains and their arrangement within the polysaccharide molecules. Polysaccharides tend to be insoluble in water and are major constituents of cell membranes. See *starch*, *glycogen*, and *dextrin*.

polyunsaturated. An organic compound, such as a *fatty acid*, in which there is more than one double-bond carbon group. The *essential fatty acids* are among the more highly unsaturated fatty acids (*linoleic, linolenic,* and *arachidonic acids*) and have two, three, and four double bonds (respectively) per molecule; hence they are said to be polyunsaturated. Polyunsaturated fats occur in all liquid vegetable oils (corn, cottonseed, safflower, soybean); in margarines containing substantial amounts of the above oils in liquid form; in fish, mayonnaise, and salad dressing and in nuts, walnuts, filberts, pecans, almonds, peanuts, and peanut butter.

polyuria. Excessive urination. One symptom of *diabetes mellitus*.

pomegranate (*Punica granatum*). The fruit of a bush or small tree with bright-green leaves and orange-red flowers. Pomegranates are one of nature's most interesting fruits, about the size of a large orange, with a vaguely six-sided shape and a hard, leathery skin which can range in color from light yellow to deep purplish red, but is most often a pinkish or brownish yellow. The flesh is a brilliant red, enveloping a large quantity of little seeds. The little flesh there is has a delicious sweet, pleasantly acid taste. Pomegranates are eaten as a fruit, in salads, and sprinkled over desserts.

pompano (*Trachinotus carolinus*). An important saltwater food fish. The pompano, related to the mackerel, reaches a length of about 18 inches and has a silvery blue skin that is highly polished with gold reflections and touches of orange on the fins. Its rich yet delicate flavor makes it loved by gourmets. A good source of protein and fat.

popover. A quick bread made from an egg-rich batter. A well-made popover is large, light, puffed on top, with firm, crisp brown walls. The center cavity is moist and yellow.

poppy seed (*Papaver somniferum*). The minute seed of an annual species of the large poppy family. The seeds make an excellent food flavoring in cooking and baking.

porgy. The name applied to various marine food and game fish of the sea bream family. One genus, *Pagrus*, is crimson with blue spots and is called the red porgy. The variety familiar in Atlantic coastal waters from Cape Cod to South Carolina belongs to the *Senostomus* genus and is more commonly known as the scup. The fish is tender, flaky, and of good flavor.

pork. The flesh of domestic swine is called pork. Although all flesh of domestic swine may properly be called pork, once pigs or hogs (the older swine) are butchered, the word "ham" is used to describe the rear-leg cuts, particularly when they are cured and/or smoked; and the word "bacon" is used to describe the side of meat, with spareribs removed, when it is cured and smoked. A very good to excellent source of high-quality protein, fair to good in *iron*, fair to good in *niacin*, fair in *riboflavin*, and very good to excellent in *thiamine*. See this item in the table under *meats*.

porphyrin. A class of pigmented compounds containing pyrrole nuclei joined in a ring structure. Any of a group of nitrogens containing organic compounds that occur in protoplasm and form the basis of animal and plant respiratory pigments obtained from *hemoglobin* and chlorophyll. See *heme*.

porridge. A dish made by boiling a grain or vegetable in water or milk to make a thickened soup to be eaten with a spoon. Today the word is used chiefly in connection with boiled grains, and although a porridge can be made from any grain, the word now is associated mostly with oatmeal.

portal circulation. Refers to a circulation of blood through the liver. Blood is brought into the liver by the portal vein and out by the hepatic vein.

positive nitrogen balance. See *nitrogen balance*.

posset. A beverage made from hot milk, curdled, with wine and lemon juice. It is sweetened with sugar or molasses and sometimes thickened with flour or bread.

posterior. Situated toward the back or at the back.

postprandial. After a meal. For example, many physiologic or chemical analyses must be done 12–18 hours postprandially, which indicates essentially overnight without food.

potassium (K). Element No. 19. At. Wt. 39.098. Potassium content of the body is about 125 g, as the potassium ion K^+, is found primarily inside the cells where it functions in association with various enzymes. It is intimately concerned with transmission of the nerve impulse, with skeletal muscle contraction, and with cardiac contraction. Excess or lack of the normal amount of potassium causes immediate malfunctioning of the heart. Daily requirements are estimated at 2–4 g per day. The average diet will readily supply this amount since potassium is widespread in vegetables, fruit, and meat. Meats and other lean-muscle tissues, milk, many fruits, especially dried dates, bananas, cantaloupes, apricots, and citrus fruits are good sources of potassium. Tomato juice and the dark-green, leafy vegetables are also high in this nutrient. Shown is the potassium content of foods which may contribute substantially to potassium intake.

Potassium in mg/100 g of food

All bran	100	Fresh fruit	120–370
Beef, mutton and poultry	225–400	Fruit juices, pure	130–225
Biscuits	110–170	Milk, fresh, whole	160
Bread, white and brown	110–225	Nuts	400–900
Breakfast cereal, various brands	110–425	Potato chips	1020
Cheese	110–200	Rice, polished	110
Chocolate milk	350	Soya flour	1660
Coffee, instant, teaspoonful		Syrup, golden	225
in cup of hot water	138	Treacle	1000
Dried fruit, various raw	700–1880	Vegetable, boiled	80–500
Eggs, fresh, whole	150	Vegetables, raw and salad	200–300
Fish, various types	225–425		

potassium bromate. Mol. Wt. 167. $KBrO_3$. Used to artifically age and improve baking properties of flour. Bromate is used at levels of 5–75 ppm. Baking converts bromate (BrO_3^-) to bromide (Br^-), which is absorbed by the body when bread is digested. Bromide circulates harmlessly in the blood and is gradually excreted in the urine.

potassium bromide. A crystalline salt (KBr) with a saline taste and used sometimes as a sedative.

potato (*Solanum tuberosum*). The white potato is a starchy white tuber of the nightshade family. The common white potato, like corn and tomatoes, originated in the Americas and is now the most important starchy food in the temperature regions of America and Europe. Potatoes contain 75%–80% water and yield from 290–380 kJ (70 to 90 kcal)/100 g. Of the energy, 7.6% comes from protein, a negligible amount from fat, and most from starch. The protein content is low, about 2 g/100 g, but potato has a high biological value when fed to humans. Potatoes are a useful source of protein tuberin and contain small, unimportant amounts of minerals and the B group of vitamins. They are a good source of potassium, but variable in *ascorbic acid* (vitamin C). The ascorbic acid content will vary from 5–50 mg/100 g since there are losses due to storage. One medium-size potato is a fair source of *ascorbic acid* (vitamin C). This can be significant when eaten in quantity. Potatoes are a fair source of *thiamine* and *niacin*. See this item in the table under *vegetables*.

potato flour or starch. A very fine flour made from potatoes ground to a pulp and freed from their fibers. The residue is flour. Potato flour is used both for cooking, as in gravies and sauces, and in stewed fruits thickened with potato flour to make a pudding, and for baking, where it gives a dry texture to cakes. Contains some protein, *calcium*, *phosphorus*, *riboflavin*, *thiamine*, *niacin*, and *ascorbic acid* (vitamin C).

potherb. Any *herb* whose leaves, stems, or blossoms are cooked like a vegetable. Some of the commonest ones are borage, chervil, chicory, lovage, sorrel, sweet cicely, and rampion. When cooking potherbs, the leaves are cooked in a similar fashion to spinach.

pot liquor. The liquid left in the pot after cooking vegetables.

pot pie. A meat or poultry pie, usually made with vegetables and potatoes and baked in an uncovered casserole with a single or double crust of pastry or biscuit dough.

pot roast. A term applied to larger cuts of meat which are cooked or braised, that is, cooked slowly in a small amount of liquid or in steam. The meat may or may not be browned in a little fat before it is braised. See this item in the table under *meats*.

poultry. All domesticated birds bred and raised for use as human food. The most common are chickens, Rock Cornish hens, ducks, turkeys, geese, guinea fowls, and pigeons, the last marketed as squabs. Other birds occasionally domesticated for the same purpose are peafowl (peacocks), quail, pheasants, and swans. Wild ducks and wild turkeys are considered game birds and not poultry. Poultry ranks as high nutritionally as any food. Since poultry contains many essential nutrients, protein being chief among them, it is recognized as one of the important members of the meat group, one of the four food groups essential for a balanced diet. (The other three are the milk, bread-cereal, and vegetable-fruit groups). In addition to its excellent qualifications as a protein food, poultry is a good source of calcium, phosphorus, and iron minerals. Important vitamins present in poultry are *riboflavin*, *thiamine*, and *niacin*.

Poultry
Composition of Foods—Edible Portion

Food and Description	Wt. GM	Approximate Measure	Food Energy CAL	Protein GM	Fat GM	Carbohydrate Total GM	Carbohydrate Fiber GM	Water GM	Minerals Calcium µG	Minerals Phosphorus µG	Minerals Iron µG	Minerals Vitamin A I.U.	Vitamins Thiamine µG	Vitamins Riboflavin µG	Vitamins Niacin µG	Vitamins Ascorbic Acid µG
Chicken, cooked																
Light meat	100	3½ ozs.	166	32	3	0	0	64	11	265	1.3	60	0.04	0.10	11.6	0
no skin, roasted, fried	100	3½ ozs.	197	32	6	1	0	60	12	280	1.3	50	0.05	0.25	12.9	0
Dark meat	100	3½ ozs.	176	28	6	0	0	64	13	229	1.7	150	0.07	0.23	5.6	0
no skin, roasted, fried	100	3½ ozs.	220	30	9	2	0	58	14	225	1.8	130	0.07	0.45	6.8	0
Canned, boneless	100	3½ ozs.	198	22	12	0	0	65	21	247	1.5	230	0.04	0.12	4.4	4
Livers, fried	100	3½ ozs.	140	22	14	2.3	0		16	240	7.4	32,200			11.8	20
Duck, domestic, flesh only	100	3½ ozs.	165	21	8	0	0	69	12	203	1.3		0.10	0.12	7.7	
Turkey, total edible roasted	100	3½ ozs.	263	27	16	0	0	55				Tr.	0.09	0.14	8.0	0
Flesh only, roasted	100	3½ ozs.	190	32	6	0	0	61	8	251	1.8		0.05	0.18	7.7	0

powdered sugar. Granular sugar (*sucrose*) that has been ground into extremely fine particles and then mixed with *cornstarch* to prevent caking.

ppm. See *part per million*.

prawn (Peneus setiferus). A shrimplike crustacean ranging in length from 1 inch to 6 inches and, in the tropics, to 2 feet. Prawns are sold as *shrimp*. The only distinction between them is that prawns are considered the large shrimp and the small shrimp are called "shrimps."

pre-beta (β) lipoproteins. The *very-low-density lipoproteins* (VLDL) carry large lipid content but include about 8–13 percent cholesterol and are formed in the liver from endogenous fat sources. See *lipoprotein*.

precipitate. When a chemical comes out of solution due to chemical or physical forces, it is said to precipitate. The curdling of milk (precipitation of casein) occurs when it is treated with acid (mixing milk with vinegar or grapefruit juice) and is an example of precipitation.

precursors. Chemical compounds or metabolites that are ultimately converted in the body to other useful chemicals or metabolites. The amino acid *phenylalanine* is converted to the hormone *epinephrine* by a series of biochemical reactions. Phenylalanine, then, is a precursor to epinephrine.

preservative. Any chemical used to increase the safety, shelf-life, or palatability of foods. There are two broad classes of preservatives, *antimicrobials* which inhibit the growth of microorganisms, and *antioxidants* which prevent rancidity and discoloration due to oxidation.

pressor amines. Amines that promote the rapid constriction of blood vessels and thus elevate the blood pressure dramatically. *Tyramine* and *histamine* are pressor amines that occur naturally in such foods as bananas and cheese. See *cheese*.

pretzel. A long roll of dough traditionally twisted into the shape of a loose knot or the letter B. There are two kinds of pretzels, hard and soft, and either salted or unsalted. Hard salted pretzels are also made in the form of sticks and bite-size balls. Small amounts of potassium, calcium, phosphorus, and vitamins, such as *ascorbic acid* (vitamin C) and *carotene* (vitamin A).

prickly pear (Opuntia). A name given to a cactus and its fruit. Some species of prickly pear have edible fruit. Among them are *O. vulgaris*, or barberry fig, and *O. tuna*, or tuna, common in the southwestern United States. The tuna varies from pear-shaped to round and is yellowish rose in color when ripe. Sweet, flavorsome, and juicy, it may be peeled, sliced, chilled, and served with lemon juice. Small amounts of potassium, calcium, phosphorus, *ascorbic acid* (vitamin C), and *carotene* (vitamin A activity).

primary structure. The sequential order of the building blocks or structural units in macromolecules without taking their three-dimensional structure into consideration, as in the sequential order of the amino acids in proteins.

principal food constituents. There are three principal constituents of foods. The first is *protein*; the second is the *carbohydrates*, a general term including sugars and starches. The third is the fats or *lipids*. Lipid is actually a general term that includes the neutral fats and fat-like substances, such as *cholesterol*.

proenzyme. An inactive form of an enzyme as, for example, pepsinogen. Proenzyme is a generic term that includes *zymogens*.

progesterone. A steroid hormone obtained from the corpus luteum, adrenals, or placenta. It is responsible for changes in uterine endometrium (the mucous membrane lining the inner surface of the uterus) in the second half of the menstrual cycle preparatory for implantation of the blastocyst, development of maternal placenta after implantation, and development of mammary glands. Used in treatment of menstrual disorders (amenorrhea, dysmenorrhea).

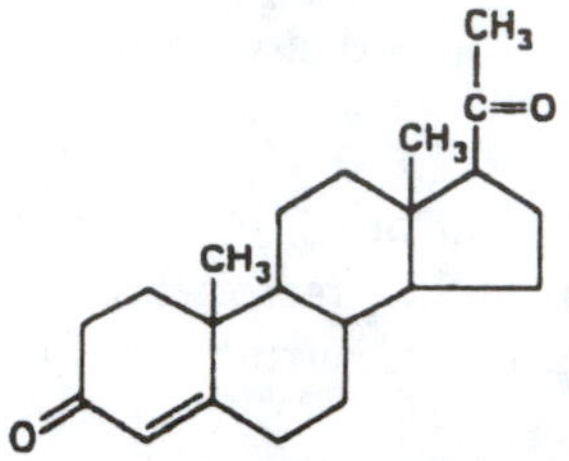

Progesterone

prolactin. See *luteotropic hormone (LTH)*.

prolamines. Major plant proteins that are insoluble in neutral solutions, but soluble in weak acids and alkalies, and present in cereals. Prolamines are insoluble in water but dissolve in alcoholic solution. On hydrolysis, they give large quantities of *proline* and ammonia. Typical prolamines are *gliadin* from wheat and *zein* from maize.

proline (Pro, P). Mol. Wt. 115. Proline is not a true amino acid since its nitrogen in the ring structure is an amino group. Because of the structure of proline, it has a special significance in protein structures. The presence of proline in an amino acid sequence prevents the formation of the *alpha* (α) *helix* at that point. Proline often occurs at points in the polypeptide chain sequence of amino acids where bends or changes of direction of chain occur. Proline and *glycine* occur in very high concentrations in collagen and give collagen its special structural features. See *collagen*.

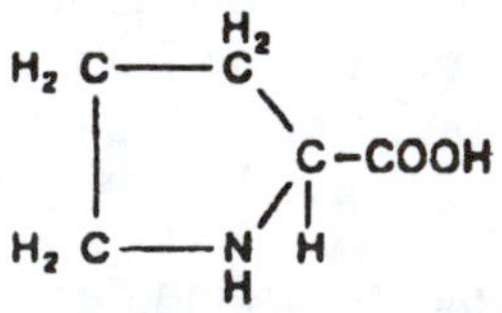

Proline (Pro, P)

prophylaxis. Prevention of disease or preventive treatments.

propionate. A salt or ester of *propionic acid*.

Propionibacteriaceae. Bacteria of the genus *Propionibacterium* are found in foods which ferment *lactic acid*, *carbohydrates*, and *polyalcohols* to *propionic* and *acetic acids* and carbon dioxide. In Swiss cheese, certain species ferment the lactates to produce the gas that aids in the formation of the holes, or "eyes," and also contributes to the flavor.

propionic acid. Mol. Wt. 74. A liquid, sharp-odored *fatty acid* found in milk and distillates of wood, coal, and petroleum.

$$CH_3 - CH_2 - COOH$$

Propionic acid

propylene glycol. Mol. Wt. 76. A humectant and one of several additions (*glycerol* and *sorbitol* are the two others) that are used in foods to help maintain the desired moisture content and texture. Manufacturers add 0.03–5% propylene glycol to candy, baked goods, icings, shredded coconut, and moist pet foods. Propylene glycol also serves as a carrier for oily flavorings and helps them dissolve in soft drinks and other water-based foods. See *alginate*.

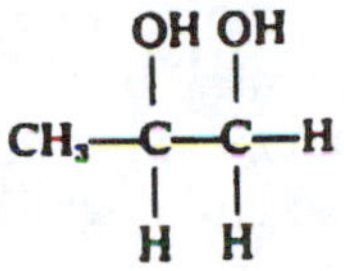

$$CH_3 - \underset{\underset{H}{|}}{\overset{\overset{OH}{|}}{C}} - \underset{\underset{H}{|}}{\overset{\overset{OH}{|}}{C}} - H$$

Propylene glycol

propyl gallate. Mol. Wt. 170. An *antioxidant* added to foods to retard spoilage of fats and oils. It may also increase slightly the shelf-life of foods. Propyl gallate is used at levels up to 0.02% (of the fat or oil content) in animal fat, vegetable oil, meat products, potato sticks, and chicken soup base, and up to 0.1% in chewing gum.

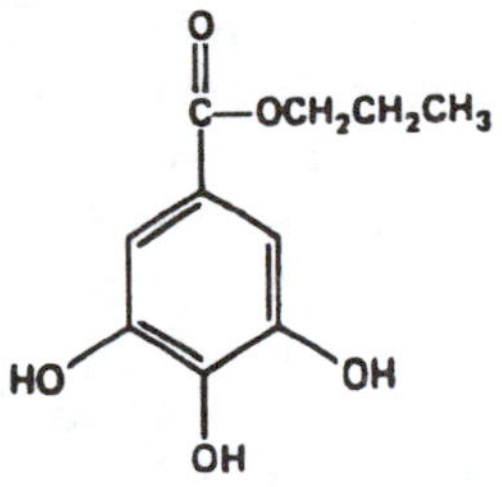

Propyl gallate

prostaglandins. Fatty acids which are thought to be formed in the cell membrane. They are extremely potent substances which produce a variety of physiologic effects in small doses. They have a very wide spectrum of action, including behavioral and central nervous system effects as well as actions which appear to mimic or inhibit many of the known hormones. It is believed that prostaglandins serve as regulators of hormonal action by modulating cyclic formations. The essential fatty acid *arachidonic acid* is a *precursor* to the prostaglandins. There are several classes of prostaglandins that depend on the hydrocarbon chain structures and the positions of the hydroxyl groups. Examples of some of the structures and classifications are given. The *thromboxanes* and *leukotrienes* are related compounds.

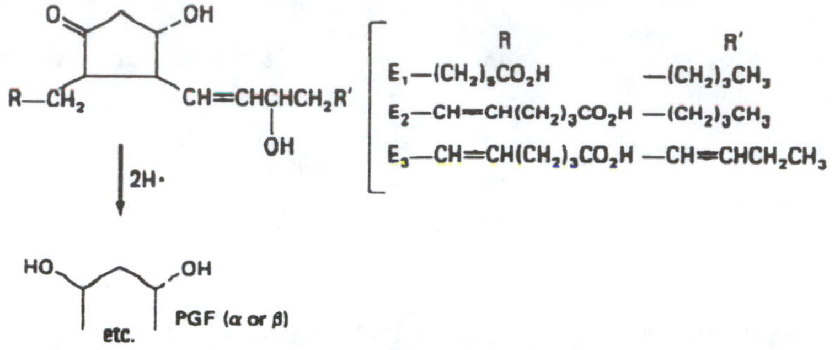

Prostaglandins

prosthetic group. A small organic group (nonprotein) attached to an *apoenzyme* (protein) and required for enzyme activity. A prosthetic group differs from a *coenzyme* only by the higher affinity for the apoenzyme. Coenzymes are more readily removed from the apoenzyme, while prosthetic groups often require chemical treatment or extreme conditions for removal. Functionally, prosthetic groups and coenzymes are similar. As examples, *flavin adenine dinucleotide* (FAD) is often considered a prosthetic group while *nicotinamide adenine dinucleotide* (NAD) is generally considered to be a coenzyme.

protamines. Basic polypeptides that are simpler than *histones, albuminoids,* or *globulins*. Protamines are soluble in water, not coagulable by heat, possess strong basic properties, and on hydrolysis yield a few amino acids, among which the basic amino acids greatly predominate.

protease. A protein-splitting enzyme. An enzyme that digests or degrades protein. Enzymes are usually named to indicate the substance in which they act. Proteolytic enzyme proteases include the proteinases, which catalyze the hydrolysis of the protein molecule into large polypeptides and the peptidases, which hydrolyze these polypeptide fragments as far down as amino acids. The preparations of proteases from microorganisms are mixtures of proteinases and peptidases with varying specificities. Proteases from microorganisms are used primarily for their proteinase activity. Bacteria proteases have been applied to meat for tenderization, and to malt beverages for clarification and maturation. Fungal proteases are active in the manufacture of soy sauce and other oriental mold-fermented foods. Proteases are sometimes added to bread dough, where along with amylases they help improve the consistency of the dough; they are added for thinning egg white so that it can be filtered before drying, and for the hydrolysis of gelatinous protein material in fish waste. Example of proteases are *pepsin, trypsin, chymotrypsin,* and *dipeptidases*, all of which aid in the digestion of protein.

protein. Proteins are high-molecular-weight *polypeptides*. Their unit structures or building blocks of proteins are the *amino acids,* and the linear linkage of these amino acids is an amide linkage called the *peptide linkage (bond)*. The peptide bonds are formed through linkage of the alpha-amino group of one amino acid with the alpha-carboxyl group of another. There are

22 amino acids which may participate in the formation of a protein, and the kind, number, and sequence of the amino acids determines the physical and chemical characteristics of a protein. The variations are enormous, and in nature the extent of that variety is evident. Some proteins are biological catalysts called enzymes; some proteins are a part of cell membranes; some proteins, such as collagen, are for structural purposes outside the cell and others are for structural purposes within the cell, such as the microtubules; some proteins act as carriers of vitamins, metals, oxygen, and a variety of metabolites. Within each of the possible activities of protein are large numbers of different proteins involved in the same general type of function. For example, there are an estimated 2000–4000 individual biochemical reactions within each cell, each different and each catalyzed by a different enzyme. Proteins are classified in several ways and some of the classifications overlap one another. The most general classification is to separate proteins into simple proteins and conjugated proteins. Simple proteins contain only amino acids. Conjugated proteins have additional nonprotein molecules as an integral part of their structure. Examples of a simple protein are serum albumin and *collagen*. Examples of conjugated proteins are *hemoglobin*, which contains a *heme* group, and *casein*, which contains phosphate groups. Proteins are also classified according to the nonprotein components. Another classification of protein is based upon its three-dimensional structure. Thus, globular proteins have a generally round shape; albumins are more elliptic; scleroproteins are fibrous in structure; and *keratins* have one very long dimension with complex intra- and intermolecular bondings. In addition to the primary structure of proteins, the peptide bonds, and the sequence of amino acids, there are three other levels of protein structure. The secondary level of structure relates to the twists and turns that the amino acids make relative to one another along the chain. The secondary structure is determined by the sequence of the amino acids and *hydrogen bonds*. The *alpha (α) helix* is an example. The tertiary or third level of structure is the twists and turns one part of the chain of amino acid makes with respect to the other part of the chain. The *beta (β) pleated sheet* is an example. The tertiary structure determines the overall shape of the molecule. Sometimes separate polypeptide chains associate with one another as a defined unit. The resulting structure is called the quartenary level of structure and each polypeptide chain is called a subunit. Hemoglobin is an example of a protein which requires a quarternary level of structure to be fully functional. Hemoglobin is composed of four subunits, two alpha (α) subunits plus two beta (β) subunits. Many enzymes require a quartenary level of structure to be functional. Listed are examples of proteins in the several different classifications mentioned, with their names, functions, and sources.

Simple Proteins

NAME		SOURCE	FUNCTION
Globular			
Albumins	Serum albumin	Blood	The albumins function as carrier proteins
	Lactalbumin	Milk	and osmotic regulators
	Ovalbumin	Eggs	
Globulins	Myosin	Muscle	A part of the contractile element of muscle
Fibrous			
Collagens	Collagen	Connective tissue, tendons	
		Elastic tissues	Structural support
Keratins	α keratins	Hair	Structural support

Conjugated Proteins

NAME	NONPROTEIN COMPONENT	SOURCE	FUNCTION
Nucleoprotein	Nucleic acid	Chromosomes	A part of the genetic apparatus
Mucoproteins	More than 4% carbohydrate	Blood, stomach, mucous linings (intrinsic factor)	Carrier proteins; protects cells
Glycoproteins	Less than 4% carbohydrate	Blood (alpha, beta, and gamma globulins)	Antibodies, enzymes
Lipoproteins	Phospholipids	Membrane	Enzymes; protection; permeability control
Chromoproteins	Heme	Blood (hemoglobin)	Carries oxygen
Metaloproteins	Iron	Blood (transferrin)	Carries iron
Phosphoproteins	Phosphate	Milk (casein)	Nutrient for offspring

Nutritionally proteins are important with respect to amount and with respect to the quality of the protein, that is, its biologic value. About 0.8 g of good-quality protein per kilogram of body weight, as a rule of thumb, is sufficient to meet all but the most stringent activity. There is evidence to show that half of that value is consistent with good health. A protein uptake that is too low will result in a *protein-calorie malnutrition* known as *marasmus*. The preferred method for determining the amount of protein intake needed is based upon the individual energy expenditure or caloric requirements per day. The table gives some examples of protein intakes recommended as adequate, based on sex, age, caloric requirements, weight, and the percent of the total caloric intake that should be protein. The quality of the protein is taken as 75 out of a possible 100 that represents as good a protein quality as is found in a well-balanced meal.

Recommended Protein Intakes

	AGE YEARS	CALORIE REQUIREMENTS KCAL/DAY	WEIGHT KG	PROTEIN GM/KG	PROTEIN GM/DAY	PROTEIN CALORIES AS PERCENT OF TOTAL CALORIES
Both sexes	1–3	1300	12	2.4	29	9.0
	4–6	1700	18	2.0	36	8.5
	7–9	2100	24	1.8	42	8.0
	10–12	2500	30	1.6	48	7.75
Females	13–15	2600	46	1.0	48	7.5
	16–19	2400	55	0.8	44	7.25
	adults	2300	55	0.75	41	7.0
Addition for pregnancy	—	—	—	—	8	—
Addition for lactation	—	—	—	—	20	—
Males	13–15	3100	44	1.3	58	7.5
	16–19	3600	63	1.0	65	7.25
	adults	3200	65	0.85	55	7.0

The quality of a protein, its *biological value*, depends upon the correct proportions of the essential amino acids to meet the demands of the body. In this regard, the hen's egg is the standard to which all other proteins are compared. It means that the addition of one or more, or a combination of essential amino acid, does not increase the ability of the protein from hen's eggs to support growth and repair of tissues at a low level of intake that still maintains *nitrogen balance*. The table gives the essential amino acid composition of some proteins.

Essential amino acid composition of egg, milk, beef, and wheat
(amino acid in mg/g total N)

	HEN'S EGG	COW'S MILK	BEEF MUSCLE	WHEAT FLOUR
Isoleucine	415	407	332	262
Leucine	553	630	515	442
Lysine	403	496	540	126
Phenylalanine	365	311	256	322
Tyrosine	262	323	212	174
Sulfur-containing amino acids	346	211	237	192
Threonine	317	292	275	174
Tryptophan	100	90	75	69
Valine	454	440	345	262

The comparative quality of the proteins of several foods is given in the table. Given is the essential amino acid that is lacking in maximum proportion—the limiting amino acid—which therefore lowers its value below that of hen's egg. Given for comparison is the *chemical source*, based on amino acid analysis of the food, and biological assessment, based on the *net protein utilization* (NPU) in an animal. The percent of the total calories that comes from protein must be considered in estimating whether or not a given food is a good protein source.

Limiting amino acid, chemical score
and NPU (Net Protein Utilization) of common foods

FOOD	LIMITING AMINO ACID	CHEMICAL SCORE	NPU
Beans	S	42	47
Beef	S	80	80
Cow's milk	S	60	75
Egg	—	100	100
Fish	Tryptophan	75	83
Maize	Tryptophan	45	56
Pork	S*	80	84
Potato	S	70	71
Rice	Lysine	75	67
Wheat flour	Lysine	50	52

*Sulfur-containing amino acids (methionine and cysteine)

The metabolism of protein is the metabolism of its building blocks, the amino acids. Internally, protein breaks down to amino acids and the body reuses them to build other proteins, or oxidizes them as a source of energy. Protein as an energy source is limited to less than 20% of the total caloric need even under conditions of starvation to death. Under normal circumstances, about 10% or less of protein (dietary plus endogenous) is oxidized for energy. Proteins (amino acids) supply about 4 calories per gram of protein. The amount of urea in the urine is a direct reflection of the number of grams of protein (as amino acids) that have

Protein in g/100 kcal of foods and
Percent contribution to total calories provided by each

VALUE OF FOODS AS A SOURCE OF PROTEIN	PROTEIN CONTENT G/100 KCAL	PERCENT KCAL IN PROTEIN
Good		
Beans and peas	6	26
Beef (thin)	10	38
Cow's milk, 5% fat	5	22
Cow's milk, skimmed	10	40
Fish, dried	15	62
Fish, fatty	11	46
Peanuts	5	19
Adequate		
Maize (whole wheat)	3	10
Millet	3	13
Potatoes	2	8
Rice	3	8
Sorghum	3	12
Wheat flour	3	13
Poor		
Cassava	1	3
Cooked bananas	1	4
Sweet potatoes	1	4
Taros	2	7

been oxidized by the body. Proteins from vegetables and from animals may or may not be of similar quality (NPU value). Most grains and vegetable proteins on an individual basis have a lower biological value than meat proteins since one or more of the essential amino acids is not contained in a high-enough proportion. However, a mixture of several vegetable proteins can raise the biological value of the mixture to the equivalent of meat or animal proteins, and some vegetable proteins, such as in rice, potatoes, and soya beans, have an NPU value almost equivalent to meat proteins. Proteins that contain all the essential amino acids in sufficient quantity and in the right combination to maintain nitrogen equilibrium are known as "complete proteins." Proteins that do not supply all the essential amino acids, and so are unable to support nitrogen equilibrium, are incomplete proteins. This deficiency may be partial or complete. A partially incomplete protein will sustain life, but will not support growth.

Protein functions: Dietary proteins furnish the amino acids for synthesis of tissue protein and other special metabolic functions. (1) Proteins as enzymes are used in repairing (anabolism) worn-out body tissue proteins resulting from the continual "wear and tear" (catabolism) going on in the body. (2) Proteins are used to build new tissue (anabolism) during growth by supplying the necessary amino acid building blocks. (3) Proteins are a source of heat and energy. They supply 4 calories per gram of protein. (4) Proteins contribute to numerous essential body secretions and fluids. Many hormones have amino acid components. (5) Proteins are important in the maintenance of normal osmotic pressure relationships among the various body fluids. The plasma proteins of blood play a vital role in these relations. (6) Proteins play a large role in the resistance of the body to disease. Antibodies to specific disease are found in part of the plasma globulin, specifically in what is known as the gamma globulin fraction of plasma. (7) Dietary proteins furnish the amino acids for a variety of other metabolic and structural functions.

Protein synthesis: Proteins are all synthesized from their building blocks, the amino acids. There is no storage of proteins or amino acids equivalent to the fat deposits for lipids or the *glycogen* reserves for carbohydrates. The synthesis of proteins requires a high expenditure of energy and involves the genes' *deoxyribonucleic acid* (DNA) for genetic direction (translation) to a *ribonucleic acid* (RNA) called *messenger-RNA* (m-RNA) that transcribes the "message" in conjunction with the *ribosomes* and selects the amino acid proper for the particular *genetic code*. The amino acids are brought to the messenger-RNA-ribosome complex by another ribonucleic acid called transfer-RNA. Each amino acid has a specific transfer-RNA which is required to transfer the amino acid to the growing polypeptide chain in proper sequence. Each of these complex reactions requires an energy expenditure. It is estimated that each cell has 2000–4000 different proteins.

Protein oxidation: Protein breakdown, its oxidation, and formation of urea, is the total of the catabolism of its individual amino acids. Cells contain *cathepsins, proteases* which digest proteins in a manner similar to those in the digestive system. The resulting individual amino acids are then oxidized by several different pathways. The oxidation of amino acids is incomplete. All of the carbons are not excreted as carbon dioxide. One carbon from each amino acid is excreted as *urea*, which also contains nitrogen and oxygen. Urea is excreted into the urine and is proportional to the amount of protein that was oxidized. Protein oxidation usually accounts for 7%–10% of the total *energy expenditure.*

protein-bound iodine of serum (PBI). A blood test which measures the levels of protein-bound iodine in the serum. The normal range is 4–8 mg per 100 cc of serum. The PBI is an index of thyroid function and a test for *hypo-* or *hyperthyroidism.*

protein-calorie malnutrition (PCM). A term used to describe several different types of deficiency conditions related to diets low in protein but with varying levels of calories from carbohydrate. The terms used to describe PCM are *kwashiorkor* and *marasmus*. Kwashiorkor results from a diet very low in protein but generally adequate in calories, mainly from carbohydrates, while marasmus results from a diet inadequate in protein and calories. See *kwashiorkor* and *marasmus.*

protein hydrolysate. A mixture of amino acids and polypeptides prepared by the digestion of protein by acids, alkalies, or proteases. Properly prepared hydrolysates may be used for either oral or parenteral administration. Some methods of hydrolysis lead to the destruction of certain *essential amino acids.*

proteinuria. Excretion of protein in the urine. It is an abnormal condition.

proteolytic. Affecting the hydrolysis of protein. See *protease.*

proteolytic enzymes. See *protease.*

prothrombin. A *proenzyme* of *thrombin* (factor II) produced in the liver. Thrombin is a blood-clotting factor that requires *vitamin K* for its formation. The function of vitamin K is to carboxylate the prothrombin so that it can be converted to thrombin by another enzyme. See *blood clotting, vitamin K,* and *thrombin.*

protoplasm. The material within the *cell* except the *nucleus*. A thick, viscous colloidal substance which constitutes the physical basis of all living activities, exhibiting the properties of assimilation, growth, motility, secretion, and reproduction. It is a complex mixture of heterogeneous substances surrounded by a chemically active membrane that regulates the interchange of substances with the surrounding medium. It possesses the physical properties of a colloidal mass, the medium dispersion being water. Protoplasm consists of inorganic substances (water, minerals, compounds) and organic substances (proteins, carbohydrates, and lipids). The principal elements present are oxygen, carbon, hydrogen, nitrogen, calcium, and phosphorus, which comprise about 99% of protoplasm. Others present in small amounts are potassium, sulfur, chlorine, sodium, magnesium, and iron together with trace elements (copper, cobalt, manganese, zinc, and others). The chemical composition is shown.

Percent chemical composition of protoplasm

Oxygen	76	Iron	0.01	Potassium	0.3
Carbon	10.5	Calcium	0.02	Sulfur	0.02
Hydrogen	10	Nitrogen	2.5	Sodium	0.5
Magnesium	0.02	Phosphorus	0.3	Chlorine	0.1

protoplast. A type or model of an organism or a bacterial or plant cell without its rigid cell wall, which depends on an isotonic or hypertonic medium to hold it together.

protoporphyrin. $C_{34}H_{34}N_4O_4$. A derivative of the *heme* in *hemoglobin* that contains four porphyrin nuclei. It forms from heme (ferriprotoporphyrin) by deletion of an atom of iron. It occurs naturally.

protovitamins. See *provitamins*.

protozoa. One-celled animals, a few of which cause illness in humans. Important diseases caused by protozoa include systemic infections such as malaria and amebic dysentery, and local infections such as trichomoniasis, which affects the external genitalia.

provitamins (protovitamins). Substances occurring in foods which are not themselves vitamins but are capable of conversion into vitamins in the body. Thus *beta* (β) *carotene* is a provitamin of vitamin A (*retinol*) since it can be converted to the active vitamin.

proximate composition. As applied to food, the term usually includes the percentage of protein, fat, total carbohydrate, ash, and water; caloric values may also be included.

prune. A dried *plum* that is rich in carbohydrates and contains a substance which is useful in stimulating the bowel. The ability of prunes and prune juice to exert a laxative effect is due to dihydroxyphenyl isatin. See this item in the table under *fruits*.

PSP test. Initials stand for phenolsulfonaphthalein, which is a dye administered directly into the vein. The purpose of the test is to estimate the ability of the kidneys to excrete the dye in a given number of hours. It is therefore a measure of kidney function.

psychic secretion. Small amounts of saliva and gastric juice are secreted all the time, but their flow is stimulated when food is present. Factors that stimulate the flow of saliva are chewing, taste, sight, smell, or even the thought of food. The latter type of stimulus causes what is known as "psychic secretion."

psyllium. Psyllium is a *fiber* that comes from the seed of a plant related to ribgrass or plantain. It is an ingredient in bulk laxatives such as Metamucil®. It has also been reported to be effective in lowering blood cholesterol with only mild side effects.

pteroylglutamic acid. A form of the vitamin *folacin*.

ptyalin. The amylase or starch-digestive enzyme that occurs in the *saliva*.

pulse. A characteristic associated with the heartbeat and the subsequent wave of expansion and recoil set up in the wall of an artery. Pulse is defined as the alternate expansion and recoil of an artery. With each heartbeat, blood is forced into the arteries causing them to dilate (expand). The arteries contract (recoil) as the blood moves further along in the circulatory system. The pulse can be felt at certain points in the body where an artery lies close to the surface. The most common location for feeling the pulse is at the wrist, proximal to the thumb (radial artery) on the palm side of the hand. Alternate locations are in front of the ear (temporal artery), at the side of the neck (carotid artery), and on the top of the foot (dorsalis pedis).

pulses (legumes). The nutrition properties of pulses resemble those of the whole cereal grains. All pulses have a higher protein content than cereals. Most contain about 20 g of protein/100 g dry weight. Pulses are rich in lysine and are good sources of the B-group vitamins (except *riboflavin*). Pulses are devoid of any *ascorbic acid* (vitamin C), although large amounts of ascorbic acid are formed on germination. See *legumes*.

pumpkin (*Cucurbita pepo*). The name of a gourd belonging to the Cucurbitaceae family which also includes the melons, cucumbers, and squash. The pumpkin's flesh is orange colored and has a distinctive sweet flavor. The word comes from the Old French *pompion*, in its turn derived from the Greek word *pepon* meaning "cooked by the sun." A good source of vitamin A, fair source of iron. See this item in the table under *vegetables*.

pumpkin spice. A blend of cinnamon, cloves, and ginger, ground together to weld the flavors permanently.

purines. Purine bases are compounds which contain heterocyclic nitrogenous ring structures. The purine derivatives in the body catabolize to *uric acid*. Purines are supplied in the diet by meats and are also synthesized in the body. Shown are the major purines and their corresponding *nucleosides* and *nucleotides*.

Major purines and corresponding nucleosides and nucleotides

PURINE	NUCLEOSIDE	NUCLEOTIDE
Adenine	Adenosine	Adenosine monophosphate (AMP) or adenylic acid
Guanine	Guanosine	Guanosine monophosphate (GMP) or guanylic acid
Hypoxanthine	Inosine	Inosine monophosphate (IMP) or inosinic acid

Meat and foods containing high concentrations of purines are to be avoided under certain conditions, as for example with *gout*. The purine and *pyrimidine* bases derive from the nucleic acids in foods. For the structures see *adenosine triphosphate, guanosine triphosphate, inosine triphosphate,* and *ribonucleotides.*

Purine in mg/100 g of foods

GROUP I (0-50 MG)	GROUP II (50-150 MG)	GROUP III (150-800 MG)
Vegetables	Meats, poultry	Sweetbreads
Fruits	Fish	Anchovies
Milk	Seafood	Sardines
Cheese	Beans, dry	Liver
Eggs	Peas, dry	Kidney
Cereals, bread	Lentils	Meat extracts
Sugar, fats	Spinach	Brains

Adapted from Turner, D.: Handbook of Diet Therapy, Ed. 5, Chicago University of Chicago Press, 1971.

purpura. Small hemorrhages in the skin and mucous membranes; they occur as a result of leakage from the capillaries into the tissue spaces of the subcutaneous tissues. If the hemorrhages are small, pinpoint in size, they are called petechiae; the larger ones, which resemble bruises, are called ecchymoses. Purpura is a symptom and may be secondary to a number of diseases including scurvy, liver disease with failure to utilize *vitamin K*, and allergy to certain drugs.

putrefaction. The decomposition of proteins by microorganisms under anaerobic conditions, resulting in the production of incompletely oxidized compounds, some of which are foul smelling.

pyelonephritis. An infection of the kidneys caused by bacterial invasion of the kidneys and urinary tract.

pyloric gland. A gland of the *stomach* near the pylorus.

pyloric stenosis. A condition in which the muscular tissue of the pylorus thickens and hardens, constricting the size of the opening from the stomach to the *duodenum*. As it progresses, partial or complete obstruction may occur. The primary symptom is projectile vomiting with no sign of nausea. See *digestive system.*

pyorrhea. If *gingivitis* is not treated, the gum tissue may gradually separate from the tooth and a pocket may form between the soft gum tissues and the hard tooth surface. Bacteria, saliva, and food debris collect in the pockets and intensify the destructive process. Pus usually forms (pyorrhea means "pus flowing"). The bone adjacent to the area disappears, more attaching tissue is lost, and the pocket deepens and widens. Eventually the tooth loosens and its movement in chewing sets up additional irritation.

pyrazines. The pyrazines are highly aromatic. There are about 50 which occur naturally in foods. They contribute the aromas to a wide variety of foods—peanuts, chocolate, potatoes, and paprika among them. The pryazine derivative occurs in chocolate.

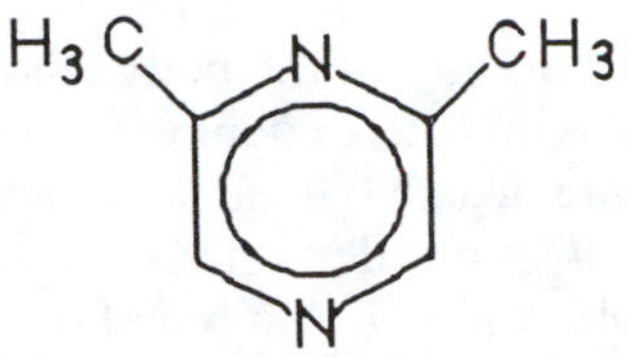

$$H_3C \quad N \quad CH_3$$

2,6 Dimethyl pryrazine

pyridine. Mol. Wt. 79. A six-membered heterocyclic nitrogenous base. It is obtained commercially from *coal tar*. The pyridine ring structure is found in the vitamin *niacin* or *nicotinamide*; in the cofactors *nicotinamide adenine dinucleotide* (NAD) and *nicotinamide adenine dinucleotide phosphate* (NADP); and in *pyridoxal phosphate* (vitamin B$_6$).

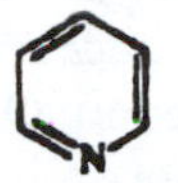

Pyridine

pyridoxal phosphate Mol. Wt. 247. The cofactor form of *pyridoxine* (vitamin B$_6$). Pyridoxal phosphate and pyridoxamine phosphate are readily interchangeable and equivalent in the body. They act as coenzymes in reactions involving the *transamination* of amino acids and function as the agents of the transfer of amino groups from an amino acid to an *alpha (α) keto acid*. In general, pyridoxal phosphate serves as a cofactor for a variety of enzymes involving the amino acids, decarboxylases (the removal of carbon dioxide), dehydrases (the removal of water), sulfhydrase (the addition of sulfhydryl groups), and many other reactions. More than 50 specific reactions of amino acids requiring pyridoxal phosphate are known. See *pyridoxine* (vitamin B$_6$).

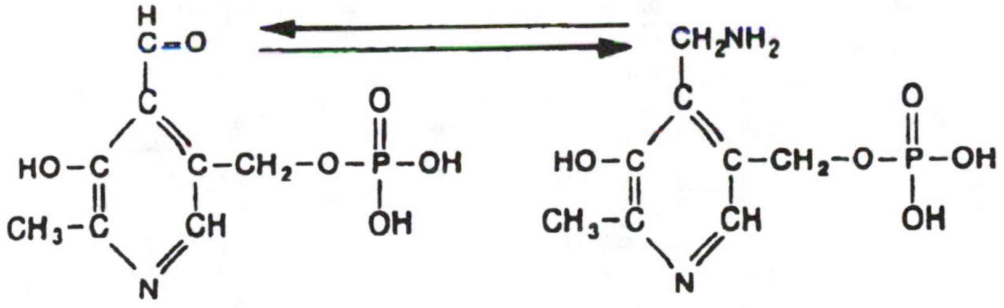

Pyridoxal phosphate   Pyridoxamine phosphate

pyridoxamine. C$_8$H1$_2$N$_2$0$_2$. A crystalline amine of the vitamin B$_6$ or *pyridoxine* group that occurs in phosphate active as a *coenzyme*.

pyridoxine (vitamin B$_6$). A generic name. Three forms of vitamin B$_6$ occur in nature: pyridoxine, pyridoxal, and pyridoxamine. In the body, the forms undergo conversion to *pyridoxal phosphate*. The most potent and active forms in body metabolism are the derivatives *pyridoxal phosphate* and pyridoxamine phosphate. The term pyridoxine, or simply vitamin B$_6$, is used to designate the entire group, as well as one of its components. Pyridoxine is a water-soluble, heat-stable vitamin that is sensitive to light and alkalies. It is absorbed in the upper portion of the small intestine and is found throughout the body tissues. In its active phosphate forms of vitamin B_6, pyridoxal phosphate is an active coenzyme in many types of reactions in amino metabolism: (1) Pyridoxal phosphate is active in *decarboxylation*; (2) pyridoxal phosphate also aids in *deamination*; (3) in *transamination* reactions (transfer of amino groups), pyridoxal phosphate acts as a coenzyme which splits off NH_2 and transfers it to a new carbon skeleton which forms a new amino acid or other compound; (4) in transulfuration (transfer of sulfur) pyridoxal phosphate aids reactions of the sulfur-containing amino acids, as in the transfer of sulfur from methionine to another amino acid (serine) to form the derivative cysteine. Pyridoxal phosphate plays a role in hemoglobin synthesis as a cofactor in the synthetic pathway to porphyrin. It has a different role as a cofactor for glycogen phosphorylase. Vitamin B_6, pyridoxine, is also involved in metabolic processes of the *central nervous system* (CNS). In severe vitamin B_6 deficiency, convulsive seizures occur. Vitamin B_6 appears to prevent uncontrolled excitation of the CNS. Vitamin B_6 deficiency is extremely rare in humans. Some years ago, an infant formula was deficient in vitamin B_6 because of the heat process used in its preparation, resulting in symptoms of vitamin B_6 deficiency. Occasionally, a vitamin B_6 deficiency is seen in chronic alcoholics. Vitamin B_6 deficiency can be prevented by 2–3 mg of vitamin B_6 daily in adults. Shown is a list of the pyridoxine (vitamin B_6) content in some common foods.

Pyridoxol   Pyridoxal   Pyridoxamine

Pyridoxine (vitamin B_6) in µg/100 g of foods

Apple	26	Halibut	110	Peas, canned	46
Asparagus, canned	30	Ham	460	Peas, dried	250
Banana	320	Heart, beef	650	Pork	500
Barley	440	Honey	15	Potatoes	200
Beans, green, canned	32	Kidney, beef	670	Raisins	94
Beef	275	Lamb	300	Rice, whole	1030
Beer	55	Lemon juice	35	Rice, white	325
Beet greens	37	Lettuce	71	Rye	340
Brains, beef	160	Liver, beef	660	Salmon, canned	450
Cabbage	200	Liver, calf's	300	Salmon, fresh	590
Cantaloupe	36	Liver, pork	440	Sardines, canned	280
Cauliflower	20	Malt extract	540	Soybeans	1000
Carrots, raw	170	Milk, whole	80	Spinach, canned	60
Cheese	98	Milk, human	13	Strawberries	44
Cod	340	Milk evaporated	30	Tomatoes	710
Corn, canned	68	Milk, dry	600	Tuna, canned	440
Corn, yellow	470	Milk, dry skim	550	Turnips	100
Corn grits	225	Molasses, blackstrap	2250	Veal	350
Cottonseed meal	1310	Oats, rolled	120	Watermelon	33
Eggs, fresh	35	Onions	63	Wheat, bran	1500
Flounder	100	Orange juice, canned	25	Wheat, germ	1200
Flour, white	130	Orange juice, fresh	40	Yams	320
Frankfurter	13	Peaches, canned	16	Yeast, baker's	650
Grapefruit juice	20	Peanuts	300	Yeast, brewer's dry	4900
Grapefruit section	110	Peas, fresh	120		

pyrimidines. Compounds which contain a heterocyclic nitrogenous ring structure. The pyrimidine derivatives in the body are catabolized to carbon dioxide and water or to beta (β)-amino isobutyric acid, which is excreted. Pyrimidines are supplied in the diet by meats and are also synthesized in the body. Shown are the major purines and their corresponding *nucleosides* and *nucleotides*.

Major pyrimidines and their corresponding nucleosides and nucleotides

PYRIMIDINE	NUCLEOSIDE	NUCLEOTIDE
Thymine	Thymidine	Thymidine monophosphate (TMP) or thymidylic acid
Pyrimidines	Uridine	Uridine monophosphate (UMP) or uridylic acid
Cystosine	Cytidine	Cytidine monophosphate (CMP) or cytidylic acid

pyrophosphate. A pyrophosphate is the salt of pyrophosphoric acid. The pyrophosphoryl group is formed by the condensation of two phosphate groups: Pyrophosphate bonds are very important in the energetics of the cell. One storage form of chemical energy in the body, *adenosine triphosphate* (ATP), has pyrophosphate bonds. The "breaking" or hydrolysis of pyrophosphate bonds is accompanied by a large release of energy which can be used for work or synthetic reactions. Often compounds containing pyrophosphate bonds are said to contain "high-energy" phosphate bonds. It is by the synthesis of the pyrophosphate bonds in ATP, using the oxidation energies from foods, that the energy of oxidation is conserved. The process is called *oxidative phosphorylation*.

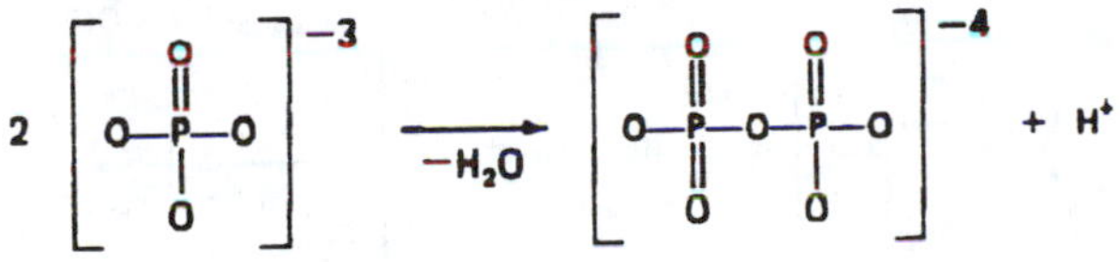

Pyrophosphate bond

pyruvic acid. Mol. Wt. 88. Pyruvic acid or pyruvate (the salt form) is the end-product of *glycolysis* (the degradation of glucose). Pyruvate is formed in the cytosol and enters the *mitochondria*, where it is oxidized completely to carbon dioxide, water, and *energy* to complete the oxidation of glucose via the *Krebs' cycle* and *oxidative phosphorylation*.

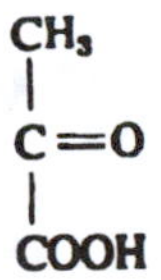

Pyruvic acid

Q

Q. The alphabetic symbol for the amino acid *glutamine* (Gln, Glx).

quince. The round to pear-shaped fruit of the *Cydonia cydonia* tree. When ripe, the fruit is rich yellow or greenish yellow with a strong odor and hard flesh. Its taste is so tart and astringent that it cannot be eaten raw. Quinces are full of natural pectin and are used for making marmalades, jellies, jams, fruit paste, butters, preserves, and syrups.

quinone. An aromatic ring structure that contains two *carbonyl groups* (>C=O) as a part of the ring. Quinones can undergo *oxidation-reduction* reactions. The oxidation-reduction reactions involve an intermediate stage called a semiquinone in which only one electron is transferred. Quinones are important in the body because *vitamin K* and coenzyme Q (*ubiquinone*), a member of the *oxidative phosphorylation* chain, are quinone derivatives.

Semi-quinone

R

R. The alphabetic symbol for the amino acid *arginine* (Arg).

rachitis. See *rickets*.

radiation. A general term for any form of radiant energy emission or divergence from luminous bodies, roentgen (x-ray) tubes, radioactive elements, and fluorescent substances. Infrared radiation is invisible heat rays beyond the red end of the visual spectrum. Ionizing radiation is radiation which either directly or indirectly induces ionization of radiation-absorbing material. Ultraviolet is radiant energy extending from 200–390 nm in the visual spectrum. It is known that some radiation kills living cells, and a practical application of this is used in food processing. Radiation used to kill microorganisms and insect pests, which inhibits the growth of sprouts on potatoes and onions and delays ripening in some fruits, is called ionizing radiation. Irradiating does not make foods radioactive. It is easier on foods than heat sterilizing, leaving them attractive with their texture undisturbed and their flavor and nutritive value altered very little, if at all. Radiation works by destroying part of the cell's machinery (the nucleic *acids*) that is involved in production and growth. In the process, it produces other substances that remain in the food after the treatment is over. These are not unlike the substances that are found in food anyway, and have been carefully studied. The FDA proposes to approve irradiation as a food-processing method and has published the regulation suggested to govern its use. See *irradiation*.

radiostol. A substance produced by the action of ultraviolet light upon *ergosterol*; it has *vitamin D* activity except for poultry.

radish (*Raphanus sativus*). The pungent fleshy root of a hardy annual plant widely used as a salad vegetable. The name radish is derived from the Latin word for "root," *radix*. Radishes come in many shapes and colors: round, long, or oblong, and white, pink, red, yellow, purple, or black. Their taste varies from mild to peppery. Depending upon the variety, they can be from one inch to two or more feet long and weigh up to several pounds apiece. See this item in the table under *vegetables*.

raffinose. A trisaccharide of *galactose*, *glucose*, and *fructose*, found in *molasses*. Present in *legumes* and responsible for *flatus*, as it is not digested in the colon but is used by colon bacteria.

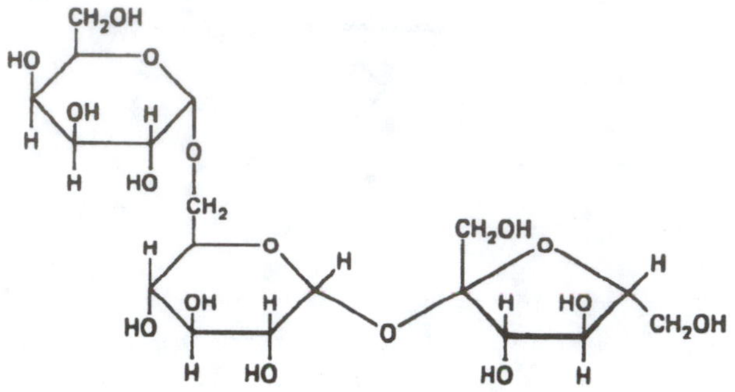

α(1→6)–D-galactosyl -α-(1→2)D-glucosyl β-D-fructoside

Raffinose

α(1→6)-D-galactosyl-α-(1→2)D-glucosyl β-D-fructoside

raisin. The name given to several varieties of grape when they are dried, either naturally in the sun or by artificial heat. When grapes are dried, their skins wrinkle, and they have a higher sugar content and a flavor quite different from that of fresh grapes. The word raisin comes from the Latin word *racemus* meaning "a cluster of grapes or berries." Varieties of grapes dried to make raisins run from dark bluish brown to golden. The two most popular varieties are muscats and sultans. When the fruit is ripe it is picked and spread out on trays to dry in the sun, and dehydrated indoors and given a sulfur treatment. This preserves the golden color. Raisins contain a variety of vitamins and minerals, especially iron. Their natural sugar content makes them an excellent sweet for children. See this item in the table under *fruits*.

rancid. Having a disagreeable *aroma* or *off-flavor*. Rancid usually describes foods with a high content of fat when oxidation of *unsaturated fatty acids* to aldehydes or hydrolysis has occurred.

rancidity. The process of becoming rancid. Rancid fats have typical rank *aromas* and *off-flavors*, changed baking properties, and other properties different from those of the original *fat*. The fats that contain *unsaturated fatty acids* are very susceptible to oxidative attack (by oxygen or light), and the *essential fatty acids* are the chief substances that are affected by rancidity. In the process of rancidification, the oxidation going on also destroys the *retinol*, *carotene* (vitamin A), and *vitamin E* which may be present, diminishing the nutrient quality of the food.

raspberry (*Rubus*). The fruit of a bush which is a member of the rose family. Raspberries grow wild in woods and are also cultivated. The berry is made up of many small drupelets. In contrast to blackberries, which retain their stems or receptacles when the fruit is picked, the stem of a raspberry separates from the berry and remains on the plant. Raspberries may be red, purple, black, or amber in color. They are a delicately flavored fruit and can be eaten raw or used for jellies, jams, puddings, pies, etc. A fair source of iron and *ascorbic acid* (vitamin C). See this item in the table under *fruits*.

ravioli. Shells or cases of noodle dough filled with meat, chicken, cheese, or spinach. Although the word is Italian, this type of food preparation is by no means a uniquely Italian dish. It occurs under different names in many lands. The Chinese know ravioli as won ton, the Jews as kreplach, and the Russians as pelmeni.

RBC. See *blood cells, red*.

RDA. See *Recommended Daily Allowances*.

receptors. (1)Free nerve endings distributed to the tongue, nasopharynx, orbit, and other mucous surfaces. Like other pain endings, their thresholds are relatively high, but the response fatigues slowly, and the receptors adapt little under most conditions of chemical stimulation. (2) "Receptors" also refers to sites on cell membrane surfaces with specific affinities for various metabolites, hormones, and other materials. Most of the hormones attach to site-specific receptors on target-cell surfaces.

Recommended Daily Allowances (RDA). The National Academy of Sciences, Washington, D.C., defines Recommended Daily Allowances as follows: "The Recommended Daily Allowances (RDA) are the levels of intake of essential nutrients considered in the judgment of the Committee on Dietary Allowances of the Food and Nutrition Board, on the basis of available scientific knowledge, to be adequate to meet the known nutritional needs of practically all healthy persons." The RDA represents the nutritional needs, over a long period of time, of population groups, expressed as a daily average. The daily values (except for energy) are thought to exceed the requirements for most individuals, although they represent a safe level of excess. The RDA is meant for healthy populations, and is based on the assumption that it will be met by a diet containing a wide variety of foods rather than by nutritional supplements (vitamins/mineral tablets) or by extensive fortification of single foods. The RDA is based on intake of nutrients in foods and has corrected, within its allowances, for less than 100% availability and less than 100% absorption of the various nutrients from a normal varied diet. See the Appendix.

reconstitute. To restore to the normal state, usually by adding water, such as reconstituting dry milk by adding water to make it fluid milk.

red blood cell (erythrocyte, red corpuscle). The red blood cell is the major cell in the blood. Men normally have about 5 million red corpuscles per milliliter (mL) and women have about 4.5 million mL. The average person has 35 trillion (35,000,000,000,000) cells. The erythrocyte is shaped like a solid doughnut and is about 7 microns (0.0003 inch) in diameter. The red blood cells make up about 45% of the total blood volume in men and about 40% in women (See *hematocrit*). The average life-span of red blood cells is about 120 days after they have been discharged from the bone marrow, where as they mature they form various stages: proerythroblasts, erythroblasts, normoblasts, and reticulocytes. The mature red blood cells has no *nucleus* or *mitochondria*. The red blood cell therefore does not divide, nor does it consume much oxygen. The most important constituent in the erythrocyte is the protein *hemoglobin*, which accounts for its red color. The *heme* moiety of hemoglobin is red and contains the reduced or ferrous iron (Fe^{+2}). The blood of the average male contains 16 g of hemoglobin in 100 mL of blood, and the blood of the average female has 14 g per 100 mL. The primary function of hemoglobin and the erythrocyte is the transport of oxygen from the lungs to other tissues. The oxygen combines with heme and does not oxidize the iron, which remains in reduced (ferrous) state. The oxygen-carrying capacity of hemoglobin is 1.34 mL of oxygen per g. Hemoglobin also acts as one of the major *buffers* of blood in maintaining the pH and is important in carrying some of the carbon dioxide (carbohemoglobin) away from the tissues to the lungs. Occasionally, the iron in the hemoglobin becomes oxidized to *methemoglobin* (ferrihemoglobin). The oxidized or ferric iron (Fe^{+3}) can be reduced by enzymes called methemoglobin reductases.

About 20 million erythrocytes are destroyed every minute. *Bile pigments, biliverdin* and *bilirubin*, green and red in color, respectively, form from the breakdown of heme and are responsible for the color of *bile*. The bile pigments are converted to stercobilin by bacterial action in the intestines, which is responsible for the brown color of *feces*.

In order for erythrocytes to be produced and maintained at normal levels, several vitamins and iron are required. The vitamins *folacin, pyridoxine*, and *cobalamin* (vitamin B_{12}) are intimately involved in erythrocyte maintenance. A deficiency of any of these nutritional factors results in nutritional anemia. Some *anemias* are genetic diseases that result in abnormal hemoglobins that may vary in shape and ability to transport oxygen, and have a shortened erythrocyte life-span, as for example sickle cell anemia.

red blood cell count. A count of blood cells to determine or test for *anemias*. See *hematocrit*.

red dye number 2 (Amaranth). A once widely used food coloring accounting for about one-third of all coloring. The dye was used in soft drinks, ice cream, pistachio nuts, candy, baked goods, pet foods, sausage, breakfast cereals, and other foods. Red No. 2 was banned by the Food and Drug Administration in 1976.

red dye number 3 (Erythrosine). A food dye used to color cherries in canned fruit cocktail, because it is insoluble in acidic solutions and therefore does not stain other fruit.

red pepper. See *pepper*.

reducing sugar. A sugar that can undergo oxidation and in turn reduces some reagents or metals. The ions of silver, bismuth, or copper are frequently used in various tests and are themselves reduced as they oxidize the sugar. The changes in color or precipitation of the metal (reduced) indicates a positive test for a reducing or an *aldehyde* group. A positive reducing sugar indicates a free aldehyde group in the sugar. The aldehyde group is oxidized to a carboxylic acid group. *Glucose* is a reducing sugar because the aldehyde group is free. The glucose in sucrose is not a reducing sugar because the aldehyde group is not free, but is involved in a chemical bonding with *fructose*.

reduction. Reduction is the opposite of *oxidation* and like oxidation can be interpreted in several ways. The addition of a hydrogen to a molecule is a reduction.

$$2H_2 \ + \ O_2 \ \longrightarrow \ 2H_2O$$
$$\text{hydrogen} \quad \text{oxygen} \qquad \text{water}$$

Reduction of hydrogen

In the example given, oxygen is reduced. Every reduction must also be accompanied by the opposite reaction, an oxidation, and in the first example hydrogen is oxidized and the oxygen is reduced to form water. In biological oxidations of food, the carbons and hydrogens are oxidized and oxygen is reduced. A more general interpretation is the addition of electrons to a molecule. For example, the iron in the cytochromes of the *terminal respiratory chain* undergoes reductions and oxidations based on the addition and removal of electrons, respectively. The reversibility of the oxidation-reduction reaction is shown in the second example. The electrons are never free. They are transferred to an electron acceptor that becomes itself reduced in the process.

$$e^- + Fe^{+3} \underset{\text{oxidation}}{\overset{\text{reduction}}{\rightleftharpoons}} Fe^{+2}$$

electron   ferric   ferrous
             iron   iron
          (oxidized)   (reduced)

Oxidation-reduction reactions

refrigeration. See *food storage*.

refuse. That portion of foods which is inedible (as bones, pits, shells), or usually discarded in preparation of food for the table (as potato parings and tough outer leaves of vegetables). In food values expressed as the "as purchased" basis, the nutrients in refuse have been disregarded.

regional enteritis. An inflammatory disease which involves the small bowel and is manifested by diarrhea, abdominal cramping, pain, fever, anemia, and weight loss. Usually the inflammation begins in the terminal *ileum* and spreads towards the *jejunum*. The inflammation frequently leads to narrowing of the bowel or stricture formation. See *digestive system*.

regurgitation. The backward flow of food; casting up of undigested food. Regurgitation also describes the backward flow of blood through the valves in the *heart* that do not close properly. See *heart valves*.

rehydration. Soaking or cooking or using other procedures to make dehydrated foods take up the water they lost during drying. See *reconstitute*.

remission. A lessening of the severity or temporary abatement of symptoms.

renal. Pertaining to the *kidney*.

renal threshold. That concentration of a given substance in the blood above which the excess will be eliminated in the *urine*. For example, when the blood glucose level exceeds about 180 mg per 100 mL of blood, the kidneys cannot reabsorb the excess, the renal threshold has been exceeded, and glucose enters the urine. This is what occurs in untreated *diabetes mellitus*.

renal tubules. See *nephron*.

renin. An enzyme produced in the kidney in response to a drop in blood pressure. Renin, a *protease*, acts on angiotensinogen in the plasma to form *angiotensin* I, which in turn is converted to angiotensin II by another plasma enzyme. The angiotensinogen comes from the liver. Angiotensin increases the blood pressure and stimulates the *adrenal glands* to produce *aldosterone*, which in turn increases water and sodium ion reabsorption in the renal tubules (*nephrons*). Do not confuse renin with *rennin*, an enzyme that curdles milk in the *gastric juice*. See *water balance*.

rennet. A combination of two enzymes or ferments, *rennin* and *pepsin*, obtained from the membranes of the stomachs of young mammals. The best quality is that from an animal so young that it has received no other food than milk, the most desirable coming from a calf's stomach. Rennet's chief importance from a food standpoint is its property of coagulating milk, and its widest food use is in the manufacture of *cheese*.

rennin. An enzyme contained in the *gastric juice* which precipitates milk in solid form (curds). Heat-treated cow's milk and human milk make for a finer, more easily digested curd than ordinary cow's milk. Rennin is especially abundant in gastric juice of babies and young animals fed on milk; it is less important in adults when the hydrochloric acid content of the gastric juice is sufficient alone to coagulate milk. Do not confuse this enzyme with *renin*, an enzyme from the kidney.

reproductive system. Consists of the testes, seminal vesicles, penis, urethra, prostate, and bulbourethral glands in the male; the ovaries, uterine tubes, uterus, vagina, and vulva in the female. All these systems are closely interrelated and dependent on each other as the reproductive machinery of animals.

requirements. Although the average minimal requirements for various nutrients cannot be stated with accuracy, certain "minimum daily requirements" for food labeling purposes have been designated in regulations for enforcement of the Federal Food and Drug and Cosmetic Act. Requirements should not be confused with the *Recommended Dietary Allowances*, though they are based on the RDA and equal the RDA for the population group likely to consume the labeled food.

residue. (1) Remainder; the contents remaining in the intestinal tract after digestion of food; includes fiber and other unabsorbed products. (2) That portion of a molecule included in another larger molecule, as a number of amino acid residues are contained in a polypeptide. (3) Resorption: A loss of substance, for example, a loss of mineral salts from bone.

respiration. In breathing, respiration is composed of two basic movements, the inspiration (intake, inhalation) of air into the lung, and expiration (exhalation) of the contents of the lung to the outside. Respiration also means the uptake or utilization of oxygen by a living system, and generally the discharge of carbon dioxide. A cell or tissue is thus considered to respire. In humans, oxygen is taken up by cells from the blood which carry oxygen from the lungs. The cells use the oxygen to oxidize the nutrients that have also been delivered to the cells by blood. The *oxidation of food, fats, carbohydrates*, and *amino acids* (proteins), results in the formation of carbon dioxide (CO_2), water, and *energy*. The water and CO_2 enter the blood and are expired through the lungs. The energy, largely chemical energy in the form of *adenosine triphosphate*, is retained by the cell for work, biosynthesis, and other functions.

respiratory acidosis. A condition when the *pH* of the blood is below 7.4 because of the high concentration of carbon dioxide (CO_2) in the blood, which forms carbonic acid (H_2CO_3). In certain diseases, such as emphysema, when CO_2 cannot be properly expelled, respiratory *acidosis* results.

respiratory alkalosis. A condition when the pH of the blood is greater than 7.4. The primary cause of respiratory *alkalosis* is hyperventilation (excessively rapid breathing) which removes the carbon dioxide (CO_2) from the blood. Hyperventilation may result from a number of causes among which are fever, hysteria, and heart failure.

respiratory chain. See *terminal respiratory chain*.

respiratory quotient (R.Q.). The determination of the R.Q. value requires the volume of oxygen consumed and the volume of carbon dioxide (CO_2) expired. The ratio of the volume of CO_2 expired to the volume of oxygen utilized is the R.Q. The respiratory quotient differs for carbohydrates, fats, and proteins because the amount of oxygen atoms and the completeness of combustion vary with each foodstuff. As an example, the R.Q. for glucose is shown. Generalized equations for the *oxidation* of other foods, fats, and proteins, can be written and the R.Q determined. The R.Q. is useful for determining a shift in the food oxidized. As more fat is oxidized, the R.Q. decreases toward a value of 0.7. Conversely, as more carbohydrate is oxidized, the R.Q. shifts toward a value of 1.0. The amount of protein oxidized is relatively constant over a wide range of conditions and does not usually contribute significantly to changes in the R.Q. value. The amount of protein oxidized for any given period of time can be determined by the amount of urea excreted for that period.

$$C_6H_{12}O_6 \;+\; 6\,O_2 \;\longrightarrow\; 6\,CO_2 \;+\; 6\,H_2O \;+\; 665 \text{ kcal/mole}$$

| glucose | oxygen | | carbon dioxide | water | energy |

(foodstuffs)

$$\frac{6 \text{ volumes of } CO_2}{6 \text{ volumes of } O_2} \;=\; \text{R.Q.} = 1.0$$

Respiratory quotient (R.Q.)

R.Q. of the Major Food Classes

Carbohydrate	1.0	Fat	0.71
Protein	0.80	Average mixed diet	0.82

respiratory system. The nose, pharynx, larynx, trachea, bronchi, and lungs. The main function is to provide oxygen for body tissues and to remove carbon dioxide. See *respiration*.

resting metabolic rate (RMR). The energy expenditure measurement under conditions similar for the basal metabolic rate but without the requirement of a 12-hour fast prior to measurement.

Because the conditions for measurement are not as strict as with the basal metabolic rate, the RMR is more frequently measured and used. See *basal metabolism* and *energy balance*.

reticular tissue. Fibrous connective *tissues* which form the supporting framework of lymph glands, liver, spleen, bone, and lungs.

reticulocyte. A young red blood cell occurring during active blood regeneration. See *collagen*.

reticuloendothelium. A system of *macrophages* concerned with *phagocytosis*, present in spleen, liver, bone marrow, connective tissue, and *lymph* nodes.

retina (eye). The back of the *eye* is lined by the retina, which consists of three main layers: (1) the innermost layer which the light first penetrates is a complex network of nerve cells and fibers which finally run together and leave the eye to form the optic nerves. (2) Behind the nerve network there is a layer of light-sensitive cells of two different types, the rods and the cones. (3) The hindmost layer, forming a backing to the rods and cones, and consisting of a black pigment called *melanin*. This absorbs any light and prevents reflection across the eye. There are about 7 million cones and 120 million rods in each eye. Most of the cones are massed together at one tiny spot, the macula, at the back of the eye, which is the central focusing point of the whole optical system of the eye. The cones are color-sensitive, with three different kinds of cone, each sensitive to either red, green, or blue. The rods contain a pigment called visual purple (*rhodopsin*) which is bleached by light at the green-violet end of the spectrum. Rhodopsin contains a vitamin A (*retinol*) derivative called 11-*cis* retinal. A deficiency of vitamin A is first manifested by a nutritional disease called night blindness (*nyctalopia*) resulting from a deficiency of the visual purple content of the rods. See *rod vision*.

retinal. The aldehyde form of vitamin A which is necessary for the synthesis of *rhodopsin* (visual purple). Light ($\lambda\nu$) causes a change in the structure of 11-*cis* retinal, after going through a series of changes. See *retinol*, *retinene*, and *rod vision*.

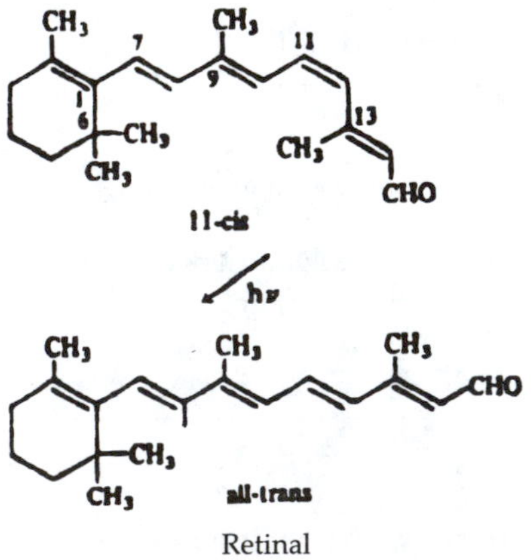

Retinal

retinene. One of a series of derivatives of vitamin A aldehyde formed as an intermediate step in bleaching or *rhodopsin* in the rods of the retina. See *retinol*, *retinene*, and *rod vision*.

retinoic acid. A derivative of vitamin A (*retinol*). The acid form of vitamin A. The exact function of this form of vitamin A is not definitely established, but it is believed that retinoic acid is involved in maintaining the health and integrity of epithelial tissue. See *retinol*, *retinene*, and *rod vision*.

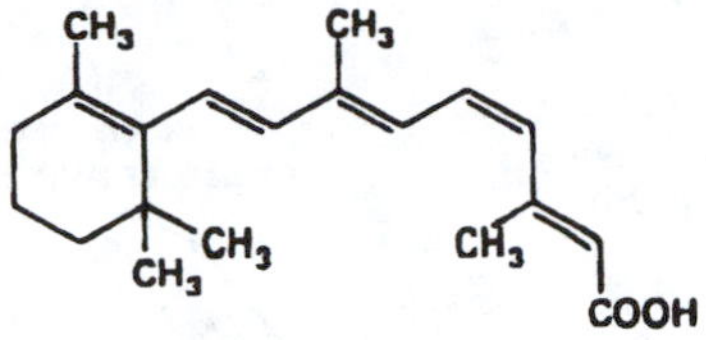

Retinoic acid

retinol (vitamin A). The form of vitamin A that occurs in the livers of animals. Retinol is the storage form of vitamin A and occurs chiefly as the retinyl ester. The principal fatty acid associated with retinyl derivative is *palmitic acid*. *Retinoic acid*, *retinal*, and *retinol* are various oxidation states of vitamin A. The conversion of retinol to retinoic acid and retinal occurs readily. *Rhodopsin* when treated with light releases all-*trans* retinal, which is an inactive form of the vitamin A (11-*cis* retinal). Conversion of all-*trans* retinal to 11-*cis* retinal can occur two ways: (1) In the retina where there is an enzyme to convert it directly or (2) the all-*trans* retinal is reduced to a retinol which is first converted to an 11-*cis* retinal in the liver and subsequently reoxidized to 11-*cis* retinal for the formation of rhodopsin in the *retina*. Vitamin A (retinol) at high levels is toxic. High levels (500,000 I.U. per day) can cause headaches, nausea, nosebleed, anorexia, and dermatitis within a few days. The *Recommended Dietary Allowance* (RDA) for vitamin A of 5000 units is liberal. While it is possible to receive toxic levels of vitamin A (*retinol*) in fish oils from shark or halibut because they contain such high concentrations (2000–100,000 units), it is doubtful that it is possible to reach toxic levels from plant sources of the vitamin, such as carrots. In plants the vitamin A activity is derived from *carotene*, which must be converted to retinol. The conversion of carotene to retinol is attended with losses due to absorption and losses occurring during the chemical conversion. As a result, carotene has one-sixth the vitamin A activity of retinol. See *vitamin toxicity*, *retinoic acid*, *carotenoids* and *retinal*.

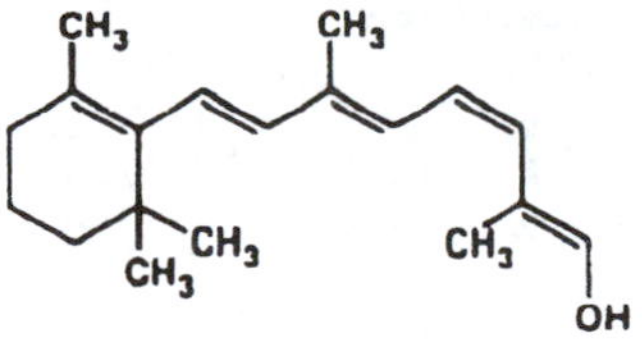

11-*cis* Retinol

A different form of the vitamin occurs in fish liver oils, vitamin A$_2$.

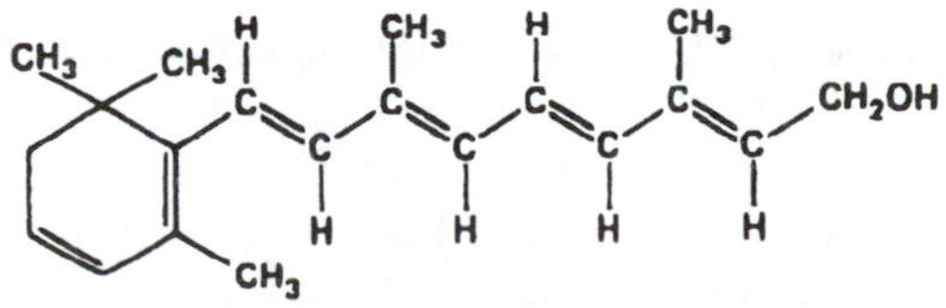

Vitamin A$_2$: predominant form in fish liver oils

The figure shows how vitamin A is involved in the visual process.

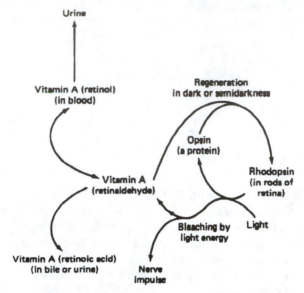

Vitamin A and the visual process

The table shows the vitamin A content or activity of various foods.

Vitamin A in *retinol equivalents* (R.E.[c])/100 g food[b]

Apricots	270	Greens, cooked		Liver	
Apricot nectar	168	Beet	510	Beef	14,000
Bok choy	310	Chard	280	Calf	7,000
Broccoli	250	Collard	700	Chicken	4,100
Butter	1000	Dandelion	1,200	Pork	3,000
Carrots	1,100	Kale	890	Lamb	15,000
Cantaloupe	340	Mustard	580	Turkey	6,000
Cheese (hard)	350	Turnip	760	Liverwurst	2,000
Fish and oils		Greens, raw		Mango	480
Cod liver oil	2,000	Endive	330	Papaya	175
Halibut liver oil	200,000	Escarole	330	Peaches	133
Shark liver oil	100,000	Romaine	190	Pumpkin	160
Swordfish	2,000	Watercress	490	Sweet potato	880[a]
Whitefish	700			Tomato, raw	135

From *Nutritive Value of American Foods in Common Units*. Agriculture Handbook No. 456, Washington, D.C., U.S. Department of Agriculture, 1975.

[a]In contrast, yams have only a trace.

[b]Based on food tables in International Units (IU), the values given are based on ß-carotene in plants and retinol in fish and meat.

[c]1 R.E. = 1 µg retinol = 6 µg ß-carotene = 3.33 IU from retinol = 10 IU from ß-carotene.

retinol equivalents (R.E.). The Food and Nutrition Board recommended the use of R.E. for vitamin A. The R.E. takes into account the losses of carotene during absorption and the losses in the conversion to *retinol*.

1 Retinol equivalent

1 µg retinol 6 µg ß-carotene	12 µg of other provitamin A carotinoids	3.33 IU activity from retinol 10 IU vitamin A activity from ß-carotene

Reye's syndrome. A poorly understood disease characterized by the sudden deterioration of the liver and the brain. Reye's syndrome in children is linked to influenza and the administration of aspirin to control the temperature.

RH factor. In addition to blood groupings and cross-matching for compatibility, the RH factor must be considered. The RH factor is carried in red cells, and about 85% of all individuals have this factor and are therefore RH positive. Individuals who do not have the RH factor are RH negative. As a general rule, RH negative blood can be given to anyone, provided it is compatible in the ABO typing system, but RH positive blood should not be given to an RH negative individual.

rhodopsin (visual purple). Rhodopsin is formed from the combination of protein opsin and 11-*cis* retinal, a derivative of vitamin A (*retinol*). When rhodopsin is exposed to light, the retinal undergoes configurational changes to all-*trans* retinal and separates from opsin, which will only combine with the 11-*cis* retinal. These changes due to light are complex and only partly understood. It is known that there are several configurational changes that occur, but the structures are not known. These reactions occur in the retina and are accompanied by nerve impulses that translate in the brain to what we know as sight. Rhodopsin is in the rods of the retina and therefore is associated with weak light (scotopic) vision. Color vision is associated with the cones in the retina, requiring more light to cause a nerve impulse, and is not so well understood as scotopic vision. See *retinene* and *rod vision*.

Rhodotorula. Red, pink, or yellow *yeasts* which may cause discoloration in foods, for example, colored spots on meats or pink areas in sauerkraut.

rhubarb (*Rheum*). A hardy perennial plant grown for its thick, succulent, leafy stalks. The plant has large clumps of broad green leaves, up to 2 feet across, growing on thick, fleshy red and green leaf stalks which average 12–18 inches in length but can be much longer. There are many varieties of rhubarb, but the only important distinction in the edible types is between forced or hothouse rhubarb and field rhubarb. The first usually has slender pink- to light-red stalks with yellow-green leaves, and the second has red stalks and green leaves. Only the leaf stalks of the rhubarb are edible. Leaves and root contain a substance that can sometimes be poisonous. Rhubarb is used in pies, desserts, jam, and wine. Fair source of β *carotene* (vitamin A activity).

Nutrients in 100 g of raw rhubarb

CALORIES KCAL	PROTEIN G	FAT G	CARBOHYDRATE G	VITAMIN A IU	ASCORBATE MG	THIAMINE µG	CALCIUM MG
16	1	Trace	4	100	9	30	78

riboflavin. Mol. Wt. 376. A vitamin of the B complex; sparingly soluble in water, decomposed by exposure to light, heat-labile in alkaline solutions but otherwise thermostable. The name "riboflavin" was adopted since the factor contains the pigment flavus and the pentose sugar D-*ribose* and is nitrogenous in nature. In pure form, it exists as fine orange-yellow crystals which are practically odorless and bitter-tasting. In water solutions, riboflavin shows a characteristic yellow-green fluorescence. Riboflavin functions biologically as the coenzymes *flavin mononucleotide* (FMN), and *flavin adenine dinucleotide* (FAD), which are components of the flavoproteins, essential to protein and energy metabolism; and it participates in cell respiration and biological oxidations. A deficiency disease, ariboflavinosis, is most frequently associated with deficiencies of other B vitamins. It is formed by all high plants, chiefly in the green leaves. These flavoproteins function in oxidative processes in living cells. They play a major role with *thiamine*-and *niacin*-containing enzymes in a long chain of oxidation-reduction reactions by which hydrogen is released and finally combines with oxygen to form water. It is one of the factors essential for successful reproduction, and it is essential for general health because it is the active constituent of several coenzymes that are essential to oxidation processes in the various body tissues. It is essential for the health of tissues of ectodermal origin such as the skin, eyes, and nerves. Free riboflavin, such as is found in some foods, must be phosphorylated in the intestinal tract before it can be absorbed. Riboflavin is widely distributed in both plant and animal tissues. Once it enters the blood, it is distributed to all cells of the body. Human requirements are now considered to be more closely related to *energy expenditure* than to protein intake; recommended daily allowances have been computed on the basis of caloric intake. Free riboflavin is excreted as such in the urine and feces. The amount of riboflavin needed is related to body size, metabolic rate, and rate of growth. Liver, milk, cheese, eggs, leafy vegetables, enriched bread, lean meat, and legumes are the foods among the richest in riboflavin. Dried yeast is a still richer source.

Riboflavin

Riboflavin in mg/100 g of food

Good and moderate sources		Oatmeal	0.2
Beef, mutton and pork, raw	0.2	Pulses, various, fresh	0.2
Brewer's yeast	2.7	Wheat and barley, whole grain	0.2
Cheese	0.4	Wheat bran, bran layer only	
Chocolate	0.2	Wheat flour, whole meal	0.5
Cocoa, powder	0.4	Wheat germ, e.g., Bernex	0.2
Eggs, fresh	0.4	Wheat germ, germ fraction steam	0.7
Fish, various, fresh and cured	0.3	heated and finely ground	0.3
Fruit, dried	0.1	Poor sources	
Green leafy vegetables	0.2	Fruits, fresh, tropical and temperate	0.05
Liver and kidney	3.0	Maize, meal	0.1
Maize, whole	0.1	Potatoes, all seasons	0.1
Milk, fresh cow's	0.2	Rice, highly milled	0.04
Millets	0.1	Rice, lightly milled	0.1
Nuts	0.2		

ribonuclease. An enzyme that hydrolyzes *ribonucleic acid* (RNA) to mononucleotides.

ribonucleic acid (RNA). A polynucleotide composed of a pyrimidine bases, cytosine and uracil; the purine bases, adenine and guanine; the sugar *ribose*; and phosphate. There are different types of RNA that have distinct structures, functions, and subcellular distributions. Messenger-RNA (mRNA) with specific enzymes copies the message from the *deoxyribonucleic acid* (DNA) genetic triplet code in the nucleus of the cell. The mRNA then enters the cytoplasm, where it combines with ribosomal RNA (rRNA) in the *ribosomes*. The ribosome mRNA complex then complexes with transfer-RNAs (tRNA) which brings amino acids to form peptide bonds. The mRNA determines the sequence and length of the *polypeptide chains*. The constituents of *nucleic acid* can be formed by the body from small compounds, and there is no specific requirement in the diet for the biosynthetic incorporation into RNA or *deoxyribonucleic acid* (DNA). The nucleotides of the ribosomal chain consist of components like those in a chain of (DNA): a phosphoric acid molecule, a distinctive sugar known as ribose, and one purine or pyrimidine. The purines are identical to those found in DNA, *adenine* and *guanine*. The pyrimidines include *cytosine*, but instead of *thymine*, the ribosomal polynucleotide chains of RNA contain the pyrimidine *uracil*. Together DNA and these forms of RNA constitute the basic tools the cells employ in making a protein according to genetic information.

ribonucleic acid polymerase (RNA-polymerase). An enzyme which catalyzes the formation of ribonucleic acids. Under the influence of RNA-polymerase, the ribonucleotides attached to the DNA by base pairings are linked together to form polynucleotides such as messenger, ribosomal, or transfer-RNA. See *deoxyribonucleic acid* (DNA).

ribonucleotides. Building blocks of the *ribonucleic acids* (RNA); each consists of sugar, ribose, a phosphate group, and a base. The dominant ribonucleotides are adenylic acid (AMP); guanylic acid (GMP); cytidylic acid (CMP); and uridylic acid (UMP). The structures are shown in the diagram. See *purines* and *pyrimidines*.

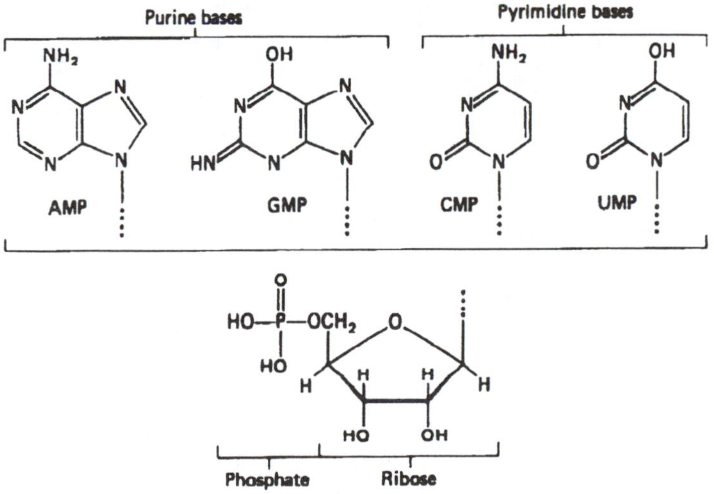

Ribonucleotides

ribose. Mol. Wt. 150. A five-carbon sugar; a constituent of nucleic acid.

α D-Ribose

ribosomes. Dense particles (*organelles*) in cell cytoplasm that are the site of protein synthesis. Cell particles composed of ribosomal *ribonucleic acid* (rRNA) and various proteins. During protein synthesis, messenger-RNA (mRNA) is bound to the ribosomes, and this is where the translation of the nucleotide sequence of mRNA to the amino acid sequence of the proteins takes place.

rice (*Oryza sativa*). A cereal grain. Rice is a major foodstuff of Asia and common in the western world. About 8% of the total energy provided by rice is protein of good quality, with a *net dietary protein* (NPU) value of about 65. The limiting essential amino acids in rice are *lysine* and *threonine*. All of the cereal grains—wheat, rice, millet, oats, and rye, as whole grains —have similar nutritive values and chemical constitutions. They have no *ascorbic acid* (vitamin C) and little or no *retinol* (vitamin A) or *carotene*. Rice, like other grains, has high concentrations of calcium and iron which are not totally available as nutrients because of the presence of *phytic acid*. The *thiamine* content of rice varies according to the degree of milling. Rice that has only the husk removed contains about 250 mg of thiamine per 100 grains; hand milling or one polishing of the rice removes half of the thiamine; and rice polished three times and ready for the market contains 70 mg of thiamine or about one-third of the original content. Washing and boiling causes further losses of the B-complex vitamins, up to 50%. Parboiled rice is steamed by a special process so that the thiamine and other vitamins and minerals are distributed throughout the kernel with only a slight loss taking place in washing and cooking. In cultures where the staple diet is rice, outbreaks of *beriberi*, a disease due to a thiamine deficiency, have occurred when highly polished rice was substituted for hand-milled rice. In modern times, beriberi is not common but not unknown in Asia. *Niacin* (4 mg per 100 g) and *riboflavin* (120 mg per 100 g) are the other B-complex vitamins present in unpolished rice. See this item in the table under *grains*.

rice, brown. The *grain* or seed of the grass *Oryza sativa*; an aquatic plant widely cultivated in warm climates on wet land. Brown rice is rich in the vitamins of the B complex, *thiamine*, *niacin*, and *riboflavin*, and in *iron* and *calcium*. It is higher in many of these vitamins and minerals than enriched, parboiled, or other processed rice.

rice flour. Ground rice made principally from the rice broken during milling. It cannot be used in breadmaking but is used commercially for making ice creams and confections. Another use is by persons on allergy diets.

rickets (rachitis). A nutritional disease resulting from a deficiency of *vitamin D* in the young. Vitamin D is a precursor to 1,25-dihydrocholecalciferol, which promotes the absorption of *calcium* from the intestine and the deposition of calcium and *phosphate* into bone. In the young, a vitamin D deficiency results in "soft" bones that grow in a distorted manner, depending on the stresses and forces placed on the growing bones by muscles or weight. Once the *bone* deformity has occurred it cannot be reversed, even though vitamin D will strengthen and harden additional bone growth. Vitamin D can be biosynthesized in the body but requires sunlight. A vitamin D deficiency in an adult results in *osteomalacia*. The deposition of calcium into bone is also under the hormonal control of *calcitonin* and *parathormone*. An intake of 300–400 I.U. per day of vitamin D is the *Recommended Dietary Allowance (RDA)* and is about three times the intake needed for satisfactory growth and calcium absorption from the intestine. Levels about three times higher than the RDA may be toxic in some individuals. Vitamin D is probably the most toxic of the vitamins. See *vitamin toxicity*.

rocambole (*Allium scorodoprasum*). A European *leek*, used like garlic but milder in flavor.

rock candy. Large, hard, clear crystals of sugar (*sucrose*), made by pouring sugar syrup cooked to a certain density into deep pans that have been laced with heavy thread on which the crystals deposit while being formed.

Rock Cornish hen. A small fowl with small bones and all white meat. It was developed from the Cornish hen, an English breed of domestic fowl with a pea comb, very close feathering, and a compact, sturdy body. Rock Cornish hens weigh from one-half to one and a quarter pounds and are broiled or roasted.

rockfish (*Sebastodes*). A saltwater food fish. The fish is sometimes mistakenly called the rock cod. Among the best-known and most valuable rockfish are the black fish, bocaccio, rasher, red rockfish, Spanish flag, yellow-backed rockfish, and yellowtail rockfish. The skin varies in color from dark gray to bright orange and the meat from almost a pure white to a deep pink. The texture and flavor of the meat of all the species seem to be the same; texture is firm, and when cooked, it is white and flaky, resembling crabmeat; flavor also resembles crabmeat and the fish is often steamed and used for salads.

rod vision. Rod vision depends on the presence of *rhodopsin* (visual purple), which in turn requires a derivative of *retinal* (vitamin A), 11-*cis retinal*. Rod vision is responsible for the ability to see in dim light. The cones, a different type of nerve cell, are responsible for the ability to see color and require an intense light to see compared to the rods. A *retinol* (vitamin A) deficiency produces night blindness (nyctalopia), an inability to see in dim light. Some individuals with nyctalopia require as much as 100 times more light than normal to see. Nyctalopia is reversed by *retinol* (vitamin A).

roe. Fish eggs still enclosed in the thin natural membrane in which they are found in the female fish are called roe or hard roe. Roe is taken from many species of fish. Shad roe is perhaps the most popular and best known. However, many different varieties are marketed, including alewife, herring, cod, mackerel, mullet, salmon, shad, and whitefish. The size of the roe varies with the fish. Shad roe is usually from 5–6 inches long, about 3 inches wide, and an inch or more thick. Soft roe or milt is the male fish's reproductive gland and is filled with secretion or is the secretion itself. It has a soft, creamy consistency and the vein must be removed before cooking. A good source of protein.

romaine (*Lactuca*). One of the principal types of lettuce, also known as Cos lettuce. Romaine has a long, narrow, cylindrical head with stiff leaves and a broad rib. The leaves are dark green on the outside, becoming a greenish-white near the center. Romaine is flavorful and crisp and lends itself to tossed salads of mixed greens. See lettuce in the table under *vegetables*.

roots and tubers. The white potato makes up an important part of the human diet, and its nutritive value is important. It contains about 20% carbohydrate, mostly starch, and 2% protein. The protein, though relatively scanty, is of high biological value. The white *potato* is primarily an energy-yielding food; it is low in fiber and highly digestible, containing a fair amount of *ascorbic acid* (vitamin C), which is best preserved in whole potatoes cooked or baked in their skins. White potatoes also supply generous amounts of potassium and small quantities of *thiamine* and *iron*. Sweet potatoes, though actually unrelated, have a composition similar to the common white potato. They are richer in carbohydrates and are noteworthy for their high β *carotene* (provitamin A) content. *Carrots* are of value primarily because of the large quantity of carotene which they contain. *Beets* and *turnips* are carbohydrate-rich foods; their leaves, however, contribute generous amounts of minerals and vitamins, including ascorbic acid. In developing countries, other roots form an even more important part of the diet, such as cassava (tapioca), yams, and colocasia (poi, taro). These are far lower in protein content and have been associated with *protein calorie malnutrition* when used as weaning foods for children.

rope. A condition in bread characterized by gelatinous threads that form in the center spore-forming bacteria (*Bacillus mesentericus, B. subtilis*) that may contaminate dough and survive the baking process. As the bacteria multiply, they digest the bread.

rosefish (Sebastes marinus). Also known as redfish, this is a saltwater food fish. When mature, it reaches a length of about 11 inches, weighs about one pound, and is bright rose-red or orange-red in color. It may be marketed as an ocean perch. The fish is fatty, with firm flesh and a bland flavor.

rose hip (Rosa). The fleshy swollen red seed capsule of any of various roses, but especially wild rose. The capsules are rich in *ascorbic acid* (vitamin C) and are used commercially in making an ascorbic acid (vitamin C) concentrate. They are also sold dried whole, cut, or powdered. Rose hips are an excellent source of *carotene* (vitamin A activity), the B complex, *tocopherol* (vitamin E), and *vitamin K*.

rosemary (Rosemarinus officinalis). A perennial evergreen shrub which grows wild in southern Europe and is cultivated throughout the rest of Europe and the United States. It reaches a height of 4–5 feet and has branching stems which bear long, thin, dark-green leaves with grayish undersides, and a strongly aromatic smell. The leaves, fresh or dried, are used as an *herb* seasoning.

rum. An alcoholic beverage distilled from the fermented products of sugar cane. There are three chief kinds of rum. The oldest type is Jamaican rum, heavy, dark, full-bodied, and usually aged in wood. Cuban rum, which is dry and light-bodied, is a relatively modern refinement. Rums more aromatic than either the Jamaican or Cuban are produced throughout the Caribbean area.

rutabaga (Brassica napobrassica). A *root* vegetable which belongs to the mustard family and is closely related to cabbage, cauliflower, brussels sprouts, kale, kohlrabi, mustard, and turnips. Rutabaga is larger than the turnip, has smooth yellowish skin and flesh, and smooth leaves. The flesh has a typical sweet flavor. There are white varieties of rutabaga, but the yellow is the best known. Some vitamin A and a small amount of *ascorbic acid* (vitamin C).

Nutrients in 100 g of raw rutabaga

CALORIES KCAL	PROTEIN G	FAT G	CARBOHYDRATE G	VITAMIN A IU	ASCORBATE MG
35	1	Trace	11	580	43

rye (*Secale cereale*). One of the cereal grains. Rye is similar to rice in composition. *Lysine* is the limiting essential amino acid in rye and it contains about 11 g of protein per 100 g of rye. The *thiamine, niacin,* and *riboflavin* content is similar to that of rice. Rye also contains no *ascorbic acid* (vitamin C) or *carotene* (vitamin A activity). The iron content is similar to that of rice, but rye is a better source of calcium. Rye also contains a small amount of the protein complex called gluten, which allows it to form a dough similar to that of wheat. Rye and wheat can be used to make breads because of their *gluten* content. The other cereal grains do not contain significant amounts of gluten. See this item in the table under *grains*.

S

S. The alphabetic symbol for the amino acid *serine* (Ser).

saccharin (ortho(*o*)-benzosulfimide). A sugar substitute that is more than 400 times sweeter than sucrose. It has no nutritive value. Congress, in November 1977, passed the Saccharin Study and Labeling Act, which imposed a two-year moratorium against any ban of the sweetener. While permitting saccharin's continued availability, the law mandated that warning labels be used to advise consumers that saccharin caused cancer in animals. The law also directed the Food and Drug Administration (FDA) to arrange further studies of carcinogens and toxic substances in foods, including saccharin, and to determine whether there were any health benefits resulting from nonnutritive sweeteners. The FDA contracted with the National Academy of Sciences (NAS) for the studies. The first NAS report, in November 1978, concluded that saccharin was a carcinogen in animals, although of low potency; that it was a potential cancer-causing agent in humans; that the impurities in saccharin were not the carcinogenic agents; and that saccharin seemed to promote the cancer-causing effects of other carcinogenic agents that might be consumed with it. The NAS's second report, in March 1979, called for an overhaul of the entire food-safety law, changes that might give the FDA a range of options in regulating substances like saccharin. Since 1977, Congress has repeatedly extended the original moratorium. Although various studies since the proposed 1977 ban have led to varying interpretations of the risks posed by saccharin, the FDA's basic position remains that the substance should not be used in food and beverages except as a tabletop sweetener.

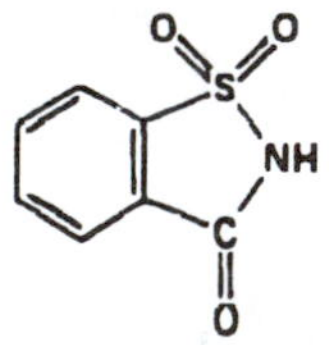

saccharin (ortho(*o*)-benzosulfimide)

Saccharomyces. A class of fungi known as yeast cells of which there are several species. In the food industry, yeast is used under anaerobic and aerobic conditions, depending upon the intention. *S. cerevisiae* or baker's yeast is used in baking under aerobic conditions. Its popular use in breads derives both from its ability to produce carbon dioxide (CO_2) and cause bread to rise and from the general taste it imparts. Strains of *S. cerevisiae* are also used under anaerobic conditions to promote the production of *ethanol* in beers and ales. In this regard, yeasts are subdivided into the "top" and "bottom" yeast. The top yeast, buoyed to the surface of the fermenting liquids by carbon dioxide (CO_2), is generally involved in making beers, and the bottom yeast, which remains at the bottom of fermenting liquids, generally is involved in making light ales and lager. The maintenance of a yeast culture is one of the great secrets of brewing because the yeasts make unpredictable genetic changes (mutate) in their characteristics. The wine industry depends on fermentation of grape juices by added yeasts and those which grow naturally on the skins of grapes.

safflower oil. An edible oil from the seeds of the safflower plant, *Carthamus tinctorius*. Safflower oil is high in *linoleic acid*, an *essential fatty acid*. Safflower oil is light, flavorless, and colorless. It does not solidify under refrigeration and is good for salad dressings and marinades, as well as for frying.

saffron (*Crocus sativus*). A small crocus, with purple flowers. There are three deep orange-yellow stigmas, or filaments, in the center of each tiny blossom. These are aromatic when dried, with a pungent taste, and are used to add flavor and color in cooking. The name saffron is an adaptation of the Arabic word *za'faran*, "yellow." The different varieties of saffron have varying degrees of pungency. Saffron gives distinctive color to breads and cakes, is used with rice dishes, and enhances cream soups, sauces, potatoes, and veal and chicken dishes.

sage (*Salvia officinalis*). There are over 500 varieties of this *herb* growing in temperature zones. The fresh or dried leaves are used in cooking for their aromatic, bitter taste. Dalmatian sage, grown in Croatia, is one of the best varieties of the plant. In addition there are the common garden sage (*S. officinalis*), white sage, Cyprus sage, meadow sage, pineapple sage, and clary sage. The name "sage" comes through French from the Latin *salvus*, meaning "safe, whole, or healthy."

sago. A starch extracted from the pithy trunks of various tropical palms, among them the sago palm. It is a basic food in the southwest Pacific, where sago meal is used for making thick soups, biscuits, and puddings. To make sago, the palm trees are felled and the trunks are cut into pieces. The bark is taken off and the inner portion is soaked in water to remove the starch. The pulpy paste that results is dried and used as sago meal. When the paste is rubbed through a sieve, pearl sago results. Sago flour is also made from the sago meal.

sake. The national alcoholic drink of Japan. Made by fermenting rice, it is yellowish-white and is often drunk warm. Its flavor lies somewhere between western beers and wines.

salami. One of a variety of *sausages* of Italian origin that can be eaten without being cooked. There are Italian, German, Hungarian, French, and kosher salamis. The word is Italian and implies "salted," meaning that the meat is preserved. Salamis differ from each other in their composition of meats, their spicing, their salting and curing, and their shape. Salami most often contains pork and some beef, although there are pure-pork and pure-beef salamis. Salamis are divided into two major groupings, hard and soft. Excellent source of protein, good source of iron, *thiamine, riboflavin*, and *niacin*.

Nutrients in 100 g of hard salami

CALORIES KCAL	PROTEIN G	FAT G	CARBOHYDRATE G	NIACIN MG	THIAMINE µG	CALCIUM MG	IRON MG
450	20	16	Trace	5	400	10	4

saliva. Secreted by the *salivary glands*, parotid, submaxillary, and sublingual, and by the numerous minute buccal glands of the mucosa of the mouth. The volume of saliva is about 1 liter per day. It consists of a large amount of water containing some glycoprotein material, *mucin*, inorganic salts, and *salivary amylase* (ptyalin). It has a specific gravity of about 1.005 and is nearly neutral in reaction (pH about 6.4 to 7.0). Substances in saliva include inorganic salts in solution, chlorides, carbonates, and phosphates of sodium, calcium, and potassium. The functions of saliva are to soften and moisten the food, assisting in *mastication* and *deglutition*; to coat the food with mucin, lubricating it and ensuring a smooth passage along the esophagus; to moisten or liquefy solid food, providing a necessary step in the process of stimulating the taste buds.

salivary amylase (ptyalin). Salivary amylase is formed in the *salivary glands* and initiates the reduction of starch into *dextrins* and *maltose* in the mouth. The process of reducing starch to maltose is a gradual one, consisting of a series of changes which take place in successive stages and result in a number of intermediate compounds. The changes due to salivary amylases are best effected at the temperature of the body, in a neutral solution, and require calcium. The time food spends in the mouth and the general bulk of food does not allow much degradation of starch by salivary amylase. In the stomach, the acid conditions denature salivary amylase, and the further degradation of starches occurs in the small intestines where several amylases reduce starches to *glucose* for absorption by the intestinal mucosa. See *digestive system*.

salivary glands (parotid glands). Salivary glands lie in the sides of the face in front of and slightly below the ears. Saliva from these glands reaches the mouth through parotid ducts, which open on the inner surfaces of the cheeks opposite the second molar teeth. There are also a pair of submaxillary glands in the angles of the lower jaws and a pair of sublingual glands under the tongue. Ducts from these glands open into the floor of the mouth beneath the tongue. Saliva from the six glands mixes with food in the mouth and softens and lubricates it. Saliva contains a digestive enzyme, *salivary amylase* (ptyalin), which acts to convert starch to sugar.

salivation. The issue of saliva into the mouth. Saliva can be stimulated to flow by a complex of physical, chemical, and psychological stimuli.

salmon (*Oncorhynchus*). Considered among the greatest of sport and food fishes. The name comes from Latin, from *salmo*, which comes from the verb for "to leap." There is one variety of Atlantic salmon, and there are five varieties of Pacific: sockeye (*O. nerka*), chinook (*O. tschawytscha*), silver (*O. kitsutch*), pink (*O. gorbuscha*), and dog (*O. keta*). In addition there is the steelhead, which is more closely related to the Atlantic than to the other Pacific salmon, and the blueblack, which is really a coho with darker markings. Salmon contain large amounts of phosphorus, potassium, some sodium, *thiamine, riboflavin*, and *niacin*, and some *carotene* (vitamin A). Canned salmon contains some calcium if the bones are eaten. See this item in the table under *fish*.

Salmonella. Infections by certain species of this bacteria are sometimes called *"food poisoning"* because the symptoms in general resemble those of staphylococcus poisoning and the outbreak is commonly explosive. The *Salmonellae* are gram-negative, nonspore-forming rods that ferment *glucose*, usually with gas, but do not ferment *lactose* or *sucrose*. They are typed on the basis of their antigen content. Humans and animals are directly or indirectly the source of the contamination of foods with *Salmonellae*. The organisms may come from actual cases of the disease or from carriers. The organisms also may come from cats, dogs, swine, and cattle. Chickens, turkeys, ducks, and geese may be infected with any of a large number of types of *Salmonella* which are found in the fecal matter, in hen's eggs, and in the flesh of dressed fowl. Meat products such as meat pies, hash, sausages, cured meats (ham, bacon, and tongue), sandwiches, chili, etc., will, when allowed to stand at room temperature over a period of time, permit growth of *Salmonellae*. See *food toxins*

Salmonellosis (food infection). About 1300 serotypes of the *Salmonella* genus have been identified, each being capable of causing infection in humans. The typhoid and paratyphoid bacilli which infect humans belong collectively to the genus *Salmonella*. They produce various infections of the intestinal tract. The types of *Salmonella* that are chiefly responsible for human disease are *S. typhi* and *S. paratyphi*. They are rod-shaped bacteria that resist cold and survive for long periods in soil, ice, water, milk, and foods. Since they do not form spores, they are easily killed by being boiled for 5 minutes or by pasteurization. Drying and direct sunlight also kill them. These organisms grow easily in simple common foods such as milk, custards, egg dishes, salad dressings, and sandwich fillings. Meat, poultry, fish, eggs, and dairy products that are eaten raw or have been inadequately heated are most frequently implicated in salmonellosis. Contaminated cake mixes, bakery foods, coloring agents, powdered yeast, and chocolate candy have also caused outbreaks of the infection. Animals, including cattle, swine, poultry, fish, dogs, and birds, harbor the organism. They are usually infected by contact of one animal with another or by animal feeds. Flies and rodents coming in contact with feces of animals or humans are responsible for contamination of food. See *food toxins*.

salsify (*Tragopogon porrifolius*). Another name for oyster plant. An elongated root eaten as a winter vegetable, boiled, baked, or in soups; the young leaves may be eaten for salad.

salt. One of a class of compounds found when the hydrogen atom of an acid radical is replaced by a metal or metal-like radical. The most common salt is *sodium chloride* (NaCl), the sodium salt of *hydrochloric acid*. Other metal or metal-like salts in food may include calcium, potassium, sodium magnesium, sulfur, manganese, iron, cobalt, zinc, and other metals. The ammonium *cation* ($NH4^+$) is a nonmetal that forms salts. They may be chlorides, sulfates, phosphates, lactates, citrates, or in combination with proteins, as in calcium caseinate. See *organic salt*.

salting out. Separation of proteins from solution by addition of high concentrations of inorganic salts, usually sodium sulfate or ammonium sulfate.

salt, iodized. Table salt (sodium chloride) to which has been added 1 part per 10,000 of iodine as potassium iodide (KI).

salt, organic. See *organic salt*.

saltpeter. The potassium salt of nitric acid. See *sodium nitrate*.

salt pork. The side of a hog, cured; it is a fattier portion with less lean than bacon. The fat is cured by the dry-salt method and is not smoked. Salt pork is used for larding. It is also used for flavoring and for adding fat to many dishes such as baked beans, clam chowder, stew, etc. Contains *niacin, thiamine,* and *riboflavin,* some calcium and potassium, and a trace of iron. Raw, 100 g = 783 calories; fried, 100 g = 341 calories.

sand dab. A small, lean, saltwater fish belonging to the flounder family. Its flesh has a delicate, subtle flavor.

saponification. The splitting of fat by an alkali, yielding *glycerol* and *soap*. This may occur during the digestion of fat. See *soap*.

saprophytic nutrition. A type of heterotrophic nutrition in which organisms absorb their required nutrients through the cell membrane following the extracellular digestion of nonliving organic material. Saprophytes differ from parasites in that the latter derive their nutrients from other living cells or tissues, sometimes at the expense of the life of the host. See *heterotrophs*.

saprophytic plants or animals. A saprophytic plant or animal (yeasts, molds, and most bacteria) is one that absorbs food materials from dead or decaying matter or from the dead parts of living plants or animals. These food materials cannot be absorbed into the body or the organism without first being digested. For this reason, saprophytes secrete extracellular digestive enzymes.

sarcolemma. A delicate membrane surrounding each striated muscle fiber.

sarcoma. A tumor that is usually malignant and derives from the proliferation of poorly differentiated cells. See *carcinoma*.

sardine. The name used to describe various small saltwater food fish, with weak bones, which can be preserved in oil. It is not the name of a specific kind of fish. Sardines include the pilchard, alewife, herring, and sprat. It is probably the French sardine, found in abundance around the island of Sardinia, from which the overall name is derived. Sardines are fatty fish. They differ according to kind, depending on locality. Sardines are an excellent source of protein and good source of *calcium, iron,* and *niacin*. See this item in the table under *fish*.

sardine oils. Obtained from fish caught in Japanese waters and off the French and Spanish coasts. Japanese and/or Korean sardine oil is manufactured from the Japanese sardine, *Sardinops melanosticta*, and the European oil from *Sardina pilchardus*. The oils have high iodine values and have been used to a limited extent as drying oils for the manufacture of paints. They are also used in the leather industry and have been *hydrogenated* for edible use.

sassafras (*Sassafras albidum* or *S. variifolium*). A tree of the laurel family, one variety of which is a native of North America. The bark is rough and gray, and the bright green leaves are of three shapes, all on the same tree. These leaves, when dried and ground, are the prime ingredients of filé, a thickening and seasoning agent which forms the base of gumbo.

satiety value. That quality of food contributing to satisfaction and resulting in a sustained sense of comfort or well-being, fullness, or gratification of appetite.

saturated fats. Fats that contain a large number of *saturated fatty acids* as a part of the fat molecule. *Unsaturated fats* (oils) contain *unsaturated fatty acids*. Saturated fat occurs in most animal fat and animal products, for example, meat—beef, veal, lamb, pork, and products such as cold meats and sausages—eggs, whole milk, lard, cheese, both sweet and sour cream, ice cream, and butter. Saturated fat also occurs in some plant products, for example, *coconut*, coconut oil, and *chocolate*. Oils may be converted to unsaturated fats by reducing the unsaturated fatty acid by a chemical process called *hydrogenation*.

saturated fatty acids (SFA). Organic acids in which the carbons contain the maximum permissible numbers of hydrogens. As a class of compounds, they have the general formula $C_nH_{2n}O_2$. *Acetic acid* (vinegar), *butyric acid*, and *stearic acid* are examples of saturated fatty acids. Some naturally occurring fatty acids are shown. See *palmitic acid*.

Naturally occuring fatty acids

COMMON NAME	CHEMICAL NAME	CHEMICAL FORMULA
Butyric	*n*-Butanoic	$C_4H_8O_2$
Caproic	*n*-Hexanoic	$C_6H_{12}O_2$
Caprylic	*n*-Octanoic	$C_8H_{16}O_2$
Capric	*n*-Decanoic	$C_{10}H_{20}O_2$
Lauric	*n*-Dodecanoic	$C_{12}H_{24}O_2$
Myristic	*n*-Tetradecanoic	$C_{14}H_{28}O_2$
Palmitic	*n*-Hexadecanoic	$C_{16}H_{32}O_2$
Stearic	*n*-Octadecanoic	$C_{18}H_{36}O_2$
Arachidic	*n*-Eicosanoic	$C_{20}H_{40}O_2$

saturation. To cause to unite with the greatest possible amount of another substance, through solution, chemical combination, or the like. A *saturated fat*, for example, is one in which the component fatty acids are completely filled or saturated with hydrogen atoms. A fatty acid is said to be saturated if all available chemical bonds of its carbon chain are filled with hydrogen. If one bond remains unfilled, it is a monounsaturated fatty acid. If two or more bonds remain unfilled, it is a polyunsaturated fatty acid. Fats of animal sources are generally more saturated than fats from plant sources.

sauerkraut. Pickled cabbage made from cabbage which has been cut fine and allowed to ferment in a brine made of its own juice, salt, and occasionally other spices. U.S. Grade A sauerkraut is white or cream-colored with long, uniform shreds, crisp firm texture, and a good flavor.

Nutrients in 100 g canned sauerkraut, solids and liquids

CALORIES KCAL	PROTEIN G	FAT G	CARBOHYDRATE G	VITAMIN A I.U.	ASCORBATE MG
18	1	0.2	4	50	14

sausage. A preparation of minced or ground meat, usually seasoned with salt and spices and stuffed into a casing. Sausages may be made of all pork, all beef, or a combination of two or more meats. They may be fresh or smoked, dry or semidry, and they may be uncooked, partially cooked, or fully cooked. The name sausage is derived from the Latin word for salt. Sausage is high in fat and contains good amounts of protein, iron, and the B vitamins. See this item in the table under *meat*.

savory (*Satureia hortensis* and *S. montana*). Two closely related herbs which belong to the mint family. The aromatic leaves of both plants are widely used for seasoning.

scallion (*Allium*). The name is given without much exactitude to several plants of the onion family: the green onion, the *shallot*, and the leek. The word scallion, like shallot, comes from the Latin name of the shallot, *A. ascalon*, which relates to the ancient city of Ascalon where it is probable that this vegetable was developed near the Mediterranean coast of Palestine and Syria. After trimming, the entire scallion is used, usually chopped or minced as a seasoning vegetable.

scallop. A group of bivalve mollusks with ribbed, rounded shells. Only the muscle which opens and closes the shell is used for eating. A good source of protein. Low in fat, scallops have some calcium, a large amount of phosphorus, traces of riboflavin and niacin.

Schizosaccharomyces. Yeasts which produce asexually by fission and form four or eight ascospores per ascus after isogamic conjugation. They have been found in tropical fruit, molasses, soil, honey, and elsewhere. A common species is *S. pombe*.

scrapple. A very solid mush made from the by-products of hog butchering. The mush is sliced and fried for a breakfast or supper dish. The basis for the making of scrapple is a broth produced by the cooking of the hog's head, liver, tongue, meaty bones, and other scraps. The meat that remains in the broth is ground, and other ground pork meat may be added. Meat and broth are then combined and seasoned, and the mixture is boiled. The mixture is normally thickened with cornmeal.

scrod (*Gadus and Melanogrammus*). A young cod or young haddock weighing from 1.5–2.5 pounds. A scrod is also a whole small cod split and boned for cooking.

scurvy. A nutritional disease caused by a lack of *ascorbic acid* (vitamin C). "A Treatise on Scurvy," written in 1773 by James Lind, recounts a classic nutritional experiment in the prevention of a nutritional disease. About 40 years later limes, which were shown to be antiscorbutic, were routinely issued to British sailors to prevent scurvy, hence the nickname "limey" for British sailors. The antiscorbutic substance in food was named vitamin C in 1920 to distinguish it from two other vitamin fractions isolated from foods, the fat-soluble *vitamin A* and the water-soluble *vitamin B*. Both vitamins A and B were later shown to consist of more than one factor. The chemical name *ascorbic acid* was suggested in 1933 by Szent-Györgyi, who also isolated sufficient quantities of the antiscorbutic substance to permit chemical analysis and synthesis by others in 1933. Besides humans and other primates, only the guinea pig and a species of fruit bat require ascorbic acid in the diet; other animals synthesize ascorbic acid from *glucose*.

sebum. The secretion of the sebaceous glands, which contains *fats, soaps, cholesterol,* protein, remnants of epithelial cells, and inorganic salts. It serves to protect the hair from becoming too dry and brittle as well as from becoming too easily saturated with moisture. Upon the surface of the skin it forms a thin protective layer, which serves to prevent undue absorption or evaporation of water from the skin. This secretion keeps the skin soft and pliable. However, this retained secretion often becomes discolored, giving rise to the condition commonly known as blackheads.

secretin. A hormone secreted by the mucosa of the small intestine, duodenum, and *jejunum* by interaction with substances present in the acid *chyme* discharged from the stomach into the duodenum. Carried by the blood to the various organs, secretin stimulates the flow of pancreatic juice and the secretion of bile and gastric enzyme pepsin, but inhibits gastric acid secretion. See *digestive hormones*.

sedatives (drugs). Drugs which have a calming, quieting effect and in large doses induce sleep. An example is phenobarbital.

selenium (Se). Element No. 34. At. Wt. 79. An essential micronutrient that is toxic at high concentrations. In terms of abundance in the earth, selenium occurs with a frequency comparable to that of gold. Certain plants can concentrate selenium (woody aster, golden weed, gray's vetch) and are responsible for alkali disease and the blind staggers in horses that graze on these plants. On the other hand, the judicious addition of selenium to the feed of lambs and calves markedly improves their health. No instance of selenium toxicity is known or has been described in humans. The amount of selenium in human blood varies greatly throughout the world from 1–10 micromoles per liter. The amount of selenium in water varies from 0.01–4 micromoles per liter of water. The content in animals also varies; therefore it is impossible to establish normal ranges of selenium in humans. Selenium is required for the activity of the enzyme glutathione peroxidase, which protects *unsaturated fatty acids* from oxidation of unsaturated bonds (*peroxidation*). It is through its protection of fatty acids from peroxidation that an associative relationship with *vitamin E* (tocopherol) occurs. Vitamin E (*tocopherol*) also protects unsaturated fatty acids from peroxidation. Selenium can also replace sulfur in some amino acids and proteins. See *minerals*.

semolina. The purified middlings (medium-size particles of ground grain) of wheat. The word is derived from the diminutive of the Italian *semola*, "bran." The best semolina, the type used in the manufacture of macaroni, spaghetti, and other pastas, is obtained in the milling of durum wheat. See *wheat* and *grains*.

sequestrant (sequestering agent). A compound capable of combining with metal ions in solution with an affinity that prevents dissociation into free ions. A sequestrant is the same a *chelate*. Sequestrants or chelates are often used in soft drinks to maintain clarity and color; in food containing unsaturated fats to prevent or slow *peroxidations* catalyzed by heavy metals; and to prevent heavy metals from making *antioxidants* ineffective by their combination with them. *Citric acid* is a naturally occurring compound that is used as an additive sequestrant in shortenings, lard, mayonnaise, soup, salad dressing, margarine, cheese, vegetable oils, pudding mixes, vinegar, and confectionary.

serine (Ser, S). Mol. Wt. 105. A nonessential *amino acid* found in proteins.

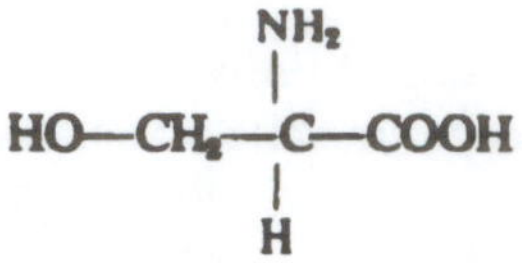

$$HO-CH_2-\overset{\displaystyle \overset{NH_2}{|}}{\underset{\displaystyle \underset{H}{|}}{C}}-COOH$$

serine (Ser, S)

serosa. The membranes lining the cavities that contain the heart, intestines, and lungs, and covering their contents.

serotonin. A chemical, 5-hydroxytryptamine (5-HT), present in platelets, gastrointestinal mucosa, mast cells and in carcinoid tumors. Serotonin is a potent vasoconstrictor.

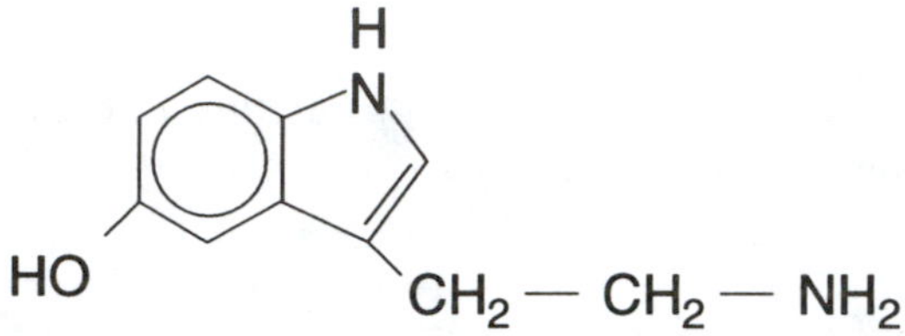

Serotonin

serum. The fluid portion of the *blood* that separates from the blood cells after clotting. It differs from *plasma* in that serum lacks the fibrinogen separated with the clot.

serum albumin. The predominant carbohydrate-free protein is albumin, which constitutes more than 50% of the total serum protein. Since serum albumin has a high affinity for free *fatty acids* and other *anions*, it binds these anions very effectively and therefore serves as a transport or carrier protein. In this manner, free fatty acids which are toxic in the free form, hemolytic and insoluble, are solubilized, removed, and transported to the liver as a soluble, nontoxic fatty acid albumin complex. Serum albumin also serves to control the *osmotic pressure* of the blood as well as maintain the *buffer* capacity of the blood *pH*. Serum albumin is approximately 69,000 in molecular weight and is a typical globular protein with a low α-helical configuration.

sesame (*Sesamum indicum*). An annual tropical and subtropical herbaceous plant. Sesame is grown for its tiny grayish-white or black seeds which have a sweet, nutty flavor and which yield a bland oil when pressed. The cake left after the oil has been expressed from the seeds has also been used for food and fodder.

sex glands or gonads. The gonads (derived from the Greek word meaning seed) consist of the testes in men and the ovaries in women. In addition to producing sperm and ova, the glands elaborate hormones that are responsible for the special male and female characteristics. The male sex glands are the two testes, which lie enclosed in the scrotal sac of the skin just below the penis and secrete semen containing the male reproductive element, the sperm. They also contain the important male sex hormone, testosterone. In the female sex glands, like the testes, the two ovaries have more than one function. They produce the ova, or eggs; they also secrete hormones needed for both reproduction and feminine characteristics. The ovaries lie in the front part of the abdomen, below the navel, and each is connected with the uterus by a fallopian tube. The ovarian hormones are estrogen and progesterone. They are produced in small amounts before puberty and after menopause, and in abundance during the childbearing years, the period when a woman has her regular monthly cycles. Menstruation involves the discharge of the extra, unused blood and tissue built up in preparation for conception.

shad (*Alosa*). An important food fish of the family *Clupeidae*, which also includes herrings. They differ from herrings chiefly in being larger and in the fact that they enter rivers to spawn. The common American shad, *A. sapidissima*, can reach a weight of 14 pounds, but the average weight ranges from 1.5–8 pounds, with 4 or 5 pounds most common. The fish has a compressed body with a rounded bluish back, and silvery sides and undersurface. It is excessively bony, but the dark-pink flesh is delicious and its roe is prized. See this item in the table under *fish*.

shaddock or pomelo (*Citris grandis*). A *citrus* fruit native to the East Indies. It is similar to the grapefruit and may be its ancestor. It grows to the size of a watermelon, weighs up to 20 pounds, and has a coarse, thick rind and reddish, aromatic, but bitter flesh.

shallot (*Allium ascalonicum*). A mild-flavored cousin of the onion, chive, garlic, and leek, which belongs to the *Liliaceae* or lily family. The shallot, *A. ascaloniecum*, derived its name from the ancient Palestinian city, Ascalon, where it was probably first grown. The shallot has a thick outer skin shading from reddish to gray, the bulb underneath greenish at the base and violet on the upper portion. It grows in clove form, with several cloves attached to a common disk. The Jersey, or "false" shallot, is of various shapes, often larger than the "true" shallot, with thin red skin and bulb sometimes white but usually all violet. The edible part of the shallot is the bulb, which after maturity and dry storage is used just as the garlic onion is used. The green tops are sometimes marketed as *scallions*. Fresh shallots are rich in *carotene* (vitamin A), *ascorbic acid* (vitamin C), and *iron*.

sheepshead. A saltwater fish, a cousin of porgies and scups. The sheepshead has large, broad incisor teeth, much like a sheep. The flesh of all sheepshead is white, tender, and pleasant. They can be fried, sauteed, or baked.

shellfish. Shellfish belong to two very large classes, the mollusks and the crustaceans, and are found in salt and fresh water. The mollusks have a soft structure and are partially or wholly enclosed in a one- or two-part shell. The former, called "univalve" mollusks, include the abalone, conch, and periwinkle. The latter, called "bivalve," include the clam, cockle, mussel, oyster, and scallop. Crustaceans are covered with a crustlike shell and have segmented bodies. Among them are the crab, crayfish, lobster, prawn, and shrimp. Shellfish are good sources of protein and iodine, and contain some amounts of the B vitamins. The crustaceans are higher in protein content than the mollusks. See items in the table under *fish*.

sherbet. A frozen dessert made of a fruit juice or puree, a sweetener, and water, to which milk, beaten egg white, gelatin, or marshmallow is added.

sherry. A Spanish apertif or dessert wine, the color varying from pale amber to dark brown and the taste from very dry to very sweet. Sherry is made differently from other wines. After the sweet juice from the pressed grapes has fermented in its own way, it is blended with many similar wines from different years. Brandy is added to the mixture and the beverage is allowed to age in special casks. Sherry improves with aging.

shigellosis. Bacillary dysentery is caused by rod-shaped bacteria of the genus *Shigella*. The *Shigella* organisms grow easily in foods, especially in milk. The boiling of food and water or pasteurization of milk kills the organisms. Several species that may cause shigellosis are spread by feces, fingers, flies, milk and food, and articles handled by unsanitary carriers.

shish kebab. A dish of meat, usually lamb, broiled or skewered. The name comes from the Turkish, *shish*, meaning "six" and *kebap*, "roast meat." Today it has come to mean as well a skewered combination of meat, fruits, and vegetables which may or may not have been marinated and seasoned with herbs and spices before broiling.

shrimp. A 10-legged (decapod) crustacean, whose comparatively small size is responsible for its name; the Middle English *shrimpe* meant "puny person" and the name is akin to the Swedish *Skrympa*, meaning "to shrink." Shrimps vary considerably in size, ranging from the great Mexican and Gulf shrimps to the tiny half-inch creatures found in the cold waters off Scandinavia. The color of shrimps also varies but is some pale shade, usually brownish red or grayish green. The bright-pink color of the shell of cooked shrimps is due to a chemical change that takes place through exposure to heat. Most shrimps available in markets are actually the abdomens and tails of shrimps, with the stalked eyes, heads, and feelers removed. The line of demarcation between shrimp, scampi, and prawns is not clearly defined. Shrimp are high in protein, low in fat. See this item in the table under *fish*.

siderosis. Term used to describe the presence of excess iron in the body, as demonstrated by the presence of an iron storage protein, *hemosiderin*, in the tissues. Siderosis may occur because of (1) an excessive iron intake, (2) excessive destruction of red cells in hemolytic conditions and after multiple blood transfusions, and (3) failure to regulate absorption. It is not clear whether a minor degree of siderosis affects health. Siderosis is one of the factors which may cause cirrhosis of the liver.

silicate. A salt or ester derived from a silicic acid, especially any of numerous insoluble, often complex metal salts that contain silicon and oxygen in the anion, and constitute the largest class of minerals.

silicon. Element No. 14. At. Wt. 28.086. A nonmetallic element found in salt. It occurs in traces in skeletal structures such as the bones and teeth.

simple sugar. See *monosaccharides*.

sitosterols. A group of similar organic compounds which occur in plants. They contain the steroid nucleus, perhydrocyclopentanophenanthrene.

skeletal muscle (striated muscle). It is skeletal muscle that constitutes what is often called flesh or meat. There are about 400 skeletal muscles made up of about 250 million individual cells called muscle fibers. They form about 30% of the total body weight. Muscle fibers are elongated structures, 1–50 millimeters long but only 0.010–0.1 millimeter in diameter, which are attached at both ends to either connective tissue or bone. The cell membrane around each muscle fiber is called the *sarcolemma*, and the fiber is full of minute protein threads (myofibrils), 1 micron in diameter. The myofibrils run along the whole length of the muscle fiber and are made up of many longitudinal strands of a protein called *myosin*. Each muscle fiber is connected to the central nervous system by a branch of a motor-nerve fiber which ends in a specialized termination called the motor end-plate. Of the three muscle types, skeletal, cardiac, and smooth, skeletal muscle acts most rapidly, completing a single contraction and relaxation in less than 0.1 second. Cardiac muscle contracts and relaxes in 1–5 seconds, and smooth muscle contracts and relaxes in periods as long as 2 minutes. Skeletal muscle is generally under voluntary control; among the exceptions is the upper third of the esophagus. All muscle attached to bones is striated muscle. Striated muscle is also attached to the tongue, the soft palate, the scalp, the pharynx, and the extrinsic eye muscles. See *meat*, *cardiac muscle*, and *smooth muscle*.

skeleton. The bone framework of animals in the phylum Chordata and the subphylum Vertebrata (vertebrates). The human skeleton contains 206 bones held together by *muscle* and *tendons*. *Cartilage* also functions as part of the framework, but is not composed of bone and is not a part of the skeleton.

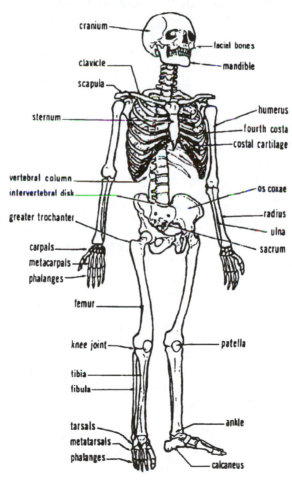

Human skeleton

Micronutrients Associated with the Skeletal System

ACTIVITY, ROLE, OR FUNCTION	MICRONUTRIENT	
INVOLVING BONE AND CARTILAGE	VITAMIN	MINERAL
Synthesize collagen	Vitamin C	Copper
Synthesize elastin		Copper
Comprise bones and teeth		Calcium, phosphorus, fluoride, magnesium, manganese, and other minerals
Harden hydroxyapatite		Fluoride
Maintain bone-forming cells	Vitamin A	Copper
Prevent rickets and softening and thinning of bones	Vitamin D	Calcium, phosphorus, fluoride

skin. The skin is called the integumentary or covering body system and serves the body in many important ways. The most obvious feature of the skin is its outward appearance. Four functions of skin are protective: as a prevention of the entrance of bacteria; regulation of body temperature through control of heat loss; sensory perception through nerve endings that transmit sensations of touch, heat, cold, and pain; excretion of body wastes through sweat. The skin has two principal layers, the *epidermis* or outer layer and the dermis, the inner layer or true skin. The epidermis and dermis are supported by a subcutaneous (under-the-skin) layer which connects the skin to underlying muscles.

skinfold test. An indirect measure of the amount of body fat can be obtained by means of the skinfold test. The clinician lifts a fold of skin from the back of the arm, back, or other locations, and measures its thickness with a caliper that applies a fixed amount of pressure. The fat attached to the skin is roughly proportional to total body fat. Triceps skinfold values of 21 mm for young women and 12 mm for young men are considered normal. Obesity is about double these measurements or about 1.5 and 1 inch, respectively, for men and women, and about ¼ inch reflects malnutrition.

skull. The skull forms the bone framework of the head and has 29 bones: 8 cranial, 14 facial, 6 ossicles (3 tiny bones in each ear), and 1 hyoid (1 single bone between the skull and neck area). The cranial bones support and protect the brain. At birth there is an opening, the fontanelle, at the top of the skull. These bones fuse together after birth in firmly united joints called sutures. The 8 cranial bones include 1 frontal, 2 parietal, 1 occipital, 2 temporal, 1 ethmoid, and 1 sphenoid. The frontal bone forms the forehead, part of the eye sockets, and part of the nose. The parietal bones form the dome of the skull and the upper side walls. The occipital bone forms the back and base of the skull. The temporal bones form the lowest part of each side of the skull and contain the essential organs of hearing and of balance in the middle and inner parts of the ear. The ethmoid and sphenoid bones complete the floor of the cranium, the ethmoid toward the front and the sphenoid toward the center. The air spaces in the frontal, ethmoid, and sphenoid bones are sinuses.

sloe (*Prunus*). The fruit of the blackthorn (*P. spinosa*) which grows wild in woods and hedges in most parts of the British Isles. The sloe, in French called *prunelle*, is edible but not usually picked to be eaten. Its chief use is to flavor sloe gin. In the United States the name sloe is also given to the fruit of the native *plum* tree (*P. americana*) which is occasionally used for jams, jellies, and conserves. The fruit of the American tree is small and bitter and generally yellow or reddish yellow in color.

small intestine. See *intestine, small*.

smell. Sensory endings for the sense of smell are located in the olfactory membrane over the surface of the superior nasal conchae (chambers) and the upper part of the septum. These sensory nerve endings are the least specialized of the special senses. To smell anything well, air is sniffed into the higher nasal chambers and thus brings the odoriferous particles in great numbers into contact with the olfactory hairs. Odors can also reach the nose by way of the mouth. Many flavors of food are really odors rather than gustatory (*taste*) sensations, and one becomes aware of them just after swallowing. Each substance smelled causes its own particular sensation, and one is able not only to recognize a multitude of distinct odors but also to distinguish individual odors in a mixed smell. The taste of any substance is usually a combination of taste and smell. See *aroma* and *flavor*.

smelt (*Osmerus*). Any of several small fish belonging to the family *Osmeridae*. Their backs are greenish and translucent, sides and belly are silvery. The name is also used for various silversides of the family *Atherinidae*, which resemble the true smelt. Their flesh is delicate, rich, and oily. Smelt contain some calcium, large amounts of phosphorus, some *thiamine*, *riboflavin*, *retinol* (vitamin A), and a small amount of *niacin*.

smoking. See *food storage*.

smooth muscle (visceral muscle). In smooth muscle, each fiber appears as a single spindle-shaped cell containing many *nuclei*. The individual muscle fibers seen in skeletal muscle are fused into a single syncytium. Smooth muscle also contains myofibril elements for contraction. The transverse striations seen in *cardiac muscle* and skeletal muscle are absent in smooth muscle, which accounts for the names "nonstriated muscle" or "plain muscle." Smooth muscles are not usually subject to voluntary (conscious) control. Contractions are slow, sustained, and sometimes rhythmic. Smooth muscle is found in the walls along the *digestive system*, the *trachea* and bronchi, the *urinary bladder*, the *gallbladder*, the urinary and genital ducts, the *uterus*, walls of *blood vessels*, the capsule of the *spleen*, the iris of the eye, and the *hair follicles* of the skin. See *meat, cardiac muscle*, and *skeletal muscle*.

snap bean. A variety of the common garden bean, which includes round, flat green, yellow or wax beans, and the so-called Italian green beans. Snap beans are also called green beans or string beans. Snap beans have small amounts of *carotene* (vitamin A), iron, and *thiamine*. Green beans have more vitamin A than yellow beans. See this item in the table under *vegetables*.

soap. A salt of a long-chain *fatty acid*. Hard soaps are sodium salts and soft soaps are potassium salts. The soaps emulsify and have a detergent activity. The carboxylate group ($-COO^-$), the anion, is balanced by an ionic bond with sodium ion (Na^+) or potassium ion (K^+). It is these parts of the soap that interact with water. The hydrocarbon chain dissolves oily material. The same principles apply to *emulsifiers*.

soda. Chemically, soda is a sodium compound of any one of many varieties. In reference to food it is most often sodium *bicarbonate* or sodium acid bicarbonate, a crystalline salt used in the manufacture of *baking powder*, carbonated beverages, and effervescent salts.

soda water (carbonated water). A beverage charged with *carbon dioxide* (CO_2) under pressure, a process which produces a liquid which bubbles, fizzes, or sparkles when opened. The term does not include beverages in which the gas is produced within the beverage by the natural process of fermentation. The carbon dioxide in soda water is produced from sodium bicarbonate by the action of sulfuric or other *acids*. Soda water is used in combination with various flavorings to produce soft drinks and combined with liquor for highballs and other alcoholic drinks.

sodium (Na). Element No. 11. At. Wt. 23. One of the two important alkali metals; potassium is the other. Sodium ions (Na^+) are chiefly in the fluids that circulate outside the cells, and only a small amount of them is inside the cells. Potassium ions (K^+) are mostly inside the cells. Sodium and potassium are vital in keeping a normal balance of water between the cells and the fluids. Sodium and potassium ions are essential for nerves to respond to stimulation, for the nerve impulses to travel to the muscles, and for the muscles to contract. All types of muscles, including the heart muscle, are influenced by sodium and potassium. Sodium and potassium also work with proteins, phosphates, and carbonates to keep a proper balance between the amount of acid and alkali in the blood. The body normally conserves its supply of sodium and potassium ions when the intake is low by reabsorption in the kidneys, which reduces the amount that is filtered in the urine. Excessive sweating can cause a major loss of sodium from the body, and so, muscle cramps. Table salt, *sodium chloride* (NaCl), is the main source of sodium in a diet, and taste and habit determine the amount eaten. Foods from animal sources, including meat, fish, poultry, milk, and cheese, contain more sodium than do foods from plant sources. Most fresh and frozen vegetables contain only small amounts of sodium unless salt is added. Beets, carrots, celery, chard, kale, beet and dandelion greens, and spinach are exceptions; they contain several times more sodium than other vegetables. Foods contain the most sodium when salt has been added to them directly or by brining or pickling, or by curing.

Sodium in g/100 g of foods

Bacon, raw	0.98	Cornflour	0.05	Oatmeal	0.03
Beef, corned	1.51	Egg, fresh, whole	0.14	Sausage, raw	1.03
Beef, pork, mutton, raw	0.08	Fruit dried, uncooked	0.06	Shellfish, fresh and canned	0.19
Biscuits, assorted	0.32	Ham, boiled, lean	2.0	Vegetables, canned	0.42
Bread, all extractions	0.53	Ice cream	0.05	Vegetables, root and green,	0.08
Cheese, cream	0.24	Margarine	0.32	cooked and raw	
Cheese, hard (cheddar, etc)	1.01	Milk, fresh, whole	0.05	Wines, ales and stout	0.03
Cornflakes	0.84				

sodium benzoate. Mol. Wt. 144. The sodium salt of benzoic acid. Sodium benzoate is a food preservative which can prevent the growth of almost all microorganisms (bacteria, fungi, and yeast), but is effective only under acidic conditions. Limited to such foods as fruit juices, carbonated drinks, pickles, salad dressing, and preserves. Used at levels of 0.05%–0.1%. Occurs naturally in many fruits and vegetables, notably cranberries (0.05–0.09%) and prunes.

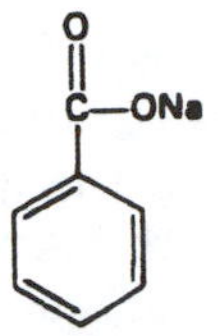

Sodium benzoate

sodium chloride (table salt). Mol. Wt. 58. The usual intake of sodium chloride is 7–15 g daily. This includes sodium chloride contained in foods, as well as that added as table salt. Deficiency of sodium chloride occurs mainly during hot weather or as a result of heavy work in a hot climate when excessive sweating takes place. The simple provision of extra salt in food or in salt tablets will prevent or correct the condition. Dehydration is generally associated with salt depletion. The blood volume is decreased, the veins collapse, the blood pressure decreases, and the pulse rate becomes rapid. Salt depletion can occur without water depletion. The condition is called "water intoxication." Large water intakes without salt cause a decreased concentration of salt in the blood that can causes *anorexia*, weakness, and mental apathy. In extreme conditions, convulsions and coma may occur. Reduced salt (sodium chloride) intake is often a recommendation in cases of severe hypertension (diastolic pressure over 120). If the sodium content is significantly lowered, there is usually a decrease in blood pressure. The table gives the approximate daily sodium chloride intakes for various sodium-restricted diets.

Daily sodium chloride intakes in g for sodium-restricted diets

Normal	9	Restricted	6	Low salt	2

sodium erythrobate. A close but nonnutritive relative of *ascorbic acid* (vitamin C). Its most important use is to brighten the pink color of frankfurters, bologna, sliced pastrami, and other cured meats to prevent that color from fading. Occasionally used as an *antioxidant* in beverages, baked goods, pimento salad, and potato salad.

sodium nitrate. Mol. Wt. 85. $NaNO_3$. The sodium salt of nitric acid (HNO_3). The potassium nitrate salt (KNO_3) is known as saltpeter. Nitrates are used as fertilizers and also as additives in cured meats such as frankfurters and bologna. Under some conditions, nitrates in food can be reduced to potentially toxic nitrites through the action of microorganisms. See *sodium nitrite*.

sodium nitrite. Mol. Wt. 69. $NaNO_2$. Sodium nitrite and sodium nitrate are used in cured meats as coloring, flavoring, and preservatives. They are present in ham, bacon, corned beef, most frankfurters, salami, liverwurst, bologna, and smoked fish. Nitrites can react with secondary amines under certain conditions, such as heat, and in the intestines, to form a class of compounds called nitrosamines ($R_2NN=O$). Dimethylnitrosamine has been shown to cause cancer in experimental animals. There is no evidence that nitrosamines cause cancer in humans, but the safety of addition of nitrites to foods such as bacon has been questioned.

sodium propionate. See *calcium proprionate* and *propionic acid*.

solute. Any solid particle that dissolves or goes into a liquid solution, usually water. Any particle that dissolves in water does in fact react with water. For example, when a solid particle of *sodium chloride* (table salt) dissolves, it interacts with water to form a hydrated sodium ion (Na^+) and hydrated chloride ions (Cl^-) which become independent in solution. Each ion is surrounded by water molecules, that is to say, each ion is hydrated.

solution. A liquid containing dissolved particles or other liquids in a homogeneous single liquid phase.

solvent. The liquid into which solids (*solutes*) dissolve.

somatotropin. See *growth hormone*.

sorbic acid. Mol. Wt. 112. Sorbic acid and its sodium and potassium salts are food additives that act as mold and yeast inhibitors. They are often added to cheeses.

$$CH_3\text{-}\overset{\overset{\displaystyle H}{|}}{C}=\overset{\overset{\displaystyle H}{|}}{C}\text{-}\overset{\overset{\displaystyle H}{|}}{C}=\overset{\overset{\displaystyle H}{|}}{C}\text{-COOH}$$

Sorbic acid

sorbitan monostearate and sorbitan monooleate. Polyoxyethylene ethers of *stearic acid* and *oleic acid* esters of *sorbitol* anhydrides. They serve as *emulsifiers* in cakes, cake icings, whipped vegetable oil toppings, frozen pudding, coconut spread, and many other foods. Used at levels up to 1%, often in combination with one of the polysorbate emulsifiers.

sorbitol (glucitol). Mol. Wt. 182. A polyalcohol made commercially by the hydrogenation (reduction) of glucose. Sorbitol is also found naturally in some fruit (such as rowanberries). It is about 60% as sweet as *sucrose* (table sugar). Sorbitol is used in the manufacture of diabetic jams, marmalade, canned fruits, fruit drinks, and chocolate. Contains 4 calories per g. Sorbitol is absorbed into the bloodstream and converted to sugar, thereby providing calories. Because sorbitol is absorbed very slowly, blood sugar levels rise only slowly. Foods sweetened with sorbitol instead of sugar provide diabetics with a relatively safe source of sweetness and energy and allow them to decrease their intake of fats. See *mannitol*.

$$HO\text{—}CH_2\text{—}\overset{\overset{\displaystyle OH}{|}}{\underset{\underset{\displaystyle H}{|}}{C}}\text{—}\overset{\overset{\displaystyle H}{|}}{\underset{\underset{\displaystyle HO}{|}}{C}}\text{—}\overset{\overset{\displaystyle OH}{|}}{\underset{\underset{\displaystyle H}{|}}{C}}\text{—}\overset{\overset{\displaystyle OH}{|}}{\underset{\underset{\displaystyle H}{|}}{C}}\text{—}CH_2OH$$

Sorbitol

sorghum. A genus of grasses with a large number of species, cultivated throughout the world for food, forage, and syrup. They are tall annuals, resembling maize. The grains are smaller and rounder than most of the true cereals such as wheat. The sorghums, although less nutritious than maize, require very little water and can be grown in regions where maize will not flourish. There are four main types of sorghums: grass, grain, broomcorn, and sugar. Grass sorghums are used entirely for hay and pasturage. The grain sorghums grown in the

United States include Durra, Milo, Shallu, Feterita, and Hegari. The grain or seed is used for livestock food and the plants for forage. Commercial uses include alcohol, beer, oil, and starch. In Asia, India, and Africa grain sorghums are a staple human food. Broomcorns, grown in the United States, have a panicle with long branches, known as the "brush." These branches are used for carpet and whisk brooms. The sugar sorghums are tall and leafy and their canelike stalk contains a sweet juice which can be boiled down into a syrup. This syrup has been used as a molasses substitute. In sorghum, the syrup is not crystallized into sugar, but rather used in a pure, concentrated form.

sorrel (dock) (*Rumex*). A hardy perennial *herb* with several varieties which differ in shape of leaves and strength of flavor. All varieties are acid to some degree. The mildest variety is dock (*R. Patientia*), also called spinach dock and herb patience dock. A tall plant, growing over 5 feet tall, its foot-long mild leaves are used in the spring as a salad green or potherb. French sorrel (*R. scutatus*) has shield-shaped leaves. It has an acid sour flavor and is used in salads. Very high in *retinol* (vitamin A), with small amounts of calcium and phosphorus and some *ascorbic acid* (vitamin C).

sour cream. In its simplest form, sour cream is unpasteurized heavy sweet cream that has been allowed to stand in a warm place until it has become sour. It varies in texture and flavor. Commercial dairy sour cream is made from sweet cream treated with lactic acid bacteria to produce a thick cream with a mild, tangy flavor. The cream is pasteurized and homogenized to distribute the fat evenly throughout. The lactic acid bacteria are then added and the cream is held at the proper temperature for a specific length of time. When the cream is ready, it is chilled to stop the action of the bacteria and then packaged. Sour cream contains sodium, calcium, phosphorus, potassium, thiamine, and *riboflavin*. Good source of *carotene* (vitamin A activity) with some *vitamin D*. See this item in the table under *milk*.

soybean (*Glycine max*). Also called soya, soy pea, soja, and soi. Found in the hairy pods of an erect bushy legume native to Asia. Soybeans contain a large proportion of assimilable protein, have a considerable fat content, and are low in carbohydrates, having no starch at all. Soybeans have been used as food in China for thousands of years. The whole dry grain contains about 40% fat. The protein of soybeans has a high quality with a *net protein utilization* (NPU) value of 65. Soybean is also a good source of B-complex vitamins. The major proteins in soybean are glycinin, phaseolin, and legumelin. The major carbohydrates are *sucrose*, *raffinose*, *stachyose*, and *pentosazon*. Soybean is now an important raw material as animal feed, as an oil in margarine, and as a flour in human foods. Soy flour is present in cereal products, sausages, biscuits, infant foods, milk substitutes, and artificial meat.

Nutrients in 100 g soybean

CALORIES KCAL	PROTEIN G	FAT G	CARBOHYDRATE G	VITAMIN A I.U.	NIACIN MG	THIAMINE µG	CALCIUM MG	IRON MG
403	34	18	34	80	5	1100	225	8

soybean oil. An oil extracted from the soybean, which contains about 18% oil by weight. Soybean oil is used in the manufacture of margarine, shortening, candy, and soap. The oil is rich in *unsaturated fatty acids*; 25% *oleic acid*, 49% *linoleic acid* (an *essential fatty acid*), and 11% linolenic acid. About 11% of the fatty acids are saturated.

soy sauce. Soy sauce is a mixture of amino acids, polypeptides, simple proteins, carbohydrates, and other degradation products obtained by a combination of mold fermentation and acid hydrolysis. More than half of the vitamins in soybeans are destroyed in the process.

spaghetti. One of the most popular members of the pasta family, spaghetti is made from a mixture of semolina, the flour that is milled from durum *wheat*, and water. The dough is passed through metal disks full of holes to emerge as slender, solid rods. The name spaghetti is Italian from the plural form of *spaghetto*, "string." Spaghetti is a fair source of iron and *thiamine*.

Nutrients in 100 g spaghetti enriched, cooked al dente

CALORIES KCAL	PROTEIN G	FAT G	CARBOHYDRATE G	CALCIUM MG
148	5	0.5	30	11

Calories in 100 g various cooked spaghetti

Cooked al dente	148
Cooked tender	111
Tomato sauce with cheese, home recipe cooked	100
Tomato sauce with cheese, canned	76

spareribs. A cut of meat consisting of the lower portion of the ribs and breastbone removed from a fresh side of pig or hog. The ribs have only a small amount of meat, but the succulence of the meat and fat makes them good eating. Spareribs are high in protein, with small amounts of calcium and iron and some phosphorus, *thiamine*, *riboflavin*, and *niacin*.

spearmint (*Mentha spicata, var. viridis*). A strong-scented perennial *herb* grown for home and culinary use. The words "mint" and "spearmint" are often used synonymously. Spearmint has dark-green lance-shape leaves and red-tinged stems. Its long, pointed flower stalks bear pale purple flowers. Either fresh or dried, the leaves add a pleasant and distinctive flavor to cranberry juice, fruit cup, and some soups; they give delicate flavor to meat ragouts or fish. Mint sauce—chopped mint and vinegar—is a popular accompaniment to roast lamb, as is mint jelly. Fruit compotes, ice cream, fruit beverages, and jellies all use mint.

specific activity (enzymes). A measure of enzyme purity. Units (usually micromoles of product produced per minute) of enzyme activity per milligram of protein. The purer the enzyme, the higher the specific activity.

specific dynamic action or effect (SDA, SDE). When food is ingested, the metabolic rate (energy expenditure) increases above that of the fasting level. The total increase due to SDA of food is about 10% per day. Each food type has a different SDA value. The SDA for protein is about 30%, carbohydrate 6%, and fat 4% of increase above the energy value of the food type ingested. The cause of metabolic rate increase is not known.

spermatozoa. The mature male sex or germ cell formed within the seminiferous tubules of the testes.

sphingolipids. A class of phospholipids that have in common a sphingosine component. The sphingolipids include *ceramides*, *sphingomyelins*, and *glycosphinolipids* (cerebrosides and gangliosides).

$$CH_3\text{-}(CH_2)_{12}-\overset{\overset{\displaystyle H}{|}}{C}=\overset{\overset{\displaystyle H}{|}}{C}-\overset{\overset{\displaystyle H}{|}}{\underset{\underset{\displaystyle OH}{|}}{C}}-\overset{\overset{\displaystyle NH_2}{|}}{CH}-CH_2\text{-}OH$$

Sphingolipid (4-sphingosine)

sphingomyelin. A phospholipid found in the brain, spinal cord, and kidney. Occurs in large amounts in the myelin sheath of nerve tissue and derives its name from this structure. The sphingomyelins contain phosphorylcholine attached to the terminal carbon atom of sphingosine and a fatty acid attached in amide linkage to the nitrogen. See *sphingolipids*.

spices. The oldest of the food additives. Spices are some part of an aromatic plant, for example, seeds, roots, stems, or barks, depending upon the plant. Herbs generally involve the entire plant. Spices were originally used to mask the odors of decaying foods in times before refrigeration. The essential oils of some spices have preservative effects (e.g., clove and cinnamon), but are used now primarily as flavoring agents. Spices are used in quantities too small to provide any nutritional value. Today the word "spice" tends to be confined to the following group of products made from various parts (most often other than the seeds or leaves) of plants grown in the tropics: allspice, red pepper, and whole chili peppers, from dried fruits; cayenne pepper, from a ground whole plant; cinnamon from bark; cloves, from dried flower buds; mace, from the dried aril of the nutmeg, which itself is the kernel of a fruit; paprika, from dried pods; pepper, from a dried berry; and saffron, from the dried stigmas of a flower. See *herbs*.

spinach (*Spinacia oleracea*). An annual potherb which originated in southwestern Asia and is grown for its green leaves. An excellent source of *retinol* (vitamin A), a very good source of *ascorbic acid* (vitamin C) and iron, and a fair source of *riboflavin*. It is low in calories. Spinach is a good source of *vitamin K*, which aids in the formation of the blood substance required for clotting. See this item in the table under *vegetables*.

spleen. The largest collection of lymphoid tissue in the body, the spleen is located high in the abdominal cavity on the left side, below the diaphragm and behind the stomach. It is somewhat long and ovoid (egg-shaped). Although it can be removed (splenectomy) without noticeable harmful effects, the spleen has useful functions, such as serving as a reservoir for blood and red blood cells.

sprat (*Clupea sprattus*). One of the smallest of the herrings, 5 inches is its normal maximum length. Sprats are caught in abundance in many parts of Europe and extensively eaten there fresh and smoked. A sprat is also called a Norwegian sardine or anchovy. In the United States, the term "sprat" is applied to the young of the common herring and to many other small fishes.

sprue. A disease endemic in many tropical regions and occurring sporadically in temperate countries, characterized by weakness, weight loss, *steatorrhea*, and various digestive disorders. It occurs in two forms, tropical and idiopathic or nontropical sprue. Cause is unknown.

squab. Any young pigeon which has not been allowed to fly. Squabs weigh about 1 pound. Good source of protein, with some phosphorus and a small amount of calcium.

squash (*Cucurbita*). A gourd fruit native to the Western Hemisphere. The two main types of squash are summer and winter squash. There are many varieties within each group, each differing in shape, size, and color. See this item in the table under *vegetables*.

squash, summer. Small, quick-growing, with thin skins and light-colored flesh. The most common varieties eaten are (1) scallop or pattypan, disk-shaped with a scalloped edge. The skin is smooth or slightly worted, pale green when young, and turns white as it matures. (2) Cocozelle, cylindrical, with smooth skin, slightly ribbed with alternate stripes of dark green and yellow. Similar to zucchini. (3) Caserta, also cylindrical but thicker than cocozelle at the tip. The skin has alternate stripes of light and dark green. (4) Chayote, pear-shaped squash about the size of an acorn squash, light green in color. It has one soft seed in the center. (5) Yellow crookneck, a squash with a curved neck, larger at the top than the base. The worted skin is light yellow in young squash, turning to a deep yellow when mature. (6) Yellow straightneck, similar to the crookneck except that the neck is straight and it grows to be much larger, 20 inches long and 4 inches thick when mature. (7) Zucchini, sometimes called marrow or Italian marrow. It is cylindrical but larger at the base. The skin has a lacy pattern of green and yellow that concentrates to give the appearance of stripes. Summer squash provides *ascorbic acid* (vitamin C), *carotene* (vitamin A activity), and *niacin*. Since summer squash is low in calories and sodium it may be used frequently in a sodium-restricted diet, reducing, or other special diets. See this item in the table under *vegetables*.

squash, winter. Winter squash has a hard, coarse, rough rind that is dark green or orange in color. There are many types of winter squash. The most common varieties are: (1) Acorn which grows to be 5–8 inches long and 4–5 inches wide. It has a thin, smooth, hard shell which is widely ribbed, and is dark green, but changes to orange during storage. The flesh is pale orange and there is a large seed cavity. (2) Buttercup has a turbanlike formation at the blossom end. The hard skin is dark green with faint gray pockmarks and stripes and the turban is light gray. The dry, sweet flesh is orange in color. (3) Butternut is cylindrical in shape with a bulblike base. The skin is smooth and hard and is a light-brown or dark-yellow color. (4) Warren turban is drum-shaped with a turbanlike formation at the blossom end. The hard, worted skin is bright orange, the blossom end slightly striped, and the turban a bluish color. (5) Hubbard is globe-shaped with a thick, tapered neck that is somewhat smaller at the blossom end. The skin may be bronze-green, blue-gray, or orange-red in color; it is hard, worted, and ridged. The flesh is yellowish orange and has a sweet taste. (6) Sugar has green or orange rind with round or oval ridges and the stem at the top. The flesh is bright orange with many seeds in the center of the pumpkin. Winter squash is an excellent source of vitamin A and has fair *ascorbic acid* (vitamin C), *riboflavin*, and *iron*. See this item in the table under *vegetables*.

stabilizers and thickeners. Stabilizing substances are added to many foods to impart smooth texture and to help maintain flavor. In chocolate milk and instant breakfasts made basically of skim milk, stabilizers thicken the milk and prevent separation of the chocolate. *Carageenan*, a seaweed derivative, is widely used in diet milk products. In commercial ice cream and other frozen desserts, stabilizers often are used to increase viscosity and to help prevent the water in the product from freezing into crystals. Flavor oils used in some cake mixes, gelatins, and pudding mixes are highly volatile and stabilizers are used to prevent flavor evaporation and deterioration. Among the thickeners often used commercially to process foods are *pectins* and *gelatins*.

stachyose. An indigestible tetrasaccharide containing *galactose*, present in beans. There is evidence that the flatulence (*flatus*) after consumption of large amounts of beans is due to stachyose and *raffinose*, a trisaccharide containing *galactose*, *glucose*, and *fructose*, which is not digested by the enzymes in the small intestine but passes to the colon where it is fermented by resident microflora. See *raffinose*.

Staphylococcus. A common type of bacteria responsible for food poisoning. Food handlers with cutaneous (skin) infections are a major source of this contamination of foods. Staphylococci grow in cream fillings, custards, puddings, hollandaise sauce and other starch, eggs, and milk-containing mixtures (meat and meat combinations will also support their growth). Rapidly growing staphylococci may spread their enterotoxin within a few hours in fertile media like cream puffs and custard pies if growth is not deterred by proper refrigeration. Warm foods or foods permitted to stand for prolonged periods at room temperature in summer months are an open invitation for this type of food poisoning. The toxin of *Staphylococcus* acts primarily on the gastrointestinal tract. Since a preformed poisonous substance, the enterotoxin, is involved, onset of symptoms after ingestion is rapid and usually occurs within about 3 hours. Symptoms are acute and include nausea, vomiting, diarrhea, intestinal cramps, headache, and an occasional fever. The attack does not last more than one day and frequently terminates within 6 hours or less.

starch. A high-molecular-weight polymer of *glucose* ranging in molecular weight from 50 thousand to several million. Starch occurs in two types of molecules; one type, *amylose*, consists of long unbranched chains that form a three-dimensional spiral. The connection between glucose units is a 1→4. The other type, amylopectin, is high-branched chains and very similar to *glycogen*, animal starch. The branching in amylopectin is less than that in glycogen. The branching is a 1→6 and the linear backbone is a 1→4, as in glycogen. In amylopectin, branching occurs at every 24–30 glucose units, in glycogen 8–12 units as in the figure. Starch in plants is laid down in "granules" coated with a cellulose-like substance. When subjected to moist heat, starch granules absorb water, swell, and rupture. After treatment, starch forms a colloidal dispersion in water and is more easily digested in this state. Starch is found stored in seeds, roots, tubers, bulbs, and to some extent in the stems and leaves of plants. It is of great importance as a constituent of many natural foods and as a source of *dextrins*, *maltose*, and *glucose*. It constitutes one-half to three-fourths of the solid matter of the ordinary cereal grains and at least three-fourths of the solids of mature potatoes. Unripe apples and bananas contain much starch, which is to a large extent changed into sugars as these fruits ripen; on the other hand, young, tender corn (maize) kernels and peas contain sugar which is transformed into starch as these seeds mature. Starch is the most important source of *carbohydrate* intake in the American diet. The cooking of starch not only improves flavor, but also softens and ruptures the starch cells which facilitate enzymatic digestive processes. The digestion of starch begins in the mouth, where salivary *amylase*, an enzyme, is secreted. Under its influence, the chains of glucose units are split into smaller fragments. Hydrolysis continues in the stomach after the food is swallowed until the stomach contents become too acid. The starch fragments and undigested starch and sugars then pass into the small intestine. There the acid is neutralized, more *amylase* is secreted into the intestine from the pancreas, and the starch is eventually broken down to maltose and *isomaltose*, disaccharides that consist of two glucose units. Maltose and isomaltose are hydrolyzed to glucose by their specific maltases.

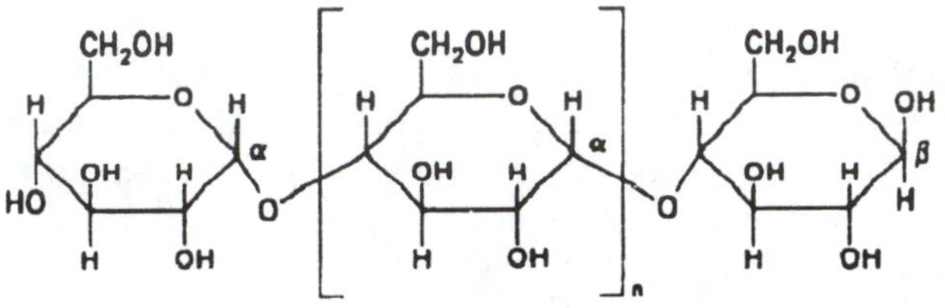

Amylose

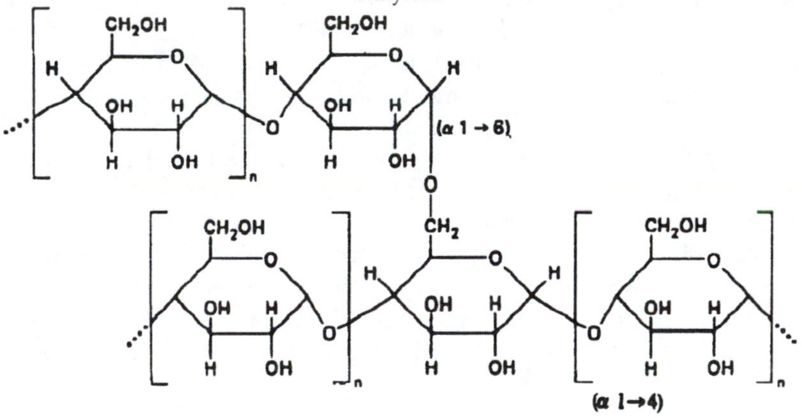

Amylopectin and glycogen

Classification and examples of starches

I. POTATO GROUP	II. LEGUMINOUS GROUP	III. WHEAT GROUP	IV. SAGO GROUP	V. RICE GROUP
Canna	Beans	Wheat	Sago	Rice
Potato	Peas	Barley	Cassava	Maize
Arrowroot	Lentils	Rye	Arum	Oats

Percentage of starch in various foods

Arrowroot	23	Corn grits, degermed, dry	78	Peas, dried	60
Bananas	22	Cornmeal, degermed, dry	78	Potatoes, uncooked	17
Beans, common	79	Lentils, raw	60	Potatoes, sweet, uncooked	26
Beans, green	61	Oatmeal, uncooked, dry	68	Rice, white, uncooked	80
Breadfruit, raw	26	Peanuts, roasted and salted	10	Rye flour, light	78
Buckwheat flour	26	Peas, canned, green, drained	17	Wheat flour, all-purpose	76
Chestnuts, dried	72				

steapsin. A lipolytic enzyme present in *pancreatic juice* that hydrolyzes *fats* to *fatty acid* and *glycerol*. The bile salts prepare the fats for the action of steapsin by emulsifying them. It is a *lipase*.

stearic acid. Mol. Wt. 284. A saturated fatty acid. The difference in consistency of various fats at room temperature is due to differences in the kinds and amounts of fatty acids that enter into their composition. *Palmitic* and stearic acids, which enter largely into the composition of solid fats, have a type formula of $C_nH_{2n}O_2$; they are said to be saturated because they cannot take up any more hydrogen.

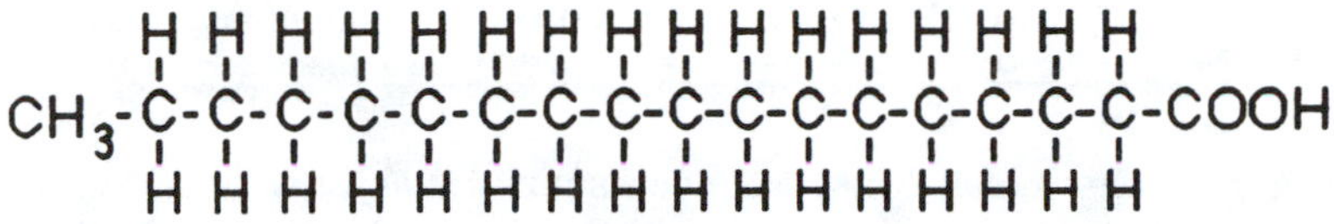

$$CH_3-\overset{\displaystyle H}{\underset{\displaystyle H}{C}}-\overset{\displaystyle H}{\underset{\displaystyle H}{C}}-\overset{\displaystyle H}{\underset{\displaystyle H}{C}}-\overset{\displaystyle H}{\underset{\displaystyle H}{C}}-\overset{\displaystyle H}{\underset{\displaystyle H}{C}}-\overset{\displaystyle H}{\underset{\displaystyle H}{C}}-\overset{\displaystyle H}{\underset{\displaystyle H}{C}}-\overset{\displaystyle H}{\underset{\displaystyle H}{C}}-\overset{\displaystyle H}{\underset{\displaystyle H}{C}}-\overset{\displaystyle H}{\underset{\displaystyle H}{C}}-\overset{\displaystyle H}{\underset{\displaystyle H}{C}}-\overset{\displaystyle H}{\underset{\displaystyle H}{C}}-\overset{\displaystyle H}{\underset{\displaystyle H}{C}}-\overset{\displaystyle H}{\underset{\displaystyle H}{C}}-\overset{\displaystyle H}{\underset{\displaystyle H}{C}}-\overset{\displaystyle H}{\underset{\displaystyle H}{C}}-COOH$$

Stearic acid

stearyl citrate. An ester of stearyl alcohol, $CH_3(CH_2)_{16}CH_2OH$, and citric acid. Stearyl citrate and isopropyl citrate protect oils by trapping metal (chelates) ions that might otherwise catalyze oxidation reactions and cause rancidity. It is a chelating agent or *sequestrant*. Stearyl citrate is used in margarine; isopropyl citrate is used in vegetable oil and other fat-containing foods. It has been found that the body converts these additives to citrate and stearyl or isopropyl alcohol, which are digestible and harmless.

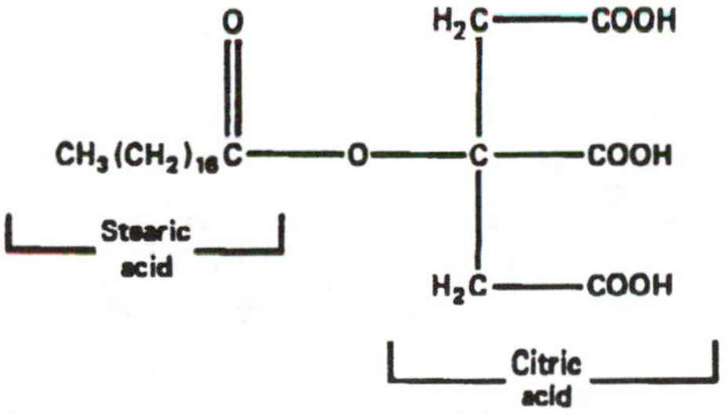

Stearyl citrate

steatorrhea. Fatty stools (*feces*) as seen in *sprue* and pancreatic diseases.

steroids. Complex molecules containing atoms arranged in four interlocking rings, three of which contain six carbon atoms each and the fourth of which contains five. The basic ring structure is a cyclopentanophenanthrene. Some steroids of biological importance are *vitamin D*, the male and female sex hormones, the adrenal cortical hormones, *bile salts*, and *cholesterol*. Cholesterol is an important structural component of nervous tissue and other tissues, and the steroid hormones are of prime importance in regulating certain phases of metabolism. See *adrenal glands*.

Cyclopentenophenanthrene

sterols. *Steroids* which possess an alcohol (−OH) group. *Cholesterol* is the most prominent member of this group found in the body, while *ergosterol* and *sitosterol* are common sterols found in plants. Sterols are widely distributed in small amounts in foods and are normal constituents of body tissues. They are concentrated especially in the liver and in lesser amounts in the blood and other tissues. Certain *hormones* formed in the *adrenal glands* and *sex glands* are also sterols.

stimulants (drugs). Drugs which cause an increase in the activity of an organ or a system. *Caffeine*, a central nervous system stimulant, decreases drowsiness and fatigue. *Digitalis*, a heart stimulant, strengthens heart muscle contraction.

stock. A liquid food made by cooking ingredients slowly for a long time so that all the essential flavor and nutrients of the ingredients are dissolved in the liquid. The solid particles remaining are discarded and the liquid may be further concentrated or clarified according to the way it is to be used.

stomach. A baglike structure about 1 foot long and 6 inches wide that can hold about 1.2 liters. It has layers of muscles that contract in different directions. As a result, the stomach can squeeze, twist, and churn food to break it up mechanically and to mix it with digestive secretions. The stomach's thick mucous lining acts as a chemical factory. It produces *hydrochloric acid* (HCl) to help in the digestion of proteins, and various enzymes to split fats and other food substances. When the stomach is filled, the pyloric sphincter closes and retains the contents until the food has been mixed with certain *digestive juices* collectively called *gastric juice*. Gastric juice has two main components, hydrochloric acid (HCl), produced by the parietal cells, and pepsin, produced by *chief cells*. The HCl in the stomach juice has three important functions: (1) It softens the connective tissues of meat. (2) It kills bacteria, destroying many potential disease-producing agents. (3) It activates at least one of the stomach enzymes, which are chemicals that convert food into soluble and absorbable substances.

strawberry (*Fragaria*). A juicy, edible fruit belonging to a member of the rose family, *Rosacae*. The fruits vary in size and color; there are whitish or yellowish fruits as well as the much more common red ones. Excellent sources of *ascorbic acid* (vitamin C). They also contain iron and other minerals. See this item in the table under *fruits*.

stricture. A narrowing of the *esophagus* resulting from acute or chronic esophagitis or secondary to a *tumor*. Difficult, painful swallowing, especially when coarse foods are swallowed, is the chief symptom.

stroke. The specific damage to the brain that results from injury to an artery either in the brain or leading to it. The artery damage deprives some of the brain of vital oxygen and other nutrients. In most cases of stroke, blood flow to part of the brain is blocked by a clot in an artery (thrombosis); another problem lies with a leaking or burst artery; or the flow is blocked by a clot coming from another area of the body and lodging in the brain (embolism). In almost every instance of blood-clot blockage, the underlying cause is *atherosclerosis* or disease of the artery wall; and in hemorrhage, the underlying cause is atherosclerosis or a combination of atherosclerosis and high *blood pressure*.

strontium (Sr). Element No. 38. At. Wt. 88. Like calcium and magnesium, strontium is a divalent alkaline earth metal and its biological behavior is in many ways similar to that of calcium. In general strontium is present in foods which are rich in calcium, especially milk and to a lesser extent fresh vegetables; it is also stored in bone.

sturgeon (*Acipenser*). Various species of fish are known as sturgeon. They are distributed throughout the coastal waters and rivers of the north temperate zone. One related genus, *Scaphirhynchae*, is recognized as a sturgeon: the shovelhead or shovelnose, a freshwater sturgeon found in the Mississippi and other North American rivers. Fresh sturgeon steak is considered a delicacy, the flavor being so distinct that it requires little seasoning. Another product of the sturgeon is isinglass, made from the swim bladder of the fish. It is used as a clarifying agent and in making jellies and glues. Sturgeon is high in protein.

subclinical disease. A disease course usually so mild that no definite symptoms can be recognized by the usual or clinical means.

subcutaneous fat. A layer of fatty tissue, directly under the skin, normally present in well-nourished individuals. The extent and thickness of this layer of fat vary considerably in different individuals, according to sex, general build, and dietary habits. Fat is a very poor conductor of heat and a good insulator, so persons with a well-developed layer of fat under the skin lose heat to the exterior much less readily than do those who have little subcutaneous fat.

substrate. A general term for a compound that is chemically altered by the action of an *enzyme*.

succinic acid. Mol. Wt. 118. $HOOC-CH_2CH_2-COOH$. A four-carbon dicarboxylic acid that is an intermediate in the *Krebs' cycle* (tricarboxylic acid cycle, Citric acid cycle).

succistearin. An *emulsifier* used to a limited extent in shortening to help make baked goods more tender. The body converts the additive to *succinic acid*, *stearic acid*, and *propylene glycol*, which may be used as sources of energy.

sucrose. Mol. Wt. 342. Sucrose is commonly known as table sugar. A disaccharide that yields *glucose* and *fructose* when hydrolyzed. Produced by squeezing the juice from sugar cane or sugar beets. This raw juice is neutralized with lime, filtered, and then subjected to vacuum evaporation to remove the excess water. After vacuum evaporation, crystals of raw sugar remain mixed with the mother liquor. The mother liquor, blackstrap molasses, is removed by centrifuging. The raw sugar is dissolved in water and decolorized by filtration through boneblack. Recrystallization is accomplished by vacuum evaporation followed by centrifuging. Sucrose includes no free keto or *aldehyde* groups, therefore it is not a reducing sugar. The average consumption is about 100 pounds of sugar per year or about 125 g per day. Large consumption of sugar (sucrose) over many years has been implicated as a cause of dental caries, heart disease, and diabetes but, except for dental caries, no firm associations have been established. The diet distribution of food consumed over the last century has varied little with respect to fat, protein, and carbohydrate. However, within the carbohydrate group, sugar has replaced starches to a large extent and represents a major dietary change. Sucrose is often used as a standard to estimate relative sweet tastes.

**Relative sweetness
of common sugars**

Fructose	110-175
Sucrose	100*
Glucose	75
Galactose	35-70
Lactose	15-30

*100 for sucrose as a base value

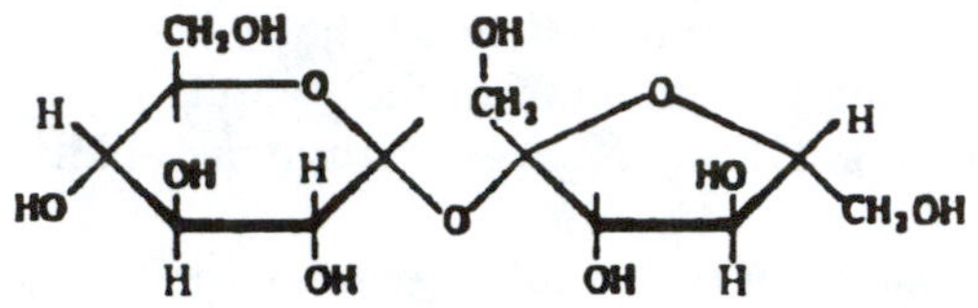

Sucrose
α-D-glucosyl-(1→2)β-fructoside

sucrose polyester (SPE). "Artificial" fat manufactured by substitution of sucrose for glycerol in the fat molecules, and thus not usable by the body.

suet. The hard fat around the kidneys and loins in beef, mutton, and other carcasses, which yields tallow. In cookery, unless the word is otherwise qualified, the reference is always to beef suet, which has a bland taste. Suet is sold in meat markets by the pound in large pieces, or sold by weight and sliced and ready to be used for barding meats.

sufu. A traditional Chinese cheese made from calcium-precipitated soybean curd by pressing it into molds to eliminate water. The pressed curd is cut into small cubes, sprayed with an acidic solution, and exposed to hot-air sterilization at 100 °C (212 °F) for 10 minutes. This minimizes bacterial contamination. These pieces are then inoculated with *Actinomucor elegans*, and the mycelium forms a mat around the particles.

sugar. A polyhydric alcohol containing three or more carbons and an aldehyde of ketone group. A sweet taste is characteristic of polyhydric alcohols. A sweet substance, capable of being crystallized, which is colorless or white when pure. It occurs in many plant juices and forms an important element of human food. Sugar as we usually think of it is, more specifically, cane sugar, which may also be called sucrose or saccharose. By extension, sugar also means any of a class of sweet, soluble compounds comprising the simpler carbohydrates. In addition to cane sugar, these carbohydrates or natural sugars are: dextrose or grape sugar, levulose or fruit sugar, lactose or milk sugar, and maltose or malt sugar. The chief sources of sugar are the sugar cane and the sugar beet. Cane sugar is made by expressing the juice from the sugar cane. The juice is then treated with lime to remove impurities, filtered, and evaporated to crystallization. In the case of beet sugar, the sugar is removed by extraction with water and carried to the refined state in one operation. There are various types of sugars: (1) Granulated sugar is the product for general use. (2) Superfine or powdered sugar is a very fine granulated sugar for use in cold drinks, for fruits and cereals, and for special cake baking. (3) Confectioners' sugar is granulated sugar that is crushed very fine and mixed with cornstarch to prevent caking. (4) Brown sugar is also called soft sugar and consists of extremely fine crystals that are covered with a film or coating of molasses. This coating gives the sugar its characteristic color and taste. (5) Maple sugar is made from the sap of the sugar maple, concentrated and crystallized into sugar. Sugar is almost 100% carbohydrate and is the most efficient source of energy that can be used by the human body. See *sucrose, glucose,* and *fructose.*

Calories in 100 g sugar	
Brown	375
White, granulated, or powdered	385

sugar-free/sugarless (food labeling). Common table sugar (sucrose), fructose, and corn syrup are among the types of calorie-containing sweeteners found in foods. A food can be labeled sugar-free and still contain calories from sugar alcohols (xylitol, sorbitol, and mannitol), provided the basis for the claim is explained. Saccharin is a nonnutritive sweetener, that is, it has no calories. Aspartame has the same calories as sugar, but is so much sweeter that only small amounts are needed to provide the desired sweetness in a product. Hence, its caloric contribution is almost negligible.

sugar substitutes. See *aspartame, cyclamates, mannitol, saccharin, sorbitol,* and *sweet.*

sulfites. Sulfites and sulfur dioxide are preserving agents against bacteria, molds, and yeasts. The toxicity level is negligible at levels generally used for preserving food color and preventing the growth of microorganisms. Some individuals are extremely sensitive to sulfites and consumption in even very small amounts can elicit an allergic response that may result in death. Sulfur dioxide is sometimes added to wines to inhibit the growth of organisms that interfere with the fermentation process.

sulfiting. Treatment of foods with sulfur dioxide or certain related compounds, sulfites. The sulfur combines with enzymes in the food and prevents them from causing quality deterioration. See *sulfur dioxide.*

sulfonamides. A group of compounds consisting of amides of sulfanilic acid derived from their parent compound, sulfanilamide. They are bacteriostatic, their action on bacteria resulting from interference with the functioning of enzyme systems necessary for normal metabolism, growth, and multiplication.

sulfur (S). Element No. 16. At. Wt. 32. Occurs principally as a constituent of the amino acids *cysteine, cystine,* and *methionine,* and is intimately associated with protein metabolism. It is present in all cells of the body but is most prevalent in the epidermal structure, keratin, and hair. Sulfur also occurs united to the carbohydrates in some instances. Food proteins contain about 1% sulfur, this amount varying with the amount of sulfur-containing amino acids. Sulfur is largely oxidized to sulfate in the liver and is excreted as inorganic and etheral sulfates in the urine. Foods that are good sources of organic sulfur include bluefish, chicken, dried beans, liver, peanuts, and turkey, but sulfur is so widespread in foods, especially protein foods, that if the protein in the diet is adequate there is little likelihood of dietary deficiencies of this element occurring.

sulfur dioxide. Mol. Wt. 64. O=S=O. See *sulfites*.

supplement, nutritional. A general term that usually refers to a concentrated source of nutrients prescribed in addition to the daily diet to increase nutrient intake. A supplement may be a food such as yeast or wheat germ, a concentrate such as cod liver oil, or a pharmaceutical preparation of vitamins or minerals.

surface active agents (surfactants). Similar to *stabilizers* and thickeners in their chemical actions. They cause two or more normally incompatible (nonpolar and polar) substances to mix. If the substances are liquids, the surface active agent is called an *emulsifier*. If the surface agent has a sufficient supply of hydroxyl groups, such as the *bile acid* or *cholic acid*, the groups form hydrogen bonds to water. Some surface active agents have hydroxyl groups and a relatively long nonpolar hydrocarbon end. Examples are diglycerides of fatty acids, monopalmitate, and sorbitan monostearate. The hydroxyl group on one end of the molecule anchors via hydrogen bonds in the water, and the nonpolar end is held by the nonpolar oils or other substances in the food. This provides tiny islands of water held to oil. These islands are distributed evenly throughout the food.

surfactant. See *emulsifiers*.

sweet. The sensation of a sweet taste is a general property of the polyalcohols. The mono- and disaccharides, *glucose, fructose,* and *sucrose* are examples of polyalcohols. The sensation of sweet taste is also obtained from a wide variety of compounds with widely varying chemical structures—polypeptides such as *aspartame*, benzene derivatives such as *saccharin*, and cyclohexanes such as *cyclamate* are examples of the structural variety. The table gives estimates of the intensity of sweet taste and the sweet taste relative to sucrose (table sugar), a common standard. The values given in the table vary considerably. The taste threshold of detection uses a common standard, sucrose, and varies from 0.01–0.04 *M*. See *mannitol, sorbitol, tongue,* and *sucrose*.

Relative sweetness of sugars

SUGAR	RECOGNITION THRESHOLD M*M*	RELATIVE SWEETNESS
Sucrose	2	100
D-Glucose	9	70
D-Fructose	5	110
Lactose	12	40
Maltose	8	50
Mannitol	—	70
Sorbitol	—	50
Xylitol	—	100

sweet basil. See *basil*.

sweetbreads. The thymus glands of lamb, veal, or young beef (under 1 year; the thymus disappears in mature beef). Sweetbreads consist of two parts: the heart sweetbread and the throat sweetbread. Lamb and veal sweetbreads are white and tender; beef sweetbreads are redder in color and a little less tender. A good source of protein.

Nutrients in 100 g calf sweetbreads, cooked, braised

CALORIES KCAL	PROTEIN G	FAT G	CARBOHYDRATE G	THIAMINE µG	CALCIUM MG	IRON MG
180	15	13	0	40	400	1

sweet cicely (*Myrrhis odorata, Osmohiza*). A perennial plant with aromatic leaves which are finely chopped in salads and stews. The leaves have a milky *anise*-like flavor. The seeds can be eaten fresh. The herb is said to improve the flavor of all other herbs with which it is combined. The seeds are especially good in beverages and cordials, fruit salads, and fruit cups.

sweeteners (nonnutritive, artificial). Artificial sweetening ingredients are *aspartame, saccharin,* sodium saccharin, sodium *cyclamates,* potassium cyclamate, calcium cyclamate, or any combination of these.

Sweet'N Low®. An artificial sweetener containing *saccharin*.

sweet potato (*Ipomoea batatas*). The enlarged or swollen roots of a perennial vine of the morning glory family. There are hundreds of varieties, with skins of many colors, although yellow tones predominate. They may be slender or globular, forked, or beet-shaped. The flesh is usually yellow-red, but some sweet potatoes are white. The majority are sweet. Some sweet potatoes have a jellylike consistency, while others are so dry that they have to be moistened with butter or a lubricant before they can be swallowed. The sweet potato is often confused with the *yam,* which it resembles. Yams, however, belong to the completely different botanical genus *Dioscorea.* Excellent source of *ascorbic acid* (vitamin C) and *carotene* (vitamin A activity). See this item in the table under *vegetables*.

swordfish (*Xiphias gladius*). An oceanic food and sport fish, which may weigh between 200–600 pounds. The swordfish is a fish of the Atlantic and Mediterranean. Occasionally it is found in the Pacific. The flesh is red, meaty, and rich. Good source of protein and vitamin A. See this item in the table under *fish*.

sympathetic nervous system. The cell bodies of the connector neurons of the sympathetic *nervous system* lie in the gray matter of the spinal cord from the levels of the eighth cervical to the second lumbar segments. The nerve fibers from these cells leave the central nervous system in the anterior nerve roots, but they split off from them to end in 22 paired sympathetic *ganglia* (collection of nerve cells), which are linked together to form the two sympathetic nerve chains running down the back wall of the cavity. These primary efferent nerve fibers are called preganglionic fibers, and they end in close approximation to numerous secondary nerve cell bodies in the sympathetic ganglia. The secondary cell bodies give rise to the secondary efferent or postganglionic nerve fibers.

syndrome. A set of symptoms occurring together. The outward signs or symptoms of a disease, for example, sneezing for hay fever, skin eruption, high fever.

synergism. The joint action of separate agents in which the total effect of their combined action is greater than the sum of their separate actions. Each agent potentiates the action of the other.

synovium. A synovial membrane, lubricated by synovial fluid or *mucin*. See *membrane*.

synthetases (synthases). A general class or group of *enzymes* that synthesizes a specific compound. For example, *fatty acid* synthase is a complex of several enzymes that leads to the synthesis of *fatty acids*. *Glycogen* synthetase is a single enzyme involved in one of several steps in the synthesis of *glycogen* (animal starch).

syrups, sugar. Highly concentrated solutions in which the sugar is unable to crystallize out owing to the presence of small quantities of other substances. They include *molasses* and golden syrup, which are by-products of the manufacture of crystalline cane sugar. These contain 20%–30% water in addition to sugar. They may also contain nutritionally insignificant amounts of calcium and iron, some of which probably come from the vessels in which they have been processed. Molasses is a popular folk remedy for the treatment of several diseases; however, there is no scientific support for its use.

systemic. Pertaining to the body as a whole.

systole. The contraction of the heart; the interval between the first and second heart sounds during which blood is forced into the aorta and pulmonary arteries. See *blood pressure* and *heart*.

systolic hypertension. A condition that may be caused either by an increase in the amount of blood pumped by the heart or by the loss of elasticity of the large arterial walls, most often due to arteriosclerosis. May be encountered by many apparently healthy people as they grow older. See *blood pressure*.

T

T. The alphabetic symbol for the *essential amino acid threonine* (Thr).

table salt. See *sodium chloride*.

tachycardia. Abnormal rapidity of *heart* action, usually defined as a heart rate over 100 beats per minute. Arrhythmias, or irregular heartbeats, are disturbances in the normal beating pattern of the heart. Normally, the heart beats at a steady 60–80 beats per minute, although it may speed up to 200 or more beats during a period of intense exercise. A number of factors can disturb the heart's normal rhythm, causing it to beat too fast (tachycardia) or too slow (bradycardia). These include cigarette smoking, anxiety, excessive caffeine, and the use of certain drugs. Most cardiac arrhythmias are temporary and benign; some however, may be life-threatening and require treatment. A common chronic arrhythmia is atrial fibrillation, in which the atria beat 400–600 times per minute. The ventricles usually beat irregularly at a rate of 170–200 times per minute in response to this rhythm. One of the most serious arrhythmias is ventricular tachycardia, in which there are three or more consecutive impulses that arise from the ventricles at a heart rate of 100 beats or more per minute.

tamarind (*Tamarindus indica*). A tall tropical shade tree native to the upper Nile region of tropical Africa and possibly southern Asia as well. Its name is derived from the Arabic *tamr hindi*, "Indian date." Tamarind pulp is used in preparing chutney, curries, and preserves. The juice is used in pickling fish and in making a syrup. This syrup, when diluted with water, makes a cold drink with a mild laxative quality.

tangelo (*Citrus*). A member of the citrus family which is a hybrid of the tangerine and grapefruit. They were crossed in 1897 to produce the new fruit. The name is derived from the words "tangerine" and "pomelo," another name by which the grapefruit is known. Tangelos have an orange rind and pale-yellow flesh with a pronounced acid flavor. Their size is medium to large. Two of the most successful varieties differ considerably in shape (pear or round) and in peel (thin and smooth or rough and thick). Tangelos are eaten out-of-hand or used in salads. They are also squeezed for juice.

tangerine (*citrus*). A citrus fruit that is a descendant of the mandarin orange. Tangerines are smaller than oranges. Like all mandarins, tangerines have thin skins which peel off readily and segments that can be easily separated from the pulp. The color of the skin is a rather intense orange-yellow, and the flavor of the fruit delicate, yet a little spicy and tart. They are named after the North African city of Tangiers, although their original home is China. Tangerines are eaten raw and are used in salads. Peeled and segmented, they can be served with a cheese tray; combined with Tokay grapes or blueberries and sprinkled with coconut; or used in a gelatin. The rind can be used grated as a flavoring. A food source of *ascorbic acid* (vitamin C). See this item in the table under *fruit*.

tannin. An acid substance found in the bark of certain plants and trees or their products, usually from nutgall (gall is a swelling of plant tissue usually due to fungi or insect parasites and sometimes forming an important source of tannin). Found in wines, coffee, and to a greater extent in tea. It is partly eliminated in the urine as gallic acid.

tapeworm. The beef tapeworm, *Taenia saginata*, and the pork tapeworm, *Taenia solium*, are transmitted by the fecal-oral route, usually in the form of mature eggs in segments of the worm. These cysts are eaten by cattle in sewage-polluted pastures or by hogs in polluted garbage. The larvae develop in the animals' intestine, then encyst in the muscle. If humans eat the infected meat raw or rare, the adult tapeworm matures in the intestine and continues its reproductive cycles.

tapioca. A farinaceous food made by heating the starch obtained from the roots of the manioc, one of the chief tropical food plants. Under the action of the heat, the starch grains burst and are converted into small, irregular masses. The product after baking to remove all moisture is flake tapioca. The pellet form or pearl tapioca is obtained by forcing the moist starch through sieves of various sizes. Granulated tapioca is also marketed in several sizes (made by grinding flake tapioca). An example of this is the quick-cooking tapioca sold in packages in food stores. Tapioca is a poor-quality food. The protein in tapioca pudding comes from milk. Tapioca contains about 0.1% protein and negligible amounts of vitamins and minerals.

Nutrients in 100 g tapioca, cooked in cream

CALORIES KCAL	PROTEIN G	FAT G	CARBOHYDRATE G
133	5	5	17

taro (*Colocasia esculenta*). A plant of the subtropics and tropics grown for its large underground tuber which has a high starch content and is very easily digested. Its large "elephant ear" leaves can be eaten as greens when young. The large starchy corms or bulbs and tubers are boiled, fried, baked, or used in soup. However, they have an acrid taste when raw. Poi, a staple food of the Pacific, particularly Hawaii, is made from the Taro root.

tarragon (*Artemisia dracunculus*). A perennial shrub-like *herb*, often called French tarragon; grows over 18 inches tall. Its dark-green leaves are long, narrow, pointed, and they are one of the most distinctive of the culinary leaf herbs. Fresh or dried, they add a slightly *anise*-like flavor to chicken livers, vegetable juices; chowders and consommes; tongue, veal, chicken, or turkey dishes; broiled fish, shellfish; scrambled eggs or omelets; and mustards and mayonnaises. Tarragon's botanical name, *dracunculus*, as well as French name, *estragon*, means "little dragon." It is said that this was chosen because of the way the roots twist about like serpents.

tartar (calculus). Light-yellow to dark-brown deposits on teeth along the gum line, which are not true stains. Tartar, properly called calculus, is made up of water, inorganic material, and organic material. It collects in layers, and as it forms it mixes with microorganisms, dead cells, and other debris in the mouth. It is made mainly of *calcium*. Tartar collects on bridges or partial dentures as well as around natural teeth. At first it is soft and may be removed by proper brushing, but as additional layers are formed it becomes hard and difficult to remove from either the natural teeth or bridges and dentures. As tartar forms, it pushes the gums away from the teeth, forming pockets in which more tartar forms. Bacteria and pus accumulate in the pockets because of gum irritation, and infection becomes more difficult to control. Tartar usually is yellowish when it begins to accumulate above the gum line. It darkens toward black (from blood pigments) as it progresses and slowly pushes the gum away from the tooth.

tartaric acid. Mol. Wt. 150. A substance that occurs naturally in grapes and other fruits and is made commercially from waste products of wine production. Tartaric acid is a constituent of grape and other artificial flavors that are used in beverages, candy, ice cream, baked goods, yogurt, and gelatin desserts. It also serves as the acid in some *baking powders*. Most of the tartaric acid ingested is destroyed in the intestines by bacteria.

$$
\begin{array}{cc}
\text{COOH} & \text{COOH} \\
| & | \\
\text{H—C—OH} & \text{HO—C—H} \\
| & | \\
\text{HO—C—H} & \text{H—C—OH} \\
| & | \\
\text{COOH} & \text{COOH} \\
\text{L-Tartaric acid} & \text{D-Tartaric acid}
\end{array}
$$

tartrate. A salt of *tartaric acid*.

taste. Sense organs for taste are taste buds located in the surface of the tongue. The primary taste (gustatory) sensations are sweet, sour, salty, and bitter. The actual sensations of taste, particularly for distinctive *flavors*, are influenced by the sense of *smell*. Taste sensation is usually dulled when nasal membranes are congested or when the nostrils are pinched shut while eating foods. Taste depends upon smell to a large extent. Impulses from taste receptors are transmitted by nerve fibers from two cranial nerves, facial and glossopharyngeal, to the temporal lobe. See *tongue, aroma, and flavor*.

taste buds. Ovoid bodies, with an external layer of supporting cells, which end in hair-like processes that project through the central taste pore. These cells are the sensory cells and the hairlike processes are stimulated by the dissolved substances. The taste buds are found on the surface of the tongue, though some are scattered over the soft palate and *epiglottis*. Taste sensitivity is caused largely by receptors on the tongue in adult humans. Sensitivity is also found on the palate (for sour and bitter) and the larynx. Strictly speaking, taste receptors give rise only to sensations of sweet, salt, sour, and bitter; the complex of the subtle sensations called "taste" in everyday speech includes smell, common chemical sensitivity, and some esthesis (feeling). A food is said to taste bland when "stinging" common chemical sensations are not present. Food tastes "flat" when one has a head cold because it is then impossible to smell food. See *tongue, aroma, and flavor*.

taurine. Mol. Wt. 125. A colorless crystalline compound of neutral reaction found in juices of muscle, especially in invertebrates, and obtained as a cleavage product of *taurocholic* acid, a *bile acid*.

$$NH_2-CH_2-CH_2-O-\overset{\overset{\displaystyle O}{\|}}{S}-OH$$

Taurine

tea (*Thea sinensis*). The name given to an evergreen shrub or small tree and the leaves of this shrub; the drink made from these leaves. The tea plant is related to the magnolia and, like its relative, would produce blossoms and grow to a great height if it were not pruned. This plant is kept to the size of a bush so the leaves may be easily plucked off as they grow. The principal difference in teas comes from the treatment of the leaves once they are picked. Black tea, by far the most popular, is made by allowing the dried and rolled tea leaves to ferment before they are fired. Green tea, produced in China, Japan, India, and Indonesia, is dried, rolled, steamed, and fired without being allowed to ferment. The leaves retain their greenish color and the resulting beverage is a greenish yellow color and rather bitter. Oolong tea, from China, Taiwan, and Japan, has leaves which are partially fermented, giving the beverage the aroma of black tea and "bite" of green tea. Besides these three main types of tea there are special teas which are scented and spiced. Tea has no nutritive value except when sugar, milk, or cream is added. Tea contains a stimulant called *theine* which is identical with caffeine in coffee.

teeth. Outgrowths of the primitive mouth (buccal) epithelium and the surrounding connective tissue. A child has a first set of 20, the deciduous teeth, which are shed and replaced by 32 permanent teeth. The fibroelastic periodontal membrane holds the teeth solidly in the sockets of the jawbones. A tooth consists of an exposed crown and one or more buried roots. The

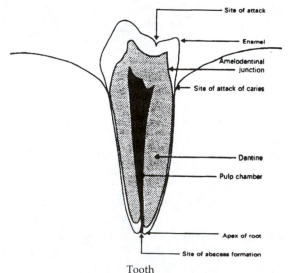

Tooth

(Davidson S., et al., *Human Nutrition and Dietetics*, 1975. Reproduction with permission of Churchill Livingstone, Edinburgh.)

junction of the crown and root, the neck, is surrounded by the gingival margins, as shown in the diagram. Enamel covers the crown, while cementum, a hardened type of bone, covers the roots. Beneath the enamel is a thick layer of dentine, another hard, calcified substance much like enamel, but very sensitive. Beneath the cementum is a thinner layer of dentine. The dentine surrounds a central cavity of the tooth which is filled with pulp. Pulp is connective tissue laced with nerves and blood vessels which supply the tooth. Dentine is the main substance of the tooth. The diagram shows a vertical section of a tooth. Certain antibiotics taken during pregnancy will show their mark on a child's teeth. Specifically, these are the three types of tetracycline (tetracycline, chlortetracycline, and oxytetracycline). These drugs travel through the mother's bloodstream. Small amounts are transferred to the unborn baby's blood and are deposited in its developing bones and teeth. The result is a yellow-gray or brownish stain on the baby's first teeth. Tetracycline can also stain the teeth of children who receive the antibiotic after birth. The discoloration, however, is not a health hazard.

teeth, nutrition. Dental caries is the most widespread of all chronic diseases. Dental decay results when oral bacteria act on teeth which are susceptible to decay. Certain microorganisms are prevalent in tooth surface areas protected from cleansing procedures. Carbohydrates, especially table sugar (*sucrose*), accumulate on the teeth, are acted upon by the organisms, and readily ferment, and the acid generated by this action penetrates the tooth enamel, thus causing tooth decay. Dental decay in susceptible teeth occurs in direct proportion to the quantity of fermentable carbohydrate in the diet, but frequency of intake and consistency (form) of the food are especially important in the decaying process. Carbohydrates that are sticky and adhere to the teeth are more destructive than those in liquid form. If they are eaten at continuous short intervals, the decay process can be practically continuous. One of the most important factors determining the resistance of a tooth to subsequent attack by *plaque* acids is a proper level of fluoride during tooth formation in the first few years of life. Fluoride is incorporated into the enamel of developing teeth, modifying the crystal structure and making them more decay-resistant. When fluoride is present in drinking water at the rate of 1 ppm, it provides the proper level of fluoride. Where there is a lack of fluoride in water, it can be prescribed as a dietary supplement during the period of tooth formation (until about 14 years of age), and will produce a level of protection similar to that of fluoridation. The supplement may take the form of drops, tablets or vitamin-fluoride combination. Fluoride has its greatest effects just before and just after the emergence of the teeth. That is why it is continued for a year after all the permanent teeth are in place. The regular use of fluoride toothpaste and mouthwashes at any age reduces decay yet further on a topical basis, such as interaction with the tooth surface.

telophase. The stage in *mitosis* in which the doubled *chromosomes* have divided and moved apart into newly forming cells.

tempeh. A method of traditional food processing developed in Southeast Asia, where dehulled *soybeans* are soaked, cooked briefly, and then inoculated with *Rhizopus oligosporms*. Within 24 to 48 hours, a continuous mat of mycelium has overgrown the beans to form a firm cake. This can be sliced or dipped in salt brine and deep-fat fried or used as chunks of protein.

tendons (sinews). White, glistening cords or bands which serve to attach the muscle to the bone. The major substance in tendon is the protein *collagen*.

terminal respiratory chain. The system responsible for the final stage of the *oxidation* of foodstuffs, fats, carbohydrates, and proteins. It is contained in the membranes of mitochondria and composed of an ordered array of cytochromes. The *cytochromes* pass the electrons removed from the foodstuffs by oxidation reactions in a sequential manner to oxygen, the cytochromes themselves undergoing *reduction* and *oxidation* in sequence. Cytochrome oxidase terminates the respiratory chain and transfers the electrons to (reduces) oxygen to form water. The sequence of electron flow is as follows: During the process of electron flow through the terminal respiratory chain, about 40% of the energy of oxidation is conserved as chemical energy, *adenosine triphosphate* (ATP), which can be used for the energy needs of cells. The remaining energy, about 60%, is converted to heat. See *oxidative phosphorylation, Krebs' cycle*, and *mitochondrion*.

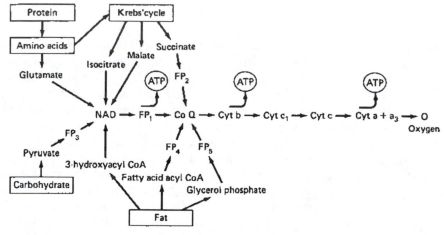

Terminal respiratory chain

terpenoids. A very large, important group of compounds which is made up of a simple repeating unit, the isoprenoid unit. This unit, by condensation, gives rise to such compounds as rubber, carotenoids, steroids, and many simpler terpenes. Isoprene, which does not occur in nature, has as its actual biologically active counterpart isopentenyl pyrophosphate, which is formed by a series of enzymatically catalyzed steps from mevalonic acid. Isopentenyl pyrophosphate undergoes further reactions to form squalene, which in turn condenses with itself to form *cholesterol*.

Terramycin®. A proprietary name for the oxy derivative of tetracycline. An antibiotic biosynthesized by *Streptomyces rimosus*. It is a broad-spectrum antibiotic effective against both gram-negative and gram-positive bacteria, *rickettsiae*, and some viruses.

testis. The male *gonad*. One of two reproductive glands, located in the scrotum, which produce the male reproductive cell or spermatozoa and the male hormone, *testosterone*.

testosterone. Mol. Wt. 288. Testicular steroid hormone synthesized from cholesterol, responsible for male secondary sex characteristics. *Progesterone* is also a precursor of testosterone. See *steroids*.

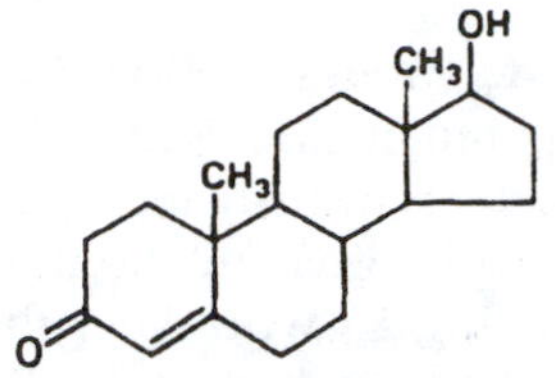

Testosterone

tetany. A disorder caused by abnormal *calcium* metabolism; fever, intermittent tonic contractions of the extremities, and muscular pain occur, and are usually caused by lowered blood calcium levels. A characteristic diagnostic sign is the inward muscular spasm of the wrist called Trousseau's sign.

tetrahydrofolic acid. Mol. Wt. 445. One of the B-complex vitamins and a specific vitamin of the general class of vitamins called *folacin*. In addition to folic acid, with only one glutamic acid group in the molecule, at least two conjugated forms of folacin exist in foods with either three or seven glutamic acid groups per molecule (folic acid glutamates). These conjugated forms serve as the major precursors of the vitamin in the diet. The coenzyme form, tetrahydrofolic acid, the most common form in the body, is also widely distributed in foods. Tetrahydrofolic acid functions prominently in one carbon metabolism, that is to say, it is this vitamin that is directly involved in the transfer of methyl ($-CH_3$), methylene ($-CH_2$), and hydroxyl methyl ($-CH_2OH$) groups to several intermediates in metabolic processes. Free, unsubstituted tetrahydrofolic acid appears to be necessary for the production of new *erythrocytes*, and through this important activity tetrahydrofolic acid is functionally associated with vitamin B_{12} (*cobalamin*). Vitamin B_{12} is able to remove the methyl ($-CH_3$) group from methyl-tetrahydrofolic acid to form free tetrahydrofolic acid, in sufficient quantity to produce new erythrocytes. In the absence of vitamin B_{12} an anemia develops known as *pernicious anemia*. See *folic acid deficiency*.

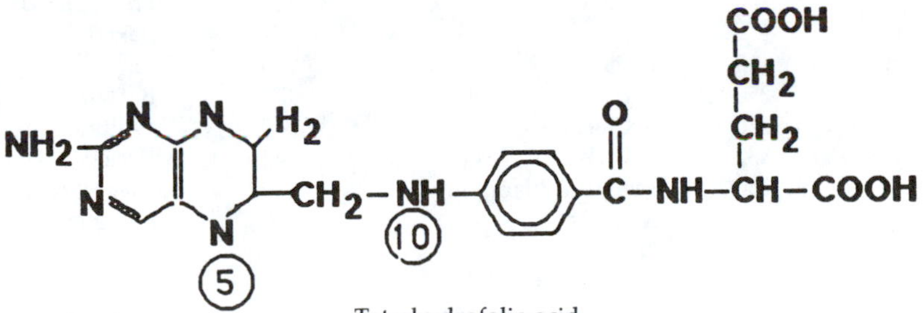

Tetrahydrofolic acid

thermogenic effect. See *specific dynamic action*.

thiaminase. Certain raw fish and seafood, particularly carp, herring, clams, and shrimp, contain the enzyme thiaminase, which is capable of splitting the vitamin *thiamine* into its two major chemical groups, thus making it inactive. The enzyme is also thought to be present in the intestinal flora of humans.

thiamine (vitamin B_1). Mol. Wt. 460. One of the B-complex vitamins. It is readily soluble in water, slightly soluble in alcohol, and insoluble in fat solvents. Thiamine may be destroyed during storage or by heating in neutral or alkaline solutions. It is quite stable in the dry state. Synthetic thiamine is usually prepared in the form of one of its salts, such as thiamine hydrochloride or thiamine mononitrate, which are more stable than the free vitamin. Thiamine plays a part in promoting appetite and better functioning of the digestive tract, effects that have an indirect influence on promoting growth. After thiamine is absorbed it is distributed widely by the blood throughout the body in all tissues and in somewhat high concentrations in such organs as the heart, liver, and kidneys. The body has limited ability to store thiamine. Tissues are depleted of their normal content of the vitamin in a relatively short period if the diet is deficient, so fresh supplies are needed regularly. The amount of thiamine required by adults varies according to size, degree of activity, dietary habits, and individual differences in how food is utilized. Daily allowances for adults according to the Food and Nutrition Board are calculated on the basis of individual calorie requirements, allowing 0.5 mg per 1000 kcal (minimum requirement is approximately 0.33 mg per 1000 kcal). The thiamine content of most fruits and vegetables, eggs, milk, and cheese does not generally exceed 100 µg per 100 g of food. The best sources of thiamine, whole grains, organ meats, pork, and legumes, are not used in quantity in most American diets. Most thiamine comes from bread and cereals, meat, fish, poultry, eggs, nuts, milk, dairy products, vegetables, and fruits.

Thiamine in µg/100 g foods as usually eaten[a]

Asparagus, cooked	160	Fish (continued)		Peas	
Avocado	110	Grouper	170	Snow	220
Bacon, fried	510	Mackerel	270	Green	280
Bamboo shoots	150	Salmon	140	Canned	100
Barley, pearled	120	fresh cooked	30	Pineapple	
Beans		canned	130	Fresh or canned	100
White	140	Shad	110	Pork	500
Red	110	Whitefish	225	Potato chips	210
Lima	180	Heart	510	Potatoes	
Bean sprouts	100	Kidney	140	French fried	120
Bread		Lamb		Baked	100
Cracked wheat	110	Liver	260	Rice	
Enriched white	250	Beef	170	Brown	90
Rye	170	Chicken	340	White	20
Pumpernickel	130	Pork		Enriched	110
Whole wheat	250	Molasses, blackstrap	110	Sausages, cold cuts	
Buckwheat,		Mussels	160	Bologna	160
whole grain	600	Nuts		Liverwurst	170
Chicken		Chestnuts	220	Minced ham	730
Dark meat	120	Filberts (hazelnuts)	460	Pork sausage	290
Giblets	170	"Indian" nuts	1280	Salami	250
Clams	100	Peanuts (roasted)	320	Scrapple	190
Collards	110	Peanut butter	120	Soybeans, cooked	310
Corn	100	Pistachio	167	Soybean sprouts	160
Eggs	110	Pignola	620	Syrup, cane	130
Fish		Walnuts	330	Wheat germ	2010
Abalone, canned	120	Oranges	100	Toasted	1650
Drum (redfish)	150	Oysters	120	Yeast, Brewer's	4280

[a]Note that products made with enriched flours: macaroni, spaghetti, and other pasta; cakes and muffins from mixes; breakfast cereals, etc., generally contain about 140 µg/100 gm of product as it is usually eaten.Do not be led astray by tables showing thiamine content of various flours or raw food.Thiamine is not stable to moist heat and much is lost in cooking and processing.Many substances which can be sources of thiamine when freshly cooked lose most of their thiamine during sterilization, if they are canned.

From *Nutritive Value of American Foods In Common Units*, Agriculture Handbook No. 456, Washington, D.C., U.S. Department of Agriculture.

Thiamine is especially involved in a *carbohydrate* metabolism. The vitamin is found in the body both in the free form and combined with phosphate as the coenzyme thiamine pyrophosphate (TPP). The coenzyme TPP combines with magnesium and specific proteins to form active enzymes, the decarboxylases. Thus, thiamine aids in the complete breakdown of carbohydrates into carbon dioxide and *acetyl coenzyme A*, releasing energy for body use. Several of the B-complex vitamins are involved. The coenzyme TPP, which contains thiamine, acts with *nicotinamide adenine dinucleotide*, which contains the vitamin *niacin*, coenzyme A, which contains the vitamin *pantothenic acid*; and *lipoic acid*. Thiamine is the active part of the coenzyme thiamine pyrophosphate shown in the diagram, made in tissue cells by the combining of thiamine with two phosphate groups. This important coenzyme is necessary for at least three different enzyme systems in mammals that are needed for the complete oxidation of carbohydrates. Two of these enzymes function by splitting off carbon dioxide from *pyruvate* in the course of oxidation in the body. Thiamine pyrophosphate is also necessary for reactions leading to production of ribose, the important pentose sugar needed by all cells in the body for the production of *nucleic acids*.

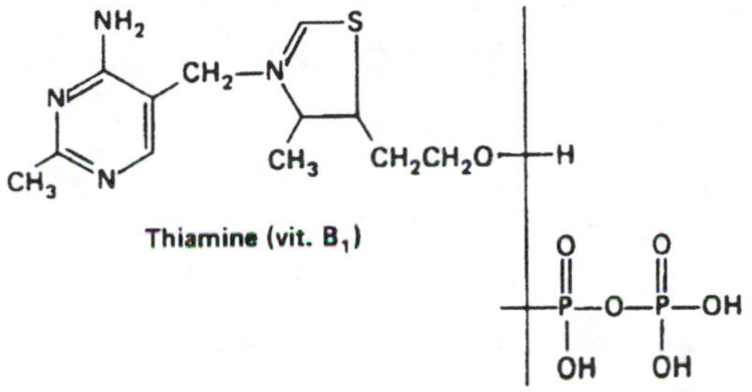

Thiamine pyrophosphate (TPP)

thiazoles. A group of heterocyclic compounds that contribute to the taste of tomatoes, wine, and green vegetables. The nutty *aroma* of fried food is due to 2, 4 dimethyl-5-vinyl-thiazole. See *flavor* and *taste*.

thickening agent. Manufacturers use thickening agents to "improve" the texture and consistency of ice cream, pudding, soft drinks, salad dressing, yogurt, soups, baby food and formula, and other foods. These chemicals control the formation of ice crystals in ice cream and other frozen foods. The thickness they create in salad dressing prevents the oil and vinegar from separating out into two layers. These additives are used to stabilize factory-made foods, that is, to keep the complex mixture of oils, acids, colors, salts, and nutrients dissolved and at the proper consistency and texture. Most thickening agents are natural carbohydrates (*agar*, *carrageenan*, *pectin*, starch, etc.) or chemically modified carbohydrates (cellulose *gum*, modified starch, etc.) They work by absorbing part of the water that is present in a food, thereby making the food thicker. See *stabilizers*.

thiocyanic acid or thiocyanate. Mol. Wt. 59. Thiocyanic acid salts (thiocyanates) are goitrogenic. They contribute to the formation of a goiter by decreasing *thyroxine* synthesis in the *thyroid* gland. The mechanism appears to be an inhibition in the synthesis of thyroxine from the thyroglobulin. The *sulfonamides* and 2-thiouracil appear to inhibit thyroxine synthesis by mechanisms similar to the thiocynates. Certain aminobenzenes also inhibit thyroxine synthesis, but the mechanism appears to be related to the formation of stable iodine derivative in the thyroid gland, thus removing the iodine normally used for thyroglobulin formation.

Thiocyanates and thiourea, other goitrogenic compounds, are found naturally in *turnips* and *cabbage*. See *thiourea* and *food toxins*.

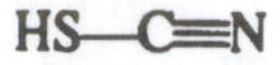

$$HS—C≡N$$

Thiocyanic acid

thiodipropionic acid. A *food additive* occasionally used in foods to prevent fats and oils from going rancid. It functions by reacting with oxygen which otherwise reacts with fat.

thiol (thioesters, polysulfides). Sulfurous compounds obtained from *cysteine, cystine*, and *methionine* by heating protein.

thiourea. Mol. Wt. 60. A goitrogenic compound that is found naturally in turnips and cabbages. Thiourea, a thiocarbamide, sulfonamides, and 2-thiouracil inhibit the synthesis of *thyroxine* in the *thyroid gland*. See *thiocyanic acid* and *food toxins*.

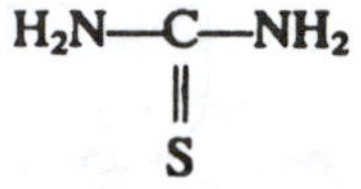

$$H_2N—C—NH_2$$
$$\|$$
$$S$$

Thiourea

thoracic cavity. In the thoracic cavity there are two pleural cavities, each containing a lung. In the space between the pleural cavities is the pericardial cavity, which contains the heart and the mediastinal region, in which are contained the trachea, esophagus, thymus gland, large blood and lymphatic vessels, lymph nodes, and nerves.

threadworm (*Strongyloides*). A parasite that produces a chronic intestinal infection with manifestations similar to hookworm infection. In heavy infections there is usually abdominal pain, watery diarrhea, loss of appetite, anemia, nausea, vomiting, and emaciation. Dithiazanine has been used for treatment.

threonine (Thr, T). Mol. Wt. 119. One of the *essential amino acids* found in proteins.

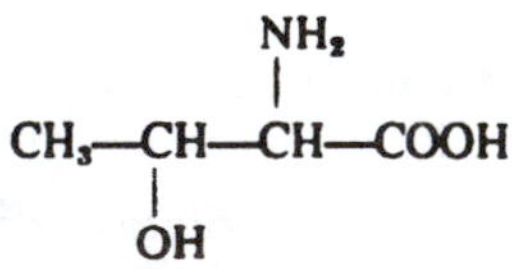

$$NH_2$$
$$|$$
$$CH_3—CH—CH—COOH$$
$$|$$
$$OH$$

Threonine (Thr, T)

thrombin. An enzyme in blood that facilitates blood clotting. *Vitamin K* is required for the production of thrombin from prothrombin. See *vitamin K*.

thrombosis. The formation, development, or existence of a blood clot or thrombus within the vascular system. The thrombus, if detached, becomes an embolus, and occludes a vessel at a distance from the original site.

thrombus. A clot in a blood vessel formed by coagulation of blood.

thromboxanes. A family of *eicosanoid hormones* that derives from the polyunsaturated fatty acid *arachidonic acid*. The other families of compounds are the *prostaglandins* and the *leukotrienes*. The thromboxanes have a variety of physiologic effects, depending upon the properties of the particular thromboxane. An example of a thromboxane structure is given.

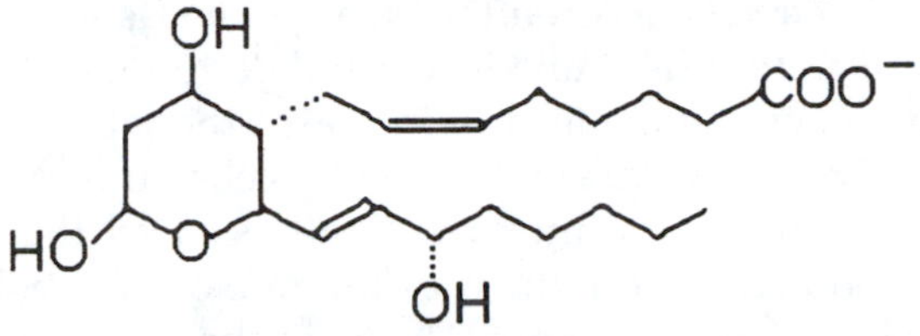

Thromboxane B$_2$

thrush. Also called moniliases, these pearly white or bluish-white patches that look like curds in the mouth are the result of infection of the fungus *Candida albicans*, a yeast. Because this same fungus can grow in the vagina, many newborn infants become infected at birth. Thrush also occurs after antibiotic therapy. This is because the antibiotic kills off, along with the disease-causing bacteria, certain useful bacteria in the mouth which normally serve to keep any fungus there under control. When these useful bacteria are killed off, the fungus thrives. Diabetics, too, are especially susceptible to thrush as part of their generally poor ability to handle any infection. The white patches also resemble leukoplakia and cheek-biting, but with thrush there are usually cracks in the corners of the mouth.

thyme (*Thymus vulgans*). There are a number of varieties of the herb. Garden and English thyme are small, bushy perennials with gray-green leaves; garden thyme's leaves are broad, while the wild or creeping thyme, *T. serpyllum*, is a firmly matted ground cover. The wild thyme's leaves may be many colors other than green. The pungent and sweetly fragrant leaves are widely used in cooking. Fresh or dried thyme flavors vegetable juices, soups, meat and poultry dishes, fish, cheese, stuffings, sauces, vegetables, cream and custard desserts, and jellies. It is a relatively powerful herb with a distinctive flavor.

thymidine. A pyrimidine *nucleoside* found in *deoxyribonucleic acid*.

thymidine pyrophosphate (TDP). An intermediate in the biosynthesis of deoxyribonucleic acid (DNA). It contains the pyridine base thymine, ribose, and pyrophosphate moiety.

thymine. A pyrimidine found in *deoxyribonucleic acid*.

thyrocalcitonin. A thyroid hormone which prohibits release of calcium from bone. See *calcitonin*.

thyroglobulin. The iodine-containing protein which is synthesized in the *thyroid gland* and can be broken down to *thyroxine* and small amounts of *triiodothyronine*.

thyroid gland. The thyroid gland is located in front of the neck and has two lobes, one on either side of the larynx. The hormone produced by the thyroid is thyroxine. This hormone is associated with the rate of metabolism, regulating heat and energy production in the body cells. Thyroid gland cells need a mineral, *iodine*, to manufacture thyroxine. Iodine is ordinarily obtained from foods included in a normal diet. Disorders of thyroid function include *hyperthyroidism*, which, when severe, causes a dangerous increase in the metabolic rate; and *hypothyroidism*, an opposite condition, which causes physical and mental sluggishness. An enlargement of the thyroid gland is called a *goiter*. When the enlargement is a nodular tumor, it is called an adenoma. The function of the thyroxine is to regulate the metabolic and oxidative rates in tissue cells of the body, including the liver. It increases the rate of glucose absorption from the intestine, increases the rate of *glucose* utilization by cells, and stimulates the growth and differentiation of tissues. In the liver it increases synthesis and the conversion of glycogen to glucose, thus raising blood sugar. It influences the rate of metabolism of lipids, proteins, carbohydrates, water, vitamins, and minerals. The most characteristic function of the thyroid gland is its ability to take up and concentrate *iodine*. The active transport of iodide is under control of the *thyroid-stimulating hormone*, which regulates thyroid function. Iodide exists in food in many forms and is readily absorbed from the intestinal lumen into the blood. In the thyroid gland, iodide is oxidized to elemental iodine, which combines with the amino acid tyrosine in thyroglobulin to form monoiodotyrosine and diiodotyrosine. The thyroid gland also stores thyroglobulin in the follicles.

thyroid hormones. Several amino acids are released from *thyroglobulin*. The most important is *thyroxine*. It normally appears in the blood and is considered to be the major hormone of the thyroid gland. Another amino acid, *triiodothyronine*, is found in the blood in extremely small amounts. It is physiologically active and considered to be a true product of the thyroid gland and one of the thyroid hormones. Thyroxine is generally referred to as T_4, and triiodothyronine is called T_3. The major function of the thyroid hormones is to control the metabolic rate. The thyroid hormones are also an important factor in growth. Nervous system activity is also influenced by the thyroid hormones.

thyroid-stimulating hormone (thyrotropin, TSH). A hormone secreted by the anterior *pituitary gland* which regulates uptake of *iodine* and synthesis of *thyroxine* by the *thyroid gland*. TSH is a polypeptide with a molecular weight of about 10,000. The major function of TSH is to stimulate the thyroid gland. TSH is thought to increase the amount of cyclic 3,5-*adenosine monophosphate* (cAMP) in the thyroid cell. The secretion of TSH is regulated in part by thyrotropin-releasing factors (TRH).

thyrotropin. See *thyroid-stimulating hormone*.

thyroxine (T_4) Mol. Wt. 777 and triiodothyronine (T_3). Mol. Wt. 651. These two hormones are extremely similar chemically and have exactly the same physiologic effect on tissues. The only difference is the speed at which the two hormones act. The most obvious effect that thyroxine has on the body is to increase the rate at which cells burn their fuel, *glucose*. As well as working in concert with *cortisol* in defending the body against stress resulting from extreme cold, thyroxine is also involved in other antistress responses. Emotional stress and severe hunger also provide an elevated thyroxine output. In general, thyroxine comes into play when there is an extra demand for energy. Thyroxine also increases the heart rate. The output of the two hormones is controlled directly by *thyroid-stimulating hormone* (TSH) secreted by the anterior pituitary. Under normal conditions the thyroid secretes about three times as much T_4 as triiodothyronine. When they are synthesized within the cells of the thyroid, the two hormones become a part of a protein (*thyroglobulin*) until they are needed. When needed, a complex reaction involving the proteolysis (hydrolysis) of thyroglobulin with the release of thyroxine takes place.

Thyroxine (T_4)

Triiodothyronine (T_3)

tin (Sn). Element No. 50. At. Wt. 119. A normal intake is probably in the range of 1.5–5 mg a day, depending on the amount of canned foods eaten. Tin is not very toxic. It has no known nutritional function.

tissue fluid. The body fluid that lies outside blood vessels and outside cells, called extravascular (outside blood vessels), or extracellular (outside cells) fluid. Living body cells contain large amounts of water and must be bathed continuously in a watery solution in order to survive and carry on their functions. The colorless and slightly salty tissue fluid is derived from the circulating blood.

tissues. The organs can be analyzed into component tissues. For example, the stomach is composed of columnar *epithelial tissue*, smooth muscle tissue, connective tissue, nerves, blood, and lymph. Microscopic study of tissues reveals that tissues are made up of smaller units or cells. Each tissue is a group of cells with more or less intercellular material. The intercellular material varies in amount and in composition and in many cases determines the nature of the tissue. *Connective tissue* is distributed throughout the body to form the supporting framework of the body and to bind together and support other tissues. It binds organs to other organs, muscles to bones, and bones to other bones. The five principal types of connective tissues are adipose, areolar, cartilage, elastic, and reticular.

1. *Adipose tissue*. A fatty connective tissue which is found under the skin and in many regions of the body. It serves as a padding around and between organs. It insulates the body, reducing heat loss, and serves as a food reserve in emergencies.

2. *Areolar tissue*. A fibrous connective tissue which forms subcutaneous layers of tissue. It fills many of the small spaces of the body and helps to hold the organs in place.

3. *Cartilage tissue*. A tough, resilient connective tissue found at the ends of the bone, between the bones, and in the nose, throat, and ears.

4. *Elastic tissue*. A fibrous connective tissue composed of elastic fibers and found in the walls of blood vessels, in the lungs, and in certain ligaments.

5. *Reticular tissue*. A fibrous connective tissue which forms the supporting framework of lymph glands, liver, spleen, bone marrow, and lungs.

Epithelial tissue forms the outer layer of skin for the protection of the body. It is also a lining tissue. As mucous membrane, it lines the nasal cavity, mouth, larynx, pharynx, trachea, stomach, and intestines. As serous membrane, it lines the abdominal, chest, and heart cavities and covers the organs that lie in these cavities. As endothelium it lines the heart and blood vessels. It lines respiratory and digestive organs for the function of protection and absorption. It helps form organs concerned with the excretion of body wastes, certain glands for the purpose of secretion, and certain sensory organs for the reception of stimuli.

TISSUE	STRUCTURE AND FUNCTION	LOCATION
1. Areolar		
Fibroblast cells	Binds organs and holds tissue fluids	Around nerves and blood vessels; under
Elastin cells	Collagen and elastin fibers provide support matrix	skin; between muscles
2. Reticular		
Phagocytic cells	Crossed fiber matrix	Lymph nodes, liver, spleen, thymus, and bone marrow
3. Adipose		
Fat cells	Insulates organs. Stores fat	Under skin. Suface of heart and other organs. Surrounds joints
4. Cartilage	Collagen and elastin fiber matrix for support	Bone surfaces, knee joints, intervertebral discs, nose, walls of respiratory passage
5. Bone		
Pourous	Hematopoiesis	Middle of flat bones and ends of long bones
Compact	Stuctural support	Outer layers of bones
6. Blood		
Red blood cells	Oxygen and nutrient transport	In plasma and within the circulatory system
Various cell types		

tobacco. Dried leaves of *Nicotiana tabacam* and other species, containing nicotine, pyridine, picoline, and colidin. Used in the form of cigars, cigarettes, pipe tobacco, snuff, and chewing tobacco. During its combustion, various products are given off, the most important being nicotine, and certain compounds which have an adverse affect on the lungs. For this reason, the use of tobacco products may be injurious to health and can lead to addiction.

tocopherol or vitamin E. Mol. Wt. 432. There are six forms of vitamin E, the alpha (α), beta (β) gamma (γ), delta (δ), epsilon (ϵ), and zeta (ζ). α-Tocopherol has the widest distribution and greatest biological activity. It is one of the *fat-soluble vitamins*. The tocopherols are sensitive to oxidation and to ultraviolet light. As *antioxidants*, the tocopherols retard oxidation of other fat-soluble vitamins and *lipoperoxidation* in adipose tissue associated with a high intake of polyunsaturated fatty acids. They may also be involved in cell respiration and in nucleoprotein synthesis. The richest sources are the vegetable oils, whole grains, and eggs; the average daily intake has been estimated at 24 mg. Human needs are related to the intake of polyunsaturated fatty acids and may vary between 10–30 mg per day for adults. Many claims have been made for vitamin E, ranging from specific aid to cardiovascular problems to a more general aid for fertility. No frank clinical condition due to a lack of vitamin E is known in humans. Vitamin E deficiencies can be demonstrated in animals, but become complicated by the fact that the symptoms differ in different animals and that the symptoms can sometimes be made to disappear by the addition of *selenium* or the sulfur amino acids. Vitamin E is not toxic. The table shows the tocopherol content in a variety of foods. For the *Recommended Dietary Allowance* see Appendix.

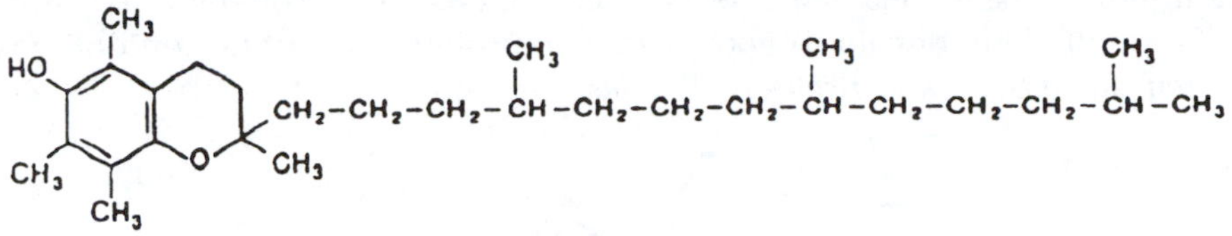

$$HO-\text{(chromanol ring, CH}_3\text{ substituents)}-CH_2-CH_2-CH_2-\overset{CH_3}{CH}-CH_2-CH_2-CH_2-\overset{CH_3}{CH}-CH_2-CH_2-CH_2-\overset{CH_3}{CH}-CH_3$$

Vitamin E (α-tocopherol)

Tocopherol in mg/100 g of foods

Fats and oils		**Meat, Fish, Poultry, and Eggs**	
Butters	1	Beef liver, broiled	1.62
Coconut oil	8	Egg	1.43
Corn oil, hydrogenated	105	Fillet of haddock, broiled	1.20
Corn oil, unhydrogenated	100	Ground beef	0.63
Cottonseed oil, hydrogenated	80	Pork chops, pan-fried	0.60
Cottonseed oil, unhydrogenated	91	**Vegetables and Fruits**	
Margarine (made with corn oil)	47	Bananas	0.42
Mayonnaise	50	Carrots	0.21
Soybean oil, hydrogenated	73	Green peas, frozen	0.65
Soybean, unhydrogenated	101	Orange juice, fresh	0.20
Cereal Grains		Potatoes, baked	0.085
White bread	0.23	Tomatoes, fresh	0.85
Whole-wheat bread	2.2		
Yellow cornmeal	3.4		

tofu. A traditional Japanese preparation made from soybean curd by coagulating soybean milk with a calcium salt. It is a white, soft, gelatinous mass containing 88% moisture, 6% protein, and 3% lipid. It is a soybean protein concentrate because soluble and insoluble carbohydrates are at least partly removed during the processing, and thus the protein content on a dry basis in tofu is higher than in the original soybean. Kori-tofu is tofu dried into a porous, spongy matrix without case hardening by the process of freezing, aging, pressing, and thawing. It has 53% protein and 9% water.

tomato (*Lycopersicon*). The fruit of a plant which grows on vines. Tomatoes come in many shapes and colors. They may be yellow, green, or whitish, or even varicolored, as well as the best-known red. They may be ribbed, round, pear-shaped, or cherry-shaped. The small green varieties are often used in pickles, while the large ripe red ones are most popular in sauces. The deep-red, pear-shaped tomato is a specialty of Italian tomato pastes. A good source of vitamins and minerals, especially *carotene* (vitamin A activity) and *ascorbic acid* (vitamin C). Tomatoes are low in calories. See this item in the table under *vegetables*.

tongue. A fibromuscular organ located partially in the oral cavity and partially in the pharynx. The root of the tongue is anchored to the hyoid bone. In addition to taste function, the tongue assists in speech, mastication, and swallowing. In mastication the tongue functions to push food between the teeth. Once the food has been broken up by the teeth, the tongue forms a *bolus*, or ball of food, which it propels into the oropharynx. The dorsum of the tongue is covered by numerous minute projections, the papillae, which vary in shape and distribution. Taste buds may be present on any of the papillae but are most numerous at the base of the palate. The tongue of beef, veal, lamb, or pork is eaten as meat. Tongue is a nourishing and appetizing food, good hot or cold. A good source of protein, high in fat content, with a good amount of *iron*, fair *niacin*, and *riboflavin*. See *taste*.

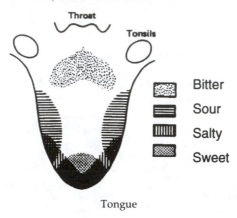

Tongue

tooth. See *teeth*.

Torulopsis. Round-to-oval, fermentative *yeasts* with multilateral budding cause trouble in breweries and spoil various foods. *T. sphaerica* ferments *lactose* and may spoil milk products. Other species can spoil sweetened condensed milk, fruit-juice concentrates, and acid foods.

toxic. Poisonous. Mutations, cancer, blindness, and liver damage are typical effects that can be caused by toxic materials. See *toxins* and *food poisoning*.

toxicity. The capacity of a chemical substance to harm living organisms. It is a general property of all matter; all substances are potentially toxic. Hazard is the capacity of a chemical to produce injury under conditions of use. Substances are hazardous only if normally consumed in quantities that can realistically be expected to cause harm. Most additives that involve risk are allowed in foods only at levels 100 times below those at which the harmful effect is known to be zero; their margin of safety is less than 1/100. In many foods, naturally occurring toxic substances may appear at a level that brings their margin of safety closer to 1/10. Even nutrients can involve risk at high dosage levels. The margin-of-safety concept also applies to nutrients when they are used as additives. Iodide (*iodine*) is added to salt to prevent iodine deficiency, but it has to be added with care because it is a deadly poison in excess. All substances can harm living things and all are hazardous when consumed in sufficiently excess quantities. See *food toxins*, and *vitamin toxicity*.

toxicity tests. (a) Acute toxicity tests reveal the effects of mammoth single doses of a chemical. Short-term toxicity tests reveal the effects of 30- to 180-day exposure to a substance with special attention usually given to liver and kidney function and blood composition. (c) Long-term toxicity tests last the lifetime of an animal (2 years in rats or mice and 7 years in dogs).

These experiments are the only kind that can reveal whether a chemical causes cancer or chronic effects. (d) Other special tests are designed to detect interference with reproduction and causation of birth defects or mutations.

toxins. Poisonous materials produced by plants or microorganisms. See *food poisoning* and *food toxins*.

trace elements. Those elements necessary in the diet in trace amounts, less than 100 g per day in humans. Among the trace elements, the range of requirements runs from milligram quantities for iron, zinc, and manganese down to microgram quantities for some of the newly discovered micronutrient elements such as *selenium, chromium*, and *vandium*. A combination total of only about 25–30 g of all trace elements (about 1 ounce) exists in the human body. There is no convenient single way to classify trace elements in nutrition because they vary so much in function, distribution, level of need, and chemical properties. The trace elements found in foods and nature are *iron, iodine, copper, manganese, zinc, fluorine, cobalt, molybdenum, selenium, chromium, nickel, tin, vanadium*, and *silicon*. Except for cobalt, all the trace elements are absorbed (or can be) in the inorganic form before being utilized by the body. Minerals present in organic forms in the food, in general, must be split off to the free inorganic form before absorption. Trace elements have no common biological role other than that they function in the body at the cellular levels, often as constituents of enzymes or an enzyme activator. Some of the trace elements have no known functions. See *minerals*.

trachea. The trachea, or windpipe, is a tube held open by cartilaginous tissue. It carries air from the larynx to the bronchi. The trachea is lined with cilia and numerous glands whose secretions provide a sticky film to keep dust and dirt out of the lungs.

tragacanth gum. A vegetable gum stabilizer that exhibits a resistance to acids which is unexcelled among vegetable gums. This property makes it the ideal *thickening agent* for foods such as vinegar-containing salad dressing. See *gums, agar, and carrageenans*.

tranquilizers (drugs). Drugs that have a sedative effect which is characterized by relief of neuromuscular tension and anxiety without producing sleep. An example is chlorpromazine hydrochloride. See *tyramine* and *food-drug interactions*.

transaminase. A class of enzymes that transfer amino ($-NH_2$) groups from one compound to another. The general reaction is as follows: The keto acid acceptors are transformed into the corresponding α-amino acids and the amino group donors become α-keto acids. Essential for these reactions is *pyridoxal phosphate* or *pyridoxamine phosphate*, the *coenzyme* forms of vitamin B_6. These reactions occur with all of the amino acids and their α-keto acid counterparts with the exception of the two essential amino acids *lysine* and *threonine*. The transaminases are specific for the amino acids and the α-keto acids. In certain diseases or abnormal conditions, the level of the transaminase activity in the blood increases and the level of certain transaminase activity is used as an aid in diagnosis, particularly in heart and liver pathologies. See *pyridoxine* (vitamin B_6) and *transamination*.

$$R_1-\overset{\overset{\displaystyle O}{\|}}{C}-COOH + R_2-\overset{\overset{\displaystyle NH_2}{|}}{CH}-COOH \underset{(B_6)}{\rightleftharpoons} R_1\overset{\overset{\displaystyle NH_2}{|}}{CH}-COOH + R_2-\overset{\overset{\displaystyle O}{\|}}{C}-COOH$$

Transaminase

transamination. The transferring of an amino group to another molecule, for example, transfer to a keto acid, thus forming another amino group. Amino acids produced by the digestion of a protein are absorbed through the intestinal wall into the blood and are transported to the liver. Certain of the amino acids are required by the cells for the synthesis of proteins, enzymes, certain hormones, and other nitrogen-containing substances. Body tissues are capable of synthesizing some amino acids (nonessential) by removing the required amino groups from other amino acids. The amino groups taken from one acid are transferred to an α-keto analogue of the amino acid to be synthesized. The transfer is called transamination. The enzymes that catalyze these reactions are called *transaminases*. Vitamin B_6 (*pyridoxine*) is a part of the coenzyme *pyridoxal phosphate* and is required for the transaminases to be active.

trans-fatty acids. The partial hydrogenation of vegetable oils transforms the fluids to solids or semisolids as in *margarine* production. In the chemical process of reducing the unsaturated double bonds, some of the unsaturated fatty acids are transformed from the *cis-* to the *trans*-isomer. Some investigations report associations of dietary trans-fatty acids and increased incidence of cardiovascular disease. See *cis-and trans-isomerism*.

transferase. An enzyme that transfers a chemical grouping from one compound to another, for example, *transaminases* transfer amino ($-NH_2$) groups and transphosphorylases transfer phosphate ($-H_2PO_4$) groups.

transferrin or siderophilin. An iron-binding protein that transports iron through blood. It is a beta (β) pseudoglobulin and occurs in blood at 0.4 mg per 100 mL of blood. Under normal conditions about 3 mg of iron is in the blood, which represents about 30% of the total transport capability of transferrin. The iron bound to transferrin must be in the oxidized state of ferric (Fe^{+3}). Ferrous (Fe^{+2}) iron will not bind. Within the cells, the iron is stored as an iron-protein complex called *hemosiderin*. The total iron in an adult male is about 700 milligrams.

***trans*-form**. The configuration of substituents around an unsaturated double bond of carbon. The opposite of the *cis*-form. See *cis- and trans-isomerism*.

transketolase. An enzyme that transfers two carbon units to other sugar intermediates. It requires the coenzyme *thiamine pyrophosphate* (TPP), which contains one of the B-complex vitamins, *thiamine* (vitamin B_1). Transketolase is necessary for the synthesis of *ribose* from *glucose*. Ribose is a five-carbon sugar required for the synthesis of the *nucleic acids, deoxyribonucleic acid* (DNA) and *ribonucleic acid* (RNA).

trehalose. A disaccharide composed of two *glucose* molecules joined at the *anomeric carbons*. It is therefore a nonreducing sugar. See *reducing sugar*. It is the principal sugar in insect blood (chemolymph). Trehalose is also present in some molds, fungi, and bacteria and is also known as "mushroom sugar." Normally only small amounts are ingested in the diet. Humans have trehalosase, an enzyme that hydrolyzes sugar.

trichinosis. An illness caused by eating raw, improperly cooked pork that is infested with *Trichinella spiralis*, a parasitic worm. Most human trichinosis results from the consumption of raw or incompletely cooked pork containing the encysted larvae. The larvae are released into the intestinal tract during digestion and invade the mucous membranes of the first part of the small intestine. Symptoms may resemble food poisoning and be followed by muscular pains, weakness, fever, and puffiness of tissues around the eyes and forehead.

triglyceride (fat, neutral fat, oil). A compound in which three *fatty acids* are esterified to a molecule of *glycerol*. The difference between a fat and an oil is that the oils contain a higher number of *unsaturated fatty acids*. Most natural triglycerides contain mixtures of fatty acids. If a triglyceride or *fat* contains only one type of fatty acid, it is named after the fatty acid; for example triolein (an oil) contains only *oleic acid* and tristearin contains only *stearic acid*. *Medium-chain triglycerides* (MCT) are used in treating various aspects of malabsorption syndromes—*sprue, steatorrhea, hyperlipoproteinemia*, among others. It has been established that medium-chain esters are absorbed by different pathways from conventional fats. Their rate of absorption and metabolism is rapid. They have a low tendency to be deposited as depot fat. It has been shown that chain lengths of C_{12} and above tend to be deposited as depot fat, but chain lengths of C_{10} and below do not. Such medium-chain triglycerides are saturated in nature, but they lower serum cholesterol levels much like the *polyunsaturated fatty acids* (oils). In animal studies, the medium-chain triglycerides demonstrate a low order of deposition of cholesterol in liver, arteries, and heart in contrast to the conventional fats and oils, saturated and unsaturated.

triiodothyronine. One of two forms of the principal hormone secreted by the thyroid gland. Chemically it is 3,5,3'-triiodothyronine (liothyronine). See *thyroxine*.

tripe. The inner lining of the stomach of beef. There are three kinds: honeycomb, pocket, and plain or smooth. Honeycomb is considered the most desirable. A good source of protein.

triphosphate. A salt or acid that contains three phosphate groups and is derived from a complex acid anhydride of orthophosphoric acid, similar to but larger than *pyrophosphate*.

triplet code. A trinucleotide. A sequence of three nucleotides in *deoxyribonucleic acid* (DNA) or *messenger-ribonucleic acid* (mRNA) that encodes an amino acid into proteins. Since there are four different nucleotides in DNA and in mRNA, there are 64 different triplet codes. This means that several of the 20 amino acids are coded for by more than one triplet. The message contained in a sequence of bases in a DNA molecule is transmitted in terms of three bases at a time, a "triplet." Each triplet calls for a particular amino acid to be incorporated into the protein for the message coded. Four different bases make up DNA molecules, and each base in each triplet can be any combination. The table shows the standard genetic code. See *deoxyribonucleic acid* and *ribonucleic acids*.

Standard triplet genetic code

CODE	AMINO ACID	CODE	AMINO ACID	CODE	AMINO ACID	CODE	AMINO ACID
UUU	Phe	UCU	Ser	UAU	Tyr	UGU	Cys
UUC	Phe	UCC	Ser	UAC	Tyr	UGC	Cys
UUA	Leu	UCA	Ser	UAA	Stop	UGA	Stop
UUG	Leu	UCG	Ser	UAG	Stop	UGG	Trp
CUU	Leu	CCU	Pro	CAU	His	CGU	Arg
CUC	Leu	CCC	Pro	CAC	His	CGC	Arg
CUA	Leu	CCA	Pro	CAA	Gln	CGA	Arg
CUG	Leu	CCG	Pro	CAG	Gln	CGG	Arg
AUU	Ile	ACU	Thr	AAU	Asn	AGU	Ser
AUC	Ile	ACC	Thr	AAC	Asn	AGC	Ser
AUA	Ile	ACA	Thr	AAA	Lys	AGA	Arg
AUG	Met	ACG	Thr	AAG	Lys	AGG	Arg
GUU	Val	GCU	Ala	GAU	Asp	GGU	Gly
GUC	Val	GCC	Ala	GAC	Asp	GGC	Gly
GUA	Val	GCA	Ala	GAA	Glu	GGA	Gly
GUG	Val	GCG	Ala	GAG	Glu	GGG	Gly

AUG is part of the initiation signal and the codon for internal methionine.

trout (*Salmo*). The name given to a large group of fishes of the family *Salmonidae*. Although most varieties are freshwater fish, a few, such as the sea trout and some of the rainbow trout, live in the sea and ascend rivers to breed. Trout vary greatly in size and coloration according to their environment. Among the most widely known are the rainbow trout (*Salmo gairdneri*), the brook or speckled trout (*Salvelinus fontinalis*), the steelhead, or salmon-trout, which is a variety of the rainbow trout; the cutthroat trout (*Salmo clarkii*) and the Dolly Varden.

trypsin. One of the first enzymes to be discovered. It has a molecular weight of about 24,000 daltons. It digests protein—for example, meat—in the small intestine. Trypsin is formed initially in the pancreas in an inactive or zymogen form as *trypsinogen*. Trypsin hydrolyzes proteins in much the same way as *chymotrypsin*, another digestive enzyme, because both compounds contain many of the same amino acids including histidine and serine in their active sites. Trypsin is highly specialized and will hydrolyze the peptide bonds at the amino acids *lysine* and *arginine*, the basic amino acid. The specificity of chymotrypsin is for *phenylalanine* and *tyrosine*, the aromatic amino acids. Trypsin also has the important function of activating chymotrypsinogen to chymotrypsin and of activating all other *zymogen* forms of the proteolytic enzymes of digestion. Trypsin itself is activated from trypsinogen by the intestinal enzyme *enterokinase*.

trypsinogen. An inactive form, a *zymogen*, of trypsin synthesized in the pancreas. During the digestive process, an enzyme, *enterokinase*, is released by the intestinal mucosa. Enterokinase removes a hexapeptide (six amino acids) from trypsinogen and it becomes active trypsin. See *trypsin* and *zymogen*.

tryptophan (Trp, W). Mol. Wt. 204. An *essential amino acid*. A constituent of body proteins, a precursor of the vitamin *niacin* and of the vasoconstrictor *serotonin*. Animal protein contains approximately 1.4% and vegetable protein 1% tryptophan. An average daily diet may provide 500–1000 mg tryptophan. The dietary tryptophan available over and above the body's requirement may be converted to niacin in a proportion of 60 mg tryptophan to 1 mg niacin.

$$CH_2-CH-COOH$$
$$NH_2$$

Tryptophan (Trp, W)

tubules. See *nephron* and *glomerulus*.

tularemia (tick fever, rabbit fever). A disease contracted by hunting and killing infected animals which are cleaned and not cooked properly; by being bitten by a blood-sucking fly or by a tick; or by drinking contaminated water. There are several types. Skin lesions such as red spots, little boils, and red lumps may appear anywhere on the body. The disease may be superficial with a small lump at the site of the cut, or an enlargement of lymph nodes regional to the cut and possible suppuration of nodes. Commonly begins suddenly with a headache, chills, fever, and prostration. Streptomycin, chloramphenicol, and the tetracycline antibiotics have been found effective in treatment.

tuna (*Thunnus*). A saltwater game fish belonging to the mackerel family. Tuna is found in almost all the seas of the temperate and warm zones of Asia, Africa, and America. In some parts of the world it can reach weights up to 1500 pounds. There are several varieties, including the albacore, bluefin, skipjack, and yellowfin. A good source of protein. Fresh, raw, 100 g = 145 calories; canned in oil, solids and liquid, 100 g = 288 calories; canned in water, solids and liquid, 100 g = 127 calories. See this item in the table under *fish*.

turkey. A native American game bird which is related to the pheasant. A good source of protein. See this item in the table under *poultry*.

turmeric. The irregularly shaped root of a tropical plant which is related to ginger. When washed, cooked, and then dried, the turmeric root has a mild aroma and a mustardlike, bitter taste. One of its characteristics is the brilliant gold color it adds to the dishes in which it is used. Turmeric is used in prepared mustards and is always present in curry powder. Turmeric flavors and colors curried meat, poultry, fish, and shellfish, deviled and creamed eggs, chicken, fish, shellfish, and egg, chicken, or potato salads.

turnip (*Brassica*). A root vegetable. There are several varieties. The flesh varies in texture; the finer-fleshed turnips are eaten as a vegetable and the coarser ones are fed to livestock. Turnips are white-fleshed. Some varieties have purple tops. Turnip tops are eaten as greens and are used for forage. The greens are an excellent source of *ascorbic acid* (vitamin C) and *carotene* (vitamin A activity), and a good source of calcium, iron, and riboflavin.

tyramine. Mol. Wt. 137. Tyramine is formed by the *decarboxylation* of *tyrosine* and is found in significant concentration in some foods. Its specific function is not known. Tyramine is a powerful vasopressor normally inactivated by the action of the enzyme *monoamine oxidase* (MAO).

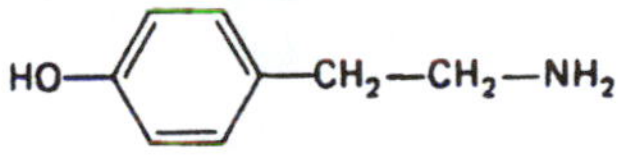

$$HO-\langle\rangle-CH_2-CH_2-NH_2$$

Tyramine

tyramine toxicity. Certain antidepressants such as isocarboxazid and phenelzine sulfate are enzyme inhibitors of monoamine oxidases (MAO) and therefore can be responsible for adverse

Tyramine in foods

Food	Tyramine mg/100 gms	Food	Tyramine mg/100 gms
Cheeses[a]		Meats	
Brie	18	Beef livers	0.5
Camembert	9	Chicken livers	0.05
Cheddar	141	Pickled herring	303
Ermanthaler	23	Other Possible Agents[b]	
Gruyère	52	Banana	
Alcoholic beverages		Cola	
Beer[a]	0.3	Coffee	
Chianti	2.5	Pineapples	
Sherry	0.4	Yeast extracts	
		Yogurt	

[a]Actual content will vary with various brands.
[b]Although the content is considered significant definitive data is not available.

food-drug interactions. Since some antidepressants inhibit MAO, they interfere with the metabolism of tyramine, and the ingestion of foods high in tyramine may lead to headaches, nausea, and hypertension. A glass of chianti or an ounce of cheese have sufficient tyramine to cause the toxic effects. Shown on page 433 is a list of foods that have significantly high concentrations of tyramine. See *food toxins* and *food-drug interactions*.

tyrosine (Tyr, Y). Mol. Wt. 181. A nonessential *amino acid* found in proteins that can be formed from the *essential amino acid phenylalanine*. Tyrosine has a "sparing" effect on phenylalanine since the presence of tyrosine in the diet decreases the amount of phenylalanine required, but can never totally replace it. Tyrosine (and therefore phenylalanine) is a precursor to the pigment *melanin*, and to *ubiquinone*, and *tyramine*.

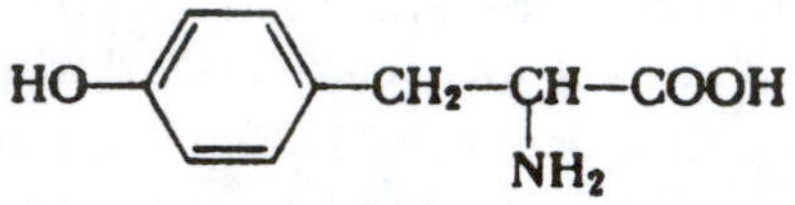

$$HO-\underset{}{\bigcirc}-CH_2-\underset{\underset{NH_2}{|}}{CH}-COOH$$

Tyrosine (Tyr, Y)

U

ubiquinone (coenzyme Q). An electron carrier in the *terminal respiratory chain*. It functions as one of a series of electron carriers in a sequential arrangement that transports electrons from foodstuffs to oxygen to form water. Ubiquinone has an isoprene side chain similar to *retinol* (vitamin A), *tocopherol* (vitamin E), and *vitamin K*. Ubiquinone occurs in the mitochondria and in the microsomes.

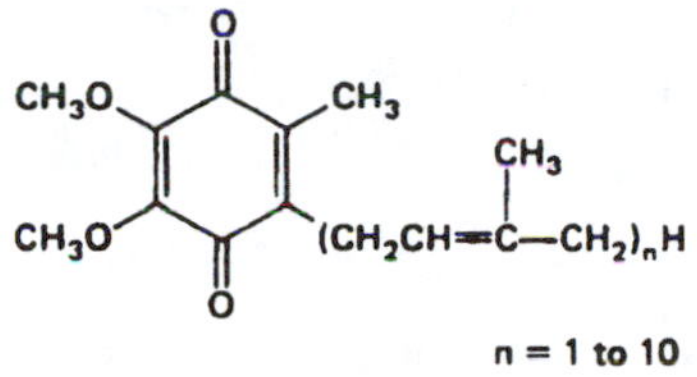

$n = 1$ to 10

Ubiquinone

ulcerative colitis. A digestive disease characterized by an inflammation, with the formation of *ulcers* in the mucosa of the colon. A digestive disorder of unknown cause which produces severe, bloody diarrhea, accompanied by fever and weight loss. Treatment consists of a bland diet, sedatives, sulfa drugs to reduce the number of bacteria in the large bowel, and drugs to reduce diarrhea.

ulcers. A *peptic ulcer* is an open lesion on the mucosa of the stomach or small intestine. When the ulcer is located in the stomach it is called a gastric ulcer; if it is located in the upper third of the small intestine, it is called a duodenal ulcer. The ulcerated area is thought to be the result of digestion of the membranous lining of the stomach or small intestine by the *gastric juices*.

ultratrace elements. See *nutrient*.

unit pattern (functional pattern). The smallest aggregate of cells which, when repeated many times, composes an organ. If the liver is studied in this way, it will be seen that the lobules (smallest macroscopic units) are composed of chains of cells with their definite supply paths of blood and lymph and bile capillaries.

unsaturated fatty acid. A *fatty acid* that has a double bond between the two carbon atoms at one or more places in the carbon chain. Examples are *oleic acid*, *linoleic acid*, and *arachidonic* *acid*. An unsaturated fat is one that contains an unsaturated fatty acid. A saturated fatty acid has no double bonds. Unsaturated fatty acids are also classified into families based on their first unsaturated carbon counting from the methyl or neutral end of the molecule. The table gives a few examples. See *oleic acid*, *saturated fatty acid*, and *lipids, classification*.

Chief sources of unsaturated fatty acids[a] in 100 g food

FOOD	% LINOLEIC ACID	% SATURATED FATTY ACID	% OLEIC ACID
Oils and fats			
Butter	2	46[b]	27
Corn	53	10	28
Cottonseed	50	25	21
Olive	7	11	76
Peanut	29	18	47
Safflower	72	8	15
Sesame	45	14	38
Soybean	52	15	20
Nuts			
Almonds	11	4	36
Brazil nuts	8	6	15
Filberts	10	3	34
Peanuts	14	11	21
Pecans	14	5	45
Pistachio	10	5	35
Walnut	40	4	10
Miscellaneous			
Chicken	1	1	1
Chick peas	2	0	2
Cornmeal	2	0	1
Margarine, liquid oil	22	15	42
Margarine, hydrogenated oil	14	18	47
Peanut butter	14	9	25
Sesame seeds	21	7	19
Sunflower seeds	30	6	9
Wheat germ	5	2	3

[a]Linoleic acid constitutes nearly all of the polyunsaturated fatty acid present. Oleic acid is monounsaturated.

[b]About 44% of this is in the form of short-chain fatty acids which are incorporated into human phospholipid.

From *Nutritive Value of American Foods in Common Units*, Agriculture Handbook No. 456, Washington, D.C., U.S. Department of Agriculture, 1975.

uracil. A *pyrimidine* base found in *ribonucleic acids*. It is the base portion of *uridine triphosphate* (UTP).

urea. Mol. Wt. 60. The major nitrogenous constituent of urine, representing between 60–90% of the total nitrogen excreted in a 24-hour period. The amount of urea excreted is proportional to the protein ingested. Protein is not completely oxidized to carbon dioxide, water, and energy, and the urea represents an end-product of that incomplete oxidation. The two nitrogen atoms are derived from aspartic acid that has been transferred (transamination) from other amino acids and ammonia in reactions of the *urea cycle*. The g urea nitrogen in a 24-hour urine collection when multiplied by the factor 6.25 g of protein per g of nitrogen yields the g of protein oxidized for that time period. See *urine*.

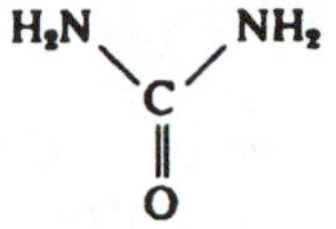

Urea

urea cycle. The biochemical series of reactions that leads to the production of urea. It is called a cycle because the amino acid *ornithine* is continually regenerated to continue the reaction series. The enzymes that constitute the cycle are partly in the *mitochondria* and partly in the *cytosol*. The series of reactions of the urea cycle are as shown.

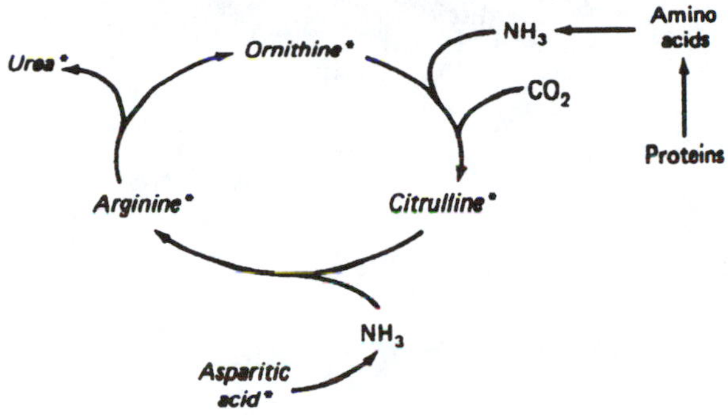

Urea cycle

urease. The first enzyme to be crystallized. It converts *urea* into ammonia and carbon dioxide.

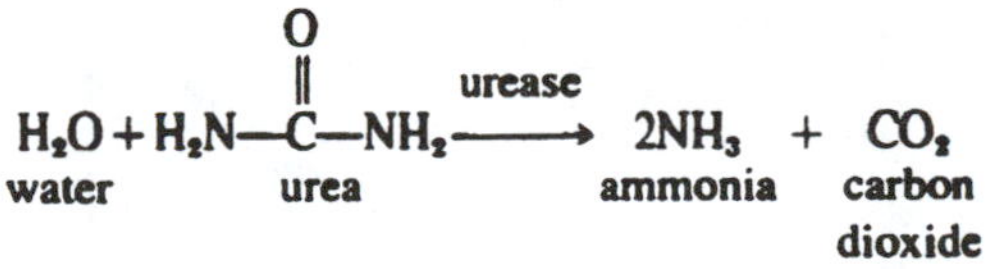

$$H_2O + H_2N-\overset{\overset{\displaystyle O}{\|}}{C}-NH_2 \xrightarrow{\text{urease}} 2NH_3 + CO_2$$

water   urea   ammonia   carbon
dioxide

Urease

uremia. Progressive degenerative changes in renal tissue bringing marked depression of kidney function. Few functioning *nephrons* remain, and these gradually deteriorate. Uremia is the term given to the symptom complex of adrenal renal insufficiency. Although the name derives from the common finding of elevated blood *urea* levels, the symptoms result not so much from urea concentrations as from disturbances in *acid-base balance* and in fluid and electrolyte metabolism and from accumulation of other obscure toxic substances not clearly defined.

ureters. The pelvis of each *kidney* is drained by a ureter, a muscular tube extending from the hilus to the posterior portion of the urinary bladder. Ureters are smooth muscles and structures, and urine is passed through each ureter by *peristalsis*. Drop by drop, urine passes into the urinary bladder. Ureters are about 15–18 inches in length and about ⅕ inch in diameter.

urethra. A canal for the discharge of urine extending from the bladder to the outside. See *urinary system*.

uric acid. Mol. Wt. 168. An acid found in *urine*, derived from the metabolism of *purines*. A chemical compound that contains nitrogen and is present in small amounts in the urine, the equivalent of 80–200 mg of urinary nitrogen in a 24-hour period. Uric acid stones occur in individuals who have an increased level of uric acid in the blood (hyperuricemia) and increased urinary excretion of uric acid. They may or may not be accompanied by symptoms of *gout*. Since uric acid is an end-product of purine metabolism, foods with a high purine content are voided. The precipitation of uric acid crystals in the urinary tract occurs most readily at a low urinary pH.

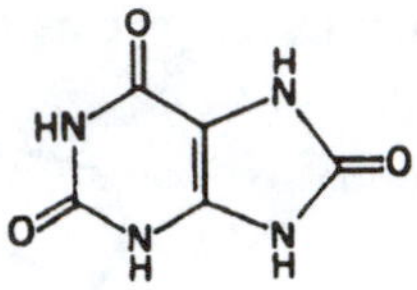

Uric acid

uridine diphosphate (UDP). See *uridine triphosphate*.

uridine monophosphate (UMP). See *uridine triphosphate*.

uridine triphosphate (UTP). Mol. Wt. 484. A high-energy phosphate compound. It is a pyrimidine nucleotide which is energetically equivalent to *adenosine triphosphate* (ATP). The synthesis of animal starch (*glycogen*) depends upon the formation of sugar derivatives of UDP. For example, the reaction that adds a *glucose* molecule to glycogen, (glucose)$_n$, is as shown:

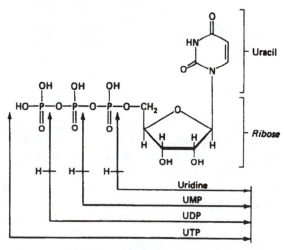

Uridine triphosphate (UTP)

$$\text{UDP-Glucose} + (\text{glucose})_n \xrightarrow[\text{synthetase}]{\text{glycogen}} (\text{glucose})_{n+1} + \text{UDP}$$

Synthesis of glycogen

urinary bladder. A muscular sac located in the lowest part of the abdominal cavity which stores urine. Normally it holds 300–500 mL. The bladder is emptied by contraction of muscles in its walls, which forces urine out through the *urethra*. See *urinary system*.

urinary system. The system involving the *kidneys*, the *ureters*, the *urinary bladder*, arteries, veins, and the *urethra*. The purpose of the urinary system is to maintain a constant composition and volume of blood and to maintain its *acid-base balance*. About 1200 mL of blood flows through the kidneys in a minute. The urinary system is a glomerular filtration of the blood that also involves secretion and absorption of specific materials in the blood. About 125 mL per minute of filtrate(urine) produces, through reabsorption, a total of about 1800 mL of urine concentrate in 24 hours. The composition of urine is similar to plasma except that it contains no proteins or large colloidal particles or glucose under normal conditions. The control of the absorption and secretions of salts and others is a complex matter involving their concentrations and hormonal influences. The resorption of water is directly controlled by the *antidiuretic hormone* (ADH). The diagram shows the urinary system. See *urine, glomerulus,* and *nephron*.

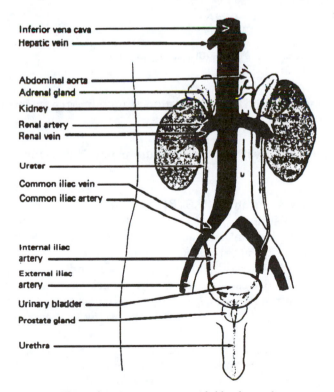

Inferior vena cava
Hepatic vein

Abdominal aorta
Adrenal gland
Kidney
Renal artery
Renal vein

Ureter

Common iliac vein
Common iliac artery

Internal iliac artery
External iliac artery
Urinary bladder
Prostate gland
Urethra

The male uringary system with blood vessels

urine. The filtrate of the urinary system. It amounts to about 1800 mL per day. The composition of urine varies depending upon composition of the diet. The table shows the components of urine and their normal ranges. *Uric acid* is an end-product of purine metabolism; *urea* is the result of protein (amino acid) oxidation; and *creatinine* is the end-product of *creatine phosphate*, a form of chemical energy in the muscles. See *urinary system* and *kidney*.

Composition of average 24-hr urine of a normal adult

COMPONENT	AMOUNT	MILLIEQUIVALENTS	U/P*
Sodium	21 g	100–200 meq	0.8–1.5
Potassium	1.5–2.0 g	35–50 meq	10–15
Magnesium	0.1–0.2 g	3–16 meq	
Calcium	0.1–0.3 g	2.5–7.5 meq	
Iron	0.2 mg		
Ammonia	0.4–1.0 g N	30–75 meq	
H$^+$	0.4–1.0 g N	4×10^{-8}–4×10^{-6} meq/L	1–100
Uric acid	0.03–0.2 g N		20
Amino acids	0.08–0.15 g N		
Hippuric acid	0.04–0.05 g N		
Chloride		10–250 meq	0.3–2
Bicarbonate		0–50 meq	0–2
Phosphate	0.7–1.6 g P	20–50 moles	25
Inorganic sulfate	0.6–1.8 g S	20–120 meq	50
Organic sulfates	0.06–0.2 g S		
Urea	6–18 g N		60
Creatinine	0.3–0.8 g N		70
Peptides	0.3–0.7 g N		

*U/P = ratio of concentration in urine (U) to that in plasma (P).

urobilin. A brain pigment formed by the oxidation of urobilinogen, a decomposition product of *bilirubin*.

urobilinogen. A colorless derivative of *bilirubin* from which it is formed by the action of intestinal bacteria.

U.S. Recommended Daily Allowances (U.S. RDA, FDA). The U.S. RDA were developed by the Food and Drug Administration (FDA) based on the recommendations of the Food and Nutrition Board. The table given in Appendix 8 contains mandatory nutrients and optional nutrients. The mandatory nutrients are protein, vitamin A (*retinol*), vitamin C (*ascorbic acid*), vitamin B, (*thiamine*), vitamin B$_2$ (*riboflavin*), *niacin*, *calcium*, and *iron* and are based upon the fact that human nutritional diseases are especially associated with deficiencies. Optional nutrients are *vitamin D*, vitamin E (α-*tocopherol*), vitamin B$_6$ (*pyridoxine*), vitamin B$_{12}$ (*cobalamin*), *phosphorous*, *iodine*, *magnesium*, *zinc*, *copper*, biotin, and *pantothenic acid*. See Appendix.

uterus. The uterus, shaped somewhat like a pear, is suspended in the pelvic cavity, supported between the bladder and the rectum by its system of eight ligaments. The normal position of the body of the uterus is anteflexion (bent forward over the bladder). The uterus is about 3 inches long and 3 inches thick at its widest part. It has a thick wall of smooth muscle and a relatively small inner cavity. During pregnancy it can increase about 20 times in size. The upper dome-shaped portion of the uterus is the fundus, the main part is the body, and the lower neck portion is the cervix. The cervix is a canal opening into the vagina. The inner lining of the uterus, the endometrium, undergoes periodic changes during the regular menstrual cycle to make the uterus ready to receive a fertilized ovum. If the ovum is not fertilized, the endometrium gets a message from hormone influences and sheds its surface cells and built-up secretions. Some of the extra blood supply, the surface cells, and uterine secretions are eliminated as menstrual flow.

V

V. The alphabetic symbol for the *essential amino acid valine* (Val).

vacuoles. Membranous sacs within the cytoplasm that contain water and dissolved substances. The cells of higher animals usually lack vacuoles. See *cell*.

valence. The power of an element or a radical to combine with (or to replace) other elements or radicals. Atoms of various elements combine in definite proportions. The valence number of an element is the number of atoms of hydrogen with which one atom of the element can combine or is equivalent.

valine (Val, V). Mol. Wt. 117. An essential amino acid. One of the amino acids found in proteins. It is classified as an aliphatic or neutral amino acid.

Valine (Val, V)

Valium®. See *diazepam*.

vanadium (V). Element No. 23. At. Wt. 51. It has been reported that vanadium reduces cholesterol production in humans. While vanadium is not yet known as an essential micronutrient for humans, it is essential in animals. It does have functions in the body, namely as a catalyst for activating enzymes that have to do with fat metabolism and certain nerve hormones called catecholamines. Vanadium is plentiful in certain foods such as seafood, soybeans, corn oil, and many vegetables.

vanilla. Any one of a group of tropical orchids. The cured seed pods of *Vanilla planifolia* contain an aromatic substance, also called vanilla, which is used as a flavoring substance. Vanillin is a crystalline compound found in vanilla pods or produced synthetically and used for flavoring foods and in pharmaceuticals.

varietal. Pertaining to differences between varieties of the same plants. Groups of plants within the same species may differ in certain characteristics. For example, different varieties of potatoes may contain widely differing levels of *ascorbic acid*. Such differences between varieties are known as varietal differences.

vascular. Full of vessels that contain a fluid. In physiology, the blood and lymph are the vessels in the body. Pertaining to or consisting of vessels.

vasoconstriction. The closing or decreased circumference of blood vessels—blood pressure is usually increased.

vasodilation. The opening up or increased circumference of blood vessels—blood pressure is usually reduced.

vasopressin. See *antidiuretic hormone.*

veal. Young beef 4–14 weeks of age. An excellent source of protein, iron, and *niacin*; a fair source of riboflavin. See this item in the table under *meats.*

vegetables. Plants cultivated for food. Some plants classified as vegetables are botanically classified under other names. For example, the tomato is really a fruit; peas and beans are seeds and are also classified as legumes; and mushrooms are fungi. Normally, vegetables include the leafy vegetables, such as spinach, lettuce, and cabbage; the stem vegetables, such as celery and asparagus; the roots and tubers, of which beets, turnips, carrots, and potatoes are examples; flower vegetables such as broccoli and cauliflower; seeds and seed pods, which include beans and peas (which are also classified under other names). Vegetables commonly include almost every part of the plant, including leaves, stems, roots, bulbs, tubers, flowers, and seeds. Mature seeds of the grasses make up the cereal group, and those of the leguminous plants make up the peas and beans. The amounts commonly consumed are not important energy-yielding foods; however, their less digestible carbohydrates (hemicellulosis and cellulose fiber) provide sufficient roughage for a normal diet. Their protein is generally of high quality though not abundant in quantity. The value of leafy vegetables lies primarily in their vitamin and mineral content. Most vegetable leaves are rich sources of *carotene* (vitamin A activity) and good sources of iron, calcium, *riboflavin*, and *folacin*. The greener the leaf, the higher the carotene content. Carotene (provitamin A) from leafy green vegetables is more readily absorbed and utilized than that from yellow ones. Fresh vegetable leaves are also good sources of *ascorbic acid* (vitamin C). The table on pages 444–449 lists the nutrient content of some common vegetables. See Appendix 9 for nutrient contents.

vegetarism. Vegetarism is the consumption of a diet composed predominantly of plant foods. Reasons for being a vegetarian are generally philosophic, religious, cultural, or health. Vegetarians are classified into several overlapping groups. Ovolacto-vegetarians use milk, milk products, and eggs, but do not eat meat, poultry, or fish. Lacto-vegetarians use milk and milk products, but exclude eggs, meat, poultry, and fish. Vegans are strict vegetarians who use no product of animal origin. Ovovegetarians eat eggs but no other animal products. Fruitarians eat chiefly fruits and nuts. Some who call themselves vegetarians eat fish and chicken, but exclude red meat. There is a wide variation in the extent to which meat and dairy products are excluded from these diets, ranging from the highest Zen macrobiotic diet, made up exclusively of cereals, to those that, while eliminating animal meat, do include animal products. The most popular of the "vegetarian diets" contain plant foods supplemented with dairy products.

One generalization which can be made about dietary deficiency is that the risk is greatest when a vegan diet is combined with additional self-imposed limitations. Such limitations

Food, Approximate Measure, and Weight (in grams)	Grams	Water percent	Food Energy calories	Protein grams	Fat grams
Vegetables and Vegetable Products					
Asparagus, green:					
Cooked, drained:					
Spears, ½-in. diam. at base — 4 spears	60	94	10	1	Trace
Pieces, 1½ to 2-in. lengths — 1 cup	145	94	30	3	Trace
Canned, solids and liquid — 1 cup	244	94	45	5	1
Beans:					
Lima, immature seeds, cooked, drained — 1 cup	170	71	190	13	1
Snap:					
Green:					
Cooked, drained — 1 cup	125	92	30	2	Trace
Canned, solids and liquid — 1 cup	239	94	45	2	Trace
Yellow or wax:					
Cooked, drained — 1 cup	125	93	30	2	Trace
Canned, solids and liquid — 1 cup	239	94	45	2	1
Sprouted mung beans, cooked, drained — 1 cup	125	91	35	4	Trace
Beets:					
Cooked, drained, peeled:					
Whole beets, 2-in. diam. — 2 beets	100	91	30	1	Trace
Diced or sliced — 1 cup	170	91	55	2	Trace
Canned, solids and liquid — 1 cup	246	90	85	2	Trace
Beet greens, leaves and stems, cooked, drained — 1 cup	145	94	25	3	Trace
Blackeye peas. See Cowpeas					
Broccoli, cooked, drained:					
Whole stalks, medium size — 1 stalk	180	91	45	6	1
Stalks cut into ½-in. pieces — 1 cup	155	91	40	5	1
Chopped, yield from 10-oz. frozen pkg. — 1⅜ cups	250	92	65	7	1
Brussels sprouts, 7–8 sprouts (1¼ to 1½ in. diam.) per cup, cooked — 1 cup	155	88	55	7	1
Cabbage:					
Common varieties:					
Raw:					
Coarsely shredded or sliced — 1 cup	70	92	15	1	Trace
Finely shredded or chopped — 1 cup	90	92	20	1	Trace
Cooked — 1 cup	145	94	30	2	Trace
Red raw, coarsely shredded — 1 cup	70	90	20	1	Trace
Savoy, raw coarsely shredded — 1 cup	70	92	15	2	Trace
Cabbage, celery or Chinese raw — 1 cup	75	95	10	1	Trace
Cabbage, spoon (or pakchoy), cooked — 1 cup	170	95	25	2	Trace
Carrots:					
Raw:					
Whole, 5½ by 1 inch, (25 thin strips) — 1 carrot	50	88	20	1	Trace
Grated — 1 cup	110	88	45	1	Trace
Cooked, diced — 1 cup	145	91	45	1	Trace
Canned, strained or chopped (baby food) — 1 ounce	28	92	10	Trace	Trace
Cauliflower, cooked, flowerbuds — 1 cup	120	93	25	3	Trace

Saturated (Total) Grams	Oleic Grams	Linoleic Grams	Carbohydrate Grams	Calcium Milligrams	Iron Milligrams	Vitamin A Value International Units	Thiamine Milligrams	Riboflavin Milligrams	Niacin Milligrams	Ascorbic Acid Milligrams
—	—	—	2	13	0.4	540	0.10	0.11	0.8	16
—	—	—	5	30	0.9	1,310	0.23	0.26	2.0	38
—	—	—	7	44	4.1	1,240	0.15	0.22	2.0	37
—	—	—	34	80	4.3	480	0.31	0.17	2.2	29
—	—	—	7	63	0.8	680	0.09	0.11	0.6	15
—	—	—	10	81	2.9	690	0.07	0.10	0.7	10
—	—	—	6	63	0.8	290	0.09	0.11	0.6	16
—	—	—	10	81	2.9	140	0.07	0.10	0.7	12
—	—	—	7	21	1.1	30	0.11	0.13	0.9	8
—	—	—	7	14	0.5	20	0.03	0.04	0.3	6
—	—	—	12	24	0.9	30	0.05	0.07	0.5	10
—	—	—	19	34	1.5	20	0.02	0.05	0.2	7
—	—	—	5	144	2.8	7,400	0.10	0.22	0.4	22
—	—	—	8	158	1.4	4,500	0.16	0.36	1.4	162
—	—	—	7	136	1.2	3,880	0.14	0.31	1.2	140
—	—	—	12	135	1.8	6,500	0.15	0.30	1.3	143
—	—	—	10	50	1.7	810	0.12	0.22	1.2	135
—	—	—	4	34	0.3	90	0.04	0.04	0.2	33
—	—	—	5	44	0.4	120	0.05	0.05	0.3	42
—	—	—	6	64	0.4	190	0.06	0.06	0.4	48
—	—	—	5	29	0.6	30	0.06	0.04	0.3	43
—	—	—	3	47	0.6	140	0.04	0.06	0.2	39
—	—	—	2	32	0.5	110	0.04	0.03	0.5	19
—	—	—	4	252	1.0	5,270	0.07	0.14	1.2	26
—	—	—	5	18	0.4	5,500	0.03	0.03	0.3	4
—	—	—	11	41	0.8	12,100	0.06	0.06	0.7	9
—	—	—	10	48	0.9	15,220	0.08	0.07	0.7	9
—	—	—	2	7	0.1	3,690	0.01	0.01	0.1	1
—	—	—	5	25	0.8	70	0.11	0.10	0.7	66

Food, Approximate Measure, and Weight (in grams)		Grams	Water Percent	Food Energy Calories	Protein Grams	Fat Grams
Celery, raw:						
Stalk, large outer, 8 by about 1½ inches, at root end	1 stalk	40	94	5	Trace	Trace
Pieces, diced	1 cup	100	94	15	1	Trace
Collards, cooked	1 cup	190	91	55	5	1
Corn sweet:						
Cooked, ear 5 by 1¾ inches	1 ear	140	74	70	3	1
Canned, solids and liquid	1 cup	256	81	170	5	2
Cowpeas, cooked immature seeds	1 cup	160	72	175	13	1
Cucumbers, 10-ounce; 7½ by about 2 inches:						
Raw, pared	1 cucumber	207	96	30	1	Trace
Raw, pared, center slice ⅛-inch thick	6 slices	50	96	5	Trace	Trace
Dandelion greens, cooked	1 cup	180	90	60	4	1
Endive, curly (including escarole)	2 ounces	57	93	10	1	Trace
Kale, leaves, including stems, cooked	1 cup	110	91	30	4	1
Lettuce, raw:						
Butterhead, as Boston types: head, 4-inch diameter	1 head	220	95	30	3	Trace
Crisphead, as Iceberg; head, 4¾ inch diameter	1 head	454	96	60	4	Trace
Looseleaf, or bunching varieties, leaves	2 large	50	94	10	1	Trace
Mushrooms, canned, solids and liquid	1 cup	244	93	40	5	Trace
Mustard greens, cooked	1 cup	140	93	35	3	1
Okra, cooked, pod 3 by ⅝ inch	8 pods	85	91	25	2	Trace
Onions:						
Mature:						
Raw, onion 2½-inch diameter	1 onion	110	89	40	2	Trace
Cooked	1 cup	210	92	60	3	Trace
Young green, small, without tops	6 onions	50	88	20	1	Trace
Parsley, raw, chopped	1 tablespoon	4	85	Trace	Trace	Trace
Parsnips, cooked	1 cup	155	82	100	2	1
Peas, green:						
Cooked	1 cup	160	82	115	9	1
Canned, solids and liquid	1 cup	249	83	165	9	1
Canned, strained (baby food)	1 ounce	28	86	15	1	Trace
Peppers, hot, red, without seeds, dried (ground chili powder, added seasonings)	1 tablespoon	15	8	50	2	2
Peppers, sweet:						
Raw, about 5 per pound:						
Green pod without stem and seeds	1 pod	74	93	15	1	Trace
Cooked, boiled, drained	1 pod	73	95	15	1	Trace
Potatoes, medium (about 3 per pound raw):						
Baked, peeled after baking	1 potato	99	75	90	3	Trace
Boiled:						
Peeled after boiling	1 potato	136	80	105	3	Trace
Peeled before boiling	1 potato	122	83	80	2	Trace

Fatty Acids										
	Unsaturated									
Saturated (Total) Grams	Oleic Grams	Linoleic Grams	Carbo-hydrate Grams	Calcium Milli-grams	Iron Milli-grams	Vitamin A Value International Units	Thiamine Milli-grams	Riboflavin Milli-grams	Niacin Milli-grams	Ascorbic Acid Milli-grams
—	—	—	2	16	0.1	100	0.01	0.01	0.1	4
—	—	—	4	39	0.3	240	0.03	0.03	0.3	9
—	—	—	9	289	1.1	10,260	0.27	0.37	2.4	87
—	—	—	16	2	0.5	6310	0.09	0.08	1.0	7
—	—	—	40	10	1.0	6690	0.07	0.12	2.3	13
—	—	—	29	38	3.4	560	0.49	0.18	2.3	28
—	—	—	7	35	0.6	Trace	0.07	0.09	0.4	23
—	—	—	2	8	0.2	Trace	0.02	0.02	0.1	6
—	—	—	12	252	3.2	21,060	0.24	0.29	—	32
—	—	—	2	46	1.0	1,870	0.04	0.08	0.3	6
—	—	—	4	147	1.3	8,140	—	—	—	68
—	—	—	6	77	4.4	2,130	0.14	0.13	0.6	18
—	—	—	13	91	2.3	1,500	0.29	0.27	1.3	29
—	—	—	2	34	0.7	950	0.03	0.04	0.2	9
—	—	—	6	15	1.2	Trace	0.04	0.60	4.8	4
—	—	—	6	193	2.5	8,120	0.11	0.19	0.9	68
—	—	—	5	78	0.4	420	0.11	0.15	0.8	17
—	—	—	10	30	0.6	40	0.04	0.04	0.2	11
—	—	—	14	50	0.8	80	0.06	0.06	0.4	14
—	—	—	5	20	0.3	Trace	0.02	0.02	0.2	12
—	—	—	Trace	8	0.2	340	Trace	0.01	Trace	7
—	—	—	23	70	0.9	50	0.11	0.12	0.2	16
—	—	—	19	37	2.9	860	0.44	0.17	3.7	33
—	—	—	31	50	4.2	1,120	0.23	0.13	2.2	22
—	—	—	3	3	0.4	140	0.02	0.02	0.4	3
—	—	—	8	40	2.3	9,750	0.03	0.17	1.3	2
—	—	—	4	7	0.5	310	0.06	0.06	0.4	94
—	—	—	3	7	0.4	310	0.05	0.05	0.4	70
—	—	—	21	9	0.7	Trace	0.10	0.04	1.7	20
—	—	—	23	10	0.8	Trace	0.13	0.05	2.0	22
—	—	—	18	7	0.6	Trace	0.11	0.04	1.4	20

Food, Approximate Measure, and Weight (in grams)		Grams	Water Percent	Food Energy Calories	Protein Grams	Fat Grams
Potatoes, medium (about 3 per pound raw):						
French-fried, piece 2 by ½ by ½ inch:						
Cooked in deep fat	10 pieces	57	45	155	2	7
Frozen, heated	10 pieces	57	53	125	2	5
Mashed:						
Milk added	1 cup	195	83	125	4	1
Milk and butter added	1 cup	195	80	185	4	8
Potato chips, medium, 2-inch diameter	10 chips	20	2	115	1	8
Pumpkin, canned	1 cup	228	90	75	2	1
Radishes, raw, small, without tops	4 radishes	40	94	5	Trace	Trace
Sauerkraut, canned, solids and liquid	1 cup	235	93	45	2	Trace
Spinach:						
Cooked	1 cup	180	92	40	5	1
Canned, drained solids	1 cup	180	91	45	5	1
Squash:						
Cooked:						
Summer, diced	1 cup	210	96	30	2	Trace
Winter, baked, mashed	1 cup	205	81	130	4	1
Sweet potatoes:						
Cooked, medium, 5 by 2 inches, weight raw about 6 ounces:						
Baked, peeled after baking	1 sweetpotato	110	64	155	2	1
Boiled, peeled after boiling	1 sweetpotato	147	71	170	2	1
Candied, 3½ by 2¼ inches	1 sweetpotato	175	60	295	2	6
Canned, vacuum or solid pack	1 cup	218	72	235	4	Trace
Tomatoes:						
Raw, approx. 3-in. diam. 2⅛ in. high; wt., 7 oz.	1 tomato	200	94	40	2	Trace
Canned, solids and liquid	1 cup	241	94	50	2	1
Tomato catsup:						
Cup	1 cup	273	69	290	6	1
Tablespoon	1 tbsp.	15	69	15	Trace	Trace
Tomato juice, canned:						
Cup	1 cup	243	94	45	2	Trace
Glass (6 fl oz.)	1 glass	182	94	35	2	Trace
Turnips, cooked, diced	1 cup	155	94	35	1	Trace
Turnips green, cooked	1 cup	145	94	30	3	Trace

Dashes in the columns for nutrients show that no suitable value could be found although there is reason to believe that a measurable amount of the nutrient may be present.

[1] Value applies to unfortified product; value for fortified low-density product would be 1500 I.U., and the fortified high-density product would be 2290 I.U.

include minimizing the variety of foods, avoiding fortified or enriched foods or appropriate vitamin-mineral supplements, and maintaining negative attitudes toward medicine. The basis for a good vegetarian diet should include a variety of plant foods, particularly those products which are rich in protein, B vitamins, iron, and fiber. Soy protein offers great potential and versatility because it can be formulated with other vegetable proteins to provide a very

| Fatty Acids | | | | | | | | | | |
| Saturated (Total) Grams | Unsaturated | | Carbo-hydrate Grams | Calcium Milli-grams | Iron Milli-grams | Vitamin A Value Interna-tional Units | Thiamine Milli-grams | Riboflavin Milli-grams | Niacin Milli-grams | Ascorbic Acid Milli-grams |
	Oleic Grams	Linoleic Grams								
2	2	4	20	9	0.7	Trace	0.07	0.04	1.8	12
1	1	2	19	5	1.0	Trace	0.08	0.01	1.5	12
—	—	—	25	47	0.8	50	0.16	0.10	2.0	19
4	3	Trace	24	47	0.8	330	0.16	0.10	1.9	18
2	2	4	10	8	0.4	Trace	0.04	0.01	1.0	3
—	—	—	18	57	0.9	14,590	0.07	0.12	1.3	12
—	—	—	1	12	0.4	Trace	0.01	0.01	0.1	10
—	—	—	9	85	1.2	120	0.07	0.09	0.4	33
—	—	—	6	167	4.0	14,580	0.13	0.25	1.0	50
—	—	—	6	212	4.7	14,400	0.03	0.21	0.6	24
—	—	—	7	52	0.8	820	0.10	0.16	1.6	21
—	—	—	32	57	1.6	8,610	0.10	0.27	1.4	27
—	—	—	36	44	1.0	8,910	0.10	0.07	0.7	24
—	—	—	39	47	1.0	11,610	0.13	0.09	0.9	25
2	3	1	60	65	1.6	11,030	0.10	0.08	0.8	17
—	—	—	54	54	1.7	17,000	0.10	0.10	1.4	30
—	—	—	9	24	0.9	1,640	0.11	0.07	1.3	[7]42
—	—	—	10	14	1.2	2,170	0.12	0.07	1.7	41
—	—	—	69	60	2.2	3,820	0.25	0.19	4.4	41
—	—	—	4	3	0.1	210	0.01	0.01	0.2	2
—	—	—	10	17	2.2	1,940	0.12	0.07	1.9	39
—	—	—	8	13	1.6	1,460	0.09	0.05	1.5	29
—	—	—	8	54	0.6	Trace	0.06	0.08	0.5	34
—	—	—	5	252	1.5	8,270	0.15	0.33	0.7	68

*Table 1, Nutritive Values of the Edible Parts of Foods, in *Nutritive Value of Foods*, Home and Garden Bulletin No. 72. United States Department of Agriculture, United States Government Printing Office, Washington, D.C., 1971.
[2]Contributed largely from beta-carotene used for coloring.

favorable essential amino acid composition of good *biological value* (BV). Many nutritionists emphasize the importance of obtaining a substantial part of protein needs from vegetable sources such as soybean products, lentils, peas, beans, and brown rice. Among meat eaters and vegetarians alike there is a high incidence of *iron deficiency anemia*, which is most likely to be seen among those who have the greatest iron needs—infants, young children, and pregnant women. Iron deficiency is probably slightly more common among vegetarians than the general public, especially those vegetarians who do not include iron-rich foods or iron supplements in their diets. *Ascorbic acid*, which is generally quite high in vegetarian diets, may help minimize iron deficiency by improving the bioavailability of plant iron. Vegetarians can suffer zinc deficiency because of low intake and the low bioavailability of plant zinc compared with animal food sources. The phytates (*phytic acid*) in whole grains may also make the zinc biochemically unavailable. Research on humans and animals shows that the blood *cholesterol* level is lower when vegetable protein is consumed than when the protein of animals is. Vegetable protein foods contain some vitamins (C and A) and minerals in greater amounts than most animal foods and provide an important fiber content. The following are several means by which the various degrees of vegetarian diets may be made nutritionally equivalent to a typical Western diet containing meat: (1) Substitute cheese, milk, and other dairy products (low fat) for meat, poultry, and fish in the diet. (2) A glass of low-fat or skim milk with an otherwise vegetarian meal will balance the plant protein eaten. (3) Combine vegetables so that the limited essential amino acid of one food complements the limited essential amino acid of the other food. Strict vegetarians, on the other hand, must be aware of the lack in their protein sources in order to balance their diets. For example, wheat is low in *lysine*, while corn is low in *tryptophan*. Combining the two to supply the protein at a meal, one can obtain the needed lysine from the corn and tryphtophan from the wheat. Vegans should also be aware that there is no plant source of the vitamin cobalamin (vitamin B_{12}) and that there are known instances where the health of newborns was compromised by the long-term strict vegetarian history of their mothers. The planning of a vegetarian diet is not difficult; it is the application of the basic concepts of good nutrition with a relatively few, but important, modifications. If one were to state the fundamental consideration, it would be to choose a wide variety of foods with a minimum number of refined products.

verbena *(Lippia citroidora)*. A perennial shrub varying greatly according to the conditions under which it is grown. The long, narrow, pointed leaves are yellow-green. Dried or fresh, the leaves have a lemony flavor and smell. They may be used to garnish fruit cups or fruit salads, or put into jellies. Lemon verbena tea is a popular herb tea.

very-low-density lipoproteins (VLDL). A class of lipoproteins that contain a greater ratio of triglycerides than low-density lipoproteins (LDL) and are the least dense lipoprotein fraction. See *lipoproteins*.

vesicles. Small bladders or bladderlike structures.

villikinin. A hormone produced by glands in the upper intestinal mucosa in response to the pressure of *chyme* entering the intestine. Villikinin stimulates alternating contractions and extensions of the villi (*villus*). This motion of the villi constantly agitates the mucosal surface, which stirs and mixes the chyme and exposes additional nutrient material for absorption.

villus. A fingerlike structure that is a part of the mucous membrane of the small *intestine* which serves to increase the efficiency of absorption of nutrients and excretion of mucous. Villi also occur in the placenta.

vinegar. Produced by the oxidation of *ethanol* to *acetic acid* by acetic acid bacteria. Any material that has undergone alcoholic fermentation can be used to produce vinegar: *wine*, fermented potatoes, or malt and cider. Vinegars are produced under aerobic conditions. Anaerobic conditions result in ethanol as an end-product, as in wines and beers. In vinegar, strength is considered as well as flavor. Vinegar's bite and sourness is in direct proportion to the amount of acetic acid in it, and a 4% vinegar will be far less pungent than one with 5% or higher. The term "40- or 50-grain strength" is used by some manufacturers instead, "grain" standing for 10 times the percent acetic acid content. The strength has no effect on the calorie count. One of the most universal of all foods, vinegar is an essential of characteristic dishes of many nations.

viosterol. A solution of irradiated *ergosterol* in oil, in which the active agent is *calciferol* (vitamin D₂).

visual purple. See *rhodopsin*. Photosensitive pigment found in the rods of the retina. Rhodopsin requires *retinol* (vitamin A) to be formed.

vitamins. Low-molecular-weight *organic* compounds required in the diet for the maintenance of good health or growth. Some dietary requirements fit this general description but are not classified as vitamins. The *essential fatty acids*, for example, were called vitamin F at one time, but the designation is no longer used, nor are they considered vitamins. Vitamins are not considered to be incorporated into the structure of the cell in general. However, since neither all of the functions nor all of the forms of all of the vitamins are presently known, some now designated as vitamins may have a structural function. Indeed, the designation of a compound as a vitamin is more of a historic classification than a highly selective category. In 1906, J. Gowland Hopkins of England showed that laboratory animals could not live on purified proteins, fats, and carbohydrates and concluded that small quantities of a vital substance were required in the diet. The vital substances or accessory factors were thought to be amines. In 1911, C. Funk called these vital amines "vitamines." Later, the "e" was dropped. The vitamins are generally classified according to their solubility, the "fat-soluble" and "water-soluble" vitamins. The use of the alphabet to designate the vitamins derives from work of McCollum and Davis at the University of Wisconsin, and Osborne and Mendel at Yale, who were isolating the factor that prevented the nutritional disease beriberi. It was recognized there were two factors in different fractions of separation procedures, a fat-soluble "fraction A" that prevented a nutritional eye disease, and a water-soluble "fraction B" that prevented beriberi. The water-soluble *antiscorbutic* factor, vitamin C (*ascorbic acid*), was recognized as distinct from the "fraction B," or vitamin B. It was soon determined that the fat-soluble A fraction contained two factors, one that prevented nutritional eye disease, vitamin A (*retinol*), and another (antirachitic) factor that prevented the nutritional disease *rickets*, *vitamin D*. The vitamin B fraction was found to be a complex of various substances, and as their structures were discovered they were given subscripts, for example, vitamin B₁, (*thiamine*), vitamin B₂ (*riboflavin*), vitamin B₆ (*pyridoxine*), and vitamin B₁₂ (*cobalamin*). The determination that these substances were vitamins occurred in laboratory animals. In humans, the avitaminoses of the water-soluble vitamins manifest themselves as *beriberi*, due to lack of thiamine; *pellagra* due to lack of niacin; *pernicious anemia*, due to lack of *cobalamin*, and *scurvy* due to lack of ascorbic acid. The avitaminoses of the fat-soluble vitamins manifest themselves as *nyctalopia* (night blindness) due to a lack of vitamin A (*retinol*); rickets due to a lack of vitamin D; and hemorrhage due to lack of *vitamin K*. No specific diseases or set of clinical symptoms in humans are associated with a lack of any of the other vitamins outside of experimental conditions. The

List of reported vitamins

vitamin A. See *retinol* A group of related vitamins

vitamin B₁. See *thiamine*.

vitamin B₂. See *riboflavin*. An obsolete term

vitamin B₃. Probably *pantothenic acid*. Necessary for growth in pigeons.

vitamin B₄. Possibly a mixture of *arginine, glycine, pryidoxine, and riboflavin*. Required in rats and chicks.

vitamin B₅. Possibly *niacin*. Needed or growth in pigeons.

vitamin B₆. See *pryidoxine*.

vitamin B₇ (vitamin I). A factor that prevents disturbances in digestion in pigeons.

vitamin B₈. *Adenylic acid* (AMP). This is not classified as a vitamin.

vitamin B₁₀. A factor for feather growth.

vitamin B₁₁. Probably vitamin B₁₂ (*cobalamin)* and *folacin*. A growth factor in chicks.

vitamin B₁₂. (colbalamin). See *folacin*.

vitamin B₁₃. An uncharacterized growth factor in rats.

vitamin B₁₄. No confirmation that vitamin B₁₄ exists.

vitamin B₁₅ (pangamic acid). Reported to facilitate oxygen uptake in rabbits.

vitamin B₁₇ (amygdalin, laetrile). See *amygdalin*.

vitamin B_c. Identical with *folacin*.

vitamin B_p. Replaceable by manganese and *choline* in chicks.

vitamin B_t (caritine). A growth factor in insects.

vitamin B_w. Identical with *biotin*.

vitamin B_x. Both *pantothenic acid* and *para-aminobenozic acid* have been given this designation.

vitamin B complex. As originally used, this term referred to the water-soluble vitamins occurring in yeast, liver, meats, and whole-grain cereals, but some of the newer B-complex vitamins, for example, *folacin* and vitamin B₁₂ (*cobalamin),* do not correspond to this distribution; includes a number of compounds which have been identified, isolated and synthesized; *thiamine, riboflavin, niacin, pyridoxine, pantothenic acid, biotin, folic acid (folacin), inositol,* and *choline*.

vitamin C. See *ascorbic acid*.

vitamin C₂ (vitamin J). A postulated antipneumonia factor.

vitamin D. See *vitamin D*.

vitamin E. See *tocopherols*.

vitamin F. An obsolete designation for the essential fatty acids, *linolenic, linokic,* and *arachidonic* acids. It was also once used for vitamin B₂ (*thiamine*).

vitamin G. An obsolete name for *riboflavin*.

vitamin H. An obsolete name for *biotin*.

vitamin I (vitamin B₇). A factor that prevents disturbances in digestion in pigeons.

vitamin J (vitamin C₂). A postulated antipeumonia factor.

vitamin K (phyloquinone, farnoquinone). See *vitamin K*.

vitamin L₁. Reported to be needed for lactation in rats.

vitamin L₂. Reported to be related to adenosine and necessary for lactation in rats.

vitamin M. An obsolete name for *folacin*.

vitamin N. A name given to extracts from the stomach and brain of animals that were reported to inhibit cancer. It is obsolete.

vitamin P (citrin). A group of bioflavinoids shown to prevent capillary fragility in animals under experimental condiitions. The flavinoids were extracted from lemon peel. The bioflavinoids are not considered vitamins.

vitamin R. A bacterial growth factor. Probably a derivative of the *folacin* group.

vitamin S. A bacterial growth factor. It is probably identical with *biotin*.

vitamin T. Reported to promote excessive growth in insects (termite factor) and to improve protein uptake in rats.

vitamin U. A bacterial growth factor. Probably a derivative of *folacin*.

vitamin V. A bacterial growth factor. Probably a derivative of *niacin, nicotinamide adenine dinucleotide* (NAD).

vitamin W. A bacterial growth factor. Probably *biotin*.

vitamin X. A bacterial growth factor. Probably *biotin*.

vitamin Y. Appears to be identical with *pyridoxine*.

---

division of the vitamins into the fat-soluble and water-soluble vitamins has more than historic significance. Certain generalities derive from the differences in solubility. In general, the fat-soluble vitamins are stored in the lipid deposits of the body, particularly in the liver. Because of their lack of solubility in water, the daily requirements for the fat-soluble vitamins are generally less stringent than for the water-soluble vitamins. In some instances, vitamins A and D, dosages can last up to several months. By the same token, in vitamin toxicity (hypervitaminosis) of the fat-soluble vitamins, the removal of the overload runs its course very slowly. The water-soluble vitamins must be replenished frequently because their solubility permits their excretion in *urine*. Exactly what is and what is not a vitamin is a source of confusion. Retinol, thiamine, pyridoxine, ascorbic acid, vitamin D, and vitamin K are definitely established vitamins in humans, and their lack in the diet leads to the associated diseases given above. All other vitamins have been demonstrated as necessary for human health under experimental conditions only, or have been demonstrated as necessary for the health of experimental animals. The extrapolations of the results in animals to humans must be done with caution. For example, vitamin C (*ascorbic acid*) is a dietary requirement for primates (humans), guinea pigs, and one species of fruit bat. All other animals are capable of the biosynthesis of ascorbic acid from *glucose*. An additional source of confusion related to the vitamins was the frequent reporting of vitamins that later proved to be combinations of known vitamins or were not determined to be vitamins in more than one species of animal. More than 50 vitamins have been reported. The trend is to designate vitamins by their chemical or generic name to circumvent the multiplicity and confusion of designations by alphabet and subscripts. See *fat-soluble vitamins* and *water-soluble vitamins*.

vitamin D. Vitamin D comprises a group of vitamin derivatives of calciferol which prevent rickets (antirachitic factors). The forms of vitamin D that are of therapeutic or nutritional importance are vitamin D_2 or ergocalciferol; vitamin D_3 or cholecalciferol; 25-hydrocholecalciferol (25 HCC); 1,25-dihydrocholecalciferol (DHCC); and 1,24,25-trihydroxycholecalciferol (THCC). All are structurally related to *cholesterol*. In addition to dietary sources for vitamin D, humans are able to biosynthesize the provitamin 7-dehydrocholesterol. Vitamins D_2 and D_3 are derived from their respective protovitamins, ergosterol, from yeast, and 7-dehydrocholesterol, in the skin, by ultraviolet irradiation. The active form of the vitamin is considered to be the 1,25-HCC with respect to intestinal *calcium* transport and bone mineral mobilization. Vitamin D increases the availability, retention, and utilization of calcium and phosphorus for proper mineralization of the skeleton. Deficiency of vitamin D is a major cause of *rickets* in the infant, and one of the causes of *osteomalacia* in the adult. The requirements of infants are generally met through the use of vitamin D milk. The needs of most adults are probably supplied by the average diet and casual exposure to sunshine. Vitamin D is absorbed in the presence of *bile*, primarily from the *jejunum* (small intestine), and is transported to the liver and then to the kidney for conversion to the active form, 1,25 dihydrocholecalciferol (1,25 DHCC). The 1,25 DHCC is carried by the bloodstream by a specific binding protein to the intestinal wall and to the bone. Reserves of vitamin D are stored as such in the liver and kidneys. After the absorption of calcium and phosphorus through the intestinal wall, vitamin D continues to work in partnership with calcium and phosphorus in the calcification aspect of bone formation. Tracer studies with radioactive isotopes have shown that 1,25-DHCC directly increases the role of mineral accretion and resorption in bone by which the tissue is built and maintained. The 1,25-DHCC activates the production of a specific protein in the intestinal wall which carries the calcium from the small intestine into the blood, thereby increasing the availability of calcium for bone deposition. In vitamin D deficiency, not only is calcium absorption from the small intestine decreased, but the mobilization of calcium from the bone is depressed, resulting in *hypocalcemia*. In addition, there is an increase in the urinary losses of phosphorus and amino acids. See *calcitonin* and *parahormone*. Sunshine is an important source of vitamin D. In the skin, a form of cholesterol, the provitamin 7-dehydrocholecalciferol, is activated to vitamin D_3 when exposed to sunlight. The natural distribution of vitamin D in common foods is limited to small, often insignificant amounts in cream, butter, eggs, and liver. For this reason it is necessary to depend upon fortified foods, fish liver oils, or concentrates for preventative and therapeutic use. Vitamin D_3 milk is produced by adding a vitamin D_3 concentrate to homogenized milk. All brands of evaporated milk also have vitamin D_3 added. Fish liver oils have a wide range of potency. Vitamin D_2, ergocalciferol, is manufactured by exposing ergosterol, a sterol found in fungi and yeasts, to ultraviolet (UV) light. Although ergocalciferol, vitamin D_2, is widely used in therapeutics, it occurs very rarely in nature. It is absent in almost all plant and animal tissues except for small amounts in certain fish liver oils. Ergosterol, from which it is derived, occurs only in plants. The fat-soluble antirachitic factor, vitamin D_2,

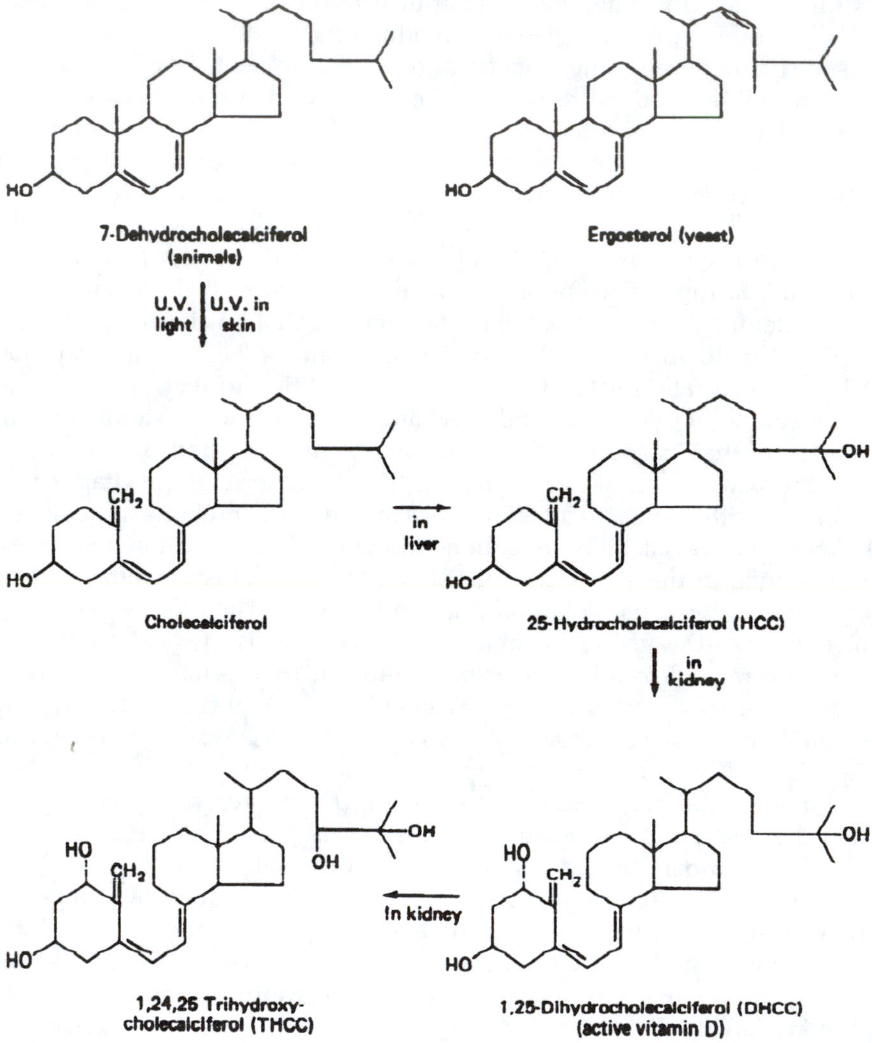

7-Dehydrocholecalciferol
(animals)

Ergosterol (yeast)

U.V. light | U.V. in skin

Cholecalciferol

in liver

25-Hydrocholecalciferol (HCC)

in kidney

1,24,25 Trihydroxy-cholecalciferol (THCC)

In kidney

1,25-Dihydrocholecalciferol (DHCC)
(active vitamin D)

Vitamin D

is obtained by ultraviolet-ray activation of 7-dehydrocholesterol. It occurs in fish liver oils and in irradiated foods of animal origin; it is termed "natural" vitamin D. Vitamin D in milk may be produced by three different methods: (1) "Fortified" milk, which is more generally distributed than other types, is that to which a vitamin D concentrate has been added. (2) "Metabolized" milk is produced by feeding cows irradiated yeast. (3) "Irradiated" milk has been exposed directly to ultraviolet rays. The standard amount used for fortification is 400 I.U. vitamin D per quart of fresh or reconstituted milk.

Vitamin D in µg/100 g of foods

FAT FISH AND THEIR OILS:		DAIRY PRODUCE:	
Cod-liver oil	475	Eggs, whole	1.4
Halibut-liver oil	5250	Eggs, yolk	7
Swordfish-liver oil	25,000	Margarine	5.5
Herring, salmon, sardine pilchard	25	Butter	1.4
		Milk	less than 0.1
		Cheese	0.3

vitamin deficiency. The absence or an inadequacy of vitamins in the human diet results in signs of poor health. Since a deficiency in a single specific vitamin is difficult to achieve even

Vitamin deficiencies and clinical symptoms

VITAMIN	SYMPTOMS
Ascorbic acid (vitamin C)	Scurvy: red, swollen, bleeding gums, perifolliculosis, poor wound healing, subcutaneous hemorrhage, swelling of joints.
Cobalamin (vitamin B$_{12}$)	Pernicious anemia. Generally due to genetic lack of *intrinsic factor*. Weakness, numbness, and dementia. Some of the symptoms (anemia) related to an induced free *folic acid* (folacin) deficiency. Dietary deficiency occasionally seen in strict vegetarians.
Folacin (folic acid)	Glossitis, gastrointestinal disturbances, diarrhea and megaloblastic anemia. The anemia is related to the type seen in *cobalamin* (vitamin B$_{12}$) deficiency.
Niacin (Nicotinic acid, nicotinamides)	Pellagra: bilateral dermatitis particularly in areas exposed to sunlight, glossitis, diarrhea, irritability, mental confusion, eventually delirium or psychotic symptoms.
Pyridoxine (vitamin B$_6$)	Convulsions have been observed in infants. Experimental deficiency in man: seborrhea dermatitis, glossitis, angular stomatitis, abnormal electroencephalogram.
Retinol (vitamin A)	Night blindness (nyctalopia), hyperkeratinization of epithelial tissues, xeophthalmia.
Riboflavin	Ariboflavinosis: cheilosis, angular stomatitis, labial dermatitis, photophobia, corneal vascularization.
Thiamine (vitamin B$_1$)	Beriberi; chiefly nervous and cardiovascular systems affected; mental confusion, muscular weakness, loss of ankle and knee jerks, painful calf muscles, peripheral paralysis, edema (wet beriberi), muscle wasting (dry beriberi), enlarged heart.
Vitamin D	Rickets in the young. Osteomalacia in adults.
Vitamin K	"Hemorrhagic disease of the newborn." Hemorrhage or slowed blood-clot times. The deficiency is sometimes associated with steatorrhea (fatty stools), diarrhea, or high-antibiotic therapy.

under experimental conditions, such an achievement in any diet is unlikely. For example, for the most part, the B-complex vitamins occur in the same foods. Therefore it is difficult to provide a diet deficient in *pyridoxine* (vitamin B$_6$) that would not also be deficient in *thiamine* (vitamin B,) and *riboflavin*. The clinical symptoms of vitamin deficiencies are not always clear or specific, partly because of problems of multiple deficiencies and partly because of the fact that many of the symptoms of the individual vitamin deficiencies overlap with one another.

For example, a dermatitis manifests itself in five different vitamin deficiencies. The known vitamin deficiencies in humans represent the clinical symptoms and the specific names given to the avitaminoses. In general, experimentally induced avitaminoses are not considered in the table. More information is given under the listing of the vitamin.

vitamin E. See *tocopherols*.

vitamin K (phyloquinone, farnoquinone). A group of fat-soluble, light-sensitive vitamins possessing a common naphthoquinone structure; natural forms include vitamin K_1 occurring in green leaves, and vitamin K_2 produced by intestinal bacteria; synthetic forms such as *menadione* are available as water-soluble esters. The major function of vitamin K is to catalyze the synthesis of normal *prothrombin* by the liver. Normal prothrombin has a terminal amino acid, gamma (γ)-carboxyglutamic acid. Vitamin K is necessary to carboxylate (add CO_2) this terminal amino acid. In the absence of vitamin K, the terminal *glutamic acid* residue in the protein is not converted to a γ-carboxyglutamyl residue and normal prothrombin is not formed. Only normal prothrombin can be converted to thrombin by the proteolytic enzyme proaccelerin or factor V. Without vitamin K the whole vital process of blood clotting cannot be initiated. Vitamin K function is therefore essential in blood coagulation for the maintenance of normal prothrombin time through its effect on prothrombin and other clotting factors. Prothrombin levels regulate the rate of blood coagulation; when they are low, the coagulation is depressed. Coumarin drugs such as *dicumarol* are anticoagulants and act as Vitamin K antagonists (*antivitamins*). They are used in anticoagulation therapy. Vitamin K deficiency, which is characterized by hemorrhagic tendencies, may result from reduced synthesis by intestinal bacteria or poor intestinal absorption; prophylaxis is achieved with 1–2 mg of vitamin K per day administered orally. It can be synthesized in the lower gastrointestinal tract by the bacterial flora. Because vitamin K is absorbed mainly from the upper section of the tract, only limited amounts are

Vitamin K_1 Mol. Wt. 450

Vitamin K_2 Mol. Wt. 580

probably absorbed. Medication such as antibiotics which reduce intestinal flora decrease the synthesis of vitamin K. Dietary sources of vitamin K are absorbed in the small intestine where fats are absorbed. Bile salts are necessary for effective absorption. The vitamin passes into the lacteals, through the thoracic duct, and into the liver. Here it functions in synthesis of the proteins, prothrombin, proconvertin factors, and the Steward factor. All these are necessary for blood clotting. Vitamin K is fairly widely distributed in foods. It appears abundantly in cauliflower, cabbage, spinach, pork liver, and soybeans and to a lesser extent in wheat and oats. The dietary vitamin K requirement is unknown and there is no United States Recommended Daily Allowance (U.S. RDA). See *blood clotting*

Vitamin K in mg/100 g of foods

Alfalfa	650	Liver, pork	175	Wheat, whole	36
Cabbage	250	Soybeans	190	Wheat bran	80
Cauliflower	275	Spinach	334	Wheat germ	37

vitamin toxicity. *Hypervitaminosis.* The water-soluble vitamins are not toxic in general. Of the fat-soluble vitamins, *retinol* and *vitamin D* can produce severe toxic symptoms. The table gives the ratio of the *Recommended Dietary Allowance* (RDA) to a toxic level in humans. The toxic level is broadly defined as a level that produces some physiologic change no matter how transient. For example, hypervitamin therapy with pyridoxine causes a flushing, itching, and warm sensation that lasts about 30 seconds. It should be borne in mind that toxicity levels vary greatly from individual to individual. In vitamin D toxicity, for example, the variations in toxic levels among individuals may be greater than tenfold.

Ratio of RDA/toxic level of vitamins

Retinol (vitamin A)	1:7,500	Niacin	1:5,000
Vitamin D	1:2,000	Pyridoxine (vitamin B_6)	1:60,000
Cobalamin (vitamin B_{12})	1:100,000	Thiamine (vitamin B_1)	1:25,000

W

W. The alphabetic symbol for the *essential amino acid tryptophan* (Trp).

walnut (*Juglans regia*). The edible nut of the fruit of the walnut tree. The most commonly known walnut is the English, or Persian, walnut. This hard-shelled nut has a wrinkled white kernel with two very irregularly shaped halves covered with a light-brown skin. The shell is thin and light tan; it is made up of two distinct halves. Walnuts have some protein, iron, and B vitamins. Walnuts are high in fat. Shelled walnuts contain about 630 calories in 100 g.

water. Mol. Wt. 18. H−O−H (H_2O). Water is the medium for transporting the food materials to be used in the body. In a state of solution or suspension, simple sugars, amino acids, fats, minerals, and vitamins are passed through the intestinal walls and are then carried to the cells by blood and lymph, the two most fluid tissues of the body. Waste products are carried and excreted in a similar manner. Oxygen and carbon dioxide are also transported by the bloodstream. After absorption much fluid reenters the alimentary tract, where it serves as a carrier of digestive enzymes. Large quantities of digestive juices are secreted daily by the body. It has been estimated that the 24-hour secretion of *saliva*, expressed in milliliters, is 500–1500; of *gastric juice*, 1000–2500; of *bile*, 100–400; and of intestinal secretions, 700–3000. Water is an efficient heat conductor and serves to maintain the uniform body temperature essential for health. As a protector of internal organs, water is indispensable; it serves as a cushion and prevents the transmission of shock from the outside. By means of the synovial fluid present in all joints, these surfaces are kept lubricated and moist; the central nervous system is bathed by the cerebospinal fluid. In terms of life need, water is second only to oxygen. The body can be deprived of oxygen for up to about 20 minutes; in rare instances can survive water deprivation for only a few days, and can live without food for weeks. When the body water loss exceeds 20%, death is likely. Water is found in all parts of the body. The water within the cells (intercellular fluid) comprises the largest part of the total amount and furnishes an aqueous medium for the chemical reactions which constantly occur. When considered in relation to total body weight, water may vary from about 40% in very obese people to 70% in very lean persons. The different parts of the body vary markedly in their water content. Muscle has about 75% water, and bone about 25%. Blood plasma and red blood cells have about 92% and 60%. *Adipose* (fat) *tissue* may vary from 10–30%. In addition to direct ingestion, water is obtained from food as a part of its content and is obtained also as a result of its metabolism. In the *oxidation* of foodstuffs to obtain *energy*, the process results in carbon dioxide, water, and energy. The table shows the water content of some common classes of food. Except for fat, pure sugar, and dry cereals, water is the major constituent of most foods.

Water content in g/100 g of foods

Meat	70	Honey	20	Coffee, roasted	5
Milk	85	Butter, Margarine	16	Milk, powdered	4
Fruits and Vegetables	80	Cereal flour	13	Oils and Fats	0
Bread	35				

The table shows the amount of water that is produced by the oxidation of the foodstuff. The oxidation of the sugar *glucose* is given as an example of how the water arises in the balanced chemical equation. See *respiratory quotient*.

Water formed in mL (g) from 100 g of oxidized food

PROTEIN	CARBOHYDRATE	FAT
107	56	41

Water is the major constituent of many foods and living organisms. It is also an integral part of the structure of many inorganic, organic, and biological compounds. The table gives the approximate water content of some foods.

Percent water of common foods

Bread	35	Fruits and Vegetables	83
Cooked cereal	85	Meat (cooked rare)	75
Dry cereal	3	Meat (cooked done)	40
Eggs	75	Milk	85

Many of the unique properties of water are due to its special structuture. The $H-O-H$ bonds form an angle of 105°, and the molecule is polarized such that there is a more negative charge associated with the oxygen than with the hydrogens, resulting in a dipole. A network of hydrogen bonds forms among the molecules, which also contributes to the special properties of water. The diagrams approximate the structure of water.

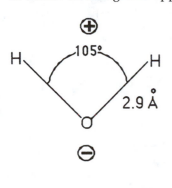

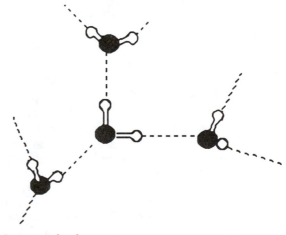

Hydrogen bonded water molecules

One of these special properties is that, unlike most substances, water expands when it freezes and the details of the structure are still not fully understood. The formation of water crystals and their expansion during the freezing process account for the alteration of the appearance and structure of some foods after freezing. See *water balance* and water *regulation*.

water balance. The total blood flow through the kidneys is about 1200 mL per minute, and the total extracellular fluid amounts to about 15 liters; about 3 liters of that total is plasma. The blood plasma and the extracellular fluid are in equilibrium with each other, and therefore an amount of blood equivalent to all the extracellular fluid can pass through the kidneys once every 15 minutes. The water and electrolyte content of the blood plasma, and therefore, indirectly, of the extracellular fluid, are closely controlled by the kidneys. Any increase of water content in the body, such as a water load by drinking, leads to the prompt production of a corresponding amount of *urine*, with a low specific gravity. Water absorption in the tubules is controlled by the *antidiuretic hormone* (ADH) of the pituitary gland, which modifies the amount of water taken up in the distal part of the renal tubule. An increase in the amount of water in the body lowers the osmotic pressure of the carotid body and reduces the production of ADH which causes an increased production of urine. See *water regulation*. The diagram shows the relationships among the various water compartments of the body and the outside world.

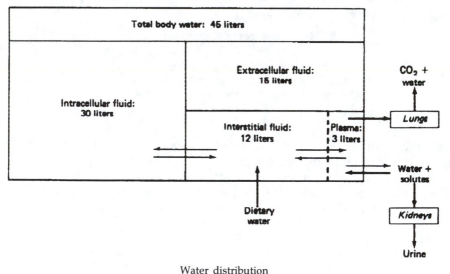

Water distribution

The typical water balance for an adult over a 24-hour period during light activity is approximately as shown:

**Water balance for adult in
24-hour period with light activity**

WATER INTAKE	ML	WATER OUTPUT	ML
Water	1200	Urine	1300
Foods	900	Feces	200
Water of oxidation	300	Perspiration	500
		Lungs	400

water chestnut (*Trapa*). The fruit of a water plant with floating leaves and small white flowers. The nutlike fruit kernel resembles a true chestnut in shape and color, but is crunchy in texture. Water chestnuts can be used in poultry, meat, seafood, and egg dishes, and adds a pleasant crispness when combined with soft foods. Raw, 100 g = 79 calories.

watercress (*Nasturtium officinale*). The most popular and widely eaten of the cresses, plants of the mustard family which includes peppergrass or garden cress, winter cress or rocket, and spring or Belle Isle cress. All have crisp green leaves and a pungent, rather bitter taste, each variety with its own characteristics. Peppergrass is sometimes sprinkled over such dishes as beet soup. All the cresses may be boiled as *potherbs*. Watercress gets its name because it grows in cold running water. The word "cress" is perhaps related to the Latin word for grass, and even further back to the Sanskrit verb meaning "to eat," especially gnawing or nibbling. Watercress is a good source of *ascorbic acid* (vitamin C) and *carotene* (vitamin A activity), and supplies a variety of minerals including iron if eaten in large amounts.

water extract. Whatever can be removed or dissolved out of a substance with water. A substance like sugar is completely soluble in water, whereas when yeast is shaken up with water only a small portion of it goes into solution. What remains is insoluble and does not pass into the water extract.

watermelon (*Citrullus vulgaris*). A member of the gourd family, most commonly a spherical fruit with pink or red flesh and many seeds. There are many varieties, among which are yellow and white watermelons as well as the red. Seeds may be white, red, brown, black, green, or speckled. The rind is usually dark green. Watermelons average 24–40 pounds, although there are some small 2-to 10-pound varieties. The flesh is sweet with a high water content. Watermelons are a good source of vitamin A activity and a fair source of *ascorbic acid* (vitamin C). See this item in the table under *fruits*.

water regulation. Water balance is regulated by several complex mechanisms. *Antidiuretic hormone* (ADH) from the posterior *pituitary* causes an increase in water absorption by the kidneys and therefore a decreased urine output. A high *osmotic pressure* (a high concentration of solutes in the blood) signals the release of ADH. Diuretics and alcohol inhibit the release of ADH from the pituitary, and increased urine output is the result. Increased urine output (diuresis) generally accompanies an increased excretion of solutes into the urine because the solutes carry the water of hydration along with them. Diuresis due to the disease *diabetes mellitus* (sugar diabetes) is due to the high blood sugar which "spills over" into the urine and carries large amounts of water of hydration. The large water loss is in turn accompanied by increased water intake (thirst or polydipsia) and the water balance is maintained. Water regulation is also intimately associated with salt (electrolyte) balance and some steroids, *aldosterone* in particular. Aldosterone and deoxycorticosterone promote the reabsorption of sodium ion (Na^+) and retention of water. The release of aldosterone by the adrenal glands is controlled indirectly by the Na^+ plasma concentration. When the Na^+ in plasma is low, the kidneys release renin, which causes the liver angiotensinogen to become angiotensin, which stimulates the adrenal glands to release aldosterone. Aldosterone can also be released by stimulation of the adrenal glands by *adrenocorticotropic hormone* (ACTH) from the pituitary. Stress can cause the release ACTH by the pituitary. The diagram shows these relationships. The female hormone *progesterone* promotes the retention of salt and water and accounts for the retention of water at certain stages of the menstrual cycle.

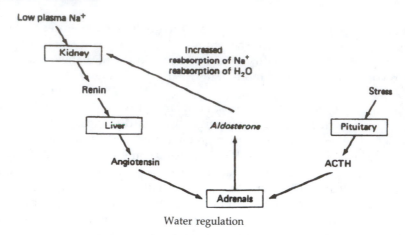

Water regulation

A change in the diet can cause a temporary retention or loss of water until a new water balance is reached. The carbohydrate content of the diet has a pronounced influence on water retention. In general, a decrease in dietary carbohydrate is accompanied by an increased loss of water. All of the diets that promise rapid weight loss are low in carbohydrates and take full advantage of the weight loss due to increased water excretion. Conversely, if the shift is to a high carbohydrate intake, the rapid increase in weight is due largely to water retention. There are several different theories as to why carbohydrates have an effect on water retention, but the mechanism is not understood clearly.

water-soluble vitamins. The water-soluble vitamins make up a large group, and all but one belong to the B complex. The remaining water-soluble vitamin is *ascorbic acid* (vitamin C). For the most part, water-soluble vitamins are not stored in the body. Excesses are largely excreted, thus eliminating the possibilities for toxicity that exist with overdoses of *fat-soluble vitamins*. At least 11 vitamins compose the B complex. Seven of them are essential in human nutrition; six are included in the allowance table of the Food and Nutrition Board. These are *thiamine* (vitamin B_1), *riboflavin, niacin, folacin, pyridoxine* (vitamin B_6), and *cobalamin* (vitamin B_{12}). All are concerned with converting the end-products of carbohydrate, fat, and protein digestion into a form of energy the body can use. They serve basically as coenzymes. The pages given contain a summary of some water-soluble vitamins.

waxes. Defined chemically as fatty acid esters of higher alcohols. Occur widely in the cuticles of leaves and fruit and in the secretions of insects, and may be mixed with very-long-chain hydrocarbon alcohols (C_{21-35}). The structure of myricyl palmitate, a major constituent of bees-wax, is given. They replace the *triglycerides* to some extent in the tissues of aquatic animals such as crustaceans. So far waxes have not been shown to be an important constituent of any of the higher land animals, nor do they contribute importantly to normal human diet.

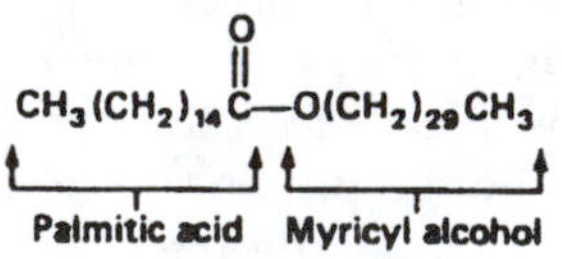

$$CH_3(CH_2)_{14}\overset{\overset{\displaystyle O}{\|}}{C}-O(CH_2)_{29}CH_3$$

Palmitic acid   Myricyl alcohol

Waxes

Summary of water-soluble vitamins

NOMEN-CLATURE	IMPORTANT SOURCES	PHYSIOLOGY AND FUNCTION	EFFECTS OF DEFICIENCY	RECOMMENDED ALLOWANCES
Ascorbic acid Vitamin C	Citrus fruits; tomatoes; melons; cabbage; broccoli; strawberries; fresh potatoes; green leafy vegetables	Very little storage in body Formation of intercellular cement substance; synthesis of collagen Absorption and use of iron Prevents oxidation of folacin	Weakened cartilage and capillary walls Cutaneous hemorrhage; sore, bleeding gums, anemia Poor wound healing Poor bone and tooth development Scurvy	Men 45 mg Women: 45 mg Pregnancy: 60 mg Lactation: 60 mg Infants: 35 mg Children under 10: 40 mg Boys and girls: 45 mg
Thiamin Vitamin B_1	Whole-grain and enriched breads, cereals, flours; organ meats, pork; other meats, poultry, fish; legumes, nuts; milk; green vegetables	Limited body storage Thiamin pyrophosphate (TPP) is coenzyme for decarboxylation and transketolation; chiefly involved in carbohydrate metabolism	Poor appetite; atony of gastrointestinal tract, constipation Mental depression, apathy, polyneuritis Cachexia, edema Cardiac failure Beriberi	Men: 1.4 mg Women: 1.0 mg Pregnancy: 1.3 mg Lactation: 1.3 mg Infants: 0.3-0.5 mg Children under 10: 0.7-1.2 mg Boys and girls: 1.1-1.5 mg
Riboflavin Vitamin B_2	Milk; organ meats; eggs; green leafy vegetables	Limited body stores, but reserves retained carefully Coenzymes for removal and transfer of hydrogen; flavin mononucleotide (FMN) and flavin adenine dinucleotide (FAD)	Cheilosis (cracks at corners of lips) Scaly desquamation around nose, ears Sore tongue and mouth Burning and itching of eyes Photophobia	Men: 1.6 mg Women: 1.2 mg Pregnancy: 1.5 mg Lactation: 1.7 mg Infants: 0.4-0.6 mg Children under 10: 0.8-1.2 mg Boys and girls: 1.3-1.8
Niacin Nicotinic acid Nicotinamide	Meat, poultry, fish; whole-grain and enriched breads, flours, cereals; nuts, legumes Tryptophan as a precursor	Coenzyme for glycolysis, fat synthesis, tissue respiration. Coenzymes NAD and NADP accept hydrogen and transfer it	Anorexia, glossitis, diarrhea Dermatitis Neurologic degeneration Pellagra	Men:18 mg Women: 13 mg Pregnancy: 15 mg Lactation: 17 mg Infants: 5-8 mg Children under 10: 16 mg Boys and girls: 14-20 mg
Vitamin B_6 Three active forms: pyridoxine, pyridoxamine pyridoxal	Meat, poultry, fish; potatoes, sweet potatoes, vegetables	Pyridoxal phosphate is coenzyme for transamination, decarboxylation, transulfuration Conversion of tryptophan to niacin; conversion of glycogen to glucose	Nervous irritability, convulsions Weakness, ataxia, abdominal pain Dermatitis; anemia	Adults: 2.0 mg Pregnancy: 2.5 mg Lactation: 2.5 mg Infants: 0.3-0.4 mg Children under 10: 0.6-1.2 mg Boys and girls: 1.6-2.0

continued

Pantothenic acid	Meat, poultry, fish; whole-grain cereals; legumes Smaller amounts in fruits, vegetables, milk	Constituent of coenzyme A: oxidation of pyruvic acid, α–ketoglutarate, fatty acids; synthesis of fatty acids, sterols, and porphyrin	Deficiency seen only with severe multiple B-complex deficits; then, gastrointestinal disturbances, neuritis, burning sensations of feet	Not known; probably about 5-10 mg
Biotin	Organ meats, egg yolks, nuts, legumes	Avidin, a protein in raw egg white, blocks absorption; large amounts of raw eggs must be eaten Coenzyme for deamination, carboxylation, and decarboxylation	Deficiency only when many raw egg whites are consumed for long periods of time Dermatitis, anorexia, hyperesthesia, anemia	Not known; probably about 5-10 mg
Vitamin B_{12} Cyanocobalamin Hydroxycobalamin	In animal foods only: organ meats, muscle meats, fish, poultry; eggs; milk	Requires intrinsic factor for absorption Biosynthesis of methyl groups Synthesis of DNA and RNA Formation of mature red blood cells	Lack of intrinsic factor leads to deficiency; pernicious anemia, following gastrectomy Macrocytic anemia Neurologic degeneration	Adults: 3 µg Pregnancy: 4 µg Lactation: 4 µg Infants: 1-2 µg Boys and girls: 3 µg
Folacin Folic acid Tetrahydrofolic acid	Organ meats, deep-green leafy vegetables; muscle meats, poultry, fish, eggs; whole-grain cereals	Active form is folinic acid; requires ascorbic acid for conversion Coenzyme for transmethylation; synthesis of nucleoproteins; maturation of red blood cells Interrelated with vitamin B_{12}	Megaloblastic anemia of infancy, pregnancy, tropical sprue	Adults: 400 µg Pregnancy: 800 µg Lactation: 600 µg Infants: 50 µg Children under 10: 100-300 µg Boys and girls: 400 mcg
Choline	Egg yolk, meat, poultry, fish, milk, whole grains	Probably not a true vitamin Donor of methyl groups: lipotropic action	Has not been observed in humans Component of acetylcholine	Not known; typical diet supplies 200-600 mg
Lipoic acid Thioctic acid Protogen		Probably not a true vitamin Coenzyme for decarboxylation of keto acids		Not known
Inositol	Widely distributed in all foods	Lipotropic agent Vitamin nature not established	Has not been observed in humans	Not known

waxy flour. A flour prepared from certain varieties of rice or corn that contains a type of starch that has waxy adhesive qualities. The flour acts as a stabilizer when it is used as an ingredient in sauces or gravies and binds the mixtures together so there is no separation when the mixtures are frozen.

Wernicke's encephalopathy. A syndrome related to *thiamine* deficiency characterized by anorexia, nystagmus, double vision, ophthalmoplegia, ataxia, loss of memory, confusion, confabulations, and hallucinations, which may progress to stupor and coma. Thiamine deficiency is largely responsible for the condition, though associated insufficiencies of other water-soluble vitamins may be involved. See *thiamine*.

wheat (*Triticum*). The grain of the grass most widely grown of the cereal *grains*. The little wheat kernels grow in beads at the top of stalks or straw. The flour made by grinding wheat grain is the best of all flours for bread making because of the presence of gluten, a form of protein that makes a soft and spongy dough. A grain of wheat has three main parts. The outer covering is the bran, the inner part is the endosperm, and the tiny nucleus within the endosperm is the germ. If the entire kernel is ground, the result is whole-wheat flour, graham flour, or entire wheat flour. If just the endosperm is used, the result is flour, wheat flour, and plain flour. Shown is a cross-section of a grain of whole wheat. The bran: The brown outer layers. This part contains (1) bulk-forming carbohydrates, (2) B vitamins, (3) minerals, especially iron. The aleurone layers: The layers located right under the bran. They are rich in (1) proteins, (2) phosphorus, a mineral.

The endosperm is the white center and consists mainly of carbohydrates (starches and sugars) and protein. The wheat proteins occupy a unique position among the cereal grains. *Gluten* or wheat protein is composed of two major proteins, gliadin (a *prolamine*) and glutenin (a *glutelin*). The combination in wheat flour gives a characteristic stickiness when mixed with water which enables the molecules to bond together under heat. This allows the wheat flour

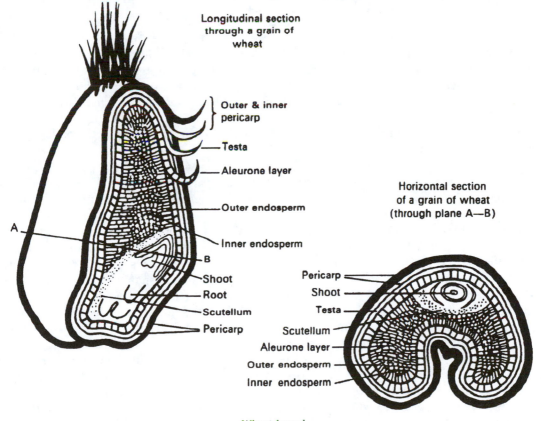

Longitudinal section
through a grain of
wheat

Outer & inner
pericarp

Testa

Aleurone layer

Outer endosperm

Inner endosperm

A

B

Shoot

Root

Scutellum

Pericarp

Horizontal section
of a grain of wheat
(through plane A—B)

Pericarp

Shoot

Testa

Scutellum

Aleurone layer

Outer endosperm

Inner endosperm

Wheat kernel

(Davidson, S., et al., *Human Nutrition and Dietetics*, 1975. Reproduced with permission of Churchill Livingstone, Edinburgh.)

dough to bake to form bread. Rye contains a small amount of gluten and it too can be made into bread. However, oats, barley, corn, rice, and millets cannot be made into rising breads. These grains or their flours can be boiled into porridges or tortillas. Wheat has a nutritive value similar to that of the other cereals. Most of the flour used today is highly refined. Milling in general consists of grinding and sifting through fine sieves in order to obtain fine, white wheat flour. The table shows the nutritive content of wheat flour relative to the percent of the whole-wheat flour in the finely milled flour. Most fine flours contain less than 70% of the whole-wheat flour.

Nutritive content of wheat flour relative to the percent of whole-wheat flour in 100 g of flour

	100	80	70	45
Fiber (gm)	2.2	0.1	trace	trace
Fat (gm)	2.5	1.4	1.2	0.9
Protein (gm)	13.6	13.2	12.8	11.8
Biotin (µg)	5	1.4	1.2	0.7
Folacin (µg)	35	13		8
Niacin (mg)	5	2	2	1
Pyridoxine (µg)	400	108	64	
Riboflavin (mg)	160	83	53	50
Thiamine (µg)	400	300	100	30

The limiting amino acid in wheat protein is *lysine*, and typical of the cereal grains it contains only a trace of *carotene* and no *ascorbic acid*. In white flour, starch is present in greater proportion and is more digestible than it is in whole-wheat flour. Therefore, it is higher in caloric value. If enriched, white flour contains added *thiamine, riboflavin, niacin,* and *iron*. Whole-wheat flour, which contains all the nutrients available in the whole grain, is high in phosphorus and potassium, and has moderate amounts of protein, niacin, thiamine, and riboflavin. See this item under *grains*.

whey. The liquid part of milk which remains after the thicker part, or *curd*, is removed. The curd is used in making cheese. Whey contains sugar, minerals, and lactalbumin. See *milk*.

whiskey or whisky. A spirit distilled from such grains as barley, rye, and corn, and subsequently refined, colored, and flavored by various processes. Each country produces a distinctive type of whiskey. The Latin term used to describe distilled spirits was *aquavitae*, "water of life." The Scotch and Irish translated it to *usquebaugh* in Gaelic. The name was later contracted to *uisge* and still later anglicized to whiskey. The four steps of whiskey production are malting, fermenting, distilling, and aging. Whiskey, strictly defined by United States federal standards, is a grain spirit, distilled at less than 190 proof and 1 day old. Thirty-three whiskey variations are listed among the United States standards, but general usage divides whiskey into two major subdivisions, straight whiskey and blended whiskey. Straight whiskey is whiskey which is unmixed with other liquors or substances, such as straight bourbon whiskey and straight rye whiskey. Federal law requires that straight whiskey be aged in new charred oak barrels for at least 2 years. A blended whiskey is a balanced blending of straight whiskeys and neutral grain spirits (a high distillate, at least 190 proof, of any fermented mash), containing at least 20% straight whiskeys and bottled at not less than 80 proof. The word "proof" applied to distilled spirits indicates the amount of alcohol in a liquor. Proof is twice the percentage of alcohol. A bonded whiskey is straight whiskey produced and bottled in accordance with the Federal Bottling-in-Bond Act. It must be at least 4 years old, must be bottled at 100 proof, must have been produced in a single distillery, by the same distiller, and be the product of a single season or year.

Calories in whiskey

TYPE OF WHISKEY	PROOF	ML (OUNCES)	CALORIES
Bourbon	86	43 (1 1/2)	125
Irish	86	43 (1 1/2)	125
Rye	86	43 (1 1/2)	125
Scotch	86	43 (1 1/2)	110

white blood cells. See *blood cells, white*.

whitefish (*Coregonus*). A fatty freshwater fish caught in North American lakes, belonging to the salmon family. Whitefish are prepared in almost any way that fish can be prepared: broiled, panfried, baked, or poached. Whitefish are very high in protein and *retinol* (vitamin A), phosphorus and potassium; have some *thiamine, riboflavin,* and *niacin*.

whitehead. See *acne*.

whiting (*Melangus melangus*). Small gray-and white-saltwater fish sometimes called kingfish or silver hake. Whiting grow to an average length of 12 inches and weight from 1–4 pound. The fish has tender white flesh, fine in texture, flaky, with a delicate flavor. It can be broiled, panfried, baked, or poached.

wild rice (*Zizania aquatica*). A native American grass that bears a grain used for food. It is a tall plant that grows in water in the western Great Lakes area and has never been domesticated. Wild rice is high in protein, phosphorus, and potassium, with some *riboflavin, thiamine,* and *niacin*.

wine. The product of the natural fermentation of the juice of the grape. The term is also used to describe beverages made from other fruit juices or vegetable juice by adding sugar and *yeast* and fermenting the mixture—examples are dandelion wine and elderberry wine. But strictly speaking, wine is the product of the vine, for grapes contain naturally all the ingredients needed for a normal fermentation of the juice. No sugar or yeast need be added. The true wine yeast is *Saccharomyces cerevisiae* var. *ellipsoideus*. The raw grape juice or *must* is high in sugar and strongly acid, an unsuitable medium for the growth of bacteria but highly suitable for yeast and molds. Fermentation is either allowed to proceed spontaneously or it is started with a must from a previously successful fermentation. The must is aerated slightly until yeast growth is vigorous and then stopped. The carbon dioxide produced by the yeast is sufficient to keep conditions anaerobic, inhibiting the growth of molds and bacteria. If anaerobic conditions are not maintained, the ethanol is oxidized further to acetic acid—the product is *vinegar*. The aging process ensues after sufficient sugar has been utilized and sufficient *alcohol* produced.

woodruff, sweet (*Asperula odorata*). A spreading plant with small white flowers whose slim yellow leaves are used to flavor beverages. The characteristic odor of its leaves is released when they are somewhat dried; they then smell like new-mown hay. The leaves may be used to flavor cold fruit drinks and wine cups.

work. The result of the utilization of *energy* to produce a change. In this sense, the use of chemical energy to produce a new compound (a synthesis) would be chemical work. Work also has a technical definition in physics restricted to linear displacement.

X

xanthelasma. A common form of xanthoma (yellow tumor). The condition occurs when there is a high level of *cholesterol* and cholesterol esters in the blood. The lesion occurs on the eyelids. The tumors are flat, soft, yellow-colored plaques of varying size. May be a forerunner of angina or high blood pressure.

xanthine. A purine formed in tissues during *nucleic acid* degradation. Xanthine derivative also occurs in plants. Three related methylated xanthines are *caffeine*, theophylline, and theobromine.

xanthomatosis. A condition in which there is a deposition of lipid in tissues usually accompanied by *hyperlipemia*. *Cholesterol* may accumulate in tumor nodules (xanthoma) in individual cells, especially histocytes and reticuloendothelial cells.

xanthoproteic test. A yellow color reaction produced when a protein is treated with concentrated nitric acid. The test is simply a nitration of the aromatic ring of certain amino acids (*tyrosine, phenylalanine,* and *tryptophan*). Recognized as the familiar nitric acid stain. The test is done on urine, and protein in urine usually indicates a dysfunction or pathology of the kidneys.

xanthosis. A yellowing of the skin seen in carotenemia resulting from ingestion of excessive quantities of carrots, squash, egg yolk, and other foods containing *carotenoids*. Condition is usually harmless but may indicate increase of lipochromes in blood due to conditions such as *hypothyroidism* or *diabetes*.

xeroderma. Dryness of the skin. Instead of the normal smooth, moist, velvet texture, the skin feels dry and often rough. On uncovering the legs, a cloud of fine, branny dandruff is often seen. Xeroderma is commonly but not constantly associated with follicular keratosis and "cracked skin."

xerophthalmia. An extreme dryness of the conjuctiva of the eye caused by lack of *retinol* (vitamin A). See *retinol*.

xylitol. Mol. Wt. 152. A five-carbon polyhydric alcohol used as a sugar substitute. Xylitol is a natural product and is metabolized and enters the five-carbon sugar metabolism by its oxidation to D-xylulose and then to D-xylulose phosphate. It is a part of the series of reactions that produces *ribose* in the pentose shunt or hexose in the monophosphate shunt. See *sorbitol*.

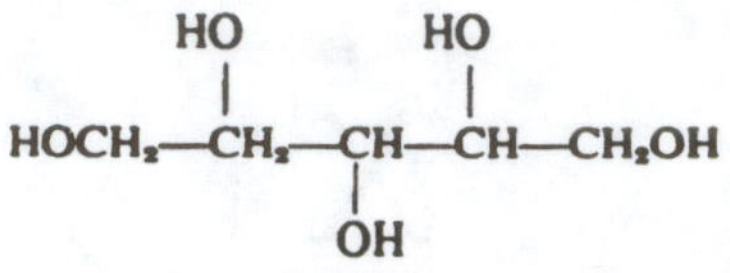

$$\underset{\text{Xylitol}}{\overset{\displaystyle \text{HO} \qquad\qquad \text{HO}}{\text{HOCH}_2-\text{CH}_2-\underset{\overset{|}{\text{OH}}}{\text{CH}}-\text{CH}-\text{CH}_2\text{OH}}}$$

Xylitol

xylose (wood sugar). Mol. Wt. 150. A five-carbon sugar that is not metabolized by the body. It occurs in wood nuts and other vegetables as a polymer class called the xylans, which occur in the cell walls of plants.

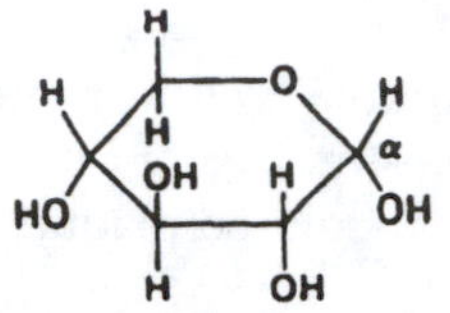

α D-xylose
(α D-xylosephyranose)

xylulose. Mol. Wt. 150. A five-carbon sugar intermediate in the pentose cycle (hexose monophosphate shunt) that leads to the biosynthesis of *ribose*.

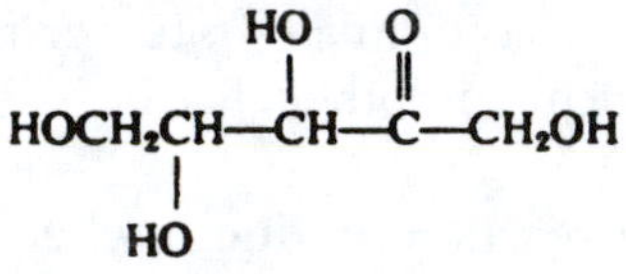

$$\underset{\text{D-xylulose}}{\text{HOCH}_2\text{CH}-\underset{\overset{|}{\text{HO}}}{\text{CH}}-\overset{\overset{\displaystyle\text{O}}{\|}}{\text{C}}-\text{CH}_2\text{OH}}$$

D-xylulose

Y

Y. The alphabetic symbol for the amino acid *tyrosine* (Tyr).

yams (*Dioscorea*). The two most important cultivated varieties are the greater yams (*D. alata*) and the lesser yams (*D. esculentia*). The yam is a thick tuber which develops at the base of the stem. There are more than 150 species, with some varieties growing up to 100 pounds; some are not larger than a small potato. The consistency varies from coarse and mealy to tender and mushy, with some crisp varieties. Like potatoes, the yam tubers are rich in starch, but also contain significant amounts of protein. Yams are often confused with *sweet potatoes* (*Ipomoea batatas*), which they resemble, but they belong to different botanical genera. Both yams and sweet potatoes are not sweet until cooked. The warming process of cooking activates the amylases and these enzymes hydrolize the starches to sugars. Raw, 100 g = 101 calories.

yeast (*Saccharomyces*). One-celled fungi widely distributed in nature. Some convert sugar in fruit juices to alcohol. Some are used to produce carbon dioxide for a leavening agent in bread making. From an industrial and technical view, the yeasts are easily the most important single group of microorganism. There are many varieties of yeast, but the most commonly used by humans are *S. cerevisiae* and its variety *ellipsoideus*. Humans have used yeast in processing food, drink, and textiles since prehistoric times. Yeasts are used in the preparation of beer, wine, cheese, butter, and flax. Yeast is an excellent source of protein and the B-complex vitamins. The table gives the nutritive value of yeast.

Nutrients in 100 g of baker's yeast

CALORIES KCAL	PROTEIN G	FAT G	CARBOHYDRATE G	NIACIN MG	THIAMINE MG	VITAMIN A IU
282	38	Trace	38	38	16	Trace

Calories in 100 g yeast

Baker's compressed	86	Brewer's dry	283
Baker's dry, active	282	Torula	277

yogurt. A semisolid milk product that has been made acid by the purposeful addition of certain bacterial cultures which have much greater acidifying power than natural ferments. Yogurt is an excellent source of the nutrients in milk for those who have developed a lactose intolerance (see *lactase*); *acidolphilous milk* (see fermented sources under *milk*) can serve a similar purpose. A good source of the B vitamins and calcium.

Nutrients in 100 g whole milk yogurt

CALORIES KCAL	PROTEIN G	FAT G	CARBOHYDRATE G	VITAMIN A IU	CALCIUM MG
62	3	3	5	140	111

Nutrients in 100 g skimmed milk yogurt

CALORIES KCAL	PROTEIN G	FAT G	CARBOHYDRATE G	VITAMIN A IU	CALCIUM MG
50	3	2	5	70	111

Z

Z. The alphabetic symbol for the amino acids *glutamic acid* (Glu) and *glutamine* (Gln, Glx).

zein. A major protein in corn. It has a low biologic value, with an *net protein utilization* (NPU) value of about 40. Zein is relatively poor in the *essential amino acids lysine* and *tryptophan*.

zinc (Zn). Element No. 30. At. Wt. 65.38. The adult human body contains about 2–3 g of zinc. Zinc is present in most tissues of the animal body. Extraordinarily high concentrations occur in choroid of the eye and in male reproductive organs. Liver, voluntary muscle, and bone contain considerably less, but more than other tissues. Most of the zinc in blood is present in the erythrocytes; almost all of the zinc occurs associated with carbonic anhydrase. Zinc is a component of a number of metalloenzymes including the pancreatic peptidases, carbonic anhydrase, alcohol dehydrogenase, and other dehydrogenases. Zinc has been found to accelerate wound healing and is necessary in humans for growth, sexual maturation, and the body synthesis of collagen tissue; in the metabolism of the all-important *nucleic acids*; and as a vital component of many enzymes which are the key to a variety of functions in human health. Many enzymes in humans have zinc as a component, or zinc activates them. Precisely how zinc works with enzymes is not known, but it is known that in almost 20 enzyme systems, functions are disturbed in zinc deficiency. Many foods are comparatively rich in zinc, such as seafood (especially oysters), liver, wheat germ, wheat bran, dried green split peas, lima beans, yeast, nuts, and milk. The table gives the zinc content of some common foods.

Zinc in 100 g of foods

applesauce	1.3	cherries	1.9	liver, pork	9	peas	13-5
barley	2.7	clams	2.0	milk, cow	1.7	potatoes	0.2
beef	2–5	corn	2.5	milk, dry skin	4.5	rice	1.5
beets	2.8	eggs, whole	5.5	oatmeal	14.0	spinach	0.6
bread, ww	3.0	egg yolk	3.3	oranges	0.1	syrup, maple	7.8
butter	0.3	herring	120	oysters	160	wheat	5.5
cabbage	0.9	lettuce	0.4	peanut butter	2.0	wheat bran	14
carrots	.0	liver, beef	0.5	pears, canned	1.6	yeast, dry	8

zucchini (*Cucurbita*). A variety of summer squash developed in Italy. It is also known as vegetable marrow or Italian marrow. Zucchini is cylindrical in shape but larger at its base than at its top. The skin has a lacy pattern of green and yellow that concentrates to give the appearance of stripes. It grows to be 10–12 inches long and 2–3 inches thick, and has pale-green flesh and a delicate flavor. Zucchini provides fair quantities of *carotene* (vitamin A activity), *ascorbic acid* (vitamin C), and small amounts of other vitamins. Cooked and drained, 100 g = 12 calories. See *squash, summer*.

zwieback. A sweet biscuit or rusk which is first baked and then sliced and toasted in the oven to make it into a kind of dry toast. The word comes from the German, and means "baked twice."

Nutrients in 100 g of zwieback

CALORIES KCAL	PROTEIN G	FAT G	CARBOHYDRATE G	VITAMIN A IU
423	11	9	74	40

zwitterion. A dipolar ion that carries both a positive and a negative charge in aqueous solution and is internally neutralized. The neutral amino acids are examples of zwitterions, because they have an *acid* group, the carboxyl group (COOH) and a basic group, the amino group (NH2). As shown, with near-neutral pHs, the zwitterion is internally neutralized.

$$H - \overset{\overset{\displaystyle H}{|}}{\underset{\underset{\displaystyle NH_3^+}{|}}{C}} - COO^-$$

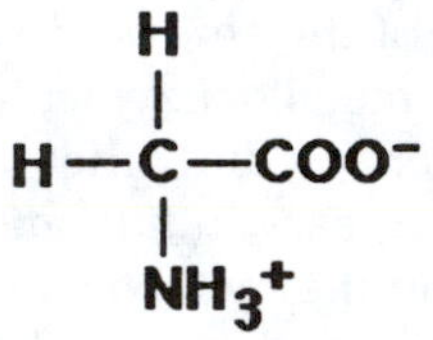

Zwitterion

zygosaccharomyces. Yeasts notable for their ability to grow in high concentrates of sugar (hence are termed osmophilic). They are involved in the spoilage of honey, syrups, and molasses and in the fermentation of soy sauce and some wines. Z. *nussbaumer* grows in honey.

zygote. The fertilized egg or the individual, resulting from the union of a sperm with an unfertilized egg.

Appendix

Common Abbreviations

AcCoA: acetyl coenzyme A
ACTH: adrenocorticotropic hormone
ADH: antidiuretic hormone
ADP: adenosine-5'-diphosphate
AMP: adenosine-5'-phosphate
ATP: adenosine-5'-triphosphate
BMR: basal metabolic rate
BUN: blood urea nitrogen
cal: calorie
cDNA: complementary deoxyribonucleic acid
CK, CPK: creatine kinase
DNA: deoxyribonucleic acid
Dopa: dioxy-or dihydroxyphenylalanine
EAA: essential amino acid
EF: extrinsic factor
EFA: essential fatty acid
FAD: flavin adenine dinucleotide oxidized form
PABA: para-amino benzoic acid
FADH$_2$: flavin adenine dinucleotide reduced form
FAO: Food and Agriculture Organization
FDA: Food and Drug Administration
FFA: free fatty acid
FMN: flavin mononucleotide
FSH: follicle-stimulating hormone
g, gm: gram (s)
GFR: glomerular filtration rate

GOT: glutamate oxalacetate transaminase
GPT: glutamate pyruvate transaminase
GTF: glucose tolerance factor
Hb: hemoglobin
HbO$_2$: oxyhemoglobin
INH: isonicotinic acid hydrazide
I.U.: international unit
J: joule
kcal: kilocalorie(s)
kg: kilogram
kJ: kilojoule
L: liter
b: pound
LCT: long-chain triglyceride
LH: luteinizing hormone
M. molar, moles per liter
MCT: medium-chain triglyceride
μg: microgram(s)
mEq: milliequivalent(s)
mg: milligram(s)
mL: milliliter(s)
mm: millimeter(s)
mRNA: messenger ribonucleic acid
N. normal, milliequivalents per liter
NAD: nicotinamide adenine dinucleotide
NADP: nicotinamide adenine dinucleotide phosphate

NEFA: nonesterified fatty acid
ng: nanogram(s)
NPN: nonprotein nitrogen
NRC: National Research Council
oz: ounce
PBI: protein-bound iodine
PCBs: polychlorinated biphenyls
pg: picogram(s)
pH: hydrogen ion concentration value
PKU: phenylketonuria
ppm: parts per million
PTH: parathyroid hormone
RDA: Recommended Dietary Allowances
RNA: ribonucleic acid

RNAse: ribonuclease
RQ: respiratory quotient
rRNA: ribosomal ribonucleic acid
TCA: tricarboxylic acid (Krebs') cycle
TPP: thiamine pyrophosphate
tRNA: transfer ribonucleic acid
TSH: thyroid-stimulating hormone
UNESCO: United Nations Educational, Scientific, and Cultural Organization
UNICEF: United Nations Children's Fund
USDA: United States Department of Agriculture
USP: United States Pharmacopeia
WHO: World Health Organization

Prefixes and Suffixes

The lists below are not intended to be complete. Many of the prefixes and suffixes are used in medicine and a medical dictionary is advised for a more comprehensive list. In the lists below, the examples given are in this text or are of common usage.

PREFIX	MEANING	EXAMPLE
A, AN	without, lack of	
A used before consonants		aphasia
AN used before vowels		anemia
AB	away from	abnormal
AD	toward, to, at	additive
ADEN, ADENO	relating to a gland	adenoid
ANA	again, back, building up	anabolism
ANTE, ANTERO	before, in front of	anterior
ANTI	against, opposed to	antigen
ARTHRO	pertaining to joints	arthritis
AUTO	self	autotrophic
BIO	pertaining to life	biochemical
BLAST, BLASTO	cell, germ	megaloblastic
CARDIO	pertaining to the heart	cardiovascular
CHOLE	pertaining to bile	cholecystokinin
CO, COM, CON	with, together	complication
CONTRA	against, opposite	contracture
CYSTO	pertaining to urinary bladder	cystitis
CYTO	pertaining to a cell	cytoplasm
DE	down, away from	deglutition
DERM, DERMATO	pertaining to the skin	dermatitis
DI	two, twice, double	disulfide
DIA	through	dialysis
DIS	reversal, separation	discharge
DYS	difficult, painful	dyspepsia
E, EC, ECTO, EX, EXO	out, outside, away from	extract
EM, EN	in	emphysema

Prefix	Meaning	Example
ENDO	within	endogenous
ENTERO	relation to the intestine	enterokinase
EPI	upon, above	epidermis
EXTRA	outside of, beyond, in addition	extracellular
GLYCO	sweetness (sugar)	glycogen
HEM, HEMO, HAEMO	some relation to the blood	hemoglobin
HETERO	other, other than, different from	heterogeneous
HISTO	some relation to tissues	histogenesis
HOMO	similarity	homeostasis
HYDRO	relation to water or hydrogen	hydrolysis
HYPER	above, over, excessive	hyperglycemia
HYPO	lack, deficiency	hypoglycemia
INFRA	below	inframandibular
INTER	between	intercellular
INTRA, INTRO	within	intracellular
LAC, LACTO	pertaining to milk	lactose
LEUCO, LEUKO	pertaining to anything white	leukocyte
MACRO	pertaining to anything large	macrocytic
MEGA, MEGALO	pertaining to anything great	megaloblastic
META	between, after, beyond—indicates changes, transformation into a succeeding stage, exchange	metabolism
MICRO	pertaining to anything small	microscopic
NEO	new, recent, young	neonatal
NEPHRO	pertaining to kidneys	nephron
NEURO	pertaining to nerves	neuralgia
ODONTO	pertaining or some relation to teeth	odontocele
OSSEO, OSSI, OSTEO	pertaining to bone	osteomalacia
PARA	beside, beyond, accessory to	parasympathetic
PATHO	pertaining to disease	pathogen
PERI	around	peristalsis
PHOTO	pertaining to light	photosynthesis
POLY	many	polysaccharide
POST	after, behind	postprandial
PRE	before	precursor
PYO	pertaining to pus	pyorrhea
SEPTI	pertaining to poison	septicemia
SUB	under, almost	subclinical
SYN	union	synthesize
THERMO	relating to heat	thermometer
TOX, TOXI, TOXICO	relating to poison	toxic
TRANS	across, through	transplant
VASO	pertaining to vessel	vasodilation

Suffix	Meaning	Example
-AC	pertaining to	hemophiliac
-AEMIA, -EMIA	denoting a condition of the blood	leukemia
-ALGIA, -ALGY	a painful condition	neuralgia
-ASE	enzyme	sucrase
-BLAST	germ, cell	myeloblast
-COCCUS	round bacterium	streptococcus
-CYTE	hollow vessels, used to denote a cell	lymphocyte
-ECTOMY	excision of	appendectomy

Suffix	Meaning	Example
-ITIS	inflammation	gastritis
-LOGY, -OLOGY	the science of	bacteriology
-LYSIS	a loosening, a dissolving	hemolysis
-OMA	morbid condition, especially a tumor	carcinoma
-OREXIA	appetite, desire	anorexia
-OSE	carbohydrate	glucose
-OSIS	a condition or process, particularly a disease condition or morbid process	xanthomatosis
-OSTOMY, -STOMY	the making of a mouth	colostomy
-OUS	full of, having, possessing	fibrous
-PHAGIA	eating	polyphagia
-PHASIA	speech	aphasia
-RRHAGIA, -RRHAGE	excessive flow	hemorrhage
-URIA	urine	polyuria

APPENDIX

3

Table of International Atomic Weights

Element	Symbol	Atomic No.	Atomic Weight	Element	Symbol	Atomic No.	Atomic Weight
Actinium	Ac	89		Gadolinium	Gd	64	157.25
Aluminum	Al	13	26.9815	Gallium	Ga	31	69.72
Americium	Am	95		Germanium	Ge	32	72.59
Antimony	Sb	51	121.75	Gold	Au	79	196.967
Argon	Ar	18	39.948	Hafnium	Hf	72	178.49
Arsenic	As	33	74.9216	Helium	He	2	4.0026
Astatine	At	85		Holmium	Ho	67	164.930
Barium	Ba	56	137.34	Hydrogen	H	1	1.00797[a]
Berkelium	Bk	97		Indium	In	49	114.82
Beryllium	Be	4	9.0122	Iodine	I	53	126.9044
Bismuth	Bi	83	208.980	Iridium	Ir	77	192.2
Boron	B	5	10.811[a]	Iron	Fe	26	55.847[b]
Bromine	Br	35	79.909[b]	Krypton	Kr	36	83.80
Cadmium	Cd	48	112.40	Lanthanum	La	57	138.91
Calcium	Ca	20	40.08	Lead	Pb	82	207.19
Californium	Cf	98		Lithium	Li	3	6.939
Carbon	C	6	12.01115[a]	Lutetium	Lu	71	174.97
Cerium	Ce	58	140.12	Magnesium	Mg	12	24.312
Cesium	Cs	55	132.905	Manganese	Mn	25	54.9380
Chlorine	Cl	17	35.453[b]	Mendelevium	Md	101	
Chromium	Cr	24	51.996[b]	Mercury	Hg	80	200.59
Cobalt	Co	27	58.9332	Molybdenum	Mo	42	95.94
Copper	Cu	29	63.54	Neodymium	Nd	60	144.24
Curium	Cm	96		Neon	Ne	10	20.183
Dysprosium	Dy	66	162.50	Neptunium	Np	93	
Einsteinium	Es	99		Nickel	Ni	28	58.71
Erbium	Er	68	167.26	Niobium	Nb	41	92.906
Europium	Eu	63	151.96	Nitrogen	N	7	14.0067
Fermium	Fm	100		Nobelium	No	102	
Fluorine	F	9	18.9984	Osmium	Os	76	190.2
Francium	Fr	87		Oxygen	O	8	15.9994[a]

Element	Symbol	Atomic No.	Atomic Weight	Element	Symbol	Atomic No.	Atomic Weight
Palladium	Pd	46	106.4	Sodium	Na	11	22.9898
Phosphorus	P	15	30.9738	Strontium	Sr	38	87.62
Platinum	Pt	78	195.09	Sulfur	S	16	32.064[a]
Plutonium	Pu	94		Tantalum	Ta	73	180.948
Polonium	Po	84		Technetium	Tc	43	
Potassium	K	19	39.102	Tellurium	Te	52	127.60
Praseodymium	Pr	59	140.907	Terbium	Tb	65	158.924
Promethium	Pm	61		Thallium	Tl	81	204.37
Protactinum	Pa	91		Thorium	Th	90	232.038
Radium	Ra	88		Thulium	Tm	69	168,934
Radon	Rn	86		Tin	Sn	50	118.69
Rhenium	Re	75	186.2	Titanium	Ti	22	47.90
Rhodium	Rh	45	102.905	Tungsten	W	74	183.85
Rubidium	Rb	37	85.47	Uranium	U	92	238.03
Ruthenium	Ru	44	101.07	Vanadium	V	23	50.942
Samarium	Sm	62	150.35	Xenon	Xe	54	131.30
Scandium	Sc	21	44.956	Ytterbium	Yb	70	173.04
Selenium	Se	34	78.96	Yttrium	Y	39	88.905
Silicon	Si	14	28.086[a]	Zinc	Zn	30	65.37
Silver	Ag	47	107.870[b]	Zirconium	Zr	40	91.22

[a] The atomic weight varies because of natural variations in the isotopic composition of the element. The observed ranges are boron, ± 0.003; carbon, ± 0.00005; hydrogen, ± 0.00001; oxygen, ± 0.0001; silicon, ± 0.001; sulfur, ± 0.003.

[b] The atomic weight is believed to have an experimental uncertainty of the following magnitude; bromine, ± 0.002; chlorine, ± 0.001; chromium, ± 0.001; iron, ± 0.003; silver, ± 0.003. For other elements the last digit given is believed to be reliable to ± 0.5.

Conversions

Weight

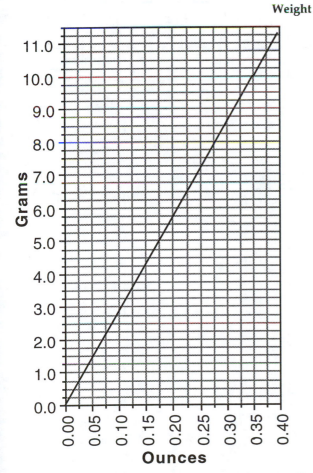

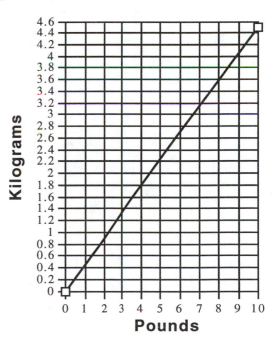

1 pound = 0.45 kilogram
1 kilogram = 2.2 pounds

1 ounce = 28 grams
1 kilogram = 2.2 pounds

Temperature
Fahrenheit-Celsius

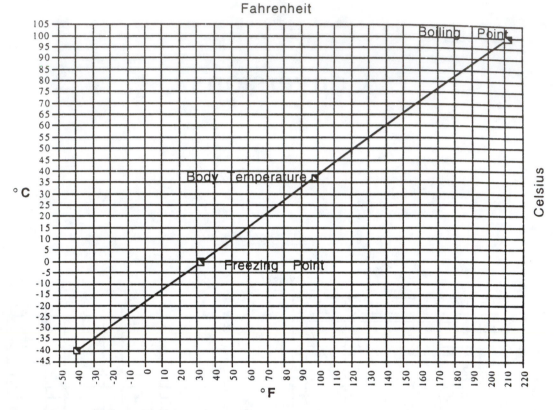

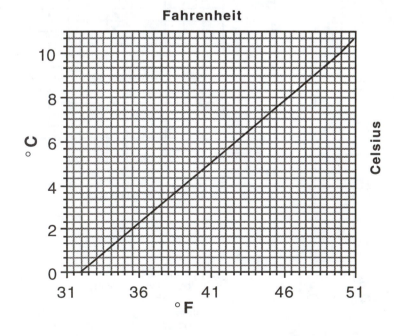

CONVERT °C TO °F

$$°F = (°C \times 9/5) + 32°$$

CONVERT °F TO °C

$$°C = 5/9 (°F - 32°)$$

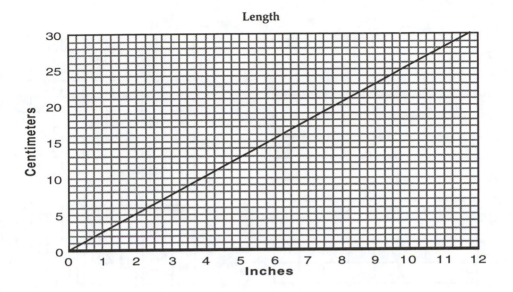

Length

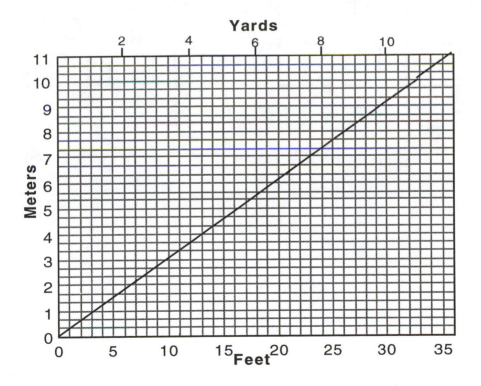

Yards

1 inch = 2.54 centimeters
1 centimeter = 0.3937 1nches

1 foot = 0.3048 meters
1 meter = 3.2808 feet
1 yard = 0.914 meter

Area

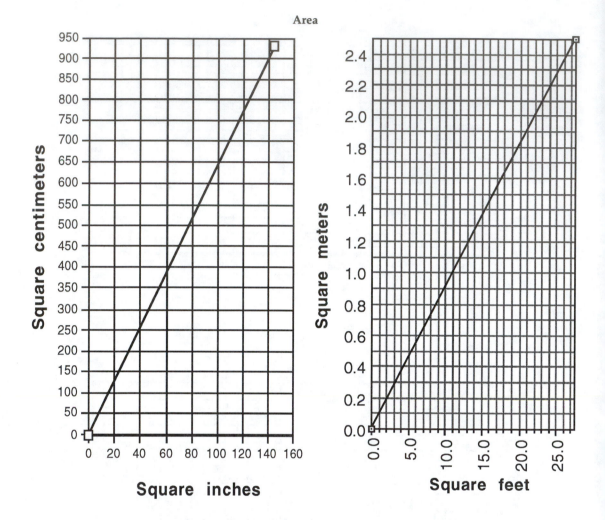

141 sq. in. = 929 sq. cm.
1 sq. in. = 6.452 sq. cm.
1 sq. cm. = 0.155 sq. in.

1 sq. yd. =0.82 sq. m.
1 sq. ft. = 0.092 sq. m.
1 sq. m. = 10.8 sq. ft.

Volume

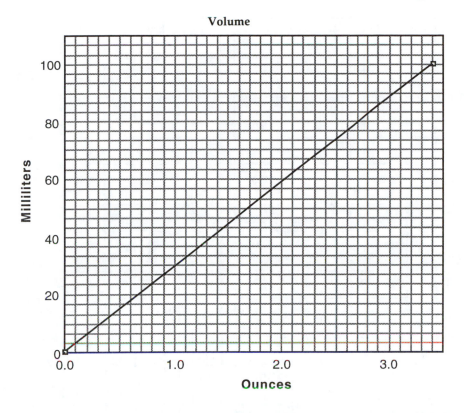

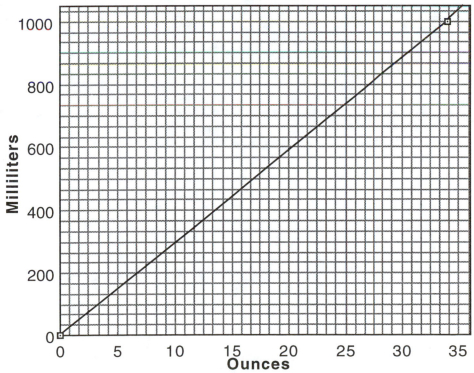

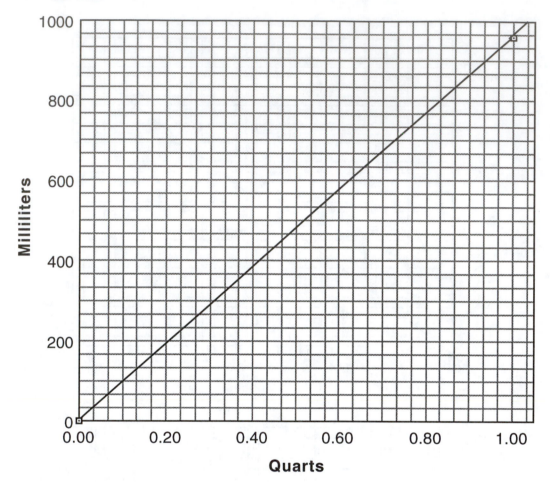

60 drops = 1 tsp   2 tbsp = 1 fluid oz   2 cups = 1 pint
        = 5 mL   = 30 mL   = 16 oz
   3 tsp = 1 tbsp   16 tbsp = 1 cup   4 cups = 1quart
        =15 mL   = 240 mL   = 960 mL

Metric Measures

If Measure Is In	Multiply By	To Find
Length		
inches	25.4	millimeters
inches	2.54	centimeters
feet	30.48	centimeters
feet	0.305	meters
centimeters	0.394	inches
meters	3.281	feet
Weight		
grains	64.799	milligrams
ounces (Av.)	28.35	grams
pounds (Av.)	454	grams
pounds	0.454	kilograms
grams	15.432	grains
grams	0.035	ounces (Av.)
grams	0.0022	pounds (Av.)
kilograms	2.205	pounds
Capacity (liquid)		
teaspoons	4.7	milliliters
tablespoons	14.1	milliliters
fluid ounces	29.573	milliliters
cups (8 ounces)	238	milliliters
pints	0.473	liters
quarts	0.946	liters
milliliters	0.034	fluid ounces
liters	1.057	quarts
Energy units		
kilocalories	4.184	kilojoules
kilojoules	0.239	kilocalories
Temperature		
Fahrenheit	subtract 32; then multiply by $\frac{5}{9}$	Celsius (Centigrade)
Celsius	multiply by $\frac{9}{5}$; then add 32	Fahrenheit

Metric equivalents
   1 kilogram (kg) = 1000 grams
   1 gram (gm) = 1000 milligrams
   1 milligram (mg) = 1000 micrograms
   1 microgram (mcg, μg, γ) = 1000 nanograms
   1 nanogram (ng) = 1000 picograms (pg)
Multiples
   deca- 10
   hecto- 10^2 (100)
   kilo- 10^3 (1000)
   mega- 10^6 (1,000,000)
Submultiples
   deci- = one tenth 10^{-1} (0.1)
   centi- = one hundredth 10^{-2} (0.01)
   milli- = one thousandth 10^{-3} (0.001)
   micro- = one millionth 10^{-6} (0.000,001)
   nano- = one billionth 10^{-9} (0.000,000,001)
   pico- = one trillionth 10^{-12} (0.000,000,000,001)

5

Greek Alphabet

The letters of the Greek alphabet are frequently employed by chemists. Many of the metabolic intermediates carry the Greek alphabet as part of the name, e.g., alpha (α) amino acid and beta (β) carotene, usually to denote the position of some substituent in the molecule. *Ortho*, *para*, and *meta* are also used to designate positions in aromatic ring compounds. *Ortho* means straight, *para* means alongside of, and *meta* means in the midst of or between.

NAME OF LETTER	CAPITAL	SMALL
alpha	A	α
beta	B	β
gamma	Γ	γ
delta	Δ	δ
epsilon	E	ϵ
zeta	Z	ζ
eta	H	η
theta	Θ	θ
iota	I	ι
kappa	K	κ
lambda	Λ	λ
mu	M	μ
nu	N	ν
xi	Ξ	ξ
omicron	O	o
pi	Π	π
rho	P	ρ
sigma	Σ	σ
tau	T	τ
upsilon	Υ	υ
phi	Φ	ϕ
chi	X	χ
psi	Ψ	ψ
omega	Ω	ω

Weight Ranges for Heights of Men and Women

HEIGHT (WITHOUT SHOES) INCHES	WEIGHT (WITHOUT CLOTHING)			HEIGHT CENTIMETERS	WEIGHT		
	LOW	MEDIAN POUNDS	HIGH		LOW	MEDIAN KILOGRAMS	HIGH
Men							
63	118	129	141	160	54	59	64
64	122	133	145	163	55	60	66
65	126	137	149	165	57	62	68
66	130	142	155	167	59	65	70
67	134	147	161	170	61	67	73
68	139	151	166	173	63	69	75
69	143	155	170	175	65	70	77
70	147	159	174	178	67	72	80
71	150	163	178	180	68	74	81
72	154	167	183	183	70	76	83
73	158	171	188	185	72	77	85
74	162	175	192	188	74	80	87
75	165	178	195	191	75	81	89
Women							
60	100	109	118	152	45	50	54
61	104	112	121	155	47	51	55
62	107	115	125	157	49	52	57
63	110	118	128	160	50	54	58
64	113	122	132	163	51	55	60
65	116	125	135	165	53	57	61
66	120	129	139	167	55	59	63
67	123	132	142	170	56	60	65
68	126	136	146	173	57	62	66
69	130	140	151	175	59	64	69
70	133	144	156	178	60	65	71
71	137	148	161	180	62	67	73
72	141	152	166	183	64	69	75

*Data for heights in inches and weights in pounds taken from: Hathaway, M. L., and Foard, E. D.: *Heights and Weights of Adults in the United States*. Home Economics Research Report No. 10, U.S. Department of Agriculture, Washington, D.C.

Conversions to centimeters and kilograms were rounded off to the nearest whole number.

Normal Constituents of Human Blood

CONSTITUENT	NORMAL RANGE		EXAMPLES OF DEVIATIONS
Physical Measurements			
Specific gravity (S)	1.025–1.029		
Bleeding time, capillary	1–3	min	
Prothrombin time (Quick, P)	10–20	sec	
Sedimentation rate (Wintrobe)			
Men	0–9	mm/hr	
Women	0–20	mm/hr	
Viscosity (water as unity) (b)	4.5–5.5		
Acid-Base Constituents			
Base, total fixed cations (Na + K + Ca + Mg) (S)	143–150	mEq/L	Low in alkali deficit; diabetic acidosis
Sodium (S)	320–335	mg/100 mL	Low in alkali deficit, diabetic acidosis, excessive fluid administration
	139–146	mEq/L	
Potassium (S)	16–22	mg/100 mL	High in acute infections, pneumonia, Addison's disease; low in diarrhea, vomiting, correction of diabetic acidosis
	4.1–5.6	mEq/L	
Calcium (S)	9–11	mg/100 mL	High with excessive vitamin D, hyperparathyroidism; low in infantile tetany, steatorrhea, severe nephritis, defective vitamin D absorption
	4.5–5.5	mEq/L	
Calcium, ionized (S)	50–60	percent	

Constituent	Normal Range		Examples of Deviations
Magnesium (S)	2–3	mg/100 mL	High in chronic nephritis, liver disease; low in uremia, tetany, severe diarrhea
	1.65–2.5	mEq/L	
Chloride (S)	340–372	mg/100 mL	High in congestive heart failure, eclampsia, nephritis
	96–105	mEq/L	
As NaCl (S)	560–614	mg/100 mL	
	96–105	mEq/L	
Phosphorus, inorganic as P (S)			
Child	4.0–6.5	mg/100 mL	High in chronic nephritis, hypoparathyroidism; low during treatment of diabetic coma, hyperparathyroidism
Adult	2.5–4.5	mg/100 mL	
Sulfates as SO_4—(S)	2.5–5.0	mg/100 mL	
	0.5–1.0	mEq/L	
Bicarbonate cation-binding power (S)	19–30	mEq/L	
Serum protein cation-binding power (S)	15.5–18.0	mEq/L	
Lactic acid (S)	10–20	mg/100 mL	
	1.1–2.2	mEq/L	
pH at 38°C (B, P, or S)	7.30–7.45		High in uncompensated alkalosis; low in uncompensated acidosis
Blood Gases			
CO_2 (venous S)	45–70	vol %	Low in primary alkali deficit, diarrhea; high in hypoventilation
	20.3–31.5	mM/L	
CO_2 content (venous B)	40–60	vol %	
	18–27	mM/L	
CO_2 tension (pCO_2) arterial blood	35–45	mm Hg	pCO_2 in venous blood is about 6 mm higher than arterial or capillary blood
Oxygen content (arterial B)	15–22	vol %	High in polycythemia; low in emphysema
Oxygen content (venous B)	11–16	vol %	
Oxygen capacity (B)	16–24	vol %	
Oxygen tension (pO_2)	85–100	mm Hg	
Carbohydrates			
Glucose			
Reducing substances (B)	90–120	mg/100 mL	High in diabetes mellitus; low in hyperinsulinism
"True"	60–85	mg/100 mL	
Glucose tolerance			
Fasting sugar	90–120	mg/100 mL	
Highest value	130–140	mg/100 mL	
Highest value reached in	45–60	minutes	

Constituent	Normal Range		Examples of Deviations
Return to fasting in	1.5–2.5	hr	
Lactose tolerance			
Fasting blood glucose (B)	90–120	mg/100 mL	In lactase deficiency
Increase in blood glucose after test dose lactose	20	mg/100 mL	the rise in blood glucose after test dose of lactose is less than 20 mg in 1 hour
Citric acid (B)	1.3–2.3	mg/100 mL	
(P)	1.6–2.7	mg/100 mL	
Lactic acid (see acid-base constituents)			
Pyruvic acid, fasting (B)	0.7–1.2	mg/100 mL	
Enzymes			
Amylase (Somogyi) (S)	60–180	units/100 mL	High in acute pancreatitis, acute appendicitis
Lactic dehydrogenase (S)	25–100	units/mL	High in myocardial infarction
Lipase (S)	0.2–1.5	units/mL	High in pancreatitis
Leucine-aminopeptidase (S)	1–3.5	units/mL	High in hemolytic anemias
Phosphatase, alkaline (Bodansky) (S) Child	4–14	units/100 mL	High in rickets, bone cancer, Paget's disease, hyperparathyroidism, vitamin D inadequacy; indicates rapid bone growth in young
Adult	1–4		
Transaminases			
Glutamic-oxalacetic (SGOT) (Karmen) (S)	10–40	units/mL	Increased within 24 hours in myocardial infarction; normal after 6 to 7 days
Glutamic-pyruvic (SGPT) (Karmen) (S)	5–35	units/mL	High in hepatic disease, and trauma after surgery
Hematologic Studies			
Cell volume	39–50	percent	High in polycythemia; low in anemia, prolonged iron deficiency
Red blood cells	4.25–5.25	million per cu mm	High in polycythemia, dehydration; low in anemia, hemorrhage
White blood cells	5000–9000	per cu mm	Increased in acute infections, leukemias
Lymphocytes	25–30	percent	
Neutrophils	60–65	percent	
Monocytes	4–8	percent	
Eosinophils	0.5–4	percent	

Constituent	Normal Range		Examples of Deviations
Basophils	0–1.5	percent	
Platelets	125,000–300,000	per cu mm	
Lipids			
Acetone (S)	0.3–2.0	mg/100 mL	High in uncontrolled diabetes and starvation
Cholesterol, total (S)	125–225	mg/100 mL	High in uncontrolled diabetes mellitus, nephrosis, hypothyroidism, hyperlipidemias
esters	50–67	percent	
free	33–50	percent	
Fatty acids, unesterified (P)	8–31	mg/100 mL	
17-Hydroxycorticosteroids (P)	10–13.5	μg/100 mL	
Lipids, total (P)	570–820	mg/100 mL	
Phospholipid (S)	150–300	mg/100 mL	
Triglycerides (S)	30–140	mg/100 mL	Increased in hyperlipidemias
Nitrogenous Constituents			
Alpha-amino acid nitrogen (S)	3.5–5.5	mg/100 mL	High in severe liver disease; low in nephrosis
Ammonia (B)	40–70	μg/100 mL	High in liver disease
Creatinine (S)	0.5–1.2	mg/100 mL	Increased in renal insufficiency
Creatinine clearance endogenous (B)	120±20	mL	Blood cleared per min by kidney; measure of glomerular filtration
Nonprotein N (NPN) (B)	25–35	mg/100 mL	High in acute glomerulonephritis, dehydration, metallic poisoning, intestinal obstruction, renal failure
Phenylalanine (S)	0.7–4	mg/100 mL	Increased in phenylketonuria
Urea nitrogen (BUN) (B)	8–18	mg/100 mL	High in renal failure, acute glomerulonephritis, mercury poisoning, dehydration; low in hepatic failure
Urea clearance (B)	75	ml/min C_m	C_m = maximal clearance
	54	ml/min C_s	C_s = standard clearance
Uric acid (S)	2–6	mg/100 mL	High in gout, nephritis, arthritis
Proteins			
Total protein (S)	6.5–7.5	gm/100 mL	High in dehydration; low in liver disease, nephrosis

Constituent	Normal Range		Examples of Deviations
Albumin (S)	3.9–4.5	gm/100 mL	Low in starvation, cirrhosis, proteinuria
Globulin (S)	2.3–3.5	gm/100 mL	High in infections, liver disease, multiple myeloma
Albumin globulin ratio	1.2–1.9		Low in liver disease, nephrosis
Fibrinogen (P)	0.2–0.5	gm/100 mL	High in infections; low in severe liver disease
Ceruloplasmin (S)	16–33	mg/100 mL	
Gamma globulin (S)	0.7–1.2	gm/100 mL	
Hemoglobin (B)			
Males	14–17	gm/100 mL	High in polycythemia; low in prolonged dietary deficiency, anemia
Females	12–16	gm/100 mL	
Vitamins			
Ascorbic acid (S)	0.3–1.4	mg/100 mL	
Folic acid (*L. casei*) (S)	6–10	ng/mL	
(*L. casei*) (B)	100–220	ng/mL	
Niacin (S)	30–150	μg/100 mL	
Riboflavin (S)	2.3–3.7	μg/100 mL	
Thiamine (B)	5.5–9.5	μg/100 mL	
Tocopherol (S)	0.6–2.0	mg/100 mL	
Vitamin A (S)	25–90	μg/100 mL	
Carotene (S)	40–125	μg/100 mL	
Vitamin B_6 (B)	1–18	μg/100 mL	
Vitamin B_{12} (S)	10–90	μg/100 mL	
Miscellaneous			
Bilirubin (S)	0–1.5	mg/100 mL	High in red cell destruction, liver disease
Icterus index	4–6	units	High in jaundice
Copper (S)	80–240	μg/100 mL	Low in anemia, Wilson's disease
Iron (S)			
Men	80–165	μg/100 mL	High in hemochromatosis, liver disease, transfusion hemosiderosis; low in iron-deficiency anemia
Women	65–130	μg/100 mL	
Iron-binding capacity (S)			
Men	250–430	μg/100 mL	High in anemia
Women	220–415	μg/100 mL	
Lead (S)	1–3	μg/100 mL	
Manganese (S)	2–5	μg/100 mL	

Constituent	Normal Range		Examples of Deviations
Protein-bound iodine (PBI) (S)	3–8	μg/100 mL	High in hyperthyroidism; low in hypothyroidism
Zinc (S)	100–140	μg/100 mL	

(B = Whole Blood, P = Plasma, S = Serum)

mL = milliliters

mg = milligrams

μg = micograms

mEq = milliequivalents

gm = grams

cu mm = cubic millimeters

$$\text{mEq per liter} = \frac{\text{mg per liter}}{\text{equivalent weight}} \quad \text{mM (millimoles) per liter} = \frac{\text{mg per liter}}{\text{molecular weight}}$$

$$\text{equivalent weight} = \frac{\text{atomic weight}}{\text{valence of element}} \quad \text{volumes per cent} = \text{mM per liter} \times 2.24$$

Sources of Data:

Oser, B. L., ed.: *Hawk's Physiological Chemistry*, 14th ed. McGraw-Hill Book Company, New York, 1965, pp. 977–79.

Robinson, H. W.: "Biochemistry," in *Rypins' Medical Licensure Examinations*, 11th ed., A. W. Wright, ed. J. B. Lippincott Company, Philadelphia, 1970, pp. 205–5.

Recommended Daily Allowances (RDA)

Food and Nutrition Board, National Academy of Sciences—National Research Council. Designed for the maintenance of good nutrition of practically all healthy people in the U.S.A.[a]

	Age (years)	Weight (kg)	Weight (lb)	Height (cm)	Height (in.)	Protein (g)	Fat-Soluble Vitamins			Water-Soluble Vitamins							Minerals					
							Vitamin A (µg R E)[b]	Vitamin D (µg)[c]	Vitamin E (mg α TE)[d]	Vitamin C (mg)	Thiamin (mg)	Riboflavin (mg)	Niacin (mg NE)[e]	Vitamin B6 (mg)	Folacin (µg)[f]	Vitamin B12 (µg)[g]	Calcium (mg)	Phosphorus (mg)	Magnesium (mg)	Iron (mg)[h]	Zinc (mg)	Iodine (µg)
Infants	0.0–0.5	6	13	60	24	kg×2.2	420	10	3	35	0.3	0.4	6	0.3	30	0.5	360	240	50	10	3	40
	0.5–1.0	9	20	71	28	kg×2.0	400	10	4	35	0.5	0.6	8	0.6	45	1.5	540	360	70	15	5	50
Children	1–3	13	29	90	35	23	400	10	5	45	0.7	0.8	9	0.9	100	2.0	800	800	150	15	10	70
	4–6	20	44	112	44	30	500	10	6	45	0.9	1.0	11	1.3	200	2.5	800	800	200	10	10	90
	7–10	28	62	132	52	34	700	10	7	45	1.2	1.4	16	1.6	300	3.0	800	800	250	10	10	120
Males	11–14	45	99	157	62	45	1000	10	8	50	1.4	1.6	18	1.8	400	3.0	1200	1200	350	18	15	150
	15–18	66	145	176	69	56	1000	10	10	60	1.4	1.7	18	2.0	400	3.0	1200	1200	400	18	15	150
	19–22	70	154	177	70	56	1000	7.5	10	60	1.5	1.7	19	2.2	400	3.0	800	800	350	10	15	150
	23–50	70	154	178	70	56	1000	5	10	60	1.4	1.6	18	2.2	400	3.0	800	800	350	10	15	150
	51+	70	154	178	70	56	1000	5	10	60	1.2	1.4	16	2.2	400	3.0	800	800	350	10	15	150
Females	11–14	46	101	157	62	46	800	10	8	50	1.1	1.3	15	1.8	400	3.0	1200	1200	300	18	15	150
	15–18	55	120	163	64	46	800	10	8	60	1.1	1.3	14	2.0	400	3.0	1200	1200	300	18	15	150
	19–22	55	120	163	64	44	800	7.5	8	60	1.1	1.3	14	2.0	400	3.0	800	800	300	18	15	150
	23–50	55	120	163	64	44	800	5	8	60	1.0	1.2	13	2.0	400	3.0	800	800	300	18	15	150
	51+	55	120	163	64	44	800	5	8	60	1.0	1.2	13	2.0	400	3.0	800	800	300	10	15	150
Pregnant						+30	+200	+5	+2	+20	+0.4	+0.3	+2	+0.6	+400	+1.0	+400	+400	+150	h	+5	+25
Lactating						+20	+400	+5	+3	+40	+0.5	+0.5	+5	+0.5	+100	+1.0	+400	+400	+150	h	+10	+50

[a] Revised 1980. The allowances are intended to provide for individual variations among most normal persons as they live in the United States under usual environmental stresses.

[b] Retinol equivalents: 1 retinol equivalent = 1 µg retinol or 6 µg beta-carotene.

[c] As cholecalciferol: 10 µg cholecalciferol = 400 I.U. of vitamin D.

[d] Alpha-tocopherol equivalents: 1 mg d-alpha-tocopherol = 1 α-TE.

[e] One (niacin equivalent) is equal to 1 mg of niacin or 60 mg of dietary tryptophan.

[f] The folacin allowances refer to dietary sources as determined by Lactobacillus casei assay after treatment with enzymes (conjugases) to make polyglutamyl forms of the vitamin available to the test organism.

[g] The recommended dietary allowance for vitamin B_{12} in infants is based on average concentration of the vitamin in human milk. The allowances after weaning are based on energy intake, as recommended by the American Academy of Pediatrics, and consideration of other factors, such as intestinal absorption.

[h] The increased requirement during pregnancy may not be met by the iron content of habitual American diets nor by the existing stores of many women; therefore, the use of 30 to 60 mg of supplemental iron is recommended. Iron needs during lactation are not substantially different from those of nonpregnant women, but continued supplementation of the mother for 2 to 3 months after parturition is advisable in order to replenish stores depleted by pregnancy.

Food and Nutrition Board, National Academy of Sciences—National Research Council.
Designed for the maintenance of good nutrition of practically all healthy people in the U.S.A. (Continued)

	Age (years)	Vitamins			Trace Elements						Electrolytes		
		Vitamin K (µg)	Pantothenic Acid (mg)	Copper (mg)	Copper (mg)	Manganese (mg)	Fluoride (mg)	Chromium (mg)	Selenium (mg)	Molybdenum (mg)	Sodium (mg)	Potassium (mg)	Chloride (mg)
Infants	0–0.5	12	35	2	0.5–0.7	0.5–0.7	0.1–0.5	0.01–0.04	0.01–0.04	0.03–0.06	115–350	350–925	275–700
	0.5–1	10–20	50	3	0.7–1.0	0.7–1.0	0.2–1.0	0.02–0.06	0.02–0.06	0.04–0.08	250–750	425–1275	400–1200
Children	1–3	15–30	65	3	1.0–1.5	1.0–1.5	0.5–1.5	0.02–0.08	0.02–0.08	0.05–0.1	325–975	550–1650	500–1500
and	4–6	20–40	85	3–4	1.5–2.0	1.5–2.0	1.0–2.5	0.03–0.12	0.03–0.12	0.06–0.15	450–1350	775–2325	700–2100
	7–10	30–60	120	4–5	2.0–2.5	2.0–3.0	1.5–2.5	0.05–0.2	0.05–0.2	0.1–0.3	600–1800	1000–3000	925–2775
Adolescents	11+	50–100	100–200	4–7	2.0–3.0	2.5–5.0	1.5–2.5	0.05–0.2	0.05–0.2	0.15–0.5	900–2700	1525–4575	1400–4200
Adults		70–140	100–200	4–7	2.0–3.0	2.5–5.0	1.5–4.0	0.05–0.2	0.05–0.2	0.15–0.5	1100–3300	1875–5625	1700–5100

[a] Because there is less information on which to base allowances, these figures are provided in the form of ranges of recommended intakes.

[b] Since the toxic levels for many trace elements may be only several times usual intakes, the upper levels for the trace elements given in the table should not be habitually exceeded.

Mineral and Vitamin Content of Foods

Sodium, Potassium, Phosphorus, Magnesium, and Zinc: Folacin, Pantothenic Acid, Vitamin B$_6$, Vitamin B$_{12}$, and Vitamin E (Values for 100 g, edible portion).

Item No.	Food	Sodium MG	Potassium MG	Phosphorus MG	Magnesium MG	Zinc MG	Folacin µG	Pantothenic Acid µG	Vitamin B6 µG	Vitamin B12 µG	Vitamin E MG
1	Almonds, dried	4	773	504	270		45	470	100	0	
2	Roasted, salted	198	773	504	—			250	95	0	
3	Apples, raw, not peeled	1	110	10	8	0.05	2	105	30	0	0.31
4	Apple brown Betty	153	100	22	—						
5	Apple juice, bottled	1	101	9	4		trace	—	30	0	
6	Applesauce, sweetened	2	65	5	5	0.1		85	30	0	
7	Apricots, raw	1	281	23	12		3	240	70	0	
8	Canned	1	234	15	7		1	92	54	0	
9	Dried, sulfured, uncooked	26	979	108	62		5[2]	753[2]	169[2]	0	
10	Cooked, sweetened	7	278	31	20						
11	Apricot nectar	trace	151	12	—						
12	Asparagus, green, cooked	1	183	50	20 (raw)		109				
13	Canned, regular pack	236	166	53	—		27	195	55	0	
14	Low sodium	3	166	53	—						
15	Frozen spears, cooked	1	238	67	14		109	410	155	0	
16	Avocado	4	604	42	45		30	1,070	420	0	
17	Bacon, cooked, drained	1,021	236	224	25		—	330 (raw)	125 (raw)	0.70 (raw)	0.53
18	Canadian, cooked	2,555	432	218	24						
	Baking powder, home use:										
19	Sodium aluminum sulfate	10,953	150	2,904							
20	Straight phosphate	8,220	170	9,438							
21	Tartrate	7,300	3,800	0							
22	Low sodium, commercial	6	10,948								
23	Low sodium, noncommercial formula		20,729								
24	Banana	1	370	26	33	0.2	10	260	510	0	0.22
25	Barley, pearled, light	3	160	189	37		—	503	224	0	
26	Bass, sea, raw	68	256	—	—			512	—	—	
	Beans, common, mature:										
27	White dry	19	1,196	425	170	2.8	125	725	560	0	0.47

28	Cooked	7	416	148	—	1.0					—
29	Canned with pork and tomato sauce	463	210	92	37			92	—	0	—
30	Red, dry	10	984	406	163		180[1]	500	441	0	
31	Cooked	3	340	140	—						
32	Beans, Lima, immature: Cooked	1	422	121	67 (raw)		34	(raw)	(raw)		
33	Canned, regular pack	236	222	70	—		13	130	90	0	
34	Low sodium	4	222	70	—						
35	Frozen, Fordhook, cooked	101	426	90	48		34	240	150	0	
36	Mature seeds, dry	4	1,529	385	180 (raw)	2.8	103	975	580	0	
37	Cooked	2	612	154	—	0.9	128				
38	Beans, Mung, sprouts, cooked	4	156	48	—		145				
39	Beans, snap, green, cooked	4	151	37	32 (raw)	0.3	28	190 (raw)	80 (raw)	0	
40	Canned, regular pack	236	95	25	14	0.3	12	75	40	0	0.03
41	Low sodium	2	95	25	—						
42	Frozen, cooked	1	152	32	21 (raw)		28	135	70	0	0.11
43	Yellow, cooked	3	151	37	—		32	250 (raw)	(raw)	0	
44	Canned, regular pack	236	95	25	—				42	0	
45	Low sodium	2	95	25	—						
46	Beef: All cuts, lean, broiled or roasted average	60	370	246	29	5.8	11	620 (raw)	435 (raw)	1.8 (raw)	0.13
47	Simmered, average	60	370	194	18	6.2					(raw)
48	Hamburger, regular, cooked	47	450	194	21		7				0.37
49	Beef, canned, roast beef	—	259	116	—						
50	Beef, corned, cooked	1,740	150	93	—				75 (with potato)	1.84 (canned)	
51	Hash, canned	540	200	67	—						—

Item No.	Food	Sodium MG	Potassium MG	Phosphorus MG	Magnesium MG	Zinc MG	Folacin µG	Pantothenic Acid µG	Vitamin B6 µG	Vitamin B12 µg	Vitamin E MG
52	Beef, dried	4,300	200	404	—			—	—	1.84	
53	Beef potpie, commercial	366	93	48	—						
54	Home recipe	284	159	71	—						
55	Beef and vegetable stew, canned	411	174	45	—			—	—	0.65	
56	Home recipe	37	250	75	—						
57	Beets, cooked	43	208	23	25 (raw)		14	150 (raw)	55 (raw)	0	
58	Canned, regular pack	236	167	18	15		3	100	50	0	
59	Low sodium	46	167	18	—						
60	Beet greens, cooked	76	332	25	106 (raw)		60	250	100 (raw)	0	
	Beverages, alcoholic										
61	Beer	7	25	30				80	60	0	
62	Gin	1	2								
63	Wine, table	5	92	10	10			30	40	0	
	Biscuits, baking powder:										
64	Enriched	626	117	175	—						
65	Self-rising flour	660[3]	64	317[3]	—						
66	Biscuit dough, commercial in cans	868	65	497	—						
67	Blackberries, raw	1	170	19	30		14	240	50	0	
68	Blueberries, raw	1	81	13	6		8	156	67	0	
69	Frozen, sweetened	1	66	11	4		8	121	54	0	
70	Bluefish, baked or broiled, prepared with butter	104	—	287	—						
71	Bouillon cube	24,000	100	—	—						
72	Bran, with sugar and malt extract	1,060	1,070	1,176	—						
73	Bran flakes (40 per cent bran)	925	—	495	—	3.6		875	384	0	
74	Bran flakes with raisins	800	—	396	—						
75	Brazil nuts	1	715	693	225		5	231	170	0	
	Breads:										
76	Boston brown	251	292	160	—						
77	Cracked wheat	529	134	128	35		25	607	92	0	

78	French or Vienna	580	90	85	22		9	378	53	0	
79	Italian	585	74	77	—		—				
80	Raisin	365	233	87	24						
81	Rye, American	557	145	147	42	1.6	16	450	100	0	0.10
82	Pumpernickel	569	454	229	71			500	160	0	
83	White, 3–4 per cent nonfat milk solids	507	105	97	22	0.6	15	430	40	trace	0.45
84	Whole-wheat bread, 2 per cent nonfat milk solids	527	273	228	78	1.8	30	760	180	0	
85	Broccoli spears, cooked	10	267	62	24 (raw)		54				
86	Frozen, cooked	12	220	58	21		54	525	170	0	
87	Brownies with nuts	251	190	148	—						
88	Brussels sprouts, cooked	10	273	72	29 (raw)		49	420 (frozen)	175 (frozen)	0	
89	Butter, salted	987	23	16	2	0.1	—	— (frozen)	3 (frozen)	trace	1.00
90	Unsalted	under 10									
91	Buttermilk	130	140	95	14		11	307	36	0.22	
92	Cabbage, raw	20	233	29	13	0.4	32[2]	205	160	0	
93	Cooked, small amount of water	14	163	20	—	0.4					
94	Cabbage, celery or Chinese	23	253	40	14						
	Cakes (home recipe)[4]										
95	Angel food	283	88	22	—						
96	Chocolate with icing	235	154	131	—			200 (commercial)	—	—	
97	Fruitcake, dark	158	496	113	—						
98	Gingerbread	237	454	65	—						
99	Plain with icing	229	114	104	—						
100	Plain without icing	300	79	102	—	0.2		—	40[5]	—	1.10
101	Poundcake, old fashioned	110	60	79	—						
102	Sponge	167	87	112	—						
	Candy:										
103	Caramels	226	192	122	—						
104	Chocolate, milk, plain	94	384	231	58						1.10
105	Fudge, plain	190	147	84	—						

Item No.	Food	Sodium MG	Potassium MG	Phosphorus MG	Magnesium MG	Zinc MG	Folacin µG	Pantothenic Acid µG	Vitamin B6 µG	Vitamin B12 µg	Vitamin E MG
106	Hard	32	4	7	trace						
107	Marshmallows	39	6	6							
108	Peanut brittle	31	151	95	—						
109	Cantaloupe	12	251	16	16		7	250	86	0	0.14
110	Carrots, raw	47	341	36	23	0.4	8	280	150	0	0.11[2]
111	Cooked	33	222	31	—	0.3					
112	Canned, regular pack	236	120	22	—	0.3	3	130	30	0	0.11
113	Low sodium	39	120	22							
114	Cashew nuts, unsalted	15	464	373	267		—	1,300	—	0	
115	Cauliflower, raw	13	295	56	24		22[22]	1,000	210	0	
116	Cooked	9	206	42	—						
117	Frozen, cooked	10	207	38	13 (raw)			540	190	0	
118	Celery, raw	126	341	28	22		7	429	60	0	0.38
119	Cooked	88	239	22							
120	Chard, Swiss, cooked	86	321	24	65 (raw)		42	172 (raw)	—	0	
	Cheese:										
121	Cheddar or American	700	82	478	45	4.0	16	500	80	1	
122	Cheddar, process	1,136[6]	80	771[6]	—		11	400	80	0.80	
123	Cottage, creamed	229	85	152	—		31	220	40	1	
124	Uncreamed	290	72	175	—						
125	Cream	250	74	95	—			270	55	0.22	
126	Parmesan	734	149	781	48			530	96	—	
127	Swiss	710	104	563	—			370	75	1.80	
128	Cherries, raw, sweet	2	191	19	14		6	261	32	0	
129	Canned, syrup pack	1	124	12	9		3	—	30	0	
130	Frozen, sweetened	2	130	15	8			83	58	0	
	Chicken, broiled:										
131	Light without skin	64	411	265	19	0.9	3	800	683	0.45	0.37
132	Dark without skin	86	321	229	—	2.8	3	1,000	325	0.40	
133	Chicken, canned, boneless	—	138	247	—			850	300	0.79	

134	Chicken potpie, frozen, commercial	411	153	50	—		28	—	0	45	0
135	Chicory	7	182	21	13			140	—	103	—
136	Chili con carne, canned with beans	531	233	126	—						
137	Chili powder with seasonings	1,574	1,000	204	169						
138	Chocolate, bitter	4	830	384	292			190	0	35	0
139	Chocolate syrup, thin	52	282	92	63	0.9					
140	Clams, raw, soft, meat only	36	235	183	—	1.5		300	98	80	
141	Hard, round, meat only	205	311	151	—	1.5					
142	Canned	—	140	137	—	1.2	2	—	—	83	—
143	Cocoa, breakfast, dry powder	6	1,522	648	420	5.6					
144	Processed with alkali	717	651	648	—						
145	Coconut, fresh, shredded	23	256	95	46		28	200	0	44	0
146	Dried, sweetened	—	353	112	77						
147	Coffee, instant, dry powder	72	3,256	383	456	0.6		400	0	32	0
148	Beverage	1	36	4	—	0.03		4	0	trace	0
149	Collards, cooked	25	234	39	57 (raw)		102	450 (frozen)	0	195 (frozen)	0
150	Cookies, plain and assorted	365	67	163	15	0.3					
151	Fig bars	252	198	60							
152	Corn, sweet, cooked	trace	165	89	48 (raw)	0.4	28[2]	540 (raw)	0	161 (raw)	
153	Canned, whole kernel, regular pack	236	97	49	19	0.4	8	220	0	200	0.5
154	Low-sodium pack	2	97	49	—						
	Corn cereals, ready to eat:										
155	Cornflakes	1,005	120	45	16	0.3	6	185	0	65	0.12
156	Cornflakes, sugar coated	775	—	24	—						
157	Corn, puffed	1,060	—	90	—			288	0	—	
158	Corn, shredded	988	—	39	—						
159	Corn, rice, and wheat flakes	950	—	120	—						
160	Corn grits, dry	1	80	73	20	0.4			0	147	0.31
161	Cooked	—	11	10	3						
162	Cornbread, southern style, degermed cornmeal	591	157	156	—						
	Cornmeal, white or yellow, dry:										
163	Whole ground	(1)	(284)	256	106	1.8		580[5]	0	250[5]	
164	Degermed, dry	1	120	99	47	0.8	7				

Item No.	Food	Sodium MG	Potassium MG	Phosphorus MG	Magnesium MG	Zinc MG	Folacin μG	Pantothenic Acid μG	Vitamin B6 μG	Vitamin B12 μg	Vitamin E MG
165	Cooked	—	16	14	7	0.1	9				
166	Cowpeas, immature, cooked	1	379	146	55		41		95 (frozen)	0.64[5]	
167	Canned, regular pack	236	352	112	—		26	162	53	0	
168	Cowpeas, dry seeds, cooked	8	229	95	230	1.2	439	1,050	562	0	
169	Crabmeat, canned	1,000	110	182	34		trace	600	300	10	
170	Crackers, graham, plain	670	384	149	51	1.1					
171	Saltines	(1,100)	(120)	90	—	0.5		—	68	0	
172	Soda	1,100	120	89	29						
173	Cranberry juice	1	10	3	—						
174	Cranberry sauce	1	30	4	2			—	22	0	
175	Cream, half-and-half	46	129	85	—						
176	Light, coffee	43	122	80	11			321	33	0.25	
177	Whipping, light	36	102	67	9			—	29	0.20	
178	Cream substitute (cream, skim milk, lactose)	575	—	—	—						
179	Cucumbers, not peeled	6	160	27	11		7	250[5]	42[5]	0	
180	Custard, baked	79	146	117	—						
181	Dandelion greens, cooked	44	232	42	36 (raw)						
182	Dates, domestic	1	648	63	58		25	780	153	0	
183	Doughnuts, cake type	501	90	190	—	0.5		387[5]	—	—	
184	Duck, flesh only, raw	74	285	(203)	—						
185	Eggplant, cooked	1	150	21	16 (raw)		10	220 (raw)	81 (raw)	0	
186	Eggs, whole	122	129	205	11	1.0	5	1,600 (raw)	110 (raw)	2.0 (raw)	0.46 (cooked)
187	White	146	139	15	9	0.02	1	200 (raw)	2 (raw)	0.10 (raw)	
188	Yolk	52	98	569	16	3.0	13	4,400	300	6	
189	Endive, curly	14	294	54	10		47	90 (canned)	20 (canned)	0	

Food item									
190 Farina, regular, dry	2	83	107	25	0.5	13	515	67	0
191 Cooked, salted	144	9	12	3	0.06				
192 Instant cooking, cooked	188	13	60	4					
193 Fats, vegetable	0	0	0	0					
194 Figs, raw	2	194	22	20		14	300	113	0
195 Canned	2	149	13	—			69	—	0
196 Dried, uncooked	34	640	77	71		32	435	175	1.2
197 Flounder, raw	78	342	195	—	0.7		850	170	0
198 Fruit cocktail	5	161	12	7				33	
199 Gelatin, dry	—	—	—	33			—	7	
200 Sweetened, ready to eat	51	—	—	—			—		
201 Goose, flesh only, raw	86	420	203	—			283		
202 Grapefruit, raw	1	135	16	12		3	120	34	0
203 Canned, sweetened	1	135	14	11			130	20	0
204 Grapefruit juice, canned	1	162	14	—		2	162	11	0
205 Frozen, diluted	1	170	17	9		1		14	0
206 Grapes, American	3	158	12	13		5	75[5]	80[5]	0
207 European	3	173	20	6					
208 Grape juice, bottled	2	116	12	12					1.3
209 Haddock, raw	61	304	197	24	0.7		130	180	
210 Fried (dipped in egg, milk, bread crumbs)	177	348	247	24					
211 Heart, beef, lean, raw	86	193	195	18			2,500	250	11
212 Cooked, braised	104	232	181	—					
213 Herring, raw, Pacific	74	420	225	—			—	—	2
214 Smoked, hard	6,231	157	—	3			500	200	7
215 Honey, strained	5	51	6	—		3	200	20	0
216 Honeydew melon	12	251	16	14		5	207	56	0
217 Ice cream, no added salt, approximately 12% fat	40	112	99	—	0.5		492	—	—
218 Ice milk, no added salt	68	195	124	—					
219 Jams and preserves	12	88	9	5				25	0
220 Jellies	17	75	7	4					0
221 Kale, cooked, leaves with stems	43	221	46	37 (raw)		70	376 (frozen)	185 (frozen)	0

Additional column (rightmost): 204 — 0.04; 209 — 0.60 (broiled); 217 — 0.06

Item No.	Food	Sodium MG	Potassium MG	Phosphorus MG	Magnesium MG	Zinc MG	Folacin µG	Pantothenic Acid µG	Vitamin B6 µG	Vitamin B12 µg	Vitamin E MG
222	Lamb, average of lean cuts, cooked	70	290	223	21	4.3	3	550 (raw)	275 (raw)	2.15 (raw)	0.16
223	Lard	0	0	0	0	0.2	—	—			
224	Lemon juice, fresh	1	141	10	8		1	103	20	0	
225	Lemonade, frozen, diluted	trace	16	1	1			11	46	0	
226	Lettuce, butterhead	9	264	26	—	0.4	25		5	0	
227	Crisphead	9	175	22	11		21[5]	200[5]	55[5]	0	0.06
228	Looseleaf	9	264	25	—	0.4	44				
229	Lime juice, fresh or canned	1	104	11	—				—	0	
230	Limeade, frozen, diluted	trace	13	1	—			314 (sweet)	(sweet)		
	Liver, cooked, fried:										
231	Beef	184	380	476	18	5.1	294 (raw)	7,700 (raw)	840 (raw)	80 (raw)	0.63 (broiled)
232	Calf	118	453	537	26	6.1		8,000 (raw)	670 (raw)	60 (raw)	
233	Pork	111	395	539	24		221	6,400 (raw)	650 (raw)	32 (raw)	
234	Lobster, canned or cooked	210	180	192	22 (raw)	2.2		1,500 (raw)	— (raw)	0.5 (raw)	
235	Macaroni, dry	2	197	162	48	1.5			64	0 (raw)	
236	Cooked, firm	1	79	65	20	0.5					
237	Tender	1	61	50	18						
238	Macaroni and cheese, baked	543	120	161	—	0.2	—				
239	Margarine, salted	987	23	16							
240	Unsalted	under 10									
241	Milk, whole	50	144	93	13	0.4	1	340	40	0.4	0.04
242	Skim	52	145	95	14	0.4	trace	370	42	0.4	
243	Dry, nonfat, instant	526	1,725	1,005	143	4.5		3,600	380	3.2	
244	Evaporated, undiluted	118	303	205	25	0.8	1	640	50	0.16	
245	Milk, goat's	34	180	106	17			320	45	0.08	
246	Milk, human	16	51	14	4			220	10	0.04	

	Milk beverages:									
247	Chocolate flavored, with skim milk	46	142	91	—		10[5]	350[5]	200[5]	0[5]	
248	Malted, with whole milk	91	200	122	—						
249	Molasses, light	15	917	45	46						
250	Blackstrap	96	2,927	84	258						
251	Muffins, corn, enriched degermed cornmeal	481	135	169	—						
252	Plain	441	125	151	—						
253	Mushrooms, raw	15	414	116	—		24	2,200	125	0	
254	Canned	400	197	68	8		4	1,000	60	0	
255	Mustard, prepared, yellow	1,252	130	73	48		60				1.75
256	Mustard greens, cooked	18	220	32	27 (raw)			164 (frozen)	133 (frozen)	0 (frozen)	1.75 (raw)
257	Nectarine	6	294	24	13		20	—	17	0	
258	Noodles, enriched, dry	5	136	183	—			—	88	trace	
259	Cooked	2	44	59	—						
260	Oatmeal, dry	2	352	405	144	3.4	30	1,500	140	0	2.27[2]
261	Cooked, salted	218	61	57	21	0.5	33				
262	Oil, vegetable	0	0	0	0	0.2	—				36.0 (corn)[7]
263	Okra, cooked	2	174	41	41 (raw)		24	215 (frozen)	45 (frozen)	0 (frozen)	
264	Olives, green	2,400	55	17	22			18	—		
265	Ripe	813	34	16	—		1	15	14	0	
266	Onions, mature, raw	10	157	36	12	0.3	11	130	130	0	
267	Cooked	7	110	29	—		10				
268	Onions, young green	5	231	39	—	0.3	14	144			
269	Oranges, peeled	1	200	20	11	0.2	5	250	60	0	
270	Orange juice, fresh	1	200	17	11	0.02	2	190	40	0	
271	Canned	1	199	18	—	0.07	2	150	35	0	
272	Frozen, diluted	1	186	16	10	0.02	2	164	28	0	
273	Oysters, eastern, raw	73	121	143	32	74.7	11 (canned)	250	50	18	0.04
274	Pancakes, buckwheat, from mix	464	245	337	—						
275	Wheat, home recipe	425	123	139	—			218			
276	Papayas, raw	3	234	16	—						

Item No.	Food	Sodium MG	Potassium MG	Phosphorus MG	Magnesium MG	Zinc MG	Folacin μG	Pantothenic Acid μG	Vitamin B6 μG	Vitamin B12 μg	Vitamin E MG
277	Parsley	45	727	63	41		38	300	164	0	
278	Parsnips, cooked	8	379	62	32		23	600[2]	90[2]	0[2]	
279	Peaches, raw	1	202	19	10 (raw)	0.2	4	170	24	0	
280	Canned	2	130	12	6	0.1	1	50	19	0	
281	Dried, sulfured, uncooked	16	950	117	48		5	—	100[2]	0[2]	
282	Cooked with sugar	4	261	32	15						
283	Frozen	2	124	13	6		4	132	18	0	
284	Peach nectar	1	78	11	—						
285	Peanuts, roasted	5	701	407	175	3.0	57	2,100	400	0	7.70 (dry)
286	Salted	418	674	401	175						
287	Peanut butter	607	670	407	173	2.9	57	—	330	0	
288	Pears, raw	2	130	11	7		2	70	17	0	
289	Canned	1	84	7	5			22	14	0	
290	Pear nectar	1	39	5	—						
291	Peas, green, cooked	1	196	99	35 (raw)	0.7	25				0.55
292	Canned, regular pack	236	96	76	20	0.8	10	150	50	0	0.02
293	Low-sodium pack	3	96	76	—						
294	Frozen, not thawed[8]	129[8]	150	90	24		25	315	130	0	0.25
295	Peas, dry, split, raw	40	895	268	180	3.2	51[2]	2,000	130	0	
296	Cooked	13	296	89	—	1.1		220	20	0	
297	Pecans	Trace	603	289	142		27	(canned) 1,707	(canned) 183	(canned) 0	
298	Peppers, sweet, green, raw	13	213	22	18		7	230	260	0	
299	Perch, ocean, Atlantic, raw	79	269	207	8						
300	Persimmons, Japanese	6	174	26	12						
301	Pickles, dill	1,428	200	21				—	7[5]	0[5]	
302	Relish, sweet	712	—	14	—						
	Pies, home recipe:										
303	Apple	301	80	22	—			110	—	0	2.50

304	Cherry	304	105	25	—	—	—	—	—	0	—
305	Custard	287	137	113	—	—	—	946	—	—	—
306	Lemon meringue	282	50	49	—	—	—	—	—	—	—
307	Mince	448	178	38	—	—	—	—	—	—	—
308	Pumpkin	214	160	69	—	—	—	519	—	—	—
309	Piecrust, baked	611	50	50	—	—	—	—	—	—	—
310	Pike, walleye, raw	51	319	214	—	—	—	—	115	—	—
311	Pineapple, raw	1	146	8	6	13	—	160	88	0	—
312	Canned	1	96	5	1	8	—	100	74	0	—
313	Pineapple juice, canned	1	149	9	1	12	—	100	96	0	—
314	Pizza, cheese, home recipe	702	130	195	—	—	—	—	—	—	—
315	Plums, raw	2	299	17	9	—	—	186	52	0	—
316	Canned, purple	1	142	10	5	1	—	72	27	0	—
317	Popcorn, salted	1,940	—	216	—	—	3.0	—	204	0	—
	Pork, fresh:										
318	Ham, lean, roasted	65	390	308	29	2 (loin)	3.1	790 (raw)	450 (raw)	0.70 (raw)	0.16 (chops, fried)
319	Picnic ham, lean, simmered	65	390	176	18	—	4.0	—	—	—	—
	Pork, cured:										
320	Ham, light cure, lean, cooked	930	326	200	20	11	4.0	675 (raw)	400 (raw)	0.60 (raw)	0.28 (fried)
321	Canned, spiced or unspiced	(1,100)	(340)	156	22 (raw)	—	—	—	—	—	—
322	Potatoes, baked	4	503	65 (raw)	7	—	0.3	—	360	233[5]	0.03
323	Boiled, unsalted	2	285	42	—	—	—	—	—	—	0.04
324	French fried	6	853	111	—	—	—	540 (frozen)	174 / 180 (frozen)	0	0.28
325	Mashed, with milk, table fat, salted	331	250	48	—	—	—	—	—	—	—
326	Potato chips	variable to 1,000	1,130	139	—	—	—	—	180	0	—
327	Pretzels	1,680[9]	130	131	5	—	—	540	540	19	6.40
328	Prunes, dried, uncooked	118	694	79	40	—	—	460[2]	240[2]	trace	0.15
329	Cooked, without sugar	4	327	37	20	—	—	—	—	0[2]	—
330	Prune juice, canned	2	235	20	10	—	—	—	—	—	—

Item No.	Food	Sodium MG	Potassium MG	Phosphorus MG	Magnesium MG	Zinc MG	Folacin µG	Pantothenic Acid µG	Vitamin B$_6$ µG	Vitamin B$_{12}$ µg	Vitamin E MG
	Pudding, home recipe:										
331	Bread with raisins	201	215	114	—						
332	Chocolate	56	171	98	—						
333	Cornstarch (blanc mange)	65	138	91	—						
334	Rennin, using mix	46	128	92	—						
335	Rice with raisins	71	177	94	—						
336	Tapioca cream	156	135	109	—						
337	Pumpkin, canned, unsalted	2	240	26	12		8	400	56	0	
					(raw)						
338	Radishes, raw	18	322	31	15		7	184	75	0	
339	Raisins, dried	27	763	101	35		10	45	240	0	
340	Raspberries, red, raw	1	168	22	20		5	240	60	0	
341	Frozen	1	100	17	—		5	270	38	0	
342	Rhubarb, cooked	2	203	15	13		4[5]	70	25	0	
								(frozen)	(frozen)		
343	Rice, white, dry	5	92	94	28	1.3	8	550	170	0	
344	Cooked, salted	374	28	28	8	0.4	16				0.18
	Rice cereals:										
345	Flakes	987	180	132	—	1.4	8	340	125	0	0.04
346	Puffed, without salt	2	100	92	—	1.4		378	75	0	
347	Rolls, commercial, plain	506	95	85	—	0.6		310	35	—	
348	Sweet	389	124	107	—						
349	Whole wheat	564	292	281	—						
350	Rutabagas, cooked	4	167	31	15		5	160[2]	100[2]	0[2]	
					(raw)						
351	Rye flour, light	1	156	185	73		16	720	90	0	
352	Rye wafers	882	600	388	—						
	Salad dressings:[10]										
353	Blue cheese	1,094	37	74							
354	Commercial, mayonnaise type	586	9	26							
355	French	1,370	79	14	10	0.2					
356	Home cooked	728	116	93							

357	Mayonnaise	597	34	28	2	0.2				
358	Thousand island	700	113	17	—					
359	Salmon, pink, raw	64	306	—	—			300	700	4	1.35 (broiled)
360	Canned	387[11]	361	286	30	0.9	1	550	300	6.89
361	Sardines, Pacific, canned in tomato sauce	400	320	478	24		1	700	160	10
362	Sauerkraut	747[12]	140	18	—			93	130	0
	Sausage:									
363	Bologna	1,300	230	128	—	1.8	—	—	100	—	0.06
364	Frankfurters, raw	1,100	220	133	—	2.0	—	430	140	1.30
365	Pork links, cooked	958	269	162	16		12	682	165	0.54	0.16 (fried)
266	Scallops, bay steamed	265	476	338	—			132 (raw)	—	1.20 (raw)	0.60 (frozen, deep fried)
367	Shad, raw	54	330	260	—			608	—	—
368	Baked, with butter or margarine	79	377	313	—					
369	Sherbet, orange	10	22	13	—					
370	Shrimp, raw	140	220	166	42	1.5		280	100	0.90
371	Canned, dry pack	—	122	263	51	2.1	2	210	60	—	(fried)
	Soup, canned, diluted with equal part water:									
372	Bean with pork	403	158	51	—					
373	Beef bouillon	326	54	13	—					
374	Beef noodle	382	32	20	—					
375	Chicken noodle	408	23	15	—					
376	Clam chowder, Manhattan type	383	75	19	—					
377	Cream soup (mushroom), prepared with milk	424	114	69	—					
378	Minestrone	406	128	24	—					
379	Pea, green	367	80	46	—					
380	Tomato	396	94	14	9					
381	Vegetable with beef broth	345	98	16	—			140	—	0
382	Spaghetti, dry	2	197	162	—			—	64	0

Item No.	Food	Sodium MG	Potassium MG	Phosphorus MG	Magnesium MG	Zinc MG	Folacin µG	Pantothenic Acid µG	Vitamin B6 µG	Vitamin B12 µg	Vitamin E MG
383	Cooked, tender	1	61	50	—						
384	Spaghetti with meatballs, canned	488	98	45	—						
385	Spaghetti in tomato sauce with cheese, home recipe	(382)	163	54	—						
386	Spinach, raw	71	470	51	88	0.8	77	300	280	0	
387	Cooked	50	324	38	—	0.7	75	75	130	0	0.02
388	Canned, regular pack	236	250	26	63	0.8	49	(frozen) 65	(frozen) 70	0	
389	Low sodium	32	250	26	—						
390	Squash, summer, cooked	1	141	25	16		11	173	63	0	
391	Winter, cooked	1	258	32	17 (raw)		12	(frozen) 282	(frozen) 91	0	
392	Strawberries, raw	1	164	21	12		9	340	55	0	0.13
393	Frozen	1	112	17	9		9	135	43	0	0.21
394	Sugar, brown	30	344	19	—						
395	Granulated	1	3	0	trace	0.06					
396	Sweet potatoes, baked	12	300	58	31 (raw)		12[5]	820 (raw)	218 (raw)	0	
397	Boiled	10	243	47	—						
398	Candied	42	190	43	—						
399	Syrup, table blend	68	4	16							
400	Tangerines, raw	2	126	18	—		7	200	67	0	
401	Tangerine juice, canned	1	178	14	—			—	32	0	
402	Tapioca, dry	3	18	18	3		6				
403	Tea, instant, dry powder	—	4,530	—	395						
404	Beverage	—	25		22	0.02					
405	Tomatoes, raw	3	244	27	14	0.2	8	330	100	0	0.40
406	Canned, regular pack	130	217	19	12	0.2	4	230	90	0	
407	Low sodium	3	217	19	—						
408	Tomato catsup, regular pack	1,042	363	50	21			—	107	0	
409	Tomato juice, canned, regular pack	200	227	18	10		7	250	192	0	0.22

410	Canned, low sodium	3	227	18	—		2				
411	Tongue, beef, braised	61	164	117	16 (raw)		8[5]				
412	Tuna, canned in oil, solids and liquid	800	301	294	—	1.0		320	425	2.20	
413	Turkey, light, roasted	82	411	(251)	28	2.1		591	—	—	
414	Dark, roasted	99	398	(251)	—	4.4		1,128	—	—	
415	Turnips, cooked, diced	34	188	24	20		4	200 (raw)	90 (raw)	0	
416	Turnip greens, canned, regular pack	236	243	30	58 (raw)		42	68	—	0	
417	Frozen, not thawed	23	188	41	—			140	100	0	
418	Veal, lean, stewed	80	500	140	—	4.2	5	1,060 (raw)	400 (raw)	1.75 (raw)	
419	Roasted	80	500	235	19	4.1					0.05 (fried)
420	Vinegar, cider	1	100	9	1			—	1[5]	0	
421	Waffles, home recipe	475	145	173	—			650	—	—	
422	Walnuts, black	3	460	570	190		77				
423	English	2	450	380	131			900	730	0	
424	Watermelon	1	100	10	8		1	300	68	0	
425	Wheat bran, crude	9	1,121	1,276	490	9.8	195				
	Wheat cereals, cooked:										
426	Wheat and malted barley, dry	1	—	350	168	3.6	33				
427	Cooked	72	trace	59	31	0.5					
428	Wheat, rolled, cooked	trace	84	76	—		49				0.61[2]
	Wheat cereals, ready to eat:										
429	Wheat flakes	1,032	—	309	—	2.3	47	469	292	0	
430	Wheat, puffed, without salt	4	340	322	—	2.6		—	170	0	
431	Wheat, shredded, plain	3	348	388	133	2.8	55	706	244	0	
	Wheat flours:										
432	All purpose or family	2	95	87	25	0.7	8	465	60	0	
433	Cake	2	95	73	—	0.3	5	320	45	0	
434	Self-rising	1,079	90[13]	466	—						
435	Whole wheat	3	370	372	113	2.4	38	1,100	340	0	
436	Wheat germ	3	827	1,118	336	14.3	305	1,200	1,150	0	
437	White sauce, medium	379	139	93	—						

ITEM No.	FOOD	SODIUM MG	POTAS-SIUM MG	PHOS-PHORUS MG	MAG-NESIUM MG	ZINC MG	FOLACIN μG	PANTOTHENIC ACID μG	VITAMIN B₆ μG	VITAMIN B₁₂ μg	VITAMIN E MG
	Yeast, bakers':										
438	Compressed	16	610	394	59			3,500	600	0	
439	Dry active	(52)	(1,291)	(1,998)				11,000	2,000	0	
440	Brewers', dry	121	1,894	1,753	231		2,022	12,000	2,500	0	
441	Yogurt, made from partially skimmed milk	51	143	94				313	46	0.11	

[1]Dashes denote lack of reliable data for a constituent believed to be present in measurable amounts.

[2]Source of data does not indicate whether raw or cooked; it is assumed that the values are for the raw food.

[3]Based on use of self-rising flour containing anhydrous monocalcium phosphate.

[4]Based on calculations using sodium aluminum sulfate powder with monocalcium phosphate monohydrate.

[5]Nature of samples not clearly defined.

[6]Values for phosphorus and sodium are based on use of 1.5 percent anhydrous disodium phosphate as the emulsifying agent. If the emulsifying agent does not contain either phosphorus or sodium, the content of these nutrients per 100 gm is sodium, 650 mg, phosphorus, 444 mg.

[7]Vitamin E in other oils as follows: cottonseed, 60.5; olive, 67.0; peanut, 61.0; safflower, 90.0; and soybean, 21.0 mg per 100 gm.

[8]Average weighted in accordance with commercial practices in freezing vegetables.

[9]Sodium content is variable. For example, very thin pretzel sticks contain about twice the average amount listed.

[10]For salad dressing without salt, sodium content is low, ranging from less than 10 mg to 50 mg per 100 gm; the amount is usually indicated on the label.

[11]If canned without salt, the sodium value is about the same as for raw salmon.

[12]Based on salt content of 1.9 percent; may vary significantly from this level.

[13]Ninety milligrams potassium per 100 gm contributed by flour. Small quantities of additional potassium may be contributed by other ingredients.

Numerical Factors: Protein, Fat, and Carbohydrate Metabolism

The factors below are determined from the metabolism of protein, fat, and carbohydrate. The protein metabolized is determined both as protein weight directly (1 g) and as 1 g of nitrogen, since urinary nitrogen is the common measure for protein. The values of grams of protein and grams of nitrogen differ by the factor 6.25 grams protein/gram of nitrogen which is based upon a 16 percent nitrogen content in the average protein.

a. "Water of Oxidation" in the table below shows the amount of water produced by the oxidation of the weight of the foodstuff given. Fat when oxidized to CO_2 + H_2O + energy gives rise to a weight of water greater than the weight of fat, i.e., 1 g fat produces 1.07 g H_2O.

b. "Gas Exchange" gives the amount of oxygen utilized per gram of foodstuff and the amount of CO_2 produced in terms of volume and weight. The "respiratory quotient" is calculated from the volume of CO_2 produced divided by the volume of O_2 metabolized.

c. "Metabolizable Energy" gives the amount of energy in the protein, fat, or carbohydrate as determined after complete metabolism. The "Gross, kcal" is the theoretical value with corrections made for incomplete oxidation. The "Metabolizable, kcal" includes a correction factor for incomplete absorption. Protein, fat, and carbohydrate have an absorption efficiency during digestion of 92 percent, 95 percent, and 97 percent, respectively.

The "Caloric Value" of protein, fat, and carbohydrate is very similar. The utilization of 1 liter of O_2 will give rise to 4.60, 4.69, and 5.05 kcal, respectively, for the oxidation of that foodstuff. The average of these values, 4.8 kcal, is the value used to determine the heat production in indirect calorimetry. The value of 4.8 kcal is called caloric equivalent.

d. "Specific dynamic action" (SDA) gives the increase in heat production that is associated with the ingestion of each type of foodstuff. Protein has the highest SDA. Some amino acids also exhibit the same effect. The quantitation of the SDA is difficult to measure in humans. A value of about 10 percent of the total calories ingested is the usual SDA for the average meal, and the SDA is generally not considered as significant in the design of meals or as a strategy for obesity.

Numerical Factors for Protein, Fat, and Carbohydrate Metabolized in the Human Body*

| | PROTEIN | | | |
ITEM AND UNITS	AS PROTEIN, 1 G	AS NITROGEN, 1 G	FAT, 1 G	CARBOHYDRATE, 1 G
a. Water of oxidation, gm	0.41	2.56	1.07	0.60
b. Gas exchange				
Oxygen, mL	966	6,030	2,019	829
Oxygen, gm	1.38	8.61	2.88	185
Carbon dioxide, mL	782	4,880	1,427	829
Carbon dioxide, gm	1.53	9.57	2.80	1.63
Respiratory quotient	0.81	0.81	0.71	1.00
c. Metabolizable energy				
Gross, kcal	4.4	27.5	9.5	4.2
Metabolizable, kcal	4.1	25.6	9.0	4.1
Caloric values				
Oxygen, 1 liter	4.60	28.7	4.69	5.05
Oxygen, 1 gm	6.07	38.0	6.70	7.21
Carbon dioxide, 1 liter	5.68	35.6	6.63	5.05
Carbon dioxide, 1 gm	11.15	69.7	13.01	9.93
d. Specific dynamic action, kcal/100 kcal	30	30	4	6

Weights of oxygen and carbon dioxide

$$1 \text{ liter } O_2 = 1.4290 \text{ gm} \quad 1 \text{ gm } O_2 = 0.6998 \text{ liter}$$
$$1 \text{ liter } CO_2 = 1.9769 \text{ gm} \quad 1 \text{ gm } CO_2 = 0.5158 \text{ liter}$$

* A. Magnus-Levy (1907).

Nomograms for Estimation of Heat Production (Metabolic Rate)

The heat production per squared meter (M^2) of body surface is very similar for all mammals. For example, the kcal/M^2/24 hr is about 1042 for humans, 1185 for the mouse, and 1142 for the average mammal. All values are within 10 percent of one another. There is no explanation for the universal nature of these values. There is also a relationship between the height (H) and weight (W) of humans and the surface area. The relationship can only be determined empirically, i.e., there is no theoretical development for an equation.

Nomogram 1 was developed from direct measurements of surface areas, heights, and weights, the approach being the empirical determination of the exponents of W and H and the factor 71.84. The measurements and information required to determine the heat production (metabolic rate) or kcal/M^2/hr are the height, weight, oxygen consumption per hour, sex, and age. As an example, the heat production of the individual below will be calculate.

Data: Sex: Female
Height: 5 ft 3 in. (160 cm)
Weight: 111 lb (50 kg)
Age: 25 yr.
Oxygen consumption: 0.20 liters/min
Conditions: At rest, 18 hr postprandial (basal conditions)

Step 1: Using Nomogram 1, the height and the body weight (shown as dots on those scales), the line joining these values intersects the center scale at 1.5 M^2, the body surface area.

Step 2: Using Nomogram 2, the surface body area (1.t M^2) and the oxygen consumption (0.20 liters/min, a determined value), the line joining these values intersects the center scale at 38 kcal/M^2/hr. This is the heat production. It is sometimes referred to as the basal metabolic rate (BMR) when measured under basal conditions, but as will be shown in Nomogram 3, the BMR is truly expressed as a percent above or below normal value (0).

Step 3: Using Nomogram 3, the heat production (38 kcal/M²/hr, the sex female, and age 25), the line joining the values intersects the center scale at +9. This means that this individual has a basal metabolic rate (BMR) of 9 percent above the normal, and she is within the accepted normal range of ±20 percent. The normal (zero percent) is a value obtained by averaging the heat productions of a large number of clinically normal individuals of a given age and sex. The normal heat production for any age and sex can be determined by pivoting a straightedge around the 0 (zero) of the center scale. It can be observed, for example, that heat production kcal/M²/hr declines with age.

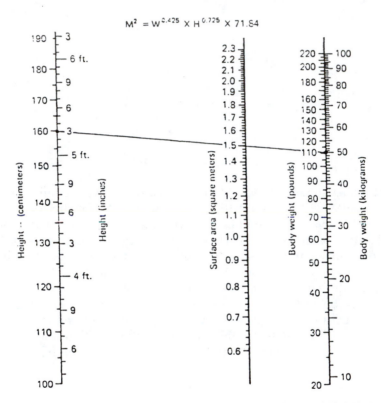

$$M^2 = W^{0.425} \times H^{0.725} \times 71.84$$

Surface area from height and weight. Nomogram constructed from the DuBois-Mech formula for surface area.

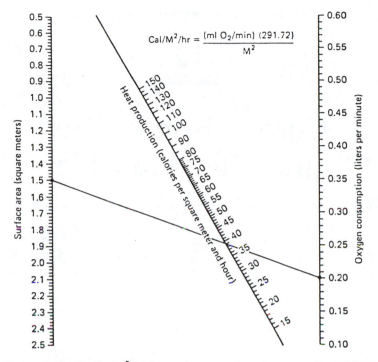

$$Cal/M^2/hr = \frac{(ml\ O_2/min)\ (291.72)}{M^2}$$

Heat production (kcal/meter^2/hr) from surface area and oxygen consumption (RQ 0.85)

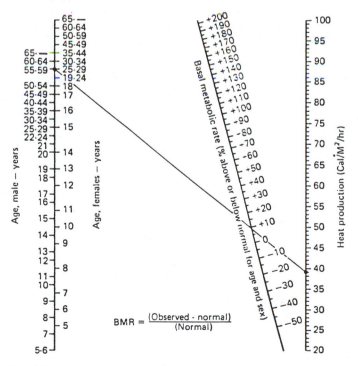

$$BMR = \frac{(Observed - normal)}{(Normal)}$$

Metabolic rate from heat production, age, and sex. The Mayo Clinic standards were employed. [*Boothby, Berkson,* and *Dunn* (1936)].

Comparison of Fats and Oils Available

Item	Calories	Cholesterol (mg)	Saturated Fat (gm)	Mono-unsaturated Fat (gm)	Poly-unsaturated Fat (gm)	Cooking Qualities
Margarines[a]						Good as table spread
Tub margarine:[b]						
With liquid safflower oil	100	0	1.5	2.5	6.7	
With liquid corn oil	100	0	2.0	3.6	5.3	
Stick margarine with						Can be used for table spread or for
liquid corn oil	100	0	2.1	4.6	4.1	cooking
Stick or tub margarine						
with partially hardened						
or hydrogenated fat	100	0	2.4	6.2	2.0	
Imitation (diet) margarine	50	0	1.0	1.8	2.5	Good as table spread
						Can be used for table spread and as salad
Mayonnaise	100	8	2.0	2.0	6.0	dressing
Oils						All-purpose cooking oil
Polyunsaturated						
Corn oil	125	0	2.0	4.0	8.0	
Cottonseed oil	125	0	4.0	3.5	6.5	Not readily available
						For salad dressings
Safflower oil	125	0	1.5	2.0	10.5	and baking
						Heavier concentrated oil (small amt.) goes a long way, good cooking oil, too
Sesame oil	125	0	2.0	6.0	6.0	heavy for baking
Soybean oil	125	0	2.0	3.5	8.5	Good for cooking

Item	Calories	Cholesterol (mg)	Saturated Fat (gm)	Mono- unsaturated Fat (gm)	Poly- unsaturated Fat (gm)	Cooking Qualities
Sunflower oil *Monounsaturated*	125	0	1.6	3.9	8.5	Cooking and salads
						Good for use in cooking or as salad
Olive oil	125	0	2.8	7.0	3.9	dressing
Peanut oil	125	0	2.0	10.0	2.0	
Saturated Products Vegetable shortening, hydrogenated	100	0	3.0	6.0	3.0	
Butter (1 tbsp.)	100	35	6.0	4.0	trace	
Lard	115	13	5.0	6.0	1.0	Limited use suggested
Coconut oil	125	0	13.0	1.0	trace	

[a] Most margarines are made from polyunsaturated oil. However, many are partly hydrogenated (saturated) so they will be solid at room temperature. Margarines sold in tub containers are more unsaturated than those sold as sticks.

[b] Ingredients here are first ingredients listed for these products on package.